MEDICAL PSYCHIATRIC PRACTICE

Volume 1

MEDICAL PSYCHIATRIC PRACTICE

Volume 1

Edited by

Alan Stoudemire, M.D.
Associate Professor of Psychiatry
Emory University School of Medicine
Atlanta, Georgia

Barry S. Fogel, M.D.
Associate Professor of Psychiatry and Human Behavior
Brown University
Providence, Rhode Island

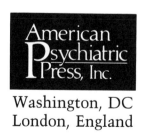

Washington, DC
London, England

Note: The authors have worked to ensure that all information in this book concerning drug dosages, schedules, and routes of administration is accurate as of the time of publication and consistent with standards set by the U.S. Food and Drug Administration and the general medical community. As medical research and practice advance, however, therapeutic standards may change. For this reason and because human and mechanical errors sometimes occur, we recommend that readers follow the advice of a physician who is directly involved in their care or the care of a member of their family.

Books published by the American Psychiatric Press, Inc., represent the views and opinions of the individual authors and do not necessarily represent the policies and opinions of the Press or the American Psychiatric Association.

This book is dedicated to the staffs of the Medical Psychiatry Unit of Emory University Hospital and the Psychiatric Medical Unit of Rhode Island Hospital.

Contents

Section V Special Topics

Contributors

David B. Abrams, Ph.D.
Associate Professor of Psychiatry and Human Behavior
Brown University
Providence, Rhode Island

Paul Camara, M.S.
Assistant Director of Chemistry and Toxicology
Roger Williams Hospital
Providence, Rhode Island

Lee S. Cohen, M.D.
Assistant Professor of Psychiatry
Harvard Medical School
Boston, Massachusetts

Paul J. Eslinger, Ph.D.
Assistant Professor of Psychiatry and Human Behavior
Brown University
Providence, Rhode Island

Carl Feinstein, M.D.
Associate Professor of Psychiatry and Human Behavior
Brown University
Clinical Director
Bradley Hospital
Providence, Rhode Island

Barry S. Fogel, M.D.
Associate Professor of Psychiatry and Human Behavior
Brown University
Providence, Rhode Island

David G. Folks, M.D.
Professor of Psychiatry and Behavioral Neurobiology
University of Alabama School of Medicine
Birmingham, Alabama

Randy S. Glassman, M.D.
Instructor in Psychiatry
Harvard Medical School
Staff Psychiatrist
Division of Psychiatry
Brigham and Women's Hospital
Boston, Massachusetts

Michael G. Goldstein, M.D.
Assistant Professor of Psychiatry
Brown University
Providence, Rhode Island

William Griffiths, Ph.D.
Clinical Associate Professor in Pathology
Brown University
Providence, Rhode Island

Lawrence R. Gulley, M.D.
Assistant Professor of Psychiatry
Emory University School of Medicine
Atlanta, Georgia

Vicki L. Heller, M.D.
Instructor in Obstetrics and Gynecology
   and Reproductive Biology
Harvard Medical School
Boston, Massachusetts

Jane Jacobs, Ed.D.
Assistant Research Professor
Center for Family Research
George Washington University Medical Center
Washington, DC

Dilip V. Jeste, M.D.
Professor of Psychiatry and Neurosciences
University of California at San Diego
Chief, Psychiatry Service
San Diego Veterans Administration Medical Center
San Diego, California

F. Cleveland Kinney, M.D., Ph.D.
Assistant Professor of Psychiatry and Behavioral Neurobiology and
  of Cell Biology
University of Alabama School of Medicine
Birmingham, Alabama

Gundy B. Knos, M.D.
Assistant Professor of Anesthesiology
Emory University School of Medicine
Atlanta, Georgia

Beryl Lawn, M.D.
Chief Resident
Department of Psychiatry
Hahnemann University School of Medicine
Philadelphia, Pennsylvania

David Levoy, M.D.
Instructor in Psychiatry
Cambridge Hospital
Harvard Medical School
Cambridge, Massachusetts

J. Wesley Libb, Ph.D.
Professor
Department of Psychiatry
University of Alabama School of Medicine
Birmingham, Alabama

M. Eileen McNamara, M.D.
Assistant Professor of Psychiatry and Human Behavior
Brown University
Providence, Rhode Island

James R. Merikangas, M.D., F.A.C.P.
Assistant Clinical Professor of Psychiatry
Yale University School of Medicine
New Haven, Connecticut

Arthur T. Meyerson, M.D.
Chairman of Psychiatry
Hahnemann University School of Medicine
Philadelphia, Pennsylvania

John M. Morihisa, M.D.
Professor and Associate Chairman for Research
Department of Psychiatry
Georgetown University School of Medicine
Washington, DC

George B. Murray, M.D.
Associate Professor of Psychiatry
Harvard Medical School
Massachusetts General Hospital
Boston, Massachusetts

Raymond Niaura, Ph.D.
Assistant Professor of Psychiatry and Human Behavior
Brown University
Providence, Rhode Island

Betty Pfefferbaum, M.D.
Professor of Psychiatry and Behavioral Sciences
University of Oklahoma College of Medicine
Oklahoma City, Oklahoma

Anne Marie Riether, M.D.
Assistant Professor of Psychiatry
Emory University School of Medicine
Atlanta, Georgia

Jerrold F. Rosenbaum, M.D.
Associate Professor of Psychiatry
Harvard Medical School
Boston, Massachusetts

Daniel D. Sewell, M.D.
Assistant Clinical Professor of Psychiatry
University of California at San Diego
San Diego, California

Elisabeth J. Shakin, M.D.
Assistant Professor of Psychiatry and Human Behavior
Jefferson Medical College
Philadelphia, Pennsylvania

Alan Stoudemire, M.D.
Associate Professor of Psychiatry
Emory University School of Medicine
Atlanta, Georgia

Paul Summergrad, M.D.
Assistant Professor of Psychiatry
Harvard Medical School
Director, Inpatient Psychiatric Service
Massachusetts General Hospital
Boston, Massachusetts

Yung-Fong Sung, M.D.
Associate Professor of Anesthesiology
Emory University School of Medicine
Atlanta, Georgia

Robert M. Swift, M.D., Ph.D.
Associate Professor of Psychiatry and Human Behavior
Brown University
Providence, Rhode Island

Troy L. Thompson II, M.D.
Professor and Chair
Department of Psychiatry and Human Behavior
Jefferson Medical College
Philadelphia, Pennsylvania

Foreword

Medical psychiatry is practiced primarily by consultation psychiatrists and psychiatrists who work in medical-psychiatry inpatient settings. Most of these workers feel, at least somewhere deep in their limbic systems, that the psychiatry they practice is a subspecialty of the broad field of medicine. They still have subscriptions to *Annals of Internal Medicine, The New England Journal of Medicine, Archives of Neurology*, and the like. They can't let go of medicine, they won't let go of medicine, and, in fact, they get inner tickles practicing it and reading about it.

However, there is an anguished side to this practice: trying to keep au courant in both psychiatry and medicine. Most tend to pick one area of medicine to be more versed in, for example, cardiology or endocrinology. They feel more comfortable with the psychiatric literature since most believe it is easier to sift through than medical literature.

Because medical psychiatrists tend to take charge of much or all of patient care, they need up-to-date medical knowledge as it impinges on their psychiatric patients. They must be apprised of new diagnostic techniques and clinical laboratory developments.

Principles of Medical Psychiatry, brought to us in 1987 by these same editors, gave us the "ground rules" and has helped shape the entity of medical psychiatry. Now we have advanced views on medical psychiatry in this present text, *Medical Psychiatric Practice*, that will generate inner tickles in all medical psychiatrists. My own knowledge base expanded from the chapters I read.

This book is not intended for those psychiatrists who in their evangelical egalitarianism (to use John Romano's words) still refer to their patients as clients. Real doctors do not have clients (from the Latin *clinare*, "to lean on," hence to seek advice from, etc.), they have patients (from the Latin *patior*, "to suffer, allow"). No client has invasive physical examinations performed on him or her. Most patients of the medical psychiatrist suffer or allow hands-on and invasive aspects of a physical examination, and thus there is a true doctor-patient relationship and not just a counselor-client verbal relationship.

Thus, the gravity of the doctor-patient relationship is another goad to the medical psychiatrist to be responsibly well informed on medical issues. The illness of the patient is in his or her hands.

Some psychiatrists thrive on responsibility, work, and pushing at the outer envelope. Reading these chapters may not make one more responsible, but it will certainly make work easier and living at the outer envelope of psychiatry more fun.

George B. Murray, M.D.

Acknowledgments

We thank the superb group of contributors who made this text possible, and appreciate the excellent assistance of the editorial advisory board for their efforts in reviewing and critiquing manuscripts for this volume.

Special thanks are also extended to our administrative assistants, Lynda Mathews and Rita St. Pierre, who, as with our other textbooks, have worked tirelessly and with remarkable dedication.

Introduction

In *Principles of Medical Psychiatry*, published in 1987, we attempted to consolidate the essential knowledge required to treat psychiatric disorders in medically ill patients. Since then, movement toward subspecialty certification in consultation-liaison psychiatry has stimulated the need to further define this knowledge base. *Medical Psychiatric Practice* builds on *Principles of Medical Psychiatry*, further delineating the information and expertise required to treat psychiatric illness in the medically ill, as well as providing information on recent developments in diagnosis and treatment in a form readily accessible to the practicing clinician.

Several factors have influenced our decision to publish a series of review volumes, of which this is the first. First, the literature concerned with the psychiatric treatment of the medically ill is extensive, expanding, and scattered in hundreds of different publications in the medical and psychiatric literature. It is virtually impossible for any busy individual practitioner to gain access to all of this literature on a regular basis, let alone to critically analyze the results of different studies. Succinct analytical reviews, with practical treatment recommendations, are needed by practitioners who daily grapple with the clinical problems of the medical-psychiatric population.

Second, psychiatrists are at times overwhelmed by the proliferation of new, expensive, and technologically sophisticated procedures for diagnostic assessment that are increasingly—and often indiscriminately—being applied to psychiatric patients. Such procedures include magnetic resonance imaging, new EEG-based procedures such as BEAM, SPECT studies, and specialized drug testing. The judicious and cost-effective use of advanced technology and special testing requires a conservative and critical approach, so that their use will not depend capriciously on local availability, reimbursement by third-party carriers, the most recent naive enthusiasm expressed in the psychiatric literature, or aggressive marketing by technology vendors.

Third, psychiatrists increasingly will function within the medical care setting to detect and manage psychiatric aspects of chronic neurological and infectious diseases, which may initially present with relatively nonspecific neuropsychiatric symptoms. The HIV epidemic and greater utilization of organ transplantation have increased the psychiatrist's role in the medical-surgical setting. Prolongation of life by high-technology procedures or immunosuppressive therapy, however, often comes at the cost of the patient's quality of life and secondary psychiatric morbidity.

Fourth, the medical research community increasingly has focused on clinical outcome studies in an effort to improve the cost-effectiveness of medical care. Associated with these efforts, the contribution of psychiatric comorbidities and complications to overall outcome has become increasingly recognized. Examples of this phenomenon are the recent Kaiser Foundation/RAND Corporation Medical Outcome Study demonstrating that ambulatory depression is a significantly disabling illness and studies of hip fracture and organ transplantation patients showing that psychiatric complications have an important influence on hospital length of stay and quality of life.

It remains to be seen whether a subspecialty of psychiatry involving the treatment of the medically ill, however named, will acquire formalized status with certification. Regardless, a precondition for any subspecialty is a clear definition of the knowledge and skills necessary for its practice. This new series, *Medical Psychiatric Practice*, attempts to meet this need.

Because psychiatry is a rapidly evolving specialty, medications, psychotherapies, disease classifications, and diagnostic technologies currently in vogue may become obsolete in the future. The discovery of new advantages, disadvantages, and limitations of treatments is inevitable and will continue to require modifications in clinical practice. Clinicians are therefore advised to use *Medical Psychiatric Practice*, as a starting point for their own critical assessment of the literature. It is our hope that Volume 1 of *Medical Psychiatric Practice* and the volumes that follow, will facilitate the integration of technical expertise with compassion in the treatment of patients burdened by the combination of medical and psychiatric illness.

Alan Stoudemire, M.D.
Barry S. Fogel, M.D.

Recent Advances in Diagnosis and Treatment

Chapter 1

Advances in Neuroimaging Technologies

John M. Morihisa, M.D.

Neuroimaging is one of the most rapidly evolving areas of research and technological innovation in the medical sciences. As with all such developing sciences, there is a continual flow of information and pragmatic application that reflects constant infusions of new knowledge in fields as diverse as software development and radiopharmaceutical manufacture. Findings in the field of clinical neuroimaging research are rapidly expanding and sometimes contradicting earlier work. As a result, no current discussion of neuroimaging technologies can be considered definitive. Not only are there no final limits to this body of knowledge, but even opinions now held with great confidence may in future years (or months) be found to be lacking or grossly incorrect. Thus, this chapter represents a temporal slice of a dynamic process.

This chapter deals with some of the newest and most promising innovations in neuroimaging and perhaps therefore those most likely to change in the future. It takes a conservative stance toward clinical applications, as this may be most useful when technology is rapidly evolving. Although much attention is attracted by visionaries that proclaim miraculous new therapeutic options before conclusive demonstration of their efficacy, a more conservative stance is less likely to raise false expectations and thereby diminish the much needed element of hope that is a source of strength for mental health professionals and the patients they treat (Morihisa 1990). This is neither a "how to" nor a "when to" chapter, but rather a "what might be" chapter. This chapter by itself cannot be used to direct clinical practice, but may help the reader envision future prospects for brain imaging in psychiatry and offer insight into some of the obstacles that must be overcome before routine clinical applications will be feasible.

A WARNING

One of the basic principles of learning new technologies (or any technique) is the understanding that for the purpose of teaching and introducing new concepts, authors often employ simplifications, reductionist generalizations, and only partially accurate metaphors. This approach has powerful heuristic value and facilitates the learner's integration of new approaches and scientific concepts. The model of understanding that is very useful for introductory teaching about a new technology is almost invariably inadequate or insufficient to use as a model for the actual interpretation of data generated by the technique. This chapter's explanations of brain imaging techniques and their potential use in psychiatry are only approximations, as are many of the other accounts of brain imaging published for general medical audiences. For example, because structural magnetic resonance imaging (MRI) scans are in large part dependent on proton density, and water is the largest contributor of protons in the brain, it is not unreasonable to think of the different patterns of the brain MRI scan as reflecting varying amounts of water content. In fact, however, the MRI scan is determined by a number of diverse variables in addition to the water content of the various structures imaged. These include not only the specific parameters of the scan but also numerous other factors, such as paramagnetic properties of hemosiderin in intracerebral hematomas (Jacobson 1988). Thus, when the readers move beyond an initial introduction to actual application of a brain imaging technique, they must return to the basic scientific principles that underlie the technique. The accurate and complete interpretation of MRI scans is a complex process that must simultaneously consider a multitude of variables. Psychiatrists endeavoring to apply MRI or other imaging techniques to practice must undertake a commitment to continual expansion and updating of their knowledge, contributed to by other articles, textbooks, and discussions with other medical and radiological consultants.

I regard these somewhat belabored cautions and disclaimers as a necessary antidote to excessive and premature enthusiasm for brain imaging as a practical clinical tool. However, despite disappointments and frustrations that imaging approaches have not been more quickly converted into useful clinical applications, there is little doubt that at least some of these techniques will eventually provide new insights that will meaningfully change the nature of diagnosis and treatment, and perhaps even the very way in which we conceptualize psychopathology.

COMPUTED TOMOGRAPHY

Computed tomography (CT) has been widely used in psychiatric research, in investigations of structural abnormalities associated with schizophrenia and other major mental disorders. Excellent synthetic reviews have emerged from this research (Coffman 1989; Jaskiw et al. 1987).

CT uses sophisticated mathematical methods to convert data generated from multiple X rays through the brain into transverse pictures of anatomic structure. CT has specifically been applied to the extensive investigation of structural associations with psychopathology, some of which were previously reported using earlier techniques such as pneumoencephalography (Weinberger and Wyatt 1982) and postmortem neuropathology. CT abnormalities reported in patients with schizophrenia have included cortical atrophy, cerebellar atrophy, and enlarged ventricles (Andreasen et al. 1982; Johnstone et al. 1976; Nasrallah et al. 1982b; Weinberger et al. 1979a; Weinberger et al. 1979b). The finding of enlarged ventricles in some patients with schizophrenia has been confirmed by the great preponderance of reports in the literature (Andreasen et al. 1982; Coffman 1989; Luchins et al. 1983; Nasrallah et al. 1982a; Pearlson et al. 1984; Weinberger et al. 1979a, 1979b).

Attempts have been made to delineate clinically relevant associations with this structural finding. It has been suggested, but has yet to be definitively demonstrated, that enlarged ventricles may be associated with impaired cognition (Johnstone et al. 1976), negative symptomatology (Pearlson et al. 1984), and response to medication (Luchins et al. 1983) and may provide a biological basis for subtyping of schizophrenia (Nasrallah et al. 1982a). However, there is as yet no general consensus concerning any definitive clinical application that these findings might have for diagnosis, prognosis, or treatment.

It has been suggested that the minority of negative studies as well as the disparity in findings concerning clinical associations may be related to variations in patient populations, differences in research methodology, and the heterogeneity of this disorder. All these are important scientific points in the evaluation of this research. However, it is essential to keep in mind that the CT findings in psychiatric investigations all consist of *statistically* significant research results that have looked, for the most part, at a *group* of schizophrenic patients compared with a *group* of control subjects. Thus, in some cases there are schizophrenic patients who do not fit the group pattern: patients with clearly demonstrated schizophrenia who do not have a particular structural abnormality. Furthermore, many of the findings reported represent subtle structural differences that clinical radiologists might not consider clearly indicative of abnormal brain structure. This in no way denigrates the potential scientific importance of these findings but rather suggests that there is a complex and perhaps multifactorial relationship between structural abnormalities and the disease process. Moreover, large ventricles are not specific to schizophrenia. They have been reported in a range of other psychiatric disorders including bipolar disorder, eating disorders, alcoholism, dementia, and normal aging (Coffman 1989; Fogel and Faust 1987). In conclusion, large ventricles are neither pathognomonic nor even characteristic of schizophrenia. They may turn out to be relevant to prognosis or treatment selection, but this has not yet been fully demonstrated.

The difficulty with interpreting CT findings of enlarged ventricles in schizophrenia exemplifies a general issue in brain imaging research: It remains extremely difficult to specify the clinical relevance and pathophysiological importance of brain imaging findings in primary psychiatric disorders, and even in the best of circumstances research reports address only that subgroup of the overall patient population in whom the evolution and presentation of the disease process has been observed. The significance of abnormal brain imaging findings requires extensive further investigation before its clinical meaning will be sufficiently clear to justify brain imaging as a routine part of our clinical approach to all psychiatric patients. The finding of enlarged ventricles on CT scans in schizophrenia has enjoyed the greatest degree of replication and relative consensus of all the findings in brain imaging. Indeed, part of the power of structural imaging research derives from the relatively static measurements that are obtained, such that some findings of in vivo CT studies may be subsequently investigated and confirmed in postmortem studies of the brain (Weinberger et al. 1982). Nonetheless, numerous questions remain to be resolved before it will translate into a routine clinical role for CT scanning in the management of schizophrenia.

Clinical Guidelines for CT in Psychiatric Patients

Clinical investigators have begun to establish some guidelines for the use of CT in the evaluation of psychiatric patients, but the body of recommendations do not represent a complete consensus nor are they all-inclusive. Fogel and Faust (1987) made a number of excellent recommendations concerning the use of brain imaging modalities in medical psychiatry, including their suggestion that the "CT scan is essential in the workup of dementia, in the evaluation of subacute mental status changes in patients with possible metastatic cancer, in patients with suspected stroke, and in head trauma patients with coma or deteriorating mental status" (p. 44). Fogel and Faust (1987) also point out that in medical psychiatric patients with disorders that have a significant rate of eventual central nervous system (CNS) involvement (e.g., lung cancer, systemic lupus erythematosus [SLE] and acquired immunodeficiency syndrome [AIDS]), the use of brain imaging procedures such as CT must be given special consideration.

Weinberger (1984) has suggested these indications for CT in a psychiatric patient: "1) confusion and/or dementia of unknown cause, 2) first episode of a psychotic disorder of unknown etiology, 3) movement disorder of uncertain etiology, 4) anorexia nervosa, 5) prolonged catatonia, and 6) first episode of a major affective disorder or personality change after age 50" (p. 1526). Weinberger (1984) points out that this list is not to be considered all-inclusive, and he provides a necessary clinical context of the characteristics of some of the relevant organic pathologic entities that can present with psychiatric symptoms and be discernible on CT. In addition, Weinberger (1984) discusses cost-benefit analysis considerations in the use of CT. It is our opinion that these recommendations should be considered in the broader context of Weinberger's entire article. In addition, since 1984 MRI has become more widely available and must be considered as an alternative or supplement to CT in the evaluation of brain structure in psychiatric patients.

Ultimately, any published guidelines for brain imaging must be considered in a greater clinical context, which includes comprehensive physical and neurological examinations, a mental status examination, and a complete history (including collateral histories). The particular pathological characteristics of the entities under suspicion will interact with the strengths and limitations of the techniques available to determine the most appropriate diagnostic tests. Test selection and interpretation often are aided by prior consultation with colleagues who have extensive expertise in the diagnosis of the specific entities under investigation.

Brain imaging studies as part of a psychiatric evaluation seldom can provide in themselves sufficient evidence for a definitive diagnosis; they usually are most helpful in providing additional information that can raise or lower suspicions concerning a particular diagnosis or set of diagnoses. It would be dangerous and naive to think that any brain imaging technique can be the sole basis for a comprehensive diagnostic evaluation. Indeed, for many brain imaging approaches, there is some controversy over whether they can yet contribute any significant additional increment of clearly interpretable information to the evaluation of many common psychiatric disorders. Nevertheless, the failure to utilize *appropriate* brain imaging investigations can impede diagnosis, particularly when the possibility of gross cerebral disease is significant. Thus, consultation with an expert—whether neurological, neuropsychiatric, or neuroradiological—frequently is the first "test" to order.

The future of CT in psychiatric research appears, in our opinion, to be less bright than that of the new structural imaging technique, magnetic resonance imaging (MRI). Drawbacks of CT include its dependence on ionizing radiation to gather data, and the limited ability of CT to provide information in multiple planes. In contrast, the excellent coronal and sagittal images now provided by MRI will likely lead to an increasing utilization of MRI techniques to address psychiatric research questions of anatomic structure, as well as structural measurements that might be desired in the clinical practice of psychiatry. It is likely that CT will most commonly be applied in clinical psychiatry to rule in or out those disease processes that are clearly associated with specific gross anatomical pathology. More subtle anatomic assessments may be possible with MRI. However, even in these instances it will be vitally important to view CT, MRI, or any brain imaging technique as only a tool to help us test our clinical hypotheses rather than as a diagnostic panacea. Fogel and Faust (1987) have suggested that the role of brain imaging in the majority of psychiatric patients may be more to provide evidence to "establish the presence of cerebral abnormality rather than make a specific pathologic diagnosis" (p. 46).

The best established applications of CT and MRI to psychiatry are as part of comprehensive evaluations of primary neurologic diseases (e.g., demyelinating disorders, brain tumor, cerebrovascular disease). The role of the psychiatrist in these disorders may be to evaluate psychiatric symptomatology that is the initial presentation of organic pathology, or to assess concomitant psychiatric symptoms that overlay and confound an already established or suspected organic process. In such discussions, the psychiatrist may need to point out to the neurologist or internist an atypical presentation of psychiatric symptomatology that suggests an organic process, or conversely to point out atypical presentations of primary psychiatric illness that may mimic neurologic disease. In many cases, definitive diagnoses cannot be made on a single assessment, and the distinction between "functional" and "organic" must be deferred. More generally, neuropsychiatric research has increasingly demonstrated the artificiality of these distinctions. Further rigid dichotomies in *clinical* thinking can actually impede a comprehensive diagnosis and effective multimodal therapy (Fogel 1990). Also, multiple disease processes may afflict an individual, so that psychiatric disorders and nonpsychiatric diseases may interact and affect the clinical manifestation of both.

MAGNETIC RESONANCE IMAGING

Magnetic resonance imaging (MRI) depends on the electromagnetic qualities of certain atoms whose nuclei generate magnetic fields and therefore may be aligned by an external magnetic field. One such atom is hydrogen. MRI systems that presently provide clinical brain structure information utilize the plentiful hydrogen of the human body. In addition to hydrogen, other atoms that align in magnetic fields include certain species of carbon, potassium, phosphorous, and sodium. Technologic advances someday may allow the development of clinical MRI approaches that utilize these atoms.

In the technique of MRI, the brain is placed in a powerful magnetic field typically 0.5–1.5 tesla in strength. This magnetic field orients all the proton nuclei of hydrogen atoms into a common alignment. These hydrogen nuclei always normally spin; however, when subjected to a powerful magnetic field, they also precess (oscillate during their normal spin) in a pattern characterized by their "Larmor frequency." The MRI contains a radio frequency transmitter that briefly broadcasts on this characteristic Larmor frequency, thereby increasing the energy of these spinning proton nuclei and deflecting their magnetic field orientation. When the Larmor frequency broadcast ends, the nuclei return to their original state. The excess energy is broadcast from the spinning nuclei and may be detected by the radio frequency receiver in the MRI apparatus. As this energy is released, the nuclei return to their original state. The Larmor frequency varies with the local environment of the hydrogen atoms. From measurements of the return over time of these hydrogen atom nuclei to their original state, and taking into account how this varies with the local environment of the hydrogen atoms, a computer creates an image of brain structure. Because the Larmor frequency also depends on the strength of the applied magnetic field, gradient magnets in the MRI system can provide the basis to link specific frequencies to specific anatomic locations. By "tuning" the transmitter and receiver, data from a specific slice of brain tissue can be collected and analyzed.

Depending on specific parameters of transmission and reception, MRI imaging can emphasize differentiation between gray and white brain matter and sharp delineation of normal anatomic structures (usually the T1-weighted scan) or, alternatively, provide the best delineation of abnormal tissues (usually the T2-weighted scan). Thus, the manner in which data have been acquired for image generation, and what data components have been emphasized, or weighted, can significantly affect both the appearance and the interpretation of the image.

CT Versus MRI

In brain imaging, the manner in which data are generated has profound implications for the potential strengths and limitations of the technique for clinical applications. In the case of MRI, the excellent differentiation between gray and white matter is clearly superior to the result from CT. Further, MRI does not depend on X rays as does CT and therefore does not have the vulnerability of CT to obstruction and artifactual distortion by bone. On the other hand, CT provides far superior visualization of bony structures and calcifications and therefore has a special role in traumatic pathology. In MRI, information is not limited to the transverse plane but also is readily available from sagittal and coronal sections. Although ingenious software applications have been developed to enhance multidimensional visualization in CT, the coronal and sagittal sections created generally are inferior to those directly produced by MRI. Compared with CT, MRI offers superior visualization of the posterior fossa, superior gray-white matter delineation, and superior delineation of pathologic changes associated with demyelinating diseases. In addition, MRI generally offers more accurate quantitative volumetric measurements than are possible with CT.

MRI does not expose the patient to ionizing radiation. However, the presence of ferromagnetic substances or devices that can be adversely affected by magnetic fields is a contraindication to MRI. For example, pacemakers and aneurysm clips are contraindicated. Because of the prolonged scan time of MRI and claustrophobic scanning conditions, psychological assessment and preparation of the patient is vital. Moreover, in the application of any brain imaging technique, the particular psychological vulnerabilities of the patient must be considered, and adequate preparation for the peculiarities of each specific test must be provided. Due to the MRI scanner design, patient monitoring and medical intervention are severely limited during the scan, so the medical stability of each patient must be carefully considered when deciding to perform MRI.

As MRI technology evolves and more is learned about its clinical application, the potential dangers and contraindications to MRI will be further elucidated. Consultation with appropriate specialists therefore is advised concerning specific potential problems in a particular case (in MRI as well as in all brain imaging modalities). Apart from effects on some magnetic objects such as clips and pacemakers, the potential adverse effects of strong magnetic fields are not known.

Perhaps one of the most striking differences from CT is MRI's potential ability to indirectly address issues of physiologic *function*, as well as changes in anatomic *structure*. Although this functional capability may be greatly enhanced with the development of MRI systems that can image additional atoms such as phosphorus-31, some functional information is already available with MRI proton imaging. This potential MRI function is illustrated by characteristic highlighting of pathological tissue in T2-weighted images, which may occur even when no gross anatomic change is visible on CT or T1-weighted MRI. (Abnormal tissue generally stands out with greater contrast in T2 versus T1 weightings.) One of the more striking clinical examples is the delineation of the CNS plaques of multiple sclerosis on T2-weighted MRI scans. However, before this advantage of MRI can be fully exploited, much more must be learned about the basic neuroscience principles underlying the behavior of water (and its component hydrogen) in normal and pathological brain tissue, including medication effects and effects of neuronal activity on the biochemical environment.

In a useful discussion of MRI of the CNS, a Council on Scientific Affairs report (Jacobson 1988) on MRI describes various clinical entities that can present with important MRI findings and directly compares

CT and MRI assessments of a range of CNS pathology. Included in this report is the suggestion that MRI is particularly useful in the investigation of diseases of demyelination and in pathology in the cervicomedullary junction and cervical spinal cord as well as in the investigation of a particular etiology of adult-onset dementia—subcortical arteriosclerotic encephalopathy, or Binswanger's disease (Kinkel et al. 1985). The utility of CT and MRI in a variety of intracranial tumors is discussed and a point is made concerning the difficulty in the MRI (T2-weighted image) delineation of meningiomas due to the similarity in signal intensity of these tumors to normal brain tissue. This report discusses the utility of CT and MRI in cerebrovascular disease and also suggests that MRI may be more able to detect lesions related to the neuropathology of SLE. This council report also warns of difficulties in the interpretation of MRI images of CNS hemorrhages and cautions in general that the theory and interpretation of MRI scans is highly complex.

Another recent and highly informative discussion of the theory underlying MRI and scan interpretation as well as the potential utility of MRI in psychiatry is available in an excellent review by Andreasen (1989). Recent research reports by her group using MRI in schizophrenia (Andreasen 1989; Andreasen et al. 1986) have tended to support some of the structural findings demonstrated by CT.

Special Problems With MRI in the Elderly

The greater sensitivity of MRI to white matter abnormalities has led to its increasing application in the evaluation of dementia and other organic mental disorders in the elderly. Unfortunately, although MRI is superior to CT in demonstrating white matter abnormalities in vascular dementia, it also frequently shows abnormalities in elderly persons with no clinical signs of either dementia or cardiovascular disease. Findings include 1) "rims"—periventricular hyperintensity on T2-weighted images; 2) "caps"—increased T2 signal around the poles of the lateral ventricles; and 3) "unidentified bright objects" (UBOs)—hyperintense bright patches in subcortical white matter on T2-weighted images (Kertesz et al. 1988).

Pathologic studies have shown that pathologically diverse processes can give rise to similar-appearing white matter densities on MRI. Hyperintense white matter foci (UBOs) may represent infarctions, areas of gliosis, or demyelinated plaques, and at times no abnormality is found at postmortem (Braffman et al. 1988). Rims of periventricular hyperintensity may be due to the reversed transependymal fluid flow of hydrocephalus (Zimmerman et al. 1986) or increased periventricular and white matter fluid due to vascular disease (Kertesz et al. 1988).

Despite the pathologic nonspecificity of white matter abnormalities on MRI, they have been shown to correlate with risk factors for cerebrovascular disease such as hypertension and diabetes (Fazekas et al. 1988; Kertesz et al. 1988). Severe rims are more likely to be associated with vascular risk factors than are mild rims; quantitation rather than mere description may be needed for greater diagnostic specificity.

Not only vascular disease but also Alzheimer's disease can produce subcortical white matter changes. Marked white matter changes are associated with more severe and rapidly progressive dementia among patients with Alzheimer's disease (Bondareff et al. 1990; Janota et al. 1989).

Quantitative assessments of white matter lesion volume by MRI have been shown to correlate with severity of cognitive impairment in a series of 19 patients with dementia, all but 1 of whom did not have a clinical diagnosis of vascular dementia (Bondareff et al. 1990). Theoretical reasons have been suggested as to why cerebral interstitial fluid might be increased by Alzheimer's disease, related to amyloid infiltration of cerebral capillaries (Glenner 1985) and "denervation microangiopathy" (Scheibel et al. 1987).

Taken together, these reports suggest that nonspecific white matter abnormalities in elderly patients may *support* a diagnosis of dementia but do not make it. Despite enthusiastic early reports (Erkinjuntti et al. 1987), these abnormalities may not reliably distinguish Alzheimer's disease from vascular dementia. Such distinctions might become more possible as quantitative methods for describing white matter changes become more standardized and better validated.

Future Prospects

The future of MRI is particularly promising due to the potential for direct imaging of energy metabolism through the use of phosphorous-31. Because organic compounds fundamental to human metabolism contain phosphorous, such as adenosine triphosphate, it is theoretically possible for MRI to provide functional data in addition to its present structural information about the CNS. This would provide an important new window on metabolic activity that might supplement, confirm, and clarify findings obtained by single photon emission computer tomography (SPECT) of regional cerebral blood flow and by positron-emission tomography (PET) of regional glucose metabolism. At present, due to current limitations in radiopharmaceutical capability, PET is the sole brain imaging technique that can directly image regional brain metabolism. The successful realization of MRI phosphorous functional imaging would provide a powerful new tool for the investigation of human regional metabolic activity.

REGIONAL CEREBRAL BLOOD FLOW

One of the earliest applications of regional cerebral blood flow (rCBF) technology was reported by Ingvar and Franzen (1974), who demonstrated abnormal frontal lobe function in patients with schizophrenia. The most recent innovations in two-dimensional rCBF studies have included improved technology with better resolution, a noninvasive approach (xenon-133 inhalational technique), and a particularly ingenious application of some recent neuroscience findings about the prefrontal cortex. Weinberger and his colleagues have reported that using a specific cognitive-activation test, the Wisconsin Card Sort, schizophrenic subjects were shown to fail to increase rCBF to the dorsolateral prefrontal cortex, whereas normal control subjects increased rCBF to this brain region when performing this test (Figure 1-1). The elegant use of this cognitive-activation test was inspired by neuroscience research (Morihisa and Weinberger 1986; Weinberger 1987; Weinberger et al. 1986) that has linked the integrity of the dorsolateral prefrontal cortex of the brain to the successful performance of cognitive tests such as the Wisconsin Card Sort. It is a fundamental design advance that allows rCBF technology to investigate the function of a specific component of the frontal lobes to better evaluate the general hypothesis of frontal lobe dysfunction in schizophrenia. In this case, a finer and more specific neuroanatomic focus on the possible pathophysiology underlying schizophrenia derives as much from the innovative application of basic neuroscience research as from an improvement in scanning technology.

This chapter has emphasized that the successful execution and interpretation of any brain imaging study is dependent on the careful consideration and control of various variables and potential confounds. This is particularly true for functional (as opposed to primarily anatomical) brain imaging approaches such as rCBF, PET, and SPECT. The work of Weinberger and his group (Berman et al. 1984; Weinberger et al. 1986) provides an example of the broad spectrum of issues that must

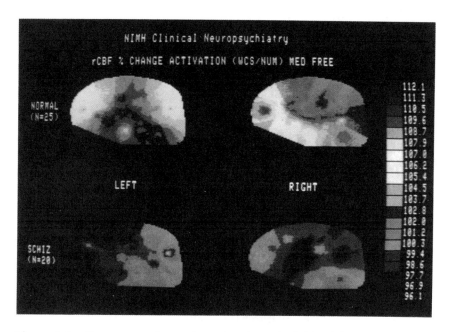

Figure 1-1. Percentage change in regional cerebral blood flow (rCBF) measurements between two test states: during cognitive activation by the performance of the Wisconsin Card Sort (WCS) compared with performance of a number-matching task (NUM; control state). Comparison is given for left and right hemispheres of normal subjects (*n* = 25) *above* and schizophrenic patients (*n* = 20) *below*. Normal control subjects significantly increase rCBF to the prefrontal cortex during the WCS, whereas schizophrenic subjects do not. (Daniel R. Weinberger, M.D., National Institute of Mental Health)

be successfully addressed to be able to interpret functional brain imaging studies. This work has included extensive studies to consider the influence of variables including medication effects, attentional differences, the psychological effects of taking an rCBF test, and practice effects. They have employed a variety of controls including both neurologic and psychiatric comparison groups and normal controls. Even with all this effort, the conclusions of their studies are based on *groups* of patients compared with control groups, and not the much more difficult interpretation of individual patients' findings.

Despite the difficulty and complexity of conducting such studies, it is our opinion that it is just such elegant and relatively specific cognitive-activation procedures that represent one of the most promising research strategies in brain imaging. Indeed, brain imaging studies in the resting alert state are subject to more confounding variables, since the unobserved and unspecified cognitive states and attentional states of subjects may vary widely.

SINGLE-PHOTON EMISSION COMPUTER TOMOGRAPHY

Single-photon emission computer tomography (SPECT) uses radiopharmaceuticals that emit gamma rays (photons) to image the human brain. Gamma detectors using sodium iodide scintillation crystals allow the SPECT system to collect data from the trajectory of single gamma rays to estimate the locus in the brain from which each gamma ray was emitted. The number of gamma rays detected from a particular locus in the brain is a reflection of the amount of radiopharmaceutical that is present there. Thus, information about the location and the amount of various radiopharmaceuticals can be used to create a picture of brain *function* (e.g., rCBF of the brain or local activity of the cholinergic neurotransmitter system).

The particular radiopharmaceutical that is chosen determines the process that may be measured. At present, various agents are available or under development, including xenon-133 for the quantitative dynamic measurement of rCBF and ^{123}I-labeled iodoamphetamine (^{123}I-IMP), which can provide qualitative assessments of rCBF. In addition, another radioxenon, xenon-127, and a technetium-labeled product, ^{99m}Tc-hexamethylpropylene amine oxime (HMPAO) have also been used to assess rCBF. The recently developed agent ^{123}I-labeled QNB (^{123}I-QNB), which binds to muscarinic acetylcholine receptors in the brain, can provide information concerning the cholinergic neurotransmitter system (Figures 1-2 and 1-3). The development of radiopharmaceuticals that can image specific neurotransmitter systems represents a new frontier of application for SPECT and may provide one of the greatest potential uses for this brain imaging modality. However, SPECT brain imaging techniques in psychiatry are as yet in the research and development phase and have yet to demonstrate a definitive application in routine clinical psychiatric practice.

Recent SPECT studies have reported some intriguing findings concerning regional blood flow differences between normal controls and various psychiatric populations (Devous 1989). For example, Holman and colleagues (Johnson et al. 1988) have reported exciting clinical correlates of IMP parietal lobe deficits in patients with Alzheimer's

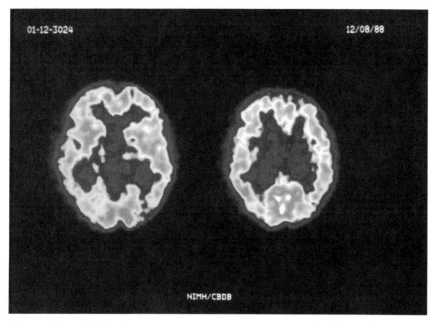

Figure 1-2. Single-photon emission computer tomography (SPECT) image of the brain of a normal control subject that investigates the cholinergic neurotransmitter system using the radiopharmaceutical ^{123}I-labeled QNB. (Daniel R. Weinberger, M.D., National Institute of Mental Health)

disease that complement research utilizing fluorine 18 2-D-deoxyglucose (FDG) PET imaging (Benson et al. 1981). This represents a promising area of research with particular hope for the potential development of a well-defined role for SPECT or PET in assisting in the early diagnostic evaluation of dementias.

In general, there is insufficient evidence that a particular constellation of SPECT findings may be considered clearly pathognomonic of any specific psychiatric disorder and consistently definitive in its diagnosis. This is exacerbated by the overlap in areas of regional dysfunction between different disease entities, and the dynamic and changing nature of the pathological processes in many clinical entities. As with the general body of brain imaging research, it remains to be shown whether SPECT findings can demonstrate the specificity and sensitivity necessary to form the scientific basis for new diagnostic or treatment approaches in psychiatry. Devous (1989) has written a thoughtful and comprehensive review of SPECT.

In the efficacious application of any brain imaging technique, care-

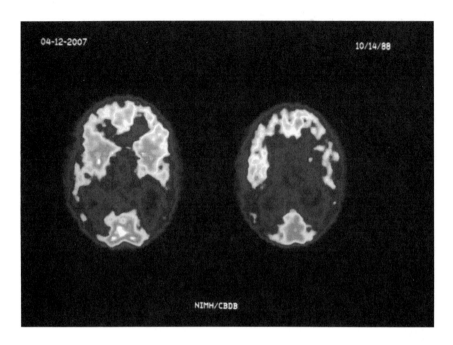

Figure 1-3.   Single-photon emission computer tomography (SPECT) image of the brain of a patient with primary degenerative dementia of the Alzheimer type, senile onset, that demonstrates differences in the cholinergic neurotransmitter system using the radiopharmaceutical ^{123}I-labeled QNB. Note focal areas of reduced activity in posterior temporal and inferior parietal cortex. (Daniel R. Weinberger, M.D., National Institute of Mental Health)

ful consideration must be given to the limitations of the specific hardware/software system that is employed. For example, in SPECT imaging, there are significant differences between the systems currently in use, ranging from early-generation machines with poor resolution, to research-grade SPECT systems with variable collimator size that have the resolution and sensitivity to conduct the most sophisticated scientific investigations of the CNS and a correspondingly greater potential to delineate organic pathology. Some SPECT research findings in psychiatry utilize these more sophisticated machines, which are available at only a few research medical centers. Although a significant number of SPECT machines are in use, the potential application of psychiatric research findings in SPECT has been limited by the scarcity of high-performance SPECT systems. The wide variety of SPECT systems makes research findings difficult to compare and problematic in clinical application in psychiatry. Thus, discussion with a brain imaging consultant must include assessment of the strengths and limitations not only of the technique but also of the particular hardware and software available at a specific institution for the evaluation of the specific clinical entity of interest. The difficulty of comparing and interpreting results from brain imaging systems with different hardware/software configurations, varying test paradigms, and differing statistical analyses is a problem that is common to all findings in this field and exacerbates the process of clinical application.

Ultimately, one of the most important variables governing our ability to effectively utilize brain imaging techniques is the depth of experience of the brain imaging team. Extensive experience with the clinical entities of interest is vital, along with expertise with the appropriate test paradigms and parameters including experience with the detection and exclusion of related artifacts. Whereas the clinical application of using PET in the evaluation of refractory focal epilepsy has been reported, there remains for most other disease entities with psychiatric presentations a much greater need for extensive further scientific investigation before clearly relevant clinical correlations may hope to be established. Indeed, the number of clinical applications for brain imaging in psychiatry that can clearly incrementally enhance the assessment of diagnosis, prognosis, or treatment of psychiatric patients over and above what already can be derived from data available before the brain imaging test is as yet disappointing.

As has been mentioned, the process of developing this research technique into a clinical tool in psychiatry will be limited by the modest resolution and sensitivity of the most commonly available SPECT systems. These earlier-generation SPECT systems generally have poorer resolution and inferior ability to provide quantitative data than are available with present-generation PET systems. Furthermore, the degree to which new radiopharmaceuticals are developed that can provide additional and more finely focused windows on brain function will ultimately determine much of the future efficacy and role of this modality.

POSITRON-EMISSION TOMOGRAPHY

Positron-emission tomography (PET) scanning images brain function via the coincident emission of pairs of diametrically opposed gamma ray photons following the annihilation in the brain of nearby electrons by positrons that are emitted from specially prepared radioisotopes that are administered to the subject. Because diametrically opposed pairs of gamma ray photons rather than single photons are detected, the relative time of detection of a gamma ray photon and its partner can be used in localizing its source. This mathematical formula for localizing radiation sources using pairs of coincident photons permits generally higher resolution three-dimensional images than standard SPECT systems. Various brain functions can be imaged depending on the radiopharmaceutical selected. For example, FDG can provide images of regional glucose metabolism in the brain. (At present, no radioisotopes to directly investigate glucose metabolism are successful in SPECT imaging. Thus, assessment of regional metabolism by SPECT must rely on indirect measures such as rCBF, which under certain pathological conditions can be different from regional glucose utilization.)

In addition, the dopamine neurotransmitter system has been investigated using positron-emitting dopamine receptor ligands: C-11-3N-methylspiperone, F-18-N-methylspiroperidol, and C-11-raclopride. Using receptor-binding radiopharmaceuticals, PET may provide functional studies of specific neurotransmitter pathways, thereby permitting in vivo investigation of brain neurotransmitter systems during normal and pathologic function. For example, Wagner and colleagues (1983) directly investigated, in vivo, the potential role of the dopamine system in the pathophysiology of schizophrenia. The development of radiopharmaceuticals is an important step in the evolution of PET research. For example, Dannals (1989), at the Johns Hopkins biomedical tracer center, reported that compounds had been labeled for the following receptors: dopamine 1, dopamine 2, benzodiazepine, muscarinic, opiate, histamine 1, and serotonin receptors.

PET and Schizophrenia

There has been a notable lack of consensus concerning the relevant metabolic and neurotransmitter findings in schizophrenia. In one of the earliest applications of PET technology, schizophrenic subjects and patients with affective disorder were shown to have abnormalities of the anterior-posterior gradient of glucose metabolism (Buchsbaum et al. 1984). Other workers demonstrated hypometabolic activity in the frontal regions of schizophrenic subjects (Wolkin et al. 1985), and "dysfunction in a prefrontal substrate of sustained attention" (Cohen et al. 1987). Under certain activation paradigms (Gur et al. 1987), laterality differences have been shown. A wide range of disparate findings have emerged from different models for data collection and analysis, and from a variety of cognitive states during the PET scan itself. Attempts to correlate these metabolic findings with clinical variables have had limited success (DeLisi et al. 1985).

PET studies have generated much greater disparity in findings among various psychiatric research groups than have SPECT studies. In part, this can be attributed to PET studies having been used more in scientifically controlled and statistically quantitated psychiatric research to date than SPECT. Unfortunately, as more studies using both SPECT and PET are reported, it can be expected that the number of disparate findings will increase, because the technology is in a constant state of evolution, because a wide range of brain functions can be assessed, and because of differences in research techniques and research study designs. Disparate findings in PET do not necessarily mean a failure to replicate or contradict results, because different studies often are not comparable in what they measure, the conditions of measurement, or the subjects studied. Further reasons are complexity of the CNS, the extensive and complicated changes that may be associated with illnesses (e.g., schizophrenia is unlikely to be solely the result of an excess of a single neurotransmitter), and the clinical heterogeneity of psychiatric illnesses. The relatively small number of patients who have been studied with PET limits the accuracy of estimates of its potential diagnostic sensitivity and specificity (Stoudemire et al. 1989). Holcomb (1989) has contributed an informative and comprehensive review of PET.

Functional brain imaging techniques such as PET have had little routine clinical utility in psychiatry. Indeed, the major applications of PET have been to investigate the possible pathophysiologic principles that might underlie psychiatric disorders rather than to make diagnoses for the individual patient. It is likely that significant diagnostic and therapeutic advances will be derived once such principles have been better delineated. Scanning paradigms will need to limit or control confounding variables and at the same time pose sufficiently focused questions concerning specific brain functions to allow reasonable interpretation.

BRAIN ELECTRICAL ACTIVITY MAPPING

Brain electrical activity mapping (BEAM) was developed by Duffy and colleagues in 1979. The first systematic scientifically controlled application of this technique in psychiatry in 1983 (Morihisa et al. 1983) demonstrated increased delta activity in schizophrenic patients compared with normal control subjects. A subsequent study by this group (Karson et al. 1987) using a different computerized EEG system to study a new group of schizophrenic patients confirmed the finding of increased delta activity. This work should be interpreted as further evidence of CNS dysfunction in schizophrenia. A preliminary study (Morihisa and McAnulty 1985) combined BEAM electrophysiological data from schizophrenic patients with structural CT data from the same schizophrenic patients. The findings suggested that it might be possible to relate gross anatomic differences measured by CT to electrophysiological differences between two groups of schizophrenic patients who differed in their CT findings of frontal atrophy. The use of multiple brain imaging modalities in concert is also one of the more promising research strategies now available. Indeed, many functional brain imaging research teams now utilize structural (e.g., MRI or CT) imaging data in the interpretation and evaluation of their functional data. Further research concerning the specificity and sensitivity of all computerized EEG and evoked-potential techniques will be required to assess their potential utility in psychiatry. Additional information concerning computerized EEG and evoked-potential mapping is available in a comprehensive review by Morihisa (1989), and a detailed critique is offered by McNamara in Chapter 5 of this volume.

Computerized EEG imaging techniques are limited by the fact that they collect two-dimensional data from scalp electrodes. A recent advance in electrophysiological investigation, magnetoencephalography (MEEG), may directly address this limitation. This technique uses a superconducting quantum interference device (SQUID) to measure the small magnetic fields generated by the electrical activity of the brain. By this technique it is possible to image the electrical activity of the brain in three dimensions. Although preliminary results have concentrated on localization of epileptic foci, MEEG may eventually have a role in demonstrating physiological correlates of mental illness, and in addressing important questions concerning the neuroanatomic origins of electrical activity detailed by surface EEG.

CONCLUSION

We have entered an exciting and very promising era in psychiatric research in which the rapid evolution of new brain imaging methods will lead to innovative applications that utilize developments in applied mathematics (increasingly elegant mathematical techniques for deriving images from masses of quantitative data), technological advances in radiopharmaceuticals and computer design, clinical research strategy (clinical subtyping of psychiatric disorders), and basic principles of neuroscience (the localization of cognitive and behavioral functions). However, in assessing the function of the CNS, we are dealing with the most complex and dynamic physiological system of the human body. Thus, it is not surprising that our brain imaging research findings have formed as yet no consistent body of work that can provide straightforward routine clinical assistance in managing psychiatric illnesses. Some findings in the field of brain imaging continue to be contradictory, to be diagnostically nonspecific, or to apply to only a specific subgroup of those afflicted by a particular disorder. Currently in psychiatry, many of these brain imaging tests appear to be most safely considered research techniques that require thoughtful and exhaustive analysis before potential correlations can even be reported in the research literature.

Although it is possible that brain imaging tests might facilitate the diagnostic process, they can seldom be considered to provide definitive diagnoses. For scientific research purposes, when a particular brain imaging technique is said to have a statistical ability to successfully sort between psychiatric patients and normal control subjects, we are actually reaffirming the likelihood that we are indeed measuring something of physiological relevance to the clinical issue being investigated. However, this is a very different step from considering a brain imaging technique a definitive method for achieving a psychiatric diagnosis in any individual patient. Even diagnostic specificity is a step removed from *incremental validity:* evidence that a particular brain imaging technique is a clearly useful adjunct to the existing process of clinical diagnosis. This is not to say that these techniques will not achieve this goal. Indeed, neuroscience research is proceeding at a pace unprecedented in medical history. It appears very likely that some brain imaging approaches will lead to important diagnostic and perhaps therapeutic tools. However, further development is required, and the complexity of psychiatric illnesses demands our respect. We cannot expect to unravel immediately the secrets of brain dysfunction with powerful technology until we better understand normal brain function and the fundamental principles of neuroscience that underlie behavior and brain physiology. Indeed, it is our opinion that one of the greatest obstacles to the successful application of brain imaging technology to the *clinical* study of psychiatric illness is our limited knowledge and understanding of *normal* brain function with all its normal variants. Until we have a better understanding of what the normal brain looks like through various brain imaging windows, we will be handicapped in our interpretation of our research findings in psychiatric illnesses.

Parallel with this limiting factor is a grave danger in this process that we may too quickly seek to depart from our present clinical rules of diagnostic assessment and place too great an emphasis on technology that has not yet been sufficiently developed. It is certainly possible that brain imaging findings might raise important questions concerning diagnosis. However, these questions should in many cases already be under consideration as part of a complete and comprehensive diagnostic workup by the clinician. Overreliance on technology that is not fully developed can breed a false confidence that undermines the most powerful diagnostic tool available to clinicians—the human mind—with its ever-questioning nature and its ability to constantly adapt to new information. Scientific researchers must investigate further the limitations as well as the apparent strengths of new brain imaging approaches before they can be placed with confidence and efficacy into our clinical armamentarium.

It would be arrogant and dangerous to think that the complex mysteries of diseases such as schizophrenia and the mood disorders will be so easily resolved that the first applications of our new technology will lead quickly to fundamental building blocks of knowledge, and that each study would move us obviously closer to a full understanding of the disease process and its treatment. The great danger of such unreasonable expectations is that inevitable disappointments will occur, risking the premature rejection of these promising techniques in their infancy, and diminishing support for scientific strategies that have slowly but surely greatly expanded our understanding of mental illness over the last half-century. The initial effect of introducing brain imaging approaches into the clinical practice of psychiatry is likely to be additional complexity in psychiatric evaluation, rather than a simplification of the diagnostic and treatment process. The recent history of immunology offers an example of continually expanding complexities with eventual, but not immediate, therapeutic benefits for many conditions. Brain imaging approaches, with all their limitations, do promise innovative new options in the diagnosis and treatment of psychiatric disorders, as well as the hope of a better understanding of the fundamental principles of neuroscience that govern all functions of the brain.

REFERENCES

Andreasen NC: Nuclear magnetic resonance imaging, in Brain Imaging: Applications in Psychiatry. Edited by Andreasen NC. Washington, DC, American Psychiatric Press, 1989, pp 67–121

Andreasen NC, Smith MR, Jacoby CJ, et al: Ventricular enlargement in schizo-phrenia: definition and prevalence. Am J Psychiatry 139:292–296, 1982

Andreasen N, Nasrallah HA, Dunn V, et al: Structural abnormalities in the frontal system in schizophrenia. Arch Gen Psychiatry 43:136–144, 1986

Benson DF, Kuhl DE, Phelps ME, et al: Positron emission computed tomog-raphy in the diagnosis of dementia (abstract). Ann Neurol 10:76, 1981

Berman KF, Weinberger DR, Morihisa JM, et al: Regional cerebral blood flow in psychiatry: application to clinical research, in Brain Imaging in Psy-chiatry. Edited by Morihisa JM. Washington, DC, American Psychiatric Press, 1984, pp 41–64

Bondareff W, Raval J, Woo B, et al: Magnetic resonance imaging and the severity of dementia in older adults. Arch Gen Psychiatry 48:47–51, 1990

Braffman BH, Zimmerman RA, Trojanowski JQ, et al: Brain MR: pathologic correlation with gross and histopathology, 2: hyperintense white-matter foci in the elderly. AJNR 9:629–636, 1988

Buchsbaum MS, DeLisi LE, Holcomb HH, et al: Anteroposterior gradients in cerebral glucose use in schizophrenia and affective disorder. Arch Gen Psychiatry 41:1159–1166, 1984

Coffman JA: Computed tomography in psychiatry, in Brain Imaging Appli-cations in Psychiatry. Edited by Andreasen NC. Washington, DC, Amer-ican Psychiatric Press, 1989, pp 1–65

Cohen RM, Semple WE, Gross M, et al: Dysfunction in a prefrontal substrate of sustained attention in schizophrenia. Life Sci 40:2031–2039, 1987

Dannals RF: Synthesis of radiotracers. Journal of Neuropsychiatry and Clinical Neuroscience 1:S14–S18, 1989

DeLisi LE, Buchsbaum MS, Holcomb HH, et al: Clinical correlates of decreased anteroposterior metabolic gradients in positron emission tomography (PET) of schizophrenic patients. Am J Psychiatry 142:78–81, 1985

Devous MD Sr: Imaging brain function by single-photon emission computer tomography, in Brain Imaging Applications in Psychiatry. Edited by An-dreasen NC. Washington, DC, American Psychiatric Press, 1989, pp 147–234

Duffy FH, Burchfiel JL, Lombroso CT: Brain electrical activity mapping (BEAM): a method for extending the clinical utility of EEG and evoked potential data. Ann Neurol 5:309–332, 1979

Erkinjuntti T, Ketonen L, Sulkava R, et al: Do white matter changes on MRI and CT differentiate vascular dementia from Alzheimer's disease? J Neurol Neurosurg Psychiatry 50:37–42, 1987

Fazekas F, Niederkorn K, Schmidt R, et al: White matter signal abnormalities in normal individuals: correlation with carotid ultrasonography, cerebral blood flow measurements, and cerebrovascular risk factors. Stroke 19:1285–1288, 1988

Fogel BS: Major depression versus organic mood disorder: a questionable distinction. J Clin Psychiatry 51:53–56, 1990

Fogel BS, Faust D: Neurologic assessment, neurodiagnostic tests, and neuropsychiatry in medical psychiatry, in Principles of Medical Psychiatry. Edited by Stoudemire A, Fogel BS. Orlando, FL, Grune & Stratton, 1987, pp 37–77

Glenner GG: On causative theories in Alzheimer's disease. Hum Pathol 16:433–435, 1985

Gur RE, Resnick SM, Alavi A, et al: Regional brain function in schizophrenia, I: a positron emission tomography study. Arch Gen Psychiatry 44:119–125, 1987

Holcomb HH, Links J, Smith C, et al: Positron emission tomography: measuring the metabolic and neurochemical characteristics of the living human nervous system, in Brain Imaging Applications in Psychiatry. Edited by Andreasen NC. Washington, DC, American Psychiatric Press, 1989, pp 235–370

Ingvar DH, Franzen G: Abnormalities of cerebral blood flow distribution in patients with chronic schizophrenia. Acta Psychiatr Scand 50:425–462, 1974

Jacobson HG: Magnetic resonance imaging of the central nervous system: Council on Scientific Affairs Report of the Panel on Magnetic Resonance Imaging. JAMA 259:1211–1222, 1988

Janota I, Mirsen TR, Hachinski VC, et al: Neuropathologic correlates of leukoaraiosis. Arch Neurol 46:1124–1128, 1989

Jaskiw GE, Andreasen NC, Weinberger DR: X-ray computed tomography and magnetic resonance imaging in psychiatry, in Psychiatry Update: American Psychiatric Association Annual Review, Vol 6. Edited by Hales RE, Frances AJ. Washington, DC, American Psychiatric Press, 1987, pp 260–299

Johnson KA, Holman BL, Mueller SP, et al: Single photon emission computed tomography in Alzheimer's disease: abnormal iofetamine I-123 uptake reflects dementia severity. Arch Neurol 45:392–396, 1988

Johnstone EC, Crow TJ, Frith CD, et al: Cerebral ventricular size and cognitive impairment in schizophrenia. Lancet 2:924–926, 1976

Karson CN, Coppola R, Morihisa JM, et al: Computed electroencephalographic activity mapping in schizophrenia. Arch Gen Psychiatry 44:514–517, 1987

Kertesz A, Black SE, Tokar G, et al: Periventricular and subcortical hyperintensities on magnetic resonance imaging. Arch Neurol 45:404–408, 1988

Kinkel WR, Jacobs L, Polachini I, et al: Subcortical arteriosclerotic encephalopathy (Binswanger's disease). Arch Neurol 42:951–959, 1985

Luchins DJ, Lewine RJ, Meltzer HY: Lateral ventricular size in the psychoses: relation to psychopathology and therapeutic and adverse response to medication. Schizophr Bull 19:518–523, 1983

Morihisa JM: Computerized EEG and evoked potential mapping, in Brain Imaging Applications in Psychiatry. Edited by Andreasen NC. Washington, DC, American Psychiatric Press, 1989, pp 123–145

Morihisa JM: Brain imaging approaches in psychiatry: early developmental considerations. J Clin Psychiatry 51 (suppl):44–46, 1990

Morihisa JM, McAnulty GB: Structure and function: brain electrical activity mapping and computerized tomography in schizophrenia. Biol Psychiatry 20:3–19, 1985

Morihisa JM, Weinberger DR: Is schizophrenia a frontal lobe disease? an organizing theory of relevant anatomy and physiology, in Can Schizophrenia Be Localized in the Brain? Edited by Andreasen NC. Washington, DC, American Psychiatric Press, 1986, pp 19–36

Morihisa JM, Duffy FH, Wyatt RJ: Brain electrical activity mapping in schizophrenic patients. Arch Gen Psychiatry 40:719–728, 1983

Nasrallah HA, Jacoby CG, McCalley-Whitters M, et al: Cerebral ventricular enlargement in subtypes of chronic schizophrenia. Arch Gen Psychiatry 39:774–777, 1982a

Nasrallah HA, McCalley-Whitters M, Jacoby CG: Cortical atrophy in schizophrenia and mania: a comparative study. J Clin Psychiatry 43:439–441, 1982b

Pearlson GD, Garbacz DJ, Breakey WR, et al: Lateral ventricular enlargement associated with persistent unemployment and negative symptoms in both schizophrenia and bipolar disorder. Psychiatry Res 12:1–9, 1984

Scheibel AB, Duong T, Tomiyasu U: Denervation microangiopathy in senile dementia, Alzheimer type. Alzheimer's Disease and Associated Disorders 1:19–37, 1987

Stoudemire A, Hill C, Gulley LR, et al: Neuropsychological and biomedical assessment of depression-dementia syndromes. The Journal of Neuropsychiatry and Clinical Neurosciences 1:347–361, 1989

Wagner HN, Burns HD, Dannals RF, et al: Imaging dopamine receptors in the human brain by positron tomography. Science 221:1264–1266, 1983

Weinberger DR: Brain disease and psychiatric illness: when should a psychiatrist order a CAT scan? Am J Psychiatry 141:1521–1527, 1984

Weinberger DR: Implications of normal brain development for the pathogenesis of schizophrenia. Arch Gen Psychiatry 44:660–669, 1987

Weinberger DR, Wyatt RJ: Brain morphology in schizophrenia: in vivo studies, in Schizophrenia as a Brain Disease. Edited by Henn FA, Nasrallah HA. New York, Oxford University Press, 1982, pp 148–175

Weinberger DR, Torrey EF, Neophytides A, et al: Lateral cerebral ventricular enlargement in chronic schizophrenia. Arch Gen Psychiatry 36:735–739, 1979a

Weinberger DR, Torrey EF, Wyatt RJ: Cerebellar atrophy in chronic schizophrenia. Lancet 1:718–719, 1979b

Weinberger DR, Luchins DJ, Morihisa JM, et al: Asymmetrical volumes of the right and left frontal and occipital regions of the human brain. Ann Neurol 11:97–100, 1982

Weinberger DR, Berman KF, Zec RF: Physiologic dysfunction of dorsolateral prefrontal cortex in schizophrenia, I: regional cerebral blood flow evidence. Arch Gen Psychiatry 43:114–124, 1986

Wolkin A, Jaeger J, Brodie JD, et al: Persistence of cerebral metabolic abnormalities in chronic schizophrenia as determined by positron emission tomography. Am J Psychiatry 142:564–571, 1985

Zimmerman RD, Fleming CA, Lee BCP, et al: Periventricular hyperintensity as seen by magnetic resonance: prevalence and significance. American Journal of Neuroradiology 7:13–20, 1986

Chapter 2

Psychopharmacology in the Medically Ill: An Update

Alan Stoudemire, M.D.
Barry S. Fogel, M.D.
Lawrence R. Gulley, M.D.

In the past few years, several new agents have been approved for the treatment of mental disorders, and a number of well-established drugs, particularly the anticonvulsants, have been used with increasing frequency for psychiatric indications. While the main thrust of psychopharmacologic research has been improved efficacy and reduced side effects in patients with primary psychiatric illness, many of the newer alternatives offer particular benefits to medically ill psychiatric patients, exemplified by the advantages of several of the newer antidepressant drugs such as fluoxetine and bupropion for depressed patients with cardiac conduction abnormalities. This chapter selectively reviews recent developments concerning psychopharmacologic treatment of psychiatric disorders in the medically ill and also discusses recent research on the application of more traditional psychotropics in this population. Topics covered include recent studies of tricyclic metabolites, lithium nephrotoxicity, and special problems with monoamine oxidase inhibitors (MAOIs) and anticonvulsants in the medically ill. Newly introduced psychotropic agents such as clozapine, fluoxetine, bupropion, buspirone, and midazolam are also discussed with respect to their use in the medically ill.

The topics covered in this chapter presume the reader's familiarity with basic principles of psychotropic drug use in the medically ill. Reviews of this material also can be found elsewhere (Stoudemire and Fogel 1987; Stoudemire et al., in press).

TRICYCLIC ANTIDEPRESSANTS

In previous publications, we and others have reviewed the cardio-vascular side effects of the tricyclic antidepressants (TCAs) (Dietch and Fine 1990; Halper and Mann 1988; Jefferson 1989; Roose et al. 1989; Stoudemire and Atkinson 1988; Stoudemire and Fogel 1987; Stoude-mire et al., in press). In these publications, the side effect profiles of the TCAs have been discussed in some detail, emphasizing their potential to cause orthostatic hypotension and quinidine-like effects. The side effect profiles of TCAs and other cyclic antidepressants are summarized in Table 2-1 (Risby et al. 1990). (In this chapter, for purposes of simplicity, the term *cyclic* antidepressants is used to refer to mono-cyclic, bicyclic, tricyclic, and tetracyclic antidepressants—basically, non-MAOI antidepressants.)

Newer antidepressants, particularly the bicyclic fluoxetine and the monocyclic bupropion, have minimal or no effects on cardiac conduction and blood pressure and appear to be safer alternatives in patients with heart block or decreased cardiac output. However, tricyclic antidepressants (TCAs) will remain the drugs of choice for many patients for some time to come, especially because data on the use of the newer agents in the medically ill are limited, and their therapeutic serum levels are not well established. Our discussion of the tricyclics focuses on the clinical significance of their hydroxylated metabolites and new information relevant to the use of tricyclics after myocardial infarction.

Hydroxylated Metabolites of TCAs

Several recent studies have assessed the contribution of the hy-droxylated metabolites of nortriptyline and desipramine to their side effects and to clinical outcome (Nelson et al. 1988a, 1988b; Nordin et al. 1987). Although therapeutic serum levels for both drugs are rea-sonably well established (50–150 ng/ml for nortriptyline and greater than 120 ng/ml for desipramine), less is known about the effects of their hydroxylated metabolites and whether their measurement is help-ful in predicting either efficacy or toxicity.

Table 2-1. Side effect profiles of the cyclic antidepressants

	Effect on serotonin reuptake	Effect on norepinephrine reuptake	Sedating effect	Anticholinergic effect	Orthostatic effect	Dosage range[a] (mg)
Amitriptyline[b]	+ + + +	+ +	+ + + +	+ + + +	+ + + +	75–300
Imipramine[b]	+ + + +	+ +	+ + +	+ + +	+ + + +	75–300
Nortriptyline	+ + +	+ + +	+ +	+ +	+	40–150
Protriptyline	+ + +	+ + + +	+ +	+ + +	+	10–60
Trazodone	+ + +	±	+ + +	±[c]	+ +	200–600
Desipramine	+ + +	+ + + +	+	+	+ +	75–300
Amoxapine[d]	+ +	+ + +	+	+ +	+ +	75–600
Maprotiline	+	+ +	+ +	+	+ +	150–200
Doxepin	+ + +	+ +	+ + +	+ +	+ +	75–300
Trimipramine[d]	+	+	+ +	+ +	+ +	50–300
Fluoxetine	+ + + +	–	–	–	–	20–60
Bupropion	–	–	–	±	–	150–450

Note. Relative potencies (some ratings are approximate) are based partly on affinities of these agents for brain receptors in competitive binding studies (Richelson E: Pharmacology of antidepressants in use in the United States. *J Clin Psychiatry* 43:4–11, 1982.) – = none. + = slight. + + = moderate. + + + = marked. + + + + = pronounced. ± = indeterminate.

[a]Dosage ranges are for treatment of major depression. Lower doses may be appropriate for other therapeutic uses.

[b]Available in injectable form.

[c]Most in vivo and clinical studies report the absence of anticholinergic effects (or no difference from placebo) with trazodone. There have been case reports, however, of apparent anticholinergic effects.

[d]Amoxapine and trimipramine have dopamine receptor blocking activity.

Source. Reprinted with permission from Risby ED, Risch SC, Stoudemire A: Mood disorders, in Clinical Psychiatry for Medical Students. Edited by Stoudemire A. Philadelphia, PA, JB Lippincott, 1990, p 187.

The major hydroxy metabolite of nortriptyline is 10-hydroxy-nortriptyline (10-OHNT). The 10-OHNT metabolite inhibits norepinephrine reuptake with about 50% of the potency of nortriptyline (Bertilsson et al. 1979; McCue et al. 1989a). The 10-OHNT metabolite has two isomers: *cis* (Z-10-OHNT) and *trans* (E-10-OHNT). The *trans* isomer comprises approximately 80% of total 10-OHNT (McCue et al. 1989a; Mellstrom et al. 1981). Although increasing age does not appear to affect plasma concentrations of nortriptyline, 10-OHNT metabolite levels do appear to increase with advancing age (Bertilsson et al. 1979; Robinson et al. 1985; Schneider et al. 1988; Young et al. 1984a).

Several groups have attempted to determine whether levels of these hydroxylated isomers are of clinical importance in predicting cardiotoxicity (Georgotas et al. 1987; McCue et al. 1989b; Schneider et al. 1988; Young et al. 1984b, 1985). Although it is well established that nortriptyline may affect cardiac conduction, it has not been clear to what extent the two isomeric forms of 10-OHNT contribute to this effect. In fact, investigations to date of the relationship of 10-OHNT isomers to cardiotoxic effects have produced conflicting results (McCue et al. 1989b).

Young and associates (1985) observed that the concentration of E-10-OHNT and the sum of nortriptyline + E-10-OHNT levels correlated with the development of prolonged cardiac conduction in a group of elderly depressed outpatients treated with nortriptyline; nortriptyline levels alone and pretreatment P-R intervals did not correlate with the development of prolonged atrioventricular (AV) conduction. Schneider and colleagues (1988) also found relationships between 10-OHNT isomers and cardiac conduction. Changes in QRS intervals were correlated with levels of nortriptyline, E-10-OHNT, Z-10-OHNT, and nortriptyline + 10-OHNT as revealed by multiple regression analyses. They also noted a trend for the Z-10-OHNT isomer concentration to be associated with increases in the QT_c interval. In animal experiments, other investigators have also observed the potential of the Z-10-OHNT isomer in high doses to cause cardiotoxicity (Pollock et al. 1987).

Although the clinical significance of hydroxylated TCA metabolites is not fully known, currently available data do not support routine measurement of the 10-OH isomeric metabolites of nortriptyline (McCue et al. 1989a). Nevertheless, the possibility of elevated levels of hydroxylated metabolites of nortriptyline, especially in elderly patients, may help explain toxicity that develops at apparently therapeutic nortriptyline serum levels (McCue et al. 1989a; Schneider et al. 1988). Hydroxymetabolites also deserve consideration as variables in treatment outcome studies of nortriptyline in depressed elderly or medically ill patients.

The hydroxylated metabolites of desipramine have also been investigated. Elderly patients are likely to have slightly higher levels of hydroxy metabolites of desipramine than younger patients, although the clinical significance of this observation, as with nortriptyline, is not fully known (Nelson et al. 1988b). For example, 2-hydroxydesipramine, the principal hydroxy metabolite of desipramine, was examined in one group of elderly patients (Kutchner et al. 1986). Prolongation of P-R intervals and increased QT_c intervals were significantly correlated with steady-state 2-OH-desipramine concentrations but not with desipramine concentrations alone. In other reports, the adverse effects of desipramine were not significantly correlated with levels of hydroxydesipramine (Nelson et al. 1982). As with nortriptyline, routine measurement of hydroxydesipramine is not supported by the literature to date. However, hydroxydesipramine levels may be useful in understanding toxicity when it occurs in patients whose serum levels of the parent compounds are within the therapeutic range.

Recent work by Baldessarini et al. (1988) suggests that hydroxymetabolites may help elucidate drug interactions. They reported that although carbamazepine usually *lowers* serum levels of parent TCA compounds, the hydroxylated metabolites of the TCAs may be *elevated* by carbamazepine, leading to clinically significant toxic effects on the ECG. One case was reported in which a patient with therapeutic serum levels of carbamazepine (9–12 ng/ml) was treated with high doses of desipramine (up to 825 mg/day), but had serum desipramine levels of less than 135 ng/ml. Despite this therapeutic serum level, the desipramine was stopped because of the development of a prolonged QRS interval. The patient was then switched to nortriptyline. In this patient (and several others treated with nortriptyline), antidepressant effects were seen at relatively low serum levels of nortriptyline (less than 50 ng/ml), apparently due to the fact that *total* TCA levels of 100–150 ng/ml were achieved when the level of 10-OHNT metabolites was added to the nortriptyline level. The relatively high 10-OHNT serum level was believed to be due to the concurrent use of carbamazepine (6–10 ng/ml). In the presence of carbamazepine, the ratio of 10-OHNT to nortriptyline was as great as 5. The authors inferred that the therapeutic effect of nortriptyline at a low blood level was due to an altered ratio of nortriptyline to 10-OHNT possibly induced by carbamazepine. They also speculated that an elevated hydroxydesipramine level had been responsible for the QRS prolongation observed in the case described earlier. Thus, measurement of hydroxylated metabolites could be relevant in understanding interactions between tricyclics and enzyme-inducing medications such as carbamazepine.

Hydroxylated TCA Metabolites in Chronic Renal Failure

Hydroxylated TCA metabolites have also been studied in patients with chronic renal failure (Lieberman et al. 1985). After initial oxidation by the hepatic microsomal mixed-function oxidase system, the tricyclics are glucuronidated and excreted in the urine (Lieberman et al. 1985). Although glucuronide-conjugated tricyclic metabolites are believed to be biologically relatively inactive, they may nevertheless alter the disposition of active forms of tricyclics by displacing active drug from protein binding sites, by competing for active transport mechanisms, or by inhibiting drug metabolism (Lieberman et al. 1985; Verbeeck 1982).

Single-dose pharmacokinetics of nortriptyline and its two major metabolites (conjugated and unconjugated forms of 10-OHNT) have been studied in chronic renal failure and hemodialysis patients (Sellers and Bendayan 1987). Although kinetics of nortriptyline in renal patients do not appear to be markedly different from those in normal subjects, conjugated forms of 10-OHNT are markedly elevated in renal disease, probably due to decreased elimination (Dawling et al. 1982).

Lieberman et al. (1985) found that the conjugated hydroxylated metabolites of TCAs were markedly elevated in hemodialysis patients by a factor of 500–1,500% compared with control patients who received equivalent oral doses. In a study of 12 dialysis patients (10 on hemodialysis and 2 on peritoneal dialysis), it was found that desipramine levels of dialysis patients were almost twice those of normal control subjects after similar oral dosage. Unconjugated 10-hydroxy desipramine metabolites in dialysis patients were twice those of control subjects. Conjugated 10-OH-desipramine metabolites, however, were almost nine times greater in dialysis patients than in control patients. Similar dramatic differences between dialysis patients and control patients were found when conjugated hydroxylated metabolites of amitriptyline were measured. Hence, although all forms of desipramine (desipramine and its conjugated and unconjugated hydroxy metabolites) were higher in dialysis patients, the most profound differences between patients and control subjects were found in the conjugated hydroxylated metabolites. Less dramatic differences were seen in the steady-state levels of the compounds amitriptyline and nortriptyline, although serum levels of these compounds were slightly higher in dialysis patients than in control subjects. However, similar marked increases were observed for the conjugated hydroxylated metabolites of amitriptyline and nortriptyline. This relative increase in conjugated metabolite levels of the TCA was explained by differences in elimination in the patients undergoing dialysis.

If conjugated hydroxylated metabolites of TCAs were biologically active, the finding that they are markedly increased in dialysis patients would help explain why some dialysis patients are hypersensitive to TCA side effects despite serum levels in the therapeutic range for the parent compounds and their demethylated metabolites. More data on the bioactivity of conjugated hydroxylated tricyclics and their influence on tricyclic protein binding are needed to test this hypothesis. Although uncontrolled studies of desipramine support its relative safety in dialysis patients (Kennedy et al. 1989), the recently reported data on tricyclic metabolites underscores the need for conservative dosing strategies and argues against excessive reliance on blood levels of the parent compound as a sole guide to dosage.

Treatment With TCAs After Myocardial Infarction

Several recent studies have added to the literature on tricyclics and the heart. One recurring theme is the antiarrhythmic action of tricyclics, previously known for imipramine and recently demonstrated for doxepin (Giardina et al. 1987), nortriptyline (Giardina et al. 1986), and desipramine (Fenster et al. 1989). In a large multicenter trial of antiarrhythmics (CAPS 1988), imipramine was included along with the antiarrhythmics encainide, flecainide, and moricizine in a placebo-controlled multicenter pilot study to evaluate their effectiveness in suppressing ventricular arrhythmias after myocardial infarction. Although imipramine had antiarrhythmic effects, its use was limited due to anticholinergic and hypotensive side effects. Although patients with left ventricular ejection fractions of less than 20% were excluded from the study, imipramine-treated patients apparently had no more trouble with subsequent congestive heart failure than placebo-treated patients in early data analyses. The CAPS study supported the efficacy of TCAs as type IA antiarrhythmics but also showed that side effects limited their clinical utility as antiarrhythmics. Nonetheless, their beneficial effect on post–myocardial infarction arrhythmias is reassuring to psychiatrists who choose to continue tricyclics after an acute myocardial infarction (Fenster et al. 1989; Giardina et al. 1987).

Several reports have documented that cardiac arrhythmias may emerge or reemerge after discontinuation of tricyclics, particularly if withdrawal is rapid (Boisvert and Chouinard 1981; Brown et al. 1978; Regan et al. 1989; Van Sweden 1988). Thus, available evidence argues against the routine abrupt discontinuation of tricyclics in patients who suffer a myocardial infarction while treated with tricyclics.

Results of animal experimentation further suggest that tricyclics may actually promote myocardial reperfusion by increasing collateral supply to the ischemic heart (Manoach et al. 1986, 1987, 1989). Manoach and colleagues have shown in experimentally induced myocardial infarction in cats that administration of a tricyclic either before or after experimental coronary artery occlusion increased retrograde perfusion of the distal component of the occluded artery and significantly decreased the volume of ischemic myocardium (Manoach et al. 1986). Although these results cannot necessarily be generalized to human clinical situations, they theoretically further support the relative safety of tricyclics in patients with recent myocardial infarction (Manoach et al. 1989) and again argue for their continuation, unless there are specific complications related to or aggravated by the tricyclic in use, such as orthostatic hypotension or tachycardia.

Prediction of TCA Serum Levels

Schneider and colleagues have developed a technique that may be helpful in predicting individual therapeutic doses of nortriptyline for relatively healthy depressed elderly outpatients. Using correlations between the nortriptyline plasma level 24 hours after a 25-mg oral nortriptyline test dose and steady-state serum levels of nortriptyline at doses of 50, 75, and 100 mg/day, a nomogram was constructed from regression equations to predict the dosage required to achieve a steady-state concentration within a 50–150 ng/ml therapeutic serum range (Schneider et al. 1987) (see Table 2-2). The study included elderly depressive patients, with a mean age of 64.7 ± 5.6 years. The subjects were relatively healthy, ambulatory outpatients, and the results cannot necessarily be generalized to older, more medically debilitated patients.

Dawling et al. (1981) studied a small sample of 10 elderly medically ill patients (mean age 82) and found that they required lower nortriptyline levels than younger healthy patients to produce therapeutic nortriptyline serum levels. Although more conservative dosages may be

Table 2-2. Suggested nortriptyline dosage guidelines in ambulatory depressed elderly patients (mean age 64.7 ± 5.6 years) based on 25-mg test dose

24-hour plasma level (ng/ml)	Suggested dosage (mg/day)
1–5	125
5–7	100
7–16	75
17–22	50
>22	<50

Source. Reprinted with permission from Schneider LS, Cooper TB, Staples FR, et al: Prediction of individual dosage of nortriptyline in depressed elderly outpatients. J Clin Psychopharmacol 7:311–314, 1987. Copyright 1987, Williams & Wilkins.

needed in elderly medically ill patients, the technique of dosage prediction may still be useful and deserves clinical validation in medically ill populations. Although a single 25-mg test dose would probably be safe for all but the most medically ill patients, a conservative 10-mg dose would be even better if a suitably modified nomogram were developed using this dosage form.

Special Reports on TCAs of Interest

Several reports continue to document the clinical efficacy of tricyclics in the management of medically ill patients with headache and other pain syndromes, even those without prominent symptoms of comorbid depression (Indaco and Carrieri 1988; Macfarlane et al. 1986; Max et al. 1987; Ziegler et al. 1987). Currently, although clinicians and many researchers persistently use amitriptyline for pain treatment, secondary tricyclics such as nortriptyline probably are equally effective and are almost always better tolerated.

A number of recent studies have documented the usefulness of TCAs in miscellaneous medical conditions. Doxepin (50–75 mg) has been found to be useful in the treatment of female bladder detrusor overactivity (Lose et al. 1989), and amitriptyline (25–75 mg) in interstitial cystitis (Hanno et al. 1989). Protriptyline in 20-mg doses has been employed in several series of patients to treat chronic lung disease with hypoxia and has been found to increase arterial oxygenation during the daytime and at night (the latter effect probably is due to suppression of rapid eye movement [REM] sleep) (Series et al. 1989; Simonds et al. 1986). In an isolated case report, amitriptyline was found to be effective in the treatment of intractable hiccups (Parvin et al. 1988).

Table 2-3.   Reported drug interactions with cyclic antidepressants (CyAds)

Medication	Effect
Type I-A antiarrhythmics (quinidine, procainamide)	May prolong cardiac conduction time
Phenothiazines	May prolong Q-T interval
Disulfiram Methylphenidate Cimetidine	Raise CyAd levels
Reserpine Guanethidine Clonidine	May decrease antihypertensive effect
Prazosin	Potentiates hypotensive effect
Warfarin	May increase prothrombin time
Oral contraceptives Ethanol Barbiturates Phenytoin	May lower CyAd levels
Parenteral sympathomimetic pressor amines (e.g., epinephrine, norepinephrine, phenylephrine)	May cause slight increases in blood pressure

Source. Reprinted with permission from Stoudemire A, Moran MG, Fogel BS: Psychotropic drug use in the medically ill: Part I. Psychosomatics 31:377–391, 1990.

Side Effects and Interactions of TCAs

Sporadic reports note an interaction between H2 (histamine) blockers and TCAs in which the H2 blockers elevate TCA levels. The combination may also carry an increased risk of psychosis and/or delirium (Miller et al. 1987). Table 2-3 summarizes clinically significant drug interactions with the cyclic antidepressants.

Of relevance to pulmonary patients, maprotiline has been reported to cause pulmonary alveolitis (Salmeron et al. 1988). The association of the yellow dye tartrazine (FD&C dye #5) contained in antidepressant compounds as a cause of allergic reactions continues to be noted (Pohl et al. 1987). Although tartrazine has been removed from most trade-name antidepressant dosage forms (e.g., Tofranil and Norpramin), it may still be found in some generic preparations of tricyclics. Patients who develop symptoms of urticaria, bronchospasm, nonthrombocytopenic purpura, angioedema, rhinitis, or anaphylaxis should be considered as possibly reacting to this dye, and patients with a history of aspirin sensitivity should not receive tartrazine-containing compounds at all.

LITHIUM

Lithium and the Kidneys

Of continuing concern with the use of lithium in the medically ill is the still-unresolved issue of long-term effects on the kidneys. A comprehensive and critical review of this area is beyond the scope of this chapter, but a few important recent articles will be mentioned. Hetmar and colleagues (1987) studied 32 patients treated with lithium for an average of 10 years and compared them with a control group of patients with mood disorders who had never been treated with lithium. Urine-concentrating ability in the lithium-treated group was less than that of the control group, but the lithium-treated group showed no further loss of urine-concentrating capacity over a follow-up period of 2 years. A single daily lithium dose was associated with significantly less polyuria than were multiple daily doses. Serum creatinine concentration was greater in lithium-treated patients than in control subjects, but both were still within normal limits. In addition, there was no evidence of deterioration in glomerular filtration rate in the lithium-treated patients at 2-year follow-up. Impairment of concentrating ability with no clinically significant change in glomerular filtration rate has been reported in other series of lithium-treated patients (Gelenberg et al. 1987). Other data suggest that lower serum lithium levels (0.7 meq/L or less) may impair concentrating ability less than higher levels (Schou and Vestergaard 1988).

Long-term exposure to lithium levels of 0.7 meq/L or less has not been definitively linked to reduced glomerular function (Schou and Vestergaard 1988). Thus, lower lithium levels and once-a-day dosing offer the potential advantages of convenience, fewer neurological side effects, and fewer effects on kidney function, both glomerular and tubular. Counterbalancing these advantages is evidence that lower serum levels of lithium may be less effective than levels maintained between 1.0 and 1.5 meq/L (Gelenberg et al. 1989), at least in younger bipolar populations.

A recently published report suggests that measurement of serum creatinine may not be an accurate substitute for the measurement of creatinine clearance, and that measurement of serum α_2-microglobulin may be superior. This test, while still under development, has been found to correlate better with creatinine clearance in lithium-treated patients than measurement of serum creatinine (Samiy and Rosnick 1987). The level of serum α_2-microglobulin, in contrast to serum creatinine, was consistently elevated when creatinine clearance was less than 70 ml/minute per 1.73 m^2 in lithium-treated patients (Samiy and Rosnick 1987). This study did not suggest, however, that lithium treatment was the reason for the decreased creatinine clearance.

α_2-Microglobulin promises to be a convenient method of monitoring small changes in creatinine clearance (Wibell 1978), and it may facilitate more definitive studies of lithium effects on glomerular function. In the meantime, the most recent summary of the available evidence suggests that lithium treatment probably does not lead to decreases in glomerular function (Schou 1989).

The nephrotic syndrome has recently been reported in a series of nine patients treated with lithium (Wood et al. 1989). Although four of the patients were relatively asymptomatic, five of the nine experienced weight gain and edema. All patients had proteinuria that varied from 7 to approximately 32 g/24 hours. Lithium discontinuation usually was followed by improvement in proteinuria, although some patients required more aggressive medical treatment with diuretics, dialysis, or prednisone. Although *routine* monitoring of the urinalysis is not recommended in patients on lithium (DasGupta and Jefferson 1990), the development of proteinuria may indicate vulnerability to the nephrotic syndrome in a small percentage of patients. Persistent proteinuria or the development of frank symptoms of the nephrotic syndrome may call for consideration of alternative antimanic drugs such as carbamazepine or valproate.

Lithium Use in Renal Transplant Recipients

Although lithium treatment is not recommended in patients with acute renal failure, there is no evidence that it is contraindicated in patients with chronic renal failure (DasGupta and Jefferson 1990). Lithium doses should be adjusted downward to accommodate decreases in creatinine clearance (Csernansky and Hollister 1985). Since it is not known if lithium accelerates the progression of certain types of renal disease, closer monitoring of renal disease is probably indicated in such patients, and alternative antimanic agents should be considered if they are not contraindicated for other reasons. The use of lithium in hemodialysis patients has been previously reviewed, and it appears to be safe and effective if lithium doses are reduced to the range of 300–600 mg and if lithium doses are given after hemodialysis (Lippman et al. 1984; Port et al. 1979; Stoudemire and Fogel 1987).

Since renal transplantation has become a relatively common procedure, clinicians increasingly will encounter patients with renal transplants requiring lithium therapy for bipolar disorder or for organic mood disorders due to steroid use. Experience with the use of lithium in transplant recipients remains quite limited, but there are a few reports of its successful implementation (Blazer et al. 1976; Koecheler et al. 1986). Koecheler recommends more conservative use of lithium in patients with cadaveric transplants because their renal function is more unstable than in patients with living related donor transplants.

Cyclosporine may elevate lithium levels by decreasing lithium's fractional excretion, so lithium doses may need to be adjusted downward in patients receiving cyclosporine (DasGupta and Jefferson 1990; Dieperink et al. 1987; Vincent et al. 1987). Close monitoring of lithium levels is essential given that the transplant's function may be unstable for weeks after transplantation.

Lithium and Diabetes

There is evidence that at least in some patients, lithium may decrease glucose tolerance (DasGupta and Jefferson 1990). However, increased glucose tolerance has also been reported as a lithium effect (Vendsborg 1979). Although some patients may have their glucose tolerance curves affected by lithium, there is no strong evidence that this is a clinically significant effect in the vast majority of patients, nor is there evidence to suggest the need for routine glucose monitoring in patients treated with lithium other than for diabetic patients with unstable control of blood glucose who undoubtedly would be monitored closely anyway (DasGupta and Jefferson 1990).

Lithium and Epilepsy

Although lithium administration has been associated with EEG changes, a recently reported series of bipolar patients treated with lithium suggests that lithium may be benign in patients with epilepsy (Shukla et al. 1988). In an open study of eight patients, lithium levels were maintained in the 0.6–1.1 meq/L range and concurrent anticonvulsants were limited to phenytoin and phenobarbital. (No patients were on carbamazepine, sodium valproate, or clonazepam.) Lithium prevented the recurrence of affective episodes without increasing seizure frequency in patients with incompletely controlled seizures and did not induce any seizures in well-controlled patients. One patient with complex partial seizures actually achieved an apparent remission in both seizure activity and mood disorder when treated with lithium alone. Although lithium should not be dismissed because of an undue concern about aggravation of seizures, the antimanic anticonvulsants carbamazepine and valproate should be considered as alternative agents for patients with concurrent bipolar disorder and epilepsy. When lithium and anticonvulsants are given simultaneously, pharmacodynamic interactions may lead to central nervous system (CNS) side effects at lithium levels within the therapeutic range (Fogel 1988), so the upper end of the therapeutic range of lithium levels usually should be avoided.

Drug Interactions With Lithium

Many commonly prescribed medications have been recently reported to affect lithium levels. The angiotensin-converting enzyme (ACE) inhibitor enalapril has been reported to elevate lithium levels to toxic range when it was added to lithium (Douste-Blazy et al. 1986; Navis et al. 1989) (Table 2-4). This same effect has also been observed with the ACE inhibitor captopril (Pulik and Lida 1988). This effect has been attributed to inhibition of the renin-angiotensin-aldosterone axis with subsequent increased sodium excretion and lithium retention, which may be increased even more if the patient is volume depleted (Navis et al. 1989). Thus, lithium dosage should be reduced, and lithium levels monitored frequently, if ACE inhibitors are to be used concurrently.

Regarding diuretics and lithium, a recent report showed that furosemide (a loop diuretic) does not increase serum lithium as much as the distal tubular diuretic hydrochlorothiazide (HCTZ) (Crabtree et al. 1989). Concurrent use of tetracycline for lithium-induced acne may slightly lower lithium levels, but the effect is of no real clinical significance (Frankhauser et al. 1988). Of a more serious nature, choreoathetosis was observed in one patient when lithium was combined with the calcium channel blocker verapamil (Helmuth et al. 1989). Other reports have also documented choreoathetosis as a sign of lithium toxicity (Reed et al. 1989), and other involuntary movements have been reported with the combined use of verapamil and lithium (Price and Giannini 1986).

Table 2-4. Reported drug interactions with lithium carbonate

Medication	Effect

Thiazide diuretics
Spironolactone
Triamterene
Enalapril
Captopril
Nonsteroidal anti-inflammatories (e.g.,
  indomethacin, ibuprofen,
  phenylbutazone, piroxicam)
	Raise Li$^+$ levels

Acetazolamide Theophylline Aminophylline	Lower Li$^+$ levels
Calcium channel blockers	May either raise or lower Li$^+$ levels, effects not clear; verapamil may cause bradycardia when used with Li$^+$
Metronidazole	May increase Li$^+$ levels; may increase chances of nephrotoxicity
Cyclosporine	May increase Li$^+$ levels

Source. Reprinted with permission from Stoudemire A, Moran MG, Fogel BS: Psychotropic drug use in the medically ill: Part II. Psychosomatics (in press).

We have previously reviewed other drug interactions with lithium, including enhanced lithium excretion with acetazolamide, theophylline, and aminophylline, all of which may lower lithium levels, and the effects of the nonsteroidal anti-inflammatory drugs (e.g., indomethacin, ibuprofen, phenylbutazone, and piroxicam), which may increase lithium levels by decreasing renal lithium clearance (Stoudemire and Fogel 1987).

The potassium-sparing diuretic amiloride helps ameliorate lithium-induced polyuria when used in doses of 10–20 mg/day (Kosten and Forrest 1986). Amiloride may, however, elevate lithium serum levels, particularly if used concurrently with HCTZ; HCTZ has been recommended for refractory lithium-induced polyuria that does not respond to amiloride alone. We have found it practical to treat lithium-induced polyuria by halving the lithium dose and giving the patient one HCTZ-amiloride (Modiuretic) tablet daily.

Finally, it has been recommended that coadministration of beta-adrenergic blockers, particularly propranolol, with lithium can decrease the renal clearance of both lithium and creatinine (Schou and Vestergaard 1987). Long-term use of propranolol alone may lower the

glomerular filtration rate. For this reason, *intermittent* use of propranolol is recommended when the drug is used to suppress lithium tremor,
and alternative agents to beta-blockers are preferable if an antihypertensive or antianginal agent is needed for a lithium-treated patient.

NEWER DRUGS

Fluoxetine

Fluoxetine, a phenylpropylamide, is a relatively new bicyclic antidepressant that is a selective inhibitor of serotonin presynaptic uptake. The drug has very little affinity for muscarinic, histaminic,
dopaminergic, or noradrenergic α_1 or α_2 receptors in vitro and in animal
experiments (Stark et al. 1985). Fluoxetine appears to augment serotonin neurotransmission. Its low affinity for other neurotransmitter
systems probably accounts for its very low incidence of anticholinergic,
antihistaminic, sedative, and hypotensive effects. In most studies, the
side effects most frequently reported have been anxiety, insomnia,
anorexia, and nausea (Feighner et al. 1988). Recently, however, Lipinski
et al. (1989) suggested that the anxiety, nervousness, and insomnia that
affect 10–15% of fluoxetine-treated patients actually represent a form
of akathisia, a side effect that may limit treatment, even if benzodiazepines or beta-blockers are coadministered to attenuate the side effect.

Although fluoxetine may cause insomnia in some patients, a substantial number of patients (10–20%) experience drowsiness or sedation with the drug (Feighner and Cohn 1985). The sedation may be
continuous, or most pronounced in the late afternoon, a pattern also
seen with MAOIs. Fluoxetine appears to be as effective as other traditional cyclic antidepressant agents in treating major depression, even
in the elderly (Feighner and Cohn 1985). The chemical structure of
fluoxetine is depicted in Figure 2-1.

Of primary interest to psychiatrists working with the elderly and
the medically ill is fluoxetine's lack of cardiac effects. Fluoxetine appears to be remarkably benign with respect to the heart (Cooper 1988).
In a comprehensive examination of the effects of fluoxetine on cardiac
conduction, Fisch (1985) examined 1,506 ECGs from 753 patients treated
with amitriptyline (54 patients), doxepin (56), imipramine (165), fluoxetine (312), and placebo (166). No appreciable changes were seen on
the ECG with the use of fluoxetine, suggesting it does not have a

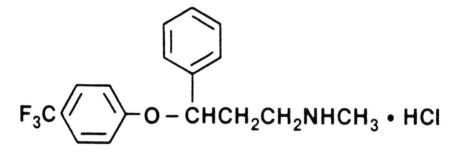

Figure 2-1. Chemical structure of fluoxetine hydrochloride.

quinidine-like effect. This observation is confirmed by its lack of cardiotoxicity in overdose. Because fluoxetine has not yet been studied in patients with advanced cardiovascular disease or those with preexisting conduction delays, its safety in this population would nevertheless still have to be considered as relative. Fluoxetine's virtual lack of anticholinergic and hypotensive effects, coupled with its benign cardiac profile, likely will make it one of the antidepressants of choice in the medically ill as well as in patients with coexistent depression and Alzheimer's disease.

Several drug interactions are relevant to medically oriented psychiatrists. Fluoxetine has been reported to prolong the half-life of diazepam and reduce its clearance, resulting in higher plasma concentrations of diazepam and a reduction in the rate of formation of the active metabolite *N*-desmethyldiazepam. However, there is no evidence that this effect has any major clinical significance as judged by results of tests of psychomotor performance (Lemberger et al. 1988). A few other agents have been studied specifically for pharmacokinetic interactions with fluoxetine; no effect on plasma half-life has been observed for warfarin, chlorothiazide, or tolbutamide (Lemberger et al. 1985).

Fluoxetine's metabolism does appear to be affected by cirrhosis, because in *stable* alcoholic cirrhosis, the elimination of fluoxetine is substantially reduced. The mean half-life of fluoxetine was 6.6 days in middle-aged patients with cirrhosis, compared to 2.2 days in age-matched control volunteers (Schenker et al. 1988). Formation of fluoxetine's principal metabolite, norfluoxetine, was delayed. These data are compatible with previous studies in which other low-clearance drugs metabolized predominantly by demethylation have shown impaired elimination in liver disease (Secor and Schenker 1987; Williams and

Mamelok 1980). It has been recommended that dosages of fluoxetine be reduced by as much as 50% in patients with liver disease, which can be accomplished practically by giving the drug on an every-other-day (or a Monday-Wednesday-Friday) schedule. Because the half-life may be even more prolonged in patients with unstable or decompensating liver disease, even lower doses may need to be given. Even under normal circumstances in healthy patients, the elimination half-life of fluoxetine is 2–3 days, and of norfluoxetine 7–9 days. Thus, less-than-daily dosage is rational, and frequently necessary, because the drug comes in only one dosage.

It is now well established that fluoxetine may increase the serum levels of tricyclics and trazodone, and if fluoxetine is *added to* the regimen of a patient with an established tricyclic level, abrupt elevation in tricyclic levels may result and cause tricyclic toxicity. In one small series of patients, after the addition of fluoxetine the ratio of antidepressant plasma level to oral dose increased from 109% to 486% in patients taking tricyclics and by 31% in a patient taking trazodone (Aranow et al. 1989). A clinically significant interaction between fluoxetine and tricyclics is now well established (Bell and Cole 1988; Downs and Downs 1989; Downs et al. 1989; Faynor and Espina 1989; Goodnick 1989; Rudorfer and Potter 1989; Vaughan 1988).

Fluoxetine infrequently provokes seizures, with the incidence of this side effect probably less than 0.2%, and similar to reported rates for seizure activity with oral tricyclics (Cooper 1988; Weber 1989). When using fluoxetine in treating known epileptic patients, care should be taken to monitor anticonvulsant levels frequently, because the frequency and magnitude of pharmacokinetic interactions between fluoxetine and anticonvulsants are not yet known.

Steiner and Fontaine (1986) reported a toxic reaction—a hyperserotonergic state—when fluoxetine was coadministered with L-tryptophan. When L-tryptophan was added to an existing regimen of fluoxetine in five patients with obsessive-compulsive disorder, the patients developed severe agitation, restlessness, insomnia, nausea, and abdominal cramps, which resolved with discontinuation of L-tryptophan (Steiner and Fontaine 1986). Similar and more severe reactions have resulted from combining MAOIs with fluoxetine (see below).

Inappropriate secretion of antidiuretic hormone has been reported as an idiosyncratic side effect of fluoxetine (Hwang and Magraw 1989), a side effect also seen occasionally and unpredictably with tricyclics and neuroleptics. The combination of fluoxetine and lithium has been reported to cause toxicity when either agent was added to a stable dose of the other (Noveske et al. 1989; Salama and Shafey 1989); symptoms were similar to those of lithium toxicity. The interaction was not due to toxic lithium levels: in one of the reported cases, the lithium level was actually decreased, and in the other, only slightly elevated.

Skin rashes occur in approximately 3% of fluoxetine-treated patients (Stark and Hardison 1985). The usual fluoxetine rash is a nonspecific maculopapular eruption typical of drug hypersensitivity; drug discontinuation is indicated when it occurs. More severe dermatologic reactions are substantially more rare, although one of the authors (B.S.F.) did observe a case of exfoliative dermatitis induced by fluoxetine among his first 50 fluoxetine-treated patients.

Bupropion

Bupropion is a new monocyclic aminoketone antidepressant that is a weak inhibitor of dopamine uptake and appears to lack direct effects on norepinephrine, serotonin, and monoamine oxidase (Ferris et al. 1983). It has a half-life of approximately 10 hours, and multiple daily doses are recommended. The drug has some structural similarities to amphetamine and diethylpropion, a sympathomimetic agent. Although bupropion has an activating effect that may be beneficial in some patients, it may induce agitation or provoke psychotic episodes (Golden et al. 1985). The psychotic reactions to bupropion reported by Golden et al. appear to be accompanied by visual and auditory hallucinations in addition to paranoia. In contrast to amphetamine-induced states, however, tactile hallucinations were absent, nor did patients display autonomic symptoms of amphetamine psychosis such as tachycardia, pupillary dilation, hypertension, sweating, nausea, or vomiting. The properties of bupropion of greatest interest to medical psychiatrists are its lack of cardiovascular toxicity and its association with seizures. The chemical structure of bupropion is depicted in Figure 2-2.

Side effects. Bupropion has an excellent side effect profile. It is essentially devoid of anticholinergic properties and has minimal effects on histamine, alpha$_1$- and alpha$_2$-adrenergic receptors. Its relative lack of sedative, anticholinergic, antihistaminic, and anti-alpha-adrenergic effects would make it particularly attractive for medically ill patients if its efficacy were conclusively demonstrated to be equal to that of more established agents.

In studies of elderly depressed patients, bupropion has shown a side effect profile comparable to placebo, with significantly less dry mouth and constipation than tricyclics such as imipramine (Branconnier et

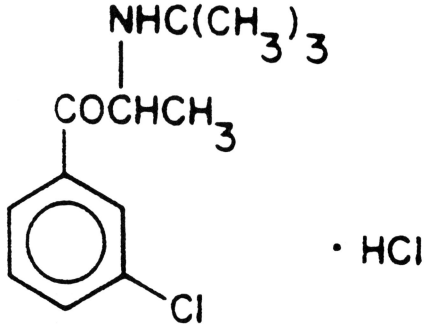

Figure 2-2.   Chemical structure of bupropion.

al. 1983a; Kane et al. 1983). Other studies have demonstrated that bupropion has not been associated with significant changes in blood pressure, heart rate, or ECG, nor has it been associated with orthostatic hypotension (Branconnier et al. 1983a, 1983b; Burroughs Wellcome Company 1989; Chouinard et al. 1981; Farid et al. 1983; Preskorn and Othmer 1984; Roose et al. 1987; Wenger and Stern 1983; Wenger et al. 1982, 1983; Zung 1983). Bupropion-treated patients have nevertheless reported symptoms of syncope, dizziness, and fainting. Syncope has been reported in 1.2% of bupropion-treated patients versus 0.5% of placebo-treated patients (Branconnier et al. 1983b).

The previously cited studies did not specifically focus on patients with concurrent advanced cardiovascular disease. However, Roose and associates (1987) compared the cardiovascular effects of bupropion with those of imipramine in a small series of depressed patients with congestive heart failure. In a randomized double-blind crossover trial, 10 depressed patients with left ventricular failure received bupropion (mean dose 445 mg/day) or imipramine (mean dose 197 mg/day). Neither bupropion nor imipramine adversely affected ejection fraction or other indices of left ventricular function. One-half of the patients treated with imipramine, however, developed severe orthostatic hypotension. Bupropion, in contrast, was well tolerated and did not cause orthostatic hypotension. Bupropion had no effect on the ECG. However, because experience with this drug in patients with preexisting heart block is limited, repeating an ECG after dosage increases in such patients would be a reasonable precaution until more systematic studies are reported.

Association of bupropion with seizures. Davidson (1989) has critically reviewed the prevalence of seizures in patients treated with bupropion and has put the issue into perspective by comparing bupropion with other available antidepressants. According to his review, there have been 37 known reports of tonic-clonic seizures in patients receiving bupropion. Patients treated for bulimia have shown the highest incidence of associated seizures (5.4%).

In patients receiving daily doses of bupropion of no more than 450 mg/day, the risk of seizures was 0.35%. This incidence was compared with estimates of the incidence of seizures with other antidepressants: 0.6–0.9% with imipramine at doses greater than 200 mg/day (Peck et al. 1983); 0.2% with maprotiline in doses of 225 mg/day or less; 3.0% with clomipramine (Trimble 1978); and 0.2% with fluoxetine. Davidson's summary estimate of the incidence of seizures in nonepileptic depressed patients on long-term (average 28 months) tricyclic treatment at an average dose of 150 mg/day was 0.5% (range 50–300 mg) (Davidson 1989; Lowry and Dunner 1980).

In the incidence estimate of 0.35% (15 of 4,240 patients), patients who received bupropion doses above 450 mg/day were excluded from the calculations (Davidson 1989). In the 15 patients who did suffer seizures at doses of less than 450 mg/day, 7 had possible predisposing factors. Three had a previous history of seizures, 1 had metastatic brain cancer, 1 was undergoing alcohol withdrawal when bupropion was administered, 1 was concomitantly receiving 450 mg/day of amitriptyline, and another patient might have been withdrawing from alprazolam. A seizure incidence of 0.35% is not meaningfully higher than the estimated incidence for full-dose tricyclics. If patients with known risk factors for seizures are eliminated, the estimated risk for bupropion would be even lower. Risk factors for seizures with bupropion (and other antidepressants) include active withdrawal from alcohol or benzodiazepines, a history of epilepsy, concurrent medications such as neuroleptics known to lower the seizure threshold, and a history of head trauma. Risk factors that may be related to bupropion-induced seizures are listed in Table 2-5.

Even patients with risk factors for bupropion-induced seizures may

Table 2-5.   Factors that may be related to bupropion-induced seizures

1. History or presence of bulimia and/or anorexia nervosa
2. Dosages in excess of 450 mg/day
3. Past history of seizures (including febrile convulsions), head injury, loss of consciousness
4. Overdose
5. Recent withdrawal from alcohol or anxiolytic drugs, especially short-acting benzodiazepines
6. Concomitant therapy with other drugs that lower seizure threshold (e.g., lithium, neuroleptics)
7. Recent or rapid dose escalation of bupropion
8. Known EEG abnormality
9. Past history or current presence of organic brain disease
10. High plasma levels of parent drug or metabolites
11. Once-daily administration of full 450-mg dose

Source. Reprinted with permission from Davidson J: Seizures and bupropion: a review. J Clin Psychiatry 50:256–261, 1989. Copyright 1989, Physicians Postgraduate Press.

still receive a bupropion trial if they give informed consent. In this situation, a relatively higher estimate of risk (e.g., 5%) should be offered to the patient, and anticonvulsant prophylaxis with phenytoin or carbamazepine should be considered, especially in patients with a definite history of seizures or with epileptiform EEGs.

There is no evidence that bupropion will aggravate seizures in well-controlled epileptic patients, if anticonvulsant levels are carefully monitored and maintained in the therapeutic range. However, because of the attention given recently to seizures related to bupropion use, the process of informed consent should be scrupulous.

Because administration of *single* doses of bupropion greater than 150 mg has been associated with seizures (independently of a total daily dose greater than 450 mg), bupropion should be given on a tid or qid schedule. Patients should be warned not to make up missed doses by doubling up on the next dose.

Buspirone

Buspirone is a relatively new nonbenzodiazepine anxiolytic that has stimulated interest among psychiatrists because of its freedom from the side effect of respiratory depression and its lack of withdrawal symptoms on discontinuation. Buspirone is an azapirone agent with a complex mechanism of action. Current data suggest that its main neuropharmacologic activity is mediated by 5-HT$_{1A}$ (serotonin) receptors. Buspirone also displays some affinity for D2 (dopamine) presynaptic autoreceptors and 5-HT$_2$ receptors (Jann 1988). Jann has proposed that buspirone inhibits the synthesis and release of serotonin by inhibiting the firing rates of serotonergic neurons in the dorsal raphe nucleus.

Buspirone's mean elimination half-life is 2.1 hours, although its metabolites may have elimination half-lives of 6–8 hours (Jann 1988). Although buspirone has significant anxiolytic activity, it is devoid of anticonvulsant, muscle relaxant, and sedative-hypnotic activity. There are no synergistic or additive effects when combining buspirone and alcohol or other sedative-hypnotics.

The pharmacokinetics of buspirone have been studied in patients with impaired liver or kidney function. In a study of 12 patients with hepatic cirrhosis, after a single 20-mg dose, the elimination half-life was 6.21 hours ± 1.79 hours in patients with cirrhosis, compared to 4.19 hours ± 0.53 hours in healthy subjects (Dalhoff et al. 1987; Goa and Ward 1986). In patients with impaired renal function, including some who were completely anuric, buspirone clearance decreased 33–50% with no correlation between the severity of renal impairment and buspirone clearance (Gammans et al. 1986). Hence, small reductions in buspirone dosage are likely to be needed in patients with hepatic and renal disease, although the reported prolongation of elimination half-life by liver or kidney failure is more likely to represent an effect of smaller magnitude than normal interindividual differences in optimal dosage. No clinically significant prolongation of buspirone pharmacokinetics in elderly patients has been observed (Gammans et al. 1989).

Drug interactions with buspirone. Buspirone does not induce or inhibit hepatic mixed oxidase enzymatic functions (Molitor et al. 1985). The ability of buspirone to displace phenytoin, warfarin, propranolol, and digoxin from protein binding has been studied in vitro (Gammans et al. 1985), and buspirone's interaction with these drugs does not appear to be clinically significant. Buspirone also appears free from interaction with antihistamines, bronchodilators, histamine (H2) receptor blockers, oral contraceptives, nonsteroidal anti-inflammatory drugs, benzodiazepine hypnotics, digitalis preparations, common antihypertensive drugs, and oral hypoglycemics (Domantay and Napoliello 1989; Levine and Napoliello 1988). Pharmacokinetic interactions between buspirone and tricyclic antidepressants have not been found (Gammans et al. 1986). However, buspirone has been observed to increase serum haloperidol concentrations (Sussman 1987). Elevations in blood pressure have been observed in patients taking buspirone with MAOIs (Knapp 1987), leading to a manufacturer's recommendation against this combination. There may be some slight prolongation in the metabolism of diazepam when concurrently used with buspirone, although this is of doubtful clinical significance (Meltzer and Fleming 1982). Some slight increase in sedation may occur if buspirone is used concurrently with diazepam (Gershon 1982).

Buspirone and pulmonary disease.   Of primary interest to medical psychiatrists is the use of buspirone in patients with pulmonary disease. Although systematic studies utilizing buspirone in the treatment of anxiety in patients with chronic obstructive pulmonary disease (COPD) have yet to be published, animal studies suggest that buspirone may serve as a respiratory stimulant. Garner and associates (1989) observed in cats that buspirone had a dose-dependent effect on respiratory output, primarily through an increase of tidal volume and respiratory frequency. The animals were also noted to have a shift in their apneic threshold to a lower level of P_{CO_2} without a change in the slope or shape of the CO_2 response curve. In contrast, benzodiazepines led to respiratory depression and a shift of the apneic threshold to a higher P_{CO_2} level. The Garner et al. study involved animal preparations (cats) in which the vagus nerve and carotid sinus nerves had been severed; applicability to humans with COPD is tempting to speculate but not conclusively established. In an open study of 82 patients, buspirone was used safely for reduction of anxiety in patients with chronic lung disease. No problems developed from using buspirone together with bronchodilators such as theophylline and terbutaline (Kiev and Domantay 1988).

Buspirone and other conditions.   Numerous reports have anecdotally suggested clinical efficacy of buspirone in various conditions other than anxiety disorders. Buspirone has been used to treat autism (Realmuto et al. 1989), for the suppression of neuroleptic-induced akathisia (D'Mello et al. 1989), and as an antidepressant (Robinson et al. 1989). A number of anecdotal reports have suggested that buspirone might also have a role in suppressing anxiety and agitation in brain-injured patients (Levine 1988) and in patients with dementia (Colenda 1988; Tiller et al. 1988). Typically, relatively low doses are needed for this antiagitation effect (5–10 mg tid). Buspirone may be helpful in smoking cessation (Gawin et al. 1989) and in premenstrual syndromes (Rickels et al. 1989; Yatham et al. 1989).

Published reports have also postulated idiosyncratic side effects of buspirone. These include a report of a 62-year-old woman on multiple medications who developed myoclonus, dystonia, and akathisia when treated with buspirone (Ritchie et al. 1988). Another report described dyskinesia precipitated by buspirone (Simpson and Singh 1988). Movement disorders have not been reported to date in patients on buspirone alone who have had no prior exposure to neuroleptics. Although some adverse effects have been reported in elderly patients, systematic studies suggest that buspirone is as well tolerated within the recommended dosage ranges in elderly patients as it is in younger patients (Robinson et al. 1988).

Although buspirone has an anxiolytic effect maximal in 4–6 weeks, some patients experience early stimulation or agitation from the drug. One of the authors (B.S.F.) has seen several of these reactions in patients with diagnoses ranging from panic disorder to depression to mental retardation. The reaction is dose dependent and can be treated by discontinuing buspirone until the agitation or insomnia resolves, then restarting the drug at a lower dosage. A reasonable approach to starting buspirone in panicky or neurologically impaired patients is to start no higher than 2.5 mg tid and warn the patient or caretaker about possible early and transient agitation. Finally, since buspirone has an antidepressant effect, it may precipitate hypomania or mania; a series of reasonably well-documented cases were recently reported (Price and Bielefeld 1989).

Clozapine

Clozapine is a novel antipsychotic with a dibenzodiazepine structure that is chemically related to the dibenzoxazepine neuroleptic loxapine. In contrast to loxapine, however, clozapine has greater alpha$_1$- and alpha$_2$-adrenergic, 5-HT$_2$, and H1 blocking potency, and stronger muscarinic anticholinergic properties. In addition, its D1 and D2 receptor affinity is relatively weak when compared with traditional neuroleptics (Kane et al. 1988), and its dopamine receptor binding is more pronounced in mesolimbic than in striatal regions (Mattes 1989). Clozapine is quickly absorbed, and peak plasma concentration is achieved after an average of 3 hours (Cheng et al. 1988). It is 94% protein-bound, has a half-life of approximately 16 hours, and is completely metabolized via demethylation and oxidation prior to excretion (Lieberman et al. 1989).

While most studies in Europe and the United States clearly support clozapine's clinical efficacy as an antipsychotic, the greatest obstacle to its widespread usage lies in its distinctive side effect profile, primarily its potential for myelosuppression. Agranulocytosis, defined as a white blood cell count less than 2,000 cells/mm^3 and a polymor-phonuclear leukocyte count of less than 500 cells/mm^3, occurs in 1–2% of patients treated with clozapine. This potentially fatal side effect is reversible if detected early. A total of 12 deaths worldwide due to agranulocytosis were reported from 1984 to 1987; there have been none reported in the United States to date. Most cases of clozapine-induced agranulocytosis occur within the first 6 months of therapy, and, if the medication is discontinued, blood counts generally normalize within 7–21 days (Lieberman et al. 1989).

Many of clozapine's other side effects are more predictable and result from its antihistaminic, anticholinergic, and antiadrenergic activity. In one recent multicenter study, the most frequent adverse side effects reported were sedation (21%), tachycardia (17%), constipation (16%), dizziness (14%), hypotension (13%), and hypersalivation (13%) (Kane et al. 1988). Although tremor, akathisia, and rigidity have been reported with clozapine treatment, these are uncommon (approximately 5%) and generally mild. Moreover, the drug does not appear to be associated with masked facies, acute dystonic reactions, and parkinsonian gait abnormalities. Indeed, improvement of both tremor and psychotic features has been reported (Ostergaard and Dupont 1988).

A recent record review of 387 inpatients, mainly with schizophrenia, who were treated with clozapine showed that severe side effects forced discontinuation of clozapine therapy in 5.9% of patients. The most common adverse reactions were sedation, EEG abnormalities, liver enzyme abnormalities, hypotension, hypersalivation, fever, ECG changes, tachycardia, gastrointestinal side effects, and delirium (Naber et al. 1989).

Friedman and Lannon reported in 1989 on the successful treatment with clozapine of psychotic symptoms in six patients with Parkinson's disease. In patients who exhibited psychotic symptoms such as auditory hallucinations and paranoia and who ranged in age from 52 to 78 years, they found that clozapine improved psychiatric symptoms without worsening motor manifestations of Parkinson's disease such as rigidity and gait disturbance. In two patients, parkinsonian symptoms actually improved. They noted that the likely explanation is that clozapine has relatively low affinity for striatal dopamine receptors. Its affinity for the D2 receptor in the caudate nucleus is only ⅕₀th that of haloperidol and ⅒th that of chlorpromazine. The patients in this case series did not develop agranulocytosis, and the major side effect encountered was hypersalivation. Psychotic symptoms were controlled with relatively low doses, ranging from 25 or 50 mg/day up to 275 mg/day (Friedman and Lannon 1989). Another case report (Roberts et al.

1989) showed similar symptomatic improvement in hallucinosis and paranoia in a 64-year-old woman with Parkinson's disease. When treated with clozapine 25 mg po qhs, not only did mental symptoms improve, but the patient's parkinsonian symptoms improved to the point where specific parkinsonian pharmacotherapy (carbidopa, levodopa, and trihexyphenidyl) could be discontinued.

Patients with Parkinson's disease may experience psychotic symptoms related either to antiparkinsonian medications or to underlying dementia. Because conventional neuroleptics typically exacerbate the motor symptoms of Parkinson's disease, patients with Parkinson's disease and psychosis have always been a difficult group to manage. Clozapine offers such patients a rational alternative to conventional neuroleptics.

One case of neuroleptic malignant syndrome (NMS) has been reported in a patient concurrently receiving clozapine and lithium (Kane et al. 1988). On the other hand, the drug has been successful in treating psychosis without recurrent NMS in a patient with a history of recurrent NMS on other neuroleptics (Stoudemire and Clayton 1989).

Clozapine lowers the seizure threshold, with the risk of seizures increasing with dosage: 1–2% at dosages below 300 mg/day, 3–4% at moderate dosages, and 5% at higher dosages of 600–900 mg/day (manufacturer's estimates). Clozapine is contraindicated in patients with myeloproliferative disorders or granulocytopenia and should not be used with other medications known to have myelosuppressive effects (e.g., carbamazepine).

If clozapine is psychiatrically indicated in a patient with epilepsy, the patient should be switched if necessary to an anticonvulsant other than carbamazepine. To minimize the risk of seizures, anticonvulsant levels should be monitored frequently during initiation of clozapine and kept at the higher end of the therapeutic range.

It is recommended that clozapine treatment be instituted at low dosages (25–50 mg on day 1) because of its potential to induce marked sedation and hypotension. The typical therapeutic range for schizophrenia in physically healthy patients is 300–500 mg/day with a maximum of 900 mg/day. Dosing should be on a bid or tid schedule (Lieberman et al. 1989). Fever up to 103°F may occur when starting clozapine and may persist with fluctuation for 4–6 weeks. Development of this fever may be managed supportively with aspirin or acetaminophen and is not in itself a reason to discontinue the drug. However, care should be taken to ensure patients are adequately hydrated and to frequently reassess patients for symptoms suggesting a nonpharmacologic reason for the fever.

Food and Drug Administration (FDA) labeling recommends that clozapine be reserved for patients who have not responded to two standard neuroleptics, and for patients with psychosis and Parkinson's disease. Clozapine is available only through a proprietary home health care pharmacy system that arranges for weekly leukocyte counts for early detection of evidence of myelosuppression. The annual cost of the drug and the obligatory monitoring system in the United States is $8,000–$9,000.

In summary, clozapine is a novel antipsychotic that has distinctive characteristics including a favorable extrapyramidal profile, no reported cases of drug-induced tardive dyskinesia, and apparent increased efficacy in refractory schizophrenia when compared with traditional neuroleptics. However, its ability to induce agranulocytosis limits its indication to subgroups of psychotic patients who are intolerant of extrapyramidal side effects or are refractory to currently available antipsychotics. At present, tardive dyskinesia in itself is not an indication for clozapine. Little is known about how clozapine interacts with other drugs, and what specific roles it may have in the medically ill population.

Conventional neuroleptics are known to have numerous interactions with drugs commonly used in the medically ill (Stoudemire and Fogel 1987). For convenience, these are listed in Table 2-6.

PSYCHOSTIMULANTS

Although use of psychostimulants in the treatment of primary depression in physically healthy patients remains controversial, their use in medically ill patients—at least for short periods of time—is relatively well accepted. The two most commonly used psychostimulants are methylphenidate and dextroamphetamine.

Dextroamphetamine is roughly twice as potent as methylphenidate, with typical therapeutic dosages of 10–20 mg/day for dextroamphetamine versus 20–40 mg/day for methylphenidate (Jenike 1985). Dextroamphetamine excretion is influenced by urinary pH, and when urine is acidic, dextroamphetamine is excreted more rapidly and largely unchanged in the urine. (Thus, ascorbic acid or cranberry juice could be used in the ambulatory treatment of mild dextroamphetamine toxicity.) Its plasma half-life is approximately 12 hours (Chiarello and Cole 1987) as opposed to the 2-hour average half-life of methylphenidate,

Table 2-6. Reported drug interactions with neuroleptics

Medication	Effect
Type I-A antiarrhythmics	Chlorpromazine/thioridazine may prolong cardiac conduction
Tricyclics Beta-blockers Chloramphenicol Disulfiram, monoamine oxidase inhibitors Acetaminophen Buspirone	May increase neuroleptic levels
Barbiturates Hypnotics Rifampin Griseofulvin Phenylbutazone Carbamazepine	Lower neuroleptic levels through induction of hepatic enzymes
Gel-type antacids with Al^+ and Mg^+	May interfere with neuroleptic absorption
Narcotics Epinephrine Enflurane Isoflurane	Potentiate hypotensive effects of neuroleptics
Prazosin Angiotensin-converting enzyme inhibitors (captopril, enalapril)	Increase hypotensive effect
Narcotics Tricyclics; barbiturates	May increase sedative effects of neuroleptics
Iproniazid	May cause encephalopathy and hepatotoxicity when used with neuroleptics
Guanethidine Clonidine	Neuroleptics may decrease blood pressure control

Source. Reprinted with permission from Stoudemire A, Moran MG, Fogel BS: Psychotropic drug use in the medically ill: Part II. Psychsomatics (in press).

which is quickly metabolized by the liver to ritalinic acid, a metabolite with little CNS activity (Goff 1986).

In addition to methylphenidate and dextroamphetamine, pemoline and diethylpropion hydrochloride (Janowsky 1988) are sympathomimetic agents that have been utilized less frequently as psychostimulants. Pemoline is structurally dissimilar to methylphenidate and the amphetamines.

Two recent literature reviews have critically examined studies on the efficacy of psychostimulants in the treatment of depression (Chiarello and Cole 1987; Satel and Nelson 1989). Satel and Nelson (1989) reviewed 16 controlled and 30 noncontrolled studies, concluding that the majority of placebo-controlled studies showed no significant advantage of stimulants over placebo in primary major depression. High response rates of placebo-treated patients have been noted in many of these studies, suggesting that uncontrolled studies should be interpreted with some skepticism. However, both reviews acknowledge potential usefulness of stimulants in certain depressive subgroups: apathetic, withdrawn geriatric patients; medically ill depressed patients who are unable to tolerate conventional antidepressants; and possibly as adjuvant therapy in patients with refractory depression.

Lingam et al. (1988) retrospectively studied the records of 25 patients with poststroke depression treated with methylphenidate at dosages of at least 20 mg/day for 5 consecutive days. These authors found "complete" recovery from depression in 52% of the patients. In a prospective study of another medically ill population, depressed cancer patients, Fernandez et al. (1987) treated 7 men and 23 women at an initial dose of 10 mg of methylphenidate tid, with 23 showing marked or moderate improvement. This study included 11 patients who were treated for 1 year at low doses of 5–10 mg/day without evidence of tolerance or abuse. One patient with dementia became more agitated and confused on the psychostimulant (Fernandez et al. 1987).

Two recent reports have targeted patients with acquired immunodeficiency syndrome (AIDS)–related depression as a medically ill depressed subgroup that may respond to psychostimulant therapy (Fernandez et al. 1988; Holmes et al. 1989). Holmes et al. (1989) prospectively studied 17 AIDS-related complex patients treated with dextroamphetamine (initial doses 5–15 mg/day) or methylphenidate (initial doses 5 mg tid). These patients had DSM-III (American Psychiatric Association 1980) diagnoses of organic mental disorder, adjustment disorder, or major depression and were treated for an average of 8 months. Treatment with either stimulant was effective in achieving a marked to moderate improvement in 79% of the patients; 89.5% showed some improvement in Clinical Global Impression ratings.

In spite of continued debate over their efficacy, psychostimulants may offer in some patients distinct advantages over traditional antidepressants. Unlike cyclic antidepressants, improvement in mood, if it occurs, is rapid, usually within the first 24–48 hours of treatment

(Woods et al. 1986). In addition, the psychostimulants are surprisingly well tolerated, even in older medically ill patients who may be unable to tolerate the anticholinergic side effects of TCAs. However, the possibilities of rebound depression after cessation of the drugs, habituation, abuse, and precipitation of paranoid reactions argue against routine usage of psychostimulants except in patients whose medical illness contraindicates use of standard antidepressants. Other chapters in this volume address the use of stimulants in patients with frontal lobe syndromes (Chapter 10), in children (Chapter 13), and in the mentally retarded (Chapter 15). For drug interactions, see Table 2-7.

MIDAZOLAM

Midazolam is a new benzodiazepine derivative that is currently approved for use as a parenteral preanesthetic in induction of general anesthesia, and for sedation before short diagnostic procedures such as endoscopy. However, its sedating and anxiolytic action, remarkably short onset and duration of action, and the option of parenteral use suggest potential uses in psychiatric patients. This notion has been bolstered by recent case reports in the psychiatric literature of its efficacy in the management of acutely agitated and psychotic patients (Bond et al. 1989; Mendoza et al. 1987).

Midazolam is highly lipophilic at physiologic pH and, unlike most benzodiazepines, is rapidly and well absorbed intramuscularly (Matson and Thurlow 1988). It has a very rapid onset of CNS effects, with sedation occurring within 5–15 minutes after intramuscular injection (3–5 minutes after intravenous administration) and reaching its peak within 30–60 minutes. The drug is rapidly displaced from benzodiazepine receptors and has a short duration of action of approximately 2 hours, with a range of 1–6 hours (Bond et al. 1989). Biologic half-life is only 1.3–2.2 hours (Beck et al. 1983). Midazolam undergoes extensive biotransformation to its major pharmacologically active metabolite, 1-hydroxymethylmidazolam, by way of microsomal oxidation. There is evidence that there are significant age-related differences in the clearance of midazolam, with decreased clearance in elderly patients, especially men (Holazo et al. 1988). Lower initial doses are therefore recommended in patients older than age 60 years. Although the drug is generally well tolerated, like other benzodiazepines, respiratory depression including apnea has been associated with its use. In addition there have been case reports of hypotension (Matson and Thurlow

1988), disinhibition of aggressive behavior (Bobo and Miwa 1988), transient paranoia and agitation (Burnakis and Berman 1989), and delirium, especially in the elderly (Patterson 1987a).

Like triazolam, another short-acting benzodiazepine, midazolam may induce amnesic episodes. Two recent reports suggest that it causes amnesia in more than 70% of patients receiving it (Dundee and Wilson 1980; White et al. 1988). This side effect may be clinically desirable in a patient undergoing an uncomfortable surgical procedure, but may be less desirable in psychiatric contexts.

Midazolam is approximately three to four times as potent per milligram as diazepam, and initial intramuscular dosage is 0.07–0.08 mg/kg, with the average dosage in a healthy adult being 5 mg, and lower dosages recommended in elderly or debilitated patients. Although dosage guidelines in the psychiatric setting are not yet clear, Bond et al. (1989) reported three case studies of use of midazolam in the treatment of mentally retarded patients with acute and refractory aggressivity and violence using 5–10 mg of midazolam administered intramuscularly. The patients (a 14-year-old girl, a 17-year-old boy, and a 26-year-old man) showed rapid improvement in aggressive behavior. Mendoza et al. in 1987 reported on three patients with acute psychotic states with hyperarousal who responded favorably when treated with lower dosages of midazolam in a psychiatric emergency room setting. The patients included a 17-year-old boy, a 38-year-old man, and a 34-year-old woman. The authors noted the onset of sedation in these patients to occur within 6–8 minutes, with sedation lasting approximately 90 minutes after a dose of 2.5–3 mg im (Mendoza et al. 1987). These clinical case reports support earlier animal work with midazolam that has shown that administration of the drug can have beneficial effects on experimentally induced aggressive rage. For example, electrical stimulation of the hypothalamus in cats can produce aggressive behavior in cats, a response that is diminished by midazolam (Pieri 1983). Wyant et al. (1990) reported a randomized single-blind comparison of 5 mg of midazolam, 250 mg of amobarbital sodium, and 10 mg of haloperidol in agitated schizophrenic patients. There were five patients in each group. Midazolam and amobarbital sodium were both more effective than haloperidol in controlling agitation over a 2-hour period.

None of the above studies were double-blind and controlled, and none involved medically ill, debilitated, or elderly patients. Moreover, midazolam is not currently FDA-approved for psychiatric indications. However, the pharmacologic properties of the drug suggest potential usage for psychiatric patients with acute psychomotor agitation or hyperarousal. A specific use may be in the emergency room, to facilitate medical assessment of patients with acute psychosis, who would otherwise be too agitated to permit examination and testing, and in whom neuroleptics are undesirable. It remains for controlled, randomized studies to provide clearer guidelines for its indications and usage in psychiatric conditions.

Reported drug interactions with benzodiazepines are listed in Table 2-7.

MONOAMINE OXIDASE INHIBITORS

MAOIs in General Anesthesia

For many years, MAOI therapy has been regarded as a relative contraindication to general anesthesia. However, in the 1980s several reports were published suggesting that general anesthesia could safely be given to patients on MAOIs, and that absolute insistence on a 2-week drug-free period was neither necessary nor always desirable (El-Ganzouri et al. 1985; Michaels et al. 1984; Stack et al. 1988; Wells and Bjorksten 1989; Wong 1986). Instead, both the urgency of the contemplated surgical procedure and the likely severity of the patient's mental and physical symptoms if MAOIs were withdrawn should be taken into account on an individual basis.

Procedures carried out safely in the presence of MAOIs have ranged from electroconvulsive therapy (ECT) (El-Ganzouri et al. 1985) to cardiac surgery (Michaels et al. 1984). Although the number of reported cases remains too small to accurately estimate the risk of anesthesia during MAOI therapy, some anesthesiologists' opinion is shifting away from an absolute requirement for MAOI discontinuation to a weighing of relative risks and benefits (Stack et al. 1988; Wells and Bjorksten 1989).

If anesthesia is to be administered to a patient on an MAOI, several issues are relevant to anesthetic and postoperative management. These have been reviewed by Janowsky and Janowsky (1985), and more recently in the above referenced articles by Stack et al. and by Wells and Bjorksten. Key points, discussed in detail in these three reviews, follow.

First, meperidine (Demerol) is absolutely contraindicated for postoperative pain, as this drug has been associated with hypertension,

Table 2-7.   Various reported drug interactions

Medication	Effect
With Benzodiazepines	
Cimetidine	May elevate serum levels of
Disulfiram	benzodiazepines metabolized
Ethanol	predominantly by oxidation
Isoniazid	
Estrogens	Tend to lower benzodiazepine levels
Cigarettes	
Methylxanthine derivatives	
Rifampin	
With Psychostimulants	
Guanethidine	Decreased antihypertensive effect
Vasopressors	Increased pressor effect
Oral anticoagulants	Increased prothrombin time
Anticonvulsants	Increased levels of phenobarbital, primidone, phenytoin
Tricyclics	Increased blood levels of cyclic antidepressants
MAOIs	Hypertension
With Carbamazepine	
Erythromycin	May raise carbamazepine levels and precipitate heart block
Antiarrhythmics	May have additive effects on cardiac conduction time
Diltiazem	May raise carbamazepine levels to toxic
Verapamil	levels
Danazol	

Source.   Reprinted with permission from Stoudemire A, Moran MG, Fogel BS: Psychotropic drug use in the medically ill: Part II. Psychosomatics (in press).

hyperpyrexia, and death in MAOI-treated patients (Denton et al. 1962; Palmer 1960; Taylor 1962). The interaction appears to be relatively specific to meperidine and possibly related to meperidine's action to block serotonin reuptake (Brown and Cass 1979; Stack et al. 1988), leading to a "serotonin syndrome" (see below). Dextromethorphan, which also blocks serotonin uptake, can produce a similar reaction when taken in high doses (Rivers and Horner 1970).

On the other hand, both morphine (Michaels et al. 1984) and fentanyl (El-Ganzouri et al. 1985; Michaels et al. 1984; Youssef and Wilkinson 1988) have been given without complication to patients on MAOIs, and codeine has been proposed as a relatively safe oral narcotic for MAOI-treated patients (Davidson et al. 1984). Nonetheless, the action of morphine and other narcotics may be more intense and prolonged in the presence of MAOIs (Stack et al. 1988), so initial dosage of narcotics should be lower than usual, and dosage should be titrated upward slowly.

If a serotonin syndrome develops because of inadvertent administration of meperidine or dextromethorphan to an MAOI-treated patient, this reaction might be treated with a serotonin-receptor blocking agent, as described below. If morphine or another narcotic produces excessive CNS depression, however, naloxone treatment is indicated.

Second, phenelzine, but not other MAOIs, has been reported to reduce pseudocholinesterase levels in some patients, and in one reported study a patient on phenelzine had prolonged apnea following a usual dose of succinylcholine (Bodley et al. 1969). Subsequent to this report, problems have not been reported either with other MAOIs or with nondepolarizing muscle relaxants such as pancuronium. However, because it has an indirect sympathomimetic effect, curare should probably be avoided in MAOI-treated patients (Stack et al. 1988). Special attention should be given to monitoring of neuromuscular function and the adequacy of respiration if succinylcholine is given to a patient on phenelzine.

Third, patients on chronic MAOI therapy are vulnerable to excessive hypertension from indirect sympathomimetics, but less likely from direct-acting drugs such as norepinephrine and isoproterenol (Elis et al. 1967; Wells and Bjorksten 1989), although mild elevations in blood pressure are possible (see Table 2-8). Therefore, if intraoperative hypotension is unresponsive to volume expansion and pressor substances are required, direct-acting sympathomimetics can be considered.

Fourth, concerns about blood pressure stability during major surgery with prolonged anesthesia can be addressed by using an indwelling arterial catheter (Wong 1986). A recent report details the prompt and successful management of intraoperative hypertensive crisis made possible by the immediate detection of the problem with an arterial line (Sides 1987). Either phentolamine or nitroprusside can be used as an intravenous hypotensive agent if arterial monitoring reveals excessive blood pressure (Janowsky and Janowsky 1985).

Fifth, regarding the specific use of ECT in MAOI-treated patients, the issue has been raised that ECT could cause greater hypertension in MAOI-treated patients because of inhibited catecholamine metab-

Table 2-8.   Reported drug interactions with monoamine oxidase inhibitors

Medication	Effect
Meperidine	Fatal reaction
L-Dopa Methyldopa Dopamine Buspirone Guanethidine Propranolol Cyclic antidepressants Carbamazepine Cyclobenzaprine	Hypertension

Direct-acting sympathomimetics
  Epinephrine
  Norepinephrine
  Isoproterenol
  Methoxamine
	Mild blood pressure elevation possible

Indirect-acting sympathomimetics
  Cocaine
  Amphetamines
  Tyramine
  Methylphenidate
  Phenethylamine
  Metaraminol
  Ephedrine
  Phenylpropanolamine
  Pseudoephedrine
  Phenylephrine
	Severe hypertension

Caffeine Theophylline Aminophylline	Mild increase in blood pressure
Hypoglycemic agents	Lower blood glucose
Anticoagulants	Prolonged prothrombin time
L-Tryptophan	Hyperreflexia, ataxia, myoclonus, delirium
Succinylcholine	Phenelzine prolongs action

Diuretics
  Propranolol
  Prazosin
  Calcium channel blockers
	Increased hypotensive effect

Source.   Reprinted with permission from Stoudemire A, Moran MG, Fogel BS: Psychotropic drug use in the medically ill: Part I. Psychosomatics 31:377–391, 1990.

olism. In fact, to our knowledge, there is no convincing evidence for greater hypertension with ECT in MAOI-treated patients, and concerns in this regard remain primarily theoretical.

MAOIs and Weight Gain

MAOIs, like other antidepressants, have been associated with weight gain (Garland et al. 1988). This side effect can be problematic in patients suffering from diabetes or hyperlipidemia, in whom weight gain may aggravate the medical problem. The association of weight gain with MAOI therapy was recently reviewed by Cantu and Korec (1988), in an informal meta-analysis of reported cases and previous reviews. They concluded that tranylcypromine, the only nonhydrazide MAOI currently approved for treating depression, is associated with a substantially lower incidence of weight gain. Its amphetamine-like properties and perhaps its inhibition of serotonin reuptake (Tuomisto and Smith 1986) may contribute to its lesser effect on weight. Tranylcypromine might then be the preferred MAOI in patients in whom weight gain would complicate management of a concurrent medical problem.

Consideration of the mechanisms of weight gain with MAOIs has led to renewed interest in earlier observations that MAOIs can potentiate insulin-induced hypoglycemia (Cooper and Ashcroft 1966). This observation suggests that close monitoring of blood glucose may be warranted in insulin-dependent diabetic patients receiving MAOIs, at least during initiation of antidepressant therapy. Specifically, insulin-dependent diabetic patients could be monitored with four-times-a-day glucose checks for a 72-hour period after initiation or dose changes in MAOI therapy to detect the need for any necessary adjustments in insulin dose.

Treatment of MAOI-Induced Orthostatic Hypotension

Although hypertensive crises may be the most feared adverse effect of MAOIs, orthostatic hypotension is a more frequent reason for MAOIs to be discontinued. Particularly in older patients who are at risk for falls, orthostatic hypotension implies a risk of injury as well as discomfort. The incidence of measurable orthostatic hypotension in older patients may approach 50% (Lazarus et al. 1986), but it is often of insufficient severity to warrant drug discontinuation. Orthostatic hypotension may develop slowly over the first few weeks of treatment, so that ongoing monitoring of blood pressure is necessary to protect patients from unpleasant surprises (Kronig et al. 1983).

Treatment of orthostatic hypotension begins with assuring adequacy of hydration, an important point in patients with poor oral intake, or in medically ill patients who may be on diuretics or salt-restricted diets because of hypertension or congestive heart failure. Whenever possible, diuretics should be reduced or discontinued, and salt intake liberalized, while carefully monitoring the patient for a recurrence of hypertension or signs of heart failure. When volume expansion alone is insufficient and MAOIs are strongly indicated psychiatrically, various measures, reported helpful in uncontrolled trials, could be considered. However, it is uncertain how truly successful these measures are over the longer term. Strategies have included the administration of fludrocortisone (Florinef) 0.1 mg/day (Simonson 1964), T_3 (Pollack and Rosenbaum 1987), and metoclopramide (Patterson 1987b). Naproxen, an anti-inflammatory drug, was recently reported to be helpful in nortriptyline-induced orthostatic hypotension (Forster 1989); its use in MAOI-induced hypotension has not been reported. Yohimbine, one proposed treatment for tricyclic-induced hypotension, has been shown to be ineffective for MAOI-induced hypotension (Lin et al. 1987).

Treatment of MAOI-Induced Hypertensive Episodes

Hypertensive episodes can occur during MAOI therapy, both from dietary indiscretions and drug interactions, and spontaneously (Fallon et al. 1988; Kahn 1988; Keck et al. 1989). Hypertensive episodes are potentially dangerous in all patients, but pose particular risk for patients on anticoagulants or with cerebrovascular disease, because of their increased risk of intracerebral hemorrhage.

Further, the risk of hypertensive episodes may persist for up to 2 months after the discontinuation of phenelzine (but not necessarily tranylcypromine). In a recent study of normal volunteers who took phenelzine for 3 weeks, reaching a maximum dose of 60 mg/day, hypertensive reactions to high-tyramine foods were seen as far removed as in the second month after phenelzine discontinuation in several patients (Bieck et al. 1989).

Recently, efforts have been made to reduce the risk of hypertensive crises by teaching patients to recognize the early signs of hypertension (i.e., headache and flushing) and providing them with an oral hypotensive "antidote" to carry with them. Although patients are still told to seek medical attention promptly for a hypertensive episode, they are spared the risk and discomfort of uncontrolled hypertension during the interval before seeing a physician. Recommended oral medications for this purpose include nifedipine 10 mg (Clary and Schweizer 1987), verapamil 80 mg (Merikangas and Merikangas 1988), chlorpromazine 25–50 mg, or thioridazine 25–50 mg (Kahn 1989). The nifedipine capsule may be chewed, with the remainder of the capsule kept under the tongue for sublingual absorption; verapamil and the phenothiazines are swallowed. A second dose of nifedipine may be taken if symptoms do not resolve in 15 or 20 minutes. Although both the phenothiazines and the calcium channel blockers are effective, the latter have the advantage of being less sedating. Kahn (1989), in discussing these strategies, advises confining them to patients who "don't panic in emergencies." However, it might be argued that since a single unnecessary dose of one of these drugs is unlikely to have a lasting adverse effect, they might be given to all patients on MAOIs, with further instruction given if they are overused. In the case of chronically ill patients cared for by family members, family caretakers should be instructed in the signs of a hypertensive reaction and be equipped with a hypotensive agent.

Diagnosis and Treatment of the "Serotonin Syndrome"

Numerous recent reports have documented a syndrome of myoclonus, ataxia, confusion, and hyperthermia occurring in association with MAOI overdose, or with MAOI drug interactions including the combination of MAOIs with tricyclics, tryptophan, fluoxetine, or meperidine (Graham and Ilett 1988; Kline et al. 1989; Sternbach 1988). Milder forms of the syndrome may occur without fever or with low-grade fever only, whereas the more severe forms may be as fulminant and fatal as NMS. Neuromuscular features of the serotonin syndrome vary from myoclonus and tremor to lead-pipe rigidity (see Chapter 12).

In cases due to drug combinations, the drug given with the MAOI is one known either to block serotonin reuptake or to increase serotonin levels. A study by Price et al. (1983) showed that the neuromuscular features of the serotonin syndrome included hyperreflexia, nystagmus, ataxia, and myoclonic jerks and could be produced in tranylcypromine-treated volunteers (dosage 10–40 mg daily) by intravenous infusion of tryptophan.

The key clinical features of the serotonin syndrome are neuromuscular excitability (myoclonus, rigidity, or hyperreflexia), signs of diffuse CNS dysfunction (nystagmus, ataxia, and/or confusion), and elevated temperature; alterations in blood pressure are not characteristic, nor is the profuse sweating so often seen in NMS. Prevention efforts should center on avoiding the offending combinations of drugs whenever possible, and using very slow upward dosage titration in those patients in whom a risky combination (e.g., TCA and MAOI) is clinically warranted. Further, TCAs should never be started in a fully MAO-inhibited patient.

Switching from fluoxetine to MAOIs is particularly problematic because of the very long and variable half-life of norfluoxetine, which can be as long as 14 days, implying that about 10 weeks would be necessary after discontinuation of fluoxetine before the metabolite's levels would become nondetectable. Although the manufacturer recommends waiting 5 weeks after discontinuing fluoxetine before starting an MAOI, a useful precaution in medically ill or elderly patients with presumptively slower metabolism is to obtain a norfluoxetine blood level and require that it be nondetectable before starting an MAOI.

Basic treatment of the serotonin syndrome begins with supportive measures, antipyretics, and discontinuation of the drugs that provoked the syndrome. However, the use of agents such as chlorpromazine or cyproheptadine that block serotonin receptors would seem rational and has been recommended anecdotally (Kahn 1989). One of the authors (B.S.F.) has successfully treated one case of the serotonin syndrome with cyproheptadine. One standard 4-mg tablet was given every hour until symptoms resolved (a total of 16 mg was needed), and additional 4-mg doses were given as needed when symptoms of neuromuscular irritability recurred. An additional 16 mg per day was given for the next 2 days, and the syndrome resolved completely. Given the extremely low toxicity of cyproheptadine, it might be considered as a treatment for the serotonin syndrome pending more definitive studies.

Interactions of MAOIs With Over-the-Counter Drugs

Although physicians who prescribe MAOIs are well aware of food-induced hypertensive crises and warn their patients accordingly, observations by Harrison et al. (1989) suggest that interactions with over-the-counter (OTC) medications may be a more common cause of hypertensive reactions in patients compliant with MAOI dietary restrictions. Major offenders are OTC cold preparations containing the

Table 2-9. Common over-the-counter (OTC) preparations that contain ingredients contraindicated for patients treated with monoamine oxidase inhibitors

OTC products containing pseudoephedrine, phenylephrine, or phenylpropanolamine

Pseudoephedrine

Actifed	Robitussin-PE
Contac	Sine-Aid
CoTylenol	Sinutab
Vicks Formula 44M	Sudafed
Vicks Formula 44D	Tylenol Maximum Strength Sinus
Vicks NyQuil	Medication

Phenylephrine

Dimetane Decongestant	Nostril
Dristan Advanced Formula	Vicks Sinex
Tablets & Coated Caplets	Robitussin Night Relief
Neo-Synephrine	

Phenylpropanolamine

Alka-Seltzer Plus	Cheracol Plus	Sine-Off
Acutrim	Coricidin	Triaminic
Allerest	Dexatrim	

OTC products for which there are prohibited combination formulations

Acceptable product	*Prohibited product*
Dimetane	Dimetane Decongestant
Robitussin	Robitussin-PE, -DM, -CF, Night Relief
Alka-Seltzer	Alka-Seltzer Plus Cold Medicine
Cheracol D Cough Formula	Cheracol Plus Head Cold/Cough Formula
Chlor-Trimeton Allergy Tablets	Chlor-Trimeton Decongestant Tablets
Sucrets Lozenges	Sucrets-Cold Decongestant Formula Lozenges
Tylenol	CoTylenol
Coricidin Tablets	Coricidin 'D' Decongestant Tablets

Source. Adapted with permission from Harrison WM, McGrath PJ, Stewart JW, et al: MAOIs and hypertensive crises: the role of OTC drugs. J Clin Psychiatry 50:64–65, 1989. Copyright 1989, Physicians Postgraduate Press.

indirect-acting sympathomimetics pseudoephedrine, phenylephrine, or phenylpropanolamine. Table 2-9 shows common OTC preparations that contain ingredients contraindicated for patients on MAOIs. A conservative approach is to inform patients taking MAOIs that they should use no OTC medication until checking with their physician; a copy of the *Physicians' Desk Reference for Nonprescription Drugs* (1990) will aid the physician in rapidly identifying which combination drugs have risky ingredients. In general, simple antihistamines and anti-cholinergics such as diphenhydramine and chlorpheniramine are safe, as long as they are not combined with sympathomimetic decongestants. The patient should be warned that similar-sounding medications may have different ingredients and different risks (Harrison et al. 1989).

Selegiline (Deprenyl)

With its recent FDA approval for the treatment of Parkinson's disease, selegiline (deprenyl), an MAO-B inhibitor, is likely to be used by psychiatrists, both for the treatment of Parkinson's disease and possibly for the (currently unapproved) indication of depression. While selegiline is a selective inhibitor of MAO-B at antiparkinsonian doses of 5 mg bid, it is a *nonselective* inhibitor (hence affecting both MAO-A and MAO-B) at higher doses such as 40–60 mg/day. Hypertensive reactions have occurred with these higher doses of selegiline (McGrath et al. 1989). Therefore, patients receiving selegiline in doses above 10 mg/day should receive the full set of warnings concerning dietary restrictions and avoidance of potentially interacting drugs.

Nonselective MAO inhibition with selegiline at doses above 10 mg/day implies that tricyclics should probably not be added in patients on established selegiline regimens of greater than 10 mg daily. However, there is no evidence that tricyclics are especially hazardous in patients on higher doses of selegiline when titrated concurrently or if the selegiline dose is 10 mg or less. Likewise, ECT would not be contraindicated by antiparkinsonian doses of selegiline. Nevertheless, because of the interindividual variability that is the rule in medically ill psychotic patients, we advise *slow* initiation of tricyclics with frequent monitoring of blood pressure.

MAOI Withdrawal

Because of concern about drug interactions, or in preparation for surgery, it is not uncommon for general medical physicians to abruptly discontinue MAOIs when patients are admitted to a general hospital for treatment of an intercurrent medical or surgical problem. Consulting psychiatrists should be aware, however, that abrupt discontinuation of MAOIs can cause various physical and mental symptoms, occasionally producing acute distress that may result in urgent psychiatric consultation. Physical symptoms may include headaches, tremors, sleep disturbance, or gastrointestinal complaints; psychiatric symptoms may include severe anxiety, agitation, delirium, or even paranoid psychosis (Dilsaver 1990). The severity of MAOI withdrawal symptoms may warrant reinstitution of the MAOI, followed by a slow taper if there are strong medical reasons for discontinuing the drug. In milder cases, symptomatic treatment of the withdrawal symptoms with other agents may suffice.

ANTICONVULSANTS

In the last several years, anticonvulsants have entered the mainstream of psychopharmacologic practice. Carbamazepine (Tegretol), valproate (Depakote, Depakene), and clonazepam (Klonopin) have all been widely employed for psychiatric indications, although they are not specifically FDA-approved as psychotropics. For a survey of the varied psychiatric uses of these anticonvulsants, including their increasingly well-documented use as alternatives or adjuncts to lithium in the treatment of bipolar disorder (Prien and Gelenberg 1989), readers are referred to the excellent recent monograph by McElroy and Pope (1988), *The Use of Anticonvulsants in Psychiatry: Recent Advances.*

Carbamazepine

Issues to be considered when prescribing carbamazepine to medically ill patients include 1) hematologic toxicity, 2) hepatic toxicity, 3) quinidine-like effects on cardiac conduction, 4) antidiuretic actions, 5) enzyme induction leading to drug-drug interactions, 6) clinical interpretation of carbamazepine blood levels, and 7) management of carbamazepine overdose. Drug interactions are summarized in Table 2-7.

Hematologic toxicity.   When carbamazepine was first introduced in the United States, the manufacturer recommended frequent blood counts because of concerns about the development of agranulocytosis. However, as evidence accumulated that these potentially fatal side effects were rare and idiosyncratic, this recommendation was dropped. Present practice regarding monitoring for hematologic interactions is based on the idea that there are two different hematologic reactions to carbamazepine. One is a predictable and often transient drop in both red and white blood cell counts; the other is a rare and idiosyncratic failure of the bone marrow that may occur at an unpredictable time after initiation of therapy. Weekly blood counts during the first month or so of therapy suffice to detect those patients with dose-related suppression of blood counts severe enough to be of clinical concern; longer-term monitoring focuses on educating patients to report for a complete blood count (CBC) if symptoms of fever or sore throat develop, suggesting the onset of neutropenia.

During the first month of therapy, a white blood cell count below 3,500 would ordinarily be an occasion for discontinuing carbamazepine. If the white count does not fall below 3,500, monthly CBCs should be continued for the next 3 months, and then may be done as indicated by symptoms or signs of anemia or neutropenia.

The situation is more complex when patients have preexisting anemia or neutropenia. In these patients, the predictable drop in red and white blood cell counts induced by carbamazepine begins from a lower baseline. However, there is no evidence that, in general, patients with preexisting blood disorders are at greater risk for the life-threatening complications of aplastic anemia and agranulocytosis. Therefore, preexisting cytopenias are relative but not absolute contraindications to carbamazepine. We recommend that hematologic consultation be obtained before initiating carbamazepine in any patient with a baseline hemoglobin below 12 or a white blood cell count below 4,000. The consultant should be asked for an individualized assessment of risk, and also for specific guidelines for monitoring and drug discontinuation if carbamazepine is begun.

Patients receiving combined therapy with lithium and carbamazepine may be at somewhat less risk for a lowering of the white blood cell count because of lithium's stimulatory effects on white blood cell production (Brewerton 1986; Vieweg et al. 1986–87).

Hepatic toxicity.   As in the case of hematologic toxicity, hepatic toxicity from carbamazepine comes in two kinds: frequent, predictable, and benign; and rare, idiosyncratic, and life threatening (Dreifuss and Langer 1987). The relatively benign form of toxicity, seen in no more than 5% of patients (Jeavons 1983), consists of mild, asymptomatic elevations of serum glutamic-oxaloacetic transaminase (SGOT) and serum glutamic-pyruvic transaminase (SGPT), usually to less than twice the upper limit of their normal values. The life-threatening toxicity is acute hepatic necrosis with liver failure, occurring in less than 1 in 10,000 carbamazepine-treated patients. Only 21 cases of this severe hepatic toxicity were reported in the first 20 years of carbamazepine's clinical use (Jeavons 1983). Severe hepatic toxicity occurs unpredictably, usually within the first month of therapy, but occasionally after several months of uneventful treatment. As with hematologic toxicity, a reasonable strategy for monitoring is to obtain weekly SGOT and SGPT determinations for the first month, and monthly determinations for the next 3 months. Elevations of SGOT and SGPT to less than twice the upper limit of normal would not necessitate discontinuation of the drug. Greater elevations would trigger either drug discontinuation or consultation with a specialist in liver diseases. In addition, patients should be warned about the rare possibility of liver failure and be told to report immediately for an examination and a full panel of liver function tests if anorexia, nausea, abdominal pain, jaundice, or a change in urine or stool color were to develop.

In regard to monitoring liver enzymes, it should be noted that GGTP (gamma-glutamyl transpeptidase) may be markedly elevated by carbamazepine as well as by other anticonvulsants, in the absence of clinical symptoms of liver disease (Jeavons 1983). An isolated elevation of GGTP, even to high levels, would indicate consultation with a gastroenterologist, but not necessarily discontinuation of the drug. A full panel of liver function tests, including a prothrombin time, should be taken into account when evaluating the significance of an elevated GGTP.

Prescription of carbamazepine for patients with preexisting liver disease has two risks. The first is that any hepatic reaction to carbamazepine will occur from a lower baseline of liver function, and the second is that carbamazepine will be metabolized more slowly, because its primary route of metabolism is hepatic. For this reason, significant liver disease is a relative contraindication to treatment with carbamazepine. Consultation from an internist or subspecialist should be obtained before prescribing carbamazepine to a patient with significant liver disease. In patients such as alcoholics who are at risk for liver disease not necessarily apparent on routine screening liver function tests, carbamazepine should be started more slowly than usual, with frequent determinations of liver enzymes, prothrombin time, and carbamazepine levels during the initiation of therapy.

Quinidine-like effects on cardiac conduction. Carbamazepine, which is similar in chemical structure to the TCAs, also has similar quinidine-like effects on the heart, with the potential for slowing conduction through the AV node, and suppressing ventricular automaticity (Benassi et al. 1987). Symptomatic heart block has been reported when carbamazepine has been given to patients with known or suspected preexisting cardiac disease (Beerman and Edhag 1978), and cardiac rhythm disturbances are a feature of severe carbamazepine overdose. Therefore, pretreatment ECGs are warranted prior to carbamazepine therapy. If the ECG shows heart block other than first-degree AV block, right bundle-branch block, left anterior hemiblock, or asymptomatic Mobitz type I (Wenckebach-type) block, carbamazepine should not be prescribed on an outpatient basis unless the patient has been cleared first by a cardiologist. In patients with benign, asymptomatic forms of heart block, a posttreatment ECG should be obtained to rule out aggravation of the heart block by carbamazepine.

Antidiuretic actions.   Carbamazepine has an antidiuretic action and is associated with both clinically significant hyponatremia and mild, asymptomatic reductions in serum sodium (Ashton et al. 1977; Flegel and Cole 1977; Kalff et al. 1984; Perucca et al. 1978; Stephens et al. 1977; Vieweg and Godleski 1988; Yassa et al. 1988). The effect is thought to be via a direct action on the renal tubules. Patients with other factors predisposing to hyponatremia, including advanced age, diuretic use, and congestive heart failure, are especially at risk. They should have electrolyte determinations weekly during the first month of carbamazepine therapy, with additional determinations done if there is any change in mental or physical status, or if there are significant changes in carbamazepine dosage or in their other medications. As with neutropenia, the antidiuretic effect of carbamazepine is attenuated when the drug is given together with lithium (Vieweg et al. 1987), because lithium makes the renal tubules less sensitive to antidiuretic hormone (White and Fetner 1975).

We offer the following suggestions for practical management of carbamazepine-induced hyponatremia: 1) If the sodium level drops below 125 meq/L in a patient treated with carbamazepine, the drug should be discontinued. 2) If the sodium level drops to between 125 and 130 meq/L, and carbamazepine appears clinically useful, other drugs that may aggravate hyponatremia, such as thiazide diuretics, should be discontinued if possible. If the sodium still persists below 130 meq/L, carbamazepine should be discontinued. 3) If the sodium level is between 130 and 135 meq/L, discontinuation of carbamazepine is not necessary, but electrolytes should be followed weekly for 1 month to assure stability of the level. Sodium should be rechecked immediately if mental status changes. 4) A workup for syndrome of inappropriate secretion of antidiuretic hormone (SIADH) should be carried out if the sodium level persists below 130 meq/L after carbamazepine discontinuation, and it is not otherwise explained (e.g., by congestive heart failure). 5) Discontinuation of long-term carbamazepine, when indicated by a low sodium level, should be gradual, to avoid withdrawal phenomena such as cholinergic rebound or seizures. 6) When carbamazepine is being used for the indication of seizures, an alternative anticonvulsant less likely to cause hyponatremia (e.g., phenytoin or valproate) should be initiated before tapering carbamazepine.

Enzyme induction leading to drug-drug interactions. Carbamazepine is known to be a potent inducer of the cytochrome P-450 system. As such, it influences the metabolism of all drugs that rely on this system for their metabolism, including carbamazepine itself. One well-known consequence of enzyme induction is the need to gradually build up carbamazepine dosage over the first few weeks of treatment to maintain a steady blood level. Two other consequences are clinically significant. The first is that the blood levels of some drugs may drop if carbamazepine is added to the regimen. This has been reported for alprazolam, with the clinically significant consequence of alprazolam withdrawal when carbamazepine was added to a steady dosage of alprazolam (Arana et al. 1988), for clonazepam (Lai et al. 1978), and for haloperidol (Arana et al. 1986). The second effect is that drug metabolites not ordinarily clinically significant might be present in larger quantities due to carbamazepine-induced induction of metabolic enzymes. (See earlier discussion in this chapter on the probable accumulation of hydroxy metabolites of desipramine causing ECG changes in a patient concurrently treated with carbamazepine [Baldessarini et al. 1988].)

A practical implication of these observations with carbamazepine is that blood levels of drugs metabolized by the liver should be determined promptly if unexpected toxicity or lack of therapeutic effect occurs in the context of concurrent carbamazepine therapy. Furthermore, toxicity in the presence of apparently therapeutic blood levels should be considered, possibly due to unusually great concentrations of unmeasured metabolites. Specifically, medically ill patients on combined carbamazepine and tricyclic therapy should have posttreatment ECGs even if tricyclic blood levels appear normal.

Clinical interpretation of blood levels. Typical normal ranges for carbamazepine blood levels in the treatment of epilepsy are 8–12 µg/ml for single-drug therapy, and 4–8 µg/ml for combined therapy with other anticonvulsants. However, when carbamazepine is used as a psychotropic, or when it is used together with other medications in medically ill patients, the interpretation of levels is subject to several caveats. First, since carbamazepine is heavily protein-bound, free carbamazepine levels, on which both therapeutic and toxic effects depend, can vary if other drugs displace carbamazepine from its protein binding sites. This has been reported for agents as ubiquitous as aspirin. Second, pharmacodynamic interactions may induce neurotoxicity of carbamazepine at therapeutic blood levels when the drug is given in conjunction with other psychotropics (Fogel 1988). This has been specifically reported for coadministration of carbamazepine with haloperidol or lithium. Third, the level of carbamazepine needed for maximum psychotropic effect may be greater than the level optimal for seizure control. Finally, usually unmeasured metabolites, such as carbamazepine 10-11-epoxide, can contribute to both therapeutic and toxic effects. While the ratio of the parent compound to the epoxide is fairly predictable among medically well persons, it may vary in the medically ill, particularly in the setting of liver disease or polypharmacy. For all these reasons, frequent clinical reassessments must supplement blood levels in evaluating carbamazepine effect. Neither free carbamazepine levels nor carbamazepine 10-11-epoxide levels are generally available, and neither can be recommended at this time for routine use as a substitute for scrupulous and frequent clinical monitoring.

Management of overdose. As carbamazepine has been more widely prescribed both as an anticonvulsant and a psychotropic, the incidence of carbamazepine overdose has been increasing. The problems of carbamazepine overdose include coma, seizures, hypotension, and cardiac arrhythmia. The general approach to supportive management is similar to that used for TCA overdose. Hemodialysis is of little use in treating carbamazepine overdose, but vigorous use of activated charcoal and laxatives is helpful, because the absorption of carbamazepine is quite slow, and much may remain in the intestine at the time the patient presents for emergency treatment (Morrow and Routledge 1989). The phenomenon of prolonged absorption can lead to a recurrence of coma following apparent recovery, due to the eventual absorption of drug remaining in the intestine (Fisher and Cysyk 1988; Sethna et al. 1989). For this reason, patients with serious carbamazepine overdose should be observed in the hospital for a full 24 hours after return of consciousness.

Valproate (Depakote, Depakene)

Valproate has been reported in mostly uncontrolled (to date) studies as effective for the treatment of bipolar disorder and as an adjunct treatment in psychotic disorders (McElroy et al. 1989). Issues to be considered when prescribing valproate to medically ill patients include

1) gastrointestinal toxicity, 2) hepatic toxicity, 3) effects on coagulation, 4) drug-drug interactions, 5) clinical interpretation of blood levels, and 6) management of overdose.

Gastrointestinal toxicity. In comparative studies of anticonvulsant side effects, the most prominent and troublesome side effect of valproate has been nausea, often accompanied by vomiting. Medically ill patients, particularly those with diseases predisposing to nausea, may be at increased risk. Depakote (divalproex sodium) is much less likely to cause gastrointestinal upset than Depakene (valproic acid), and more frequent dosing is sometimes better tolerated than larger doses taken fewer times per day. Occasional patients will do better on valproic acid syrup. However, regardless of the preparation used, a substantial proportion of patients will simply be unable to tolerate the drug.

Hepatic toxicity. Shortly after valproate was first introduced, there were several deaths from acute hepatic necrosis, and as of 1988, approximately 100 fatalities had been reported from valproate-induced liver failure (Scheffner et al. 1988). This has led to considerable caution in the use of the drug for fear of this reaction. As experiences accumulate, however, it appears that hepatic necrosis is a major risk only for children under age 2 years, particularly those given multiple-drug therapy for epilepsy. The incidence of hepatic necrosis in adults receiving valproate is well under 1 in 10,000 (Eadie et al. 1988) and may be as low as 1 in 50,000. In 95% of reported cases, patients developed symptoms within the first 6 months of therapy (Scheffner et al. 1988). Given this very infrequent occurrence of life-threatening hepatic toxicity, routine long-term monitoring of liver function tests does not seem necessary. Periodic liver function tests for the first 6 months are a reasonable precaution, however, and patients should be warned of the early signs of liver disease and be told to report immediately for repeat testing of liver function should those signs develop during valproate therapy. A much more common, though benign, hepatic effect of valproate is an increase in serum ammonia level, due to valproate's inhibition of urea synthesis (Cotariu and Zaidman 1988; Hjelm et al. 1986; Kugoh et al. 1986). This elevation in serum ammonia is usually asymptomatic; the effect, however, can be of major concern in individuals with preexisting liver disease, and especially those in whom there is a history of hepatic encephalopathy. Significant liver disease is a relative contraindication to valproate therapy, and close monitoring of liver enzymes and of serum ammonia would be an appropriate precaution with alcoholic patients suspected to have subclinical cirrhosis of the liver. Consultation with an internist or subspecialist would be advisable before starting valproate in a patient with known liver disease.

Effects on coagulation.   Valproate therapy can increase the prothrombin time, decrease fibrinogen levels, and reduce the platelet count. These findings, one or more of which may occur in as many as one-third of patients receiving valproate (Rochel and Ehrenthal 1983), rarely lead to clinically significant bleeding. However, valproate-treated patients should definitely have a full coagulation panel, including a platelet count, PT and PTT, before undergoing elective surgery or dental work, and patients with preexisting anticoagulant therapy or bleeding diatheses require especially close monitoring during initiation of valproate therapy.

Drug-drug interactions.   In contrast to carbamazepine, which is an enzyme inducer, valproate inhibits liver enzymes that metabolize drugs. Therefore, it can prolong the half-life of other drugs with mainly hepatic metabolism. This effect has been documented for diazepam, which has a prolonged half-life in the presence of valproate. In general, the coadministration of long-acting benzodiazepines with valproate may be problematic, both because of the prolongation of benzodiazepine metabolism and because of additive sedation and ataxia. If a benzodiazepine must be given to a patient on valproate, lorazepam is not likely to interact significantly. The full range of drugs that might have altered metabolism in the presence of valproate is not known, so the possibility of drug accumulation should be considered with other drugs that rely primarily on hepatic metabolism.

Interactions of valproate with other anticonvulsants have been studied extensively (Bourgeois 1988). Carbamazepine, phenytoin, and phenobarbital all can lower valproate levels (May and Rambeck 1985). On the other hand, valproate increases levels of phenobarbital by inhibiting its metabolism (Redenbaugh et al. 1980) and raises the free fraction of phenytoin by displacing the drug from protein binding sites. This phenomenon can lead to phenytoin toxicity at apparently "therapeutic" phenytoin levels (Bruno et al. 1980). Of even greater interest to psychiatrists who might be using valproate together with carbamazepine for treatment-refractory mania is the observation that valproate raises the concentration of the carbamazepine 10-11-epoxide metabolite (Pisani et al. 1986). This metabolite, not usually measured, has additive toxicity with carbamazepine (Bourgeois and Wad 1984).

Thus, when valproate is given concurrently, carbamazepine may produce toxicity at apparently therapeutic levels because of an increased level of its 10-11-epoxide metabolite.

Aspirin in usual antipyretic doses may raise both total and free valproate levels, because of both metabolite enzyme inhibition and displacement of valproate from protein binding sites. Significant toxicity may result (Goulden et al. 1987). Therefore, alternative agents such as acetaminophen would be preferable for treating fever or minor pain in patients treated with valproate.

Pharmacodynamic interactions have been reported between valproate and neuroleptics, with the development of an encephalopathic syndrome with diffuse EEG slowing (Van Sweden and Van Moffaert 1985) or increased parkinsonism (Puzynski and Klosiewicz 1984).

Clinical interpretation of blood levels.   Therapeutic blood levels for valproate in the treatment of epilepsy are usually reported as 50–100 μg/ml. The work of McElroy and colleagues (1989) suggests that effective blood levels for bipolar disorder are similar, and that little clinical effect is seen with blood levels less than 50 μg/ml. Toxic effects are frequently seen with levels greater than 100 μg/ml, so the therapeutic index is quite low. Because of individual variations in metabolism of valproate, blood levels should be obtained routinely during upward titration of valproate dosage, to ensure that the blood level is indeed adequate and to avoid toxicity. Both the McLean Hospital (Boston) experience and our own suggest that even within the therapeutic range there may be a specific threshold at which therapeutic effects begin. For example, one of the authors (B.S.F.) treated a patient who had complete relief of bulimia from valproate at a level of 80 μg/ml but no relief at 70 μg/ml.

Considering the relationship between blood levels and toxicity, it should be noted that toxicity may develop at apparently therapeutic levels when the patient is on multiple drugs, whereas levels above the usual therapeutic range may be tolerated in the context of single-drug therapy.

Management of overdose.   Because valproate is not toxic to the heart, patients receiving aggressive support have tolerated massive valproate overdoses, including ingestions of greater than 50 g. Current recommendations for managing valproate overdose focus on supportive therapy. Although gastric lavage might be considered early in the course of the overdose, it is unlikely to be of much help later because absorption of valproate is fairly rapid. One intriguing case report (Alberto et al. 1989) suggests that coma due to valproate overdose might be reversible by naloxone, because of the latter's effects on gamma-aminobutyric acid (GABA) receptors. Given the low toxicity of naloxone and its empirical use in overdoses of unknown agents, it would be an appropriate consideration as adjunctive therapy even when a patient was known to have taken valproate rather than a narcotic.

Clonazepam

Issues to be considered when prescribing clonazepam to medically ill patients include 1) consequences of its relatively long half-life and hepatic metabolism, 2) drug-drug interactions, and 3) its effects on respiratory drive.

Consequences of clonazepam's long half-life and hepatic metabolism. Clonazepam is a long-acting benzodiazepine, with a half-life in healthy adults of 20–58 hours. The primary route of metabolism is the liver. In elderly patients or individuals with impaired hepatic function due to primary liver disease, congestive heart failure, or metabolic inhibition by other drugs, clonazepam may have an even longer half-life. Therefore, it may take well over a week for steady-state levels to be reached. The prescription of a standing dose of clonazepam might be well tolerated in a patient on the first day or two of therapy, but later result in ataxia, sedation, falling, confusion, or stupor as the drug further accumulates.

For this reason, patients receiving clonazepam in the setting of advanced age, primary or secondary liver disease, or other metabolic-inhibiting drugs (although note that the clonazepam-valproate compound is contraindicated in epileptic patients) should receive very low initial doses, with up to 2 weeks between upward increments in dosage. Rapid loading with clonazepam to treat acute mania, as suggested by Chouinard (1987), could be problematic in these patients.

Another implication of clonazepam's relatively long half-life is the potential for withdrawal symptoms occurring despite what would seem to be a gradual schedule of drug discontinuation. Wong and Tiessen (1989) reported a patient without a prior seizure history who had a withdrawal seizure when clonazepam was withdrawn by 0.5 mg every 4 days. In a series of 40 epileptic children withdrawn from long-term clonazepam, Specht et al. (1989) reported withdrawal symptoms in 47.5% of patients when clonazepam was withdrawn at a rate of 0.003–0.16 mg/kg per day (equivalent to 0.2 mg/day or faster in a 70-kg adult).

These reports suggest that withdrawal from long-term clonazepam therapy should be even slower. When circumstances permit, we taper clonazepam as slowly as 0.25 mg every 2 weeks in patients who have had months or years of clonazepam therapy.

Drug-drug interactions. Clonazepam, when added to therapeutic levels of lithium, has been reported to produce a reversible neurotoxic syndrome with ataxia and dysarthria (Koczeroinski et al. 1989); the mechanism was presumably pharmacodynamic rather than via increased lithium levels. The report of additive toxicity should be taken in the context of additive therapeutic effects, as reported by Chouinard (1987, 1988), who did not find an unacceptable rate of adverse interaction, and who argues that lithium-neuroleptic combinations may be more dangerous. In general, the literature suggests that all reported combinations of multiple antimanic agents have both greater toxicity and greater effectiveness for selected treatment-refractory patients than single agents.

Effects on respiratory drive. Like other benzodiazepines, clonazepam decreases hypoxic respiratory drive. Therefore, it is relatively contraindicated in patients with COPD, who are at risk for carbon dioxide retention. When clonazepam is considered for a patient with COPD, baseline blood gases should be obtained; the drug should not be given if there is CO_2 retention at baseline. Even if baseline blood gases are normal, a follow-up blood gas would be a reasonable precaution in clonazepam-treated patients with significant impairment in pulmonary function.

CONCLUSION AND FUTURE PROSPECTS

Specific assessments of psychotropic agents in medically ill populations have been increasing in conjunction with the generally greater willingness of psychiatrists to use pharmacologic therapies for psychopathology in the medically ill. The next step—development of psychotropics specifically for the psychiatric complications of medical illness—has yet to occur; it is still the case that better drugs for the psychiatric disorders of the medically ill are a by-product of manufacturers' development of safer and more effective agents for primary psychiatric illnesses.

We plan to review psychopharmacology in the medically ill in the

subsequent volumes of this series. Over the next several years, we
expect developments in the following areas: 1) more specific trials of
the newer antidepressants and antianxiety drugs in medically ill populations; 2) further studies, and probably FDA approval of a selective
MAO-A inhibitor, an alternative serotonin reuptake inhibitor, and a
new nonbenzodiazepine anxiolytic; 3) increasing use, and more systematic study, of anticonvulsants for psychiatric problems in both
physically well and physically ill patients; 4) broader clinical experience with clomipramine and clozapine, both of which have recent FDA
approval and therefore are available for use in physically ill patients;
5) more widespread use, and perhaps more systematic study, of stimulants, following several favorable reviews and open studies; and
6) development of drugs that palliate the cognitive and memory disorders of dementia.

As the range of therapies broadens, indications for pharmacotherapy will increase, and drug choice is likely to become a more
complex task.

REFERENCES

Alberto G, Erickson T, Popiel R, et al: Central nervous system manifestations
of a valproic acid overdose responsive to naloxone. Ann Emerg Med 18:889–
891, 1989

American Psychiatric Association: Diagnostic and Statistical Manual of Mental Disorders, 3rd Edition. Washington, DC, American Psychiatric Association, 1980

Arana GW, Goff DC, Friedman H, et al: Does carbamazepine-induced reduction
of plasma haloperidol levels worsen psychotic symptoms? Am J Psychiatry
143:650–651, 1986

Arana GW, Epstein S, Molloy M, et al: Carbamazepine-induced reduction of
plasma alprazolam concentrations: a clinical case report. J Clin Psychiatry
49:448–449, 1988

Aranow RB, Hudson JI, Pope HG, et al: Elevated antidepressant plasma levels
after addition of fluoxetine. Am J Psychiatry 146:911–913, 1989

Ashton MG, Ball SG, Thomas TH, et al: Water intoxication associated with
carbamazepine treatment. Br Med J 1:1134–1135, 1977

Baldessarini RJ, Teicher MH, Cassidy JW, et al: Anticonvulsant cotreatment
may increase toxic metabolites of antidepressants and other psychotropic
drugs (letter). J Clin Psychopharmacol 8:381–382, 1988

Beck H, Salom M, Holzer J: Midazolam dosage studies in institutionalized geriatric patients. Br J Pharmacol 16:133S–137S, 1983

Beerman B, Edhag O: Depressive effects of carbamazepine on idioventricular rhythm in man. Br Med J 2:171–172, 1978

Bell IR, Cole JO: Fluoxetine induces elevation of desipramine level and exacerbation of geriatric nonpsychotic depression. J Clin Psychopharmacol 8:447–448, 1988

Benassi E, Bo GP, Cocito L, et al: Carbamazepine and cardiac conduction disturbances. Ann Neurol 22:280–281, 1987

Bertilsson L, Mellstrom B, Sjoqvist F: Pronounced inhibition of noradrenaline uptake by 10-hydroxymetabolite of nortriptyline. Life Sci 25:1285–1292, 1979

Bieck PR, Firkusny L, Schick C, et al: Monoamine oxidase inhibition by phenelzine and brofaromine in healthy volunteers. Clin Pharmacol Ther 45:260–269, 1989

Blazer DG, Petrie WM, Wilson WP: Affective psychoses following renal transplant. Diseases of the Nervous System 37:663–667, 1976

Bobo BL, Miwa LJ: Midazolam disinhibition reaction. Drug Intell Clin Pharm 22:725, 1988

Bodley RP, Halwax K, Potts L: Low serum cholinesterase levels complicating treatment with phenelzine. Br Med J 3:510–512, 1969

Boisvert D, Chouinard G: Rebound cardiac arrhythmia after withdrawal from imipramine: a case report. Am J Psychiatry 138:985, 1981

Bond WS, Mandos LA, Kurtz MB: Midazolam for aggressivity and violence in three mentally retarded patients. Am J Psychiatry 146:925–926, 1989

Bourgeois BFD: Pharmacologic interactions between valproate and other drugs. Am J Med 84 (suppl 1A):29–33, 1988

Bourgeois BFD, Wad N: Individual and combined antiepileptic and neurotoxic activity of carbamazepine and carbamazepine-10, 11-epoxide in mice. J Pharmacol Exp Ther 231:411–415, 1984

Branconnier RJ, Cole JO, Ghazvinian S, et al: Clinical pharmacology of bupropion and imipramine in elderly depressives. J Clin Psychiatry 44:130–133, 1983a

Branconnier RJ, Cole JO, Oxenkrug GF, et al: Cardiovascular effects of imipramine and bupropion in aged depressed patients. Psychopharmacol Bull 19:658–662, 1983b

Brewerton TD: Lithium counteracts carbamazepine-induced leukopenia while increasing its therapeutic effect. Biol Psychiatry 21:677–685, 1986

Brown GM, Stancer HC, Moldofsky H, et al: Withdrawal from long-term high-dose desipramine therapy. Arch Gen Psychiatry 35:1261–1264, 1978

Brown TCK, Cass NM: Beware—the use of MAO inhibitors is increasing again. Anaesth Intensive Care 7:65–68, 1979

Bruno J, Gallo JM, Lee CS, et al: Interactions of valproic acid with phenytoin. Neurology 30:1233–1236, 1980

Burnakis TG, Berman DE: Hostility and hallucinations as a consequence of midazolam administration. Drug Intell Clin Pharm 23:671–672, 1989

Burroughs Wellcome Company: Wellbutrin (bupropion hydrochloride) tablets insert. Research Triangle Park, NC, June 1989

Cantu TG, Korek JS: Monoamine oxidase inhibitors and weight gain. Drug Intell Clin Pharm 22:755–759, 1988

CAPS (Cardiac Arrhythmic Pilot Study) Investigators: Effects of encainide, flecainide, imipramine and moricizine on ventricular arrhythmias during the year after acute myocardial infarction. Am J Cardiol 61:501–509, 1988

Cheng YF, Lundberg T, Bondesson U, et al: Clinical pharmacokinetics of clozapine in chronic schizophrenia. Eur J Clin Pharmacol 34:445–449, 1988

Chiarello RJ, Cole JO: The use of psychostimulants in general psychiatry. Arch Gen Psychiatry 44:286–295, 1987

Chouinard G: Clonazepam in acute and maintenance treatment of bipolar affective disorder. J Clin Psychiatry 48(10) (suppl):29–37, 1987

Chouinard G: The use of benzodiazepines in the treatment of manic-depressive illness. J Clin Psychiatry 49(11) (suppl):15–20, 1988

Chouinard G, Annable L, Langlois R: Absence of orthostatic hypotension in depressed patients treated with bupropion. Prog Neuro-psychopharmacol 5:483–490, 1981

Clary C, Schweizer E: Treatment of MAOI hypertensive crisis with sublingual nifedipine. J Clin Psychiatry 48:249–250, 1987

Colenda CC: Buspirone in treatment of agitated demented patient. Lancet 1:1169, 1988

Cooper AJ, Ashcroft G: Potentiation of insulin hypoglycemia by MAOI antidepressant drugs. Lancet 1:407–409, 1966

Cooper GL: The safety of fluoxetine—an update. Br J Psychiatry 153 (suppl 3):77–86, 1988

Cotariu D, Zaidman JL: Valproic acid and the liver. Clin Chem 34:890–897, 1988

Crabtree BL, Mack JE, Johnson CD, et al: Effects of HCTZ versus furosemide on serum lithium (abstract). 1989 APA Annual Meeting Syllabus, p 150

Csernansky JG, Hollister LE: Using lithium in patients with cardiac and renal disease. Hospital Formulary 20:726–735, 1985

Dalhoff K, Poulsen HE, Garred P, et al: Buspirone pharmacokinetics in patients with cirrhosis. Br J Clin Pharmacol 24:547–550, 1987

DasGupta K, Jefferson JW: The use of lithium in the medically ill. Gen Hosp Psychiatry 12:83–97, 1990

Davidson J: Seizures and bupropion: a review. J Clin Psychiatry 50:256–261, 1989

Davidson J, Zung WW, Walker JI: Practical aspects of MAO inhibitor therapy. J Clin Psychiatry 45:81–84, 1984

Dawling S, Crome P, Heyer EJ: Nortriptyline therapy in elderly patients: dosage prediction from plasma concentration at 24 hours after a single 50 mg dose. Br J Psychiatry 139:413–419, 1981

Dawling S, Lynn K, Rosser R, et al: Nortriptyline metabolism in chronic renal failure: metabolite elimination. Clin Pharmacol Ther 32:322–329, 1982

Denton PH, Borell VM, Edwards NV: Dangers of monoamine oxidase inhibitors. Br Med J 2:1752–1753, 1962

Dieperink H, Leyssac PP, Kemp E, et al: Nephrotoxicity of cyclosporin A in humans: effects on glomerular filtration and tubular reabsorption rates. Eur J Clin Invest 17:493–496, 1987

Dietch JT, Fine M: The effect of nortriptyline in elderly patients with cardiac conduction disease. J Clin Psychiatry 51:65–67, 1990

Dilsaver SC: Heterocyclic antidepressant, monoamine oxidase inhibitor and neuroleptic withdrawal phenomena. Prog Neuro-Psychopharmacol Biol Psychiatry 14:137–161, 1990

D'Mello DA, McNeil JA, Harris W: Buspirone suppression of neuroleptic-induced akathisia: multiple case reports. J Clin Psychopharmacol 9:151–152, 1989

Domantay AG, Napoliello MJ: Buspirone for elderly anxious patients: a review of clinical studies. Family Practice Recertification 11 (suppl 9):17–23, 1989

Douste-Blazy PH, Rostin M, Livarek B, et al: Angiotensin converting enzyme inhibitors and lithium treatment (letter). Lancet 1:1448, 1986

Downs JM, Downs AD: Effects of fluoxetine on metabolism of tricyclic antidepressants in the lungs. Am J Psychiatry 146:814–815, 1989

Downs JM, Downs AD, Rosenthal TL, et al: Increased plasma tricyclic antidepressant concentrations in two patients concurrently treated with fluoxetine. J Clin Psychiatry 50:226–227, 1989

Dreifuss FE, Langer DH: Hepatic considerations in the use of antiepileptic drugs. Epilepsia 28 (suppl 2):S23–S29, 1987

Dundee JW, Wilson DB: Amnesic action of midazolam. Anaesthesia 35:459–461, 1980

Eadie MJ, Hooper WD, Dickinson RG: Valproate-associated hepatotoxicity and its biochemical mechanisms. Med Toxicol Adverse Drug Exp 3:85–106, 1988

El-Ganzouri AR, Ivankovich AD, Braverman B, et al: Monoamine oxidase inhibitors: should they be discontinued preoperatively? Anesth Analg 64:592–596, 1985

Elis J, Laurence DR, Mattie H, et al: Modification by monoamine oxidase inhibitors of the effect of some sympathomimetics on the blood pressure. Br Med J 2:75–78, 1967

Fallon B, Foote B, Walsh BT, et al: 'Spontaneous' hypertensive episodes with monoamine oxidase inhibitors. J Clin Psychiatry 49:163–165, 1988

Farid FF, Wenger TL, Tsai SY, et al: Use of bupropion in patients who exhibit orthostatic hypotension on tricyclic antidepressants. J Clin Psychiatry 44:170–173, 1983

Faynor SM, Espina V: Fluoxetine inhibition of imipramine metabolism. Clin Chem 35:1180, 1989

Feighner JP, Cohn JB: Double-blind comparative trials of fluoxetine and doxepin in geriatric patients with major depressive disorder. J Clin Psychiatry 46:20–25, 1985

Feighner JP, Boyer WF, Meredith CH, et al: An overview of fluoxetine in geriatric depression. Br J Psychiatry 153 (suppl 3):105–108, 1988

Fenster PE, Bressler R, Kipps J: Antiarrhythmic efficacy of desipramine. J Clin Pharmacol 29:114–117, 1989

Fernandez F, Adams F, Holmes VF, et al: Methylphenidate for depressive disorders in cancer patients. Psychosomatics 28:455–461, 1987

Fernandez F, Levy JK, Galizzi H: Response of HIV-related depression to psychostimulants: case reports. Hosp Community Psychiatry 39:628–631, 1988

Ferris RM, Cooper BR, Maxwell RA: Studies of bupropion's mechanism of antidepressant activity. J Clin Psychiatry 44:74–78, 1983

Fisch C: Effect of fluoxetine on the electrocardiogram. J Clin Psychiatry 46:42–44, 1985

Fisher RS, Cysyk B: A fatal overdose of carbamazepine: case report and review of literature. J Toxicol Clin Toxicol 26:477–486, 1988

Flegel KM, Cole CH: Inappropriate antidiuresis during carbamazepine treatment. Ann Intern Med 87:722–723, 1977

Fogel BS: Combining anticonvulsants with conventional psychopharmacologic agents, in Use of Anticonvulsants in Psychiatry: Recent Advances. Edited by McElroy SL, Pope HG. Clifton, NJ, Oxford Health Care, Inc., 1988, pp 77–94

Forster HS: Naproxen reversal of nortriptyline-induced orthostatic hypotension (letter to the editor). J Clin Psychiatry 50:356, 1989

Frankhauser MP, Lindon JL, Connolly B, et al: Evaluation of lithium-tetracycline interaction. Clin Pharm 7:314–317, 1988

Friedman JH, Lannon MC: Clozapine in the treatment of psychosis in Parkinson's disease. Neurology 39:1219–1221, 1989

Gammans RE, Bullen WW, Briner L, et al: The effects of buspirone binding of digoxin, Dilantin, propranolol and warfarin to human plasma. Fed Proc 44:1123, 1985

Gammans RE, Mayol RF, Labudde JA: Metabolism and disposition of buspirone. Am J Med 80:41–51, 1986

Gammans RE, Westrick ML, Shea JP, et al: Pharmacokinetics of buspirone in elderly subjects. J Clin Pharmacol 29:72–78, 1989

Garland EJ, Remick RA, Zis A: Weight gain with antidepressants and lithium. J Clin Psychopharmacol 8:323–330, 1988

Garner SJ, Eldridge FL, Wagner PG, et al: Buspirone, an anxiolytic drug that stimulates respiration. Am Rev Respir Dis 139:946–950, 1989

Gawin F, Compton M, Byck R: Buspirone reduces smoking. Arch Gen Psychiatry 46:288–289, 1989

Gelenberg AJ, Wojcik JD, Falk WE, et al: Effects of lithium on the kidney. Acta Psychiatr Scand 75:29–34, 1987

Gelenberg AJ, Kane JM, Keller MB, et al: Comparison of standard and low serum levels of lithium for maintenance treatment of bipolar disorder. N Engl J Med 321:1489–1493, 1989

Georgotas A, McCue RE, Friedman E, et al: Electrocardiographic effects of nortriptyline, phenelzine, and placebo under optimal treatment conditions. Am J Psychiatry 144:798–801, 1987

Gershon S: Drug interactions in controlled clinical trials. J Clin Psychiatry 43:95–98, 1982

Giardina EGV, Barnard T, Johnson L, et al: The antiarrhythmic effect of nortriptyline in cardiac patients with ventricular premature depolarizations. J Am Coll Cardiol 7:1363–1369, 1986

Giardina EV, Cooper TB, Suckow R, et al: Cardiovascular effects of doxepin in cardiac patients with ventricular arrhythmias. Clin Pharmacol Ther 42:20–27, 1987

Goa KL, Ward A: Buspirone: a preliminary review of its pharmacological properties and therapeutic efficacy as an anxiolytic. Drugs 32:114–129, 1986

Goff DC: The stimulant challenge test in depression. J Clin Psychiatry 47:538–543, 1986

Golden RN, James SP, Sherer MA, et al: Psychoses associated with bupropion treatment. Am J Psychiatry 142:1459–1462, 1985

Goodnick PJ: Influence of fluoxetine on plasma levels of desipramine. Am J Psychiatry 146:552, 1989

Goulden KJ, Dooley JM, Camfield PR, et al: Clinical valproate toxicity induced by acetylsalicylic acid. Neurology 37:1392–1394, 1987

Graham PM, Ilett KF: Danger of MAOI therapy after fluoxitine withdrawal. Lancet 2:1255–1256, 1988

Halper JP, Mann JJ: Cardiovascular effects of antidepressant medications. Br J Psychiatry 153 (suppl 3):87–98, 1988

Hanno PM, Buehler J, Wein AJ: Use of amitriptyline in the treatment of interstitial cystitis. J Urol 141:846–848, 1989

Harrison WM, McGrath PJ, Stewart JW, et al: MAOIs and hypertensive crisis: the role of OTC drugs. J Clin Psychiatry 50:64–65, 1989

Helmuth D, Ljaljevic Z, Ramirez L, et al: Choreoathetosis induced by verapamil and lithium treatment (letter). J Clin Psychopharmacol 9:454–455, 1989

Hetmar O, Clemmesen L, Ladefoged J, et al: Lithium: long-term effects on the kidney, III: prospective study. Acta Psychiatr Scand 75:251–258, 1987

Hjelm M, Oberholzer V, Seakins J, et al: Valproate-induced inhibition of urea synthesis and hyperammonaemia in healthy subjects. Lancet 2:859, 1986

Holazo AA, Winkler MB, Patel IH: Effects of age, gender and oral contraceptives on intramuscular midazolam pharmacokinetics. J Clin Pharmacol 28:1040–1045, 1988

Holmes VF, Fernandez F, Levy JK: Psychostimulant response in AIDS-related complex patients. J Clin Psychiatry 50:5–8, 1989

Hwang AS, Magraw RM: Syndrome of inappropriate secretion of antidiuretic hormone due to fluoxetine (letter). Am J Psychiatry 146:399, 1989

Indaco A, Carrieri P: Amitriptyline in the treatment of headache in patients with Parkinson's disease: a double-blind placebo-controlled study. Neurology 38:1720–1722, 1988

Jann MW: Buspirone: an update on a unique anxiolytic agent. Pharmacotherapy 8:100–116, 1988

Janowsky DS: Reply. J Clin Psychopharmacol 8:450, 1988

Janowsky EC, Janowsky DS: What precautions should be taken if a patient on an MAOI is scheduled to undergo anesthesia? J Clin Psychopharmacol 5:128–129, 1985

Jeavons PM: Hepatotoxicity in antiepileptic drugs, in Chronic Toxicity of Antiepileptic Drugs. Edited by Oxley J, Janz D, Meinardi H. New York, Raven Press, 1983, pp 1–46

Jefferson JW: Cardiovascular effects and toxicity of anxiolytics and antidepressants. J Clin Psychiatry 50:368–378, 1989

Jenike M: Handbook of Geriatric Psychopharmacology. Littleton, MA, PSG, 1985, pp 73–87

Kahn D: Mysterious MAOI hypertensive episodes. J Clin Psychiatry 49:38–39, 1988

Kahn DA: The transition to and from monoamine oxidase inhibitors in clinical practice: warnings and recommendations. Currents in Affective Illness 8:5–14, 1989

Kalff R, Houtkooper MA, Meyer JWA, et al: Carbamazepine and serum sodium levels. Epilepsia 25:390–397, 1984

Kane JM, Cole K, Sarantakos S, et al: Safety and efficacy of bupropion in elderly patients: preliminary observations. J Clin Psychiatry 44:134–136, 1983

Kane J, Honigfeld G, Singer J, et al: Clozapine for the treatment-resistant schizophrenic: a double blind comparison with chlorpromazine. Arch Gen Psychiatry 45:789–796, 1988

Keck PE, Vuckovik A, Pope HG, et al: Acute cardiovascular response to monoamine oxidase inhibitors: a prospective assessment. J Clin Psychopharmacol 9:203–206, 1989

Kennedy SH, Craven JL, Roin GM: Major depression in renal dialysis patients: an open trial of antidepressant therapy. J Clin Psychiatry 50:60–63, 1989

Kiev A, Domantay AG: A study of buspirone coprescribed with bronchodilators in 82 anxious ambulatory patients. J Asthma 25:281–284, 1988

Kline SS, Mauro LS, Scala-Barnett DM, et al: Serotonin syndrome versus neuroleptic malignant syndrome as a cause of death. Clin Pharm 8:510–514, 1989

Knapp JE: Monoamine Oxidase Inhibitor Interaction Information: Medical Update. Evansville, IN, Mead Johnson, 1987

Koczeroinski D, Kennedy SH, Swinson RP: Clonazepam and lithium—a toxic combination in the treatment of mania? Int Clin Psychopharmacol 4:195–199, 1989

Koecheler JA, Canafax DM, Simmons RL, et al: Lithium dosing in renal allograft recipients with changing renal function. Drug Intell Clin Pharm 20:623–624, 1986

Kosten TR, Forrest JN: Treatment of severe lithium-induced polyuria with amiloride. Am J Psychiatry 143:1563–1568, 1986

Kronig MH, Roose SP, Walsh BT, et al: Blood pressure effects of phenelzine. J Clin Psychopharmacol 3:307–310, 1983

Kugoh T, Yamamoto M, Hosokawa K: Blood ammonia level during valproic acid therapy. Jpn J Psychiatry Neurol 40:663–668, 1986

Kutchner SP, Reid K, Dubbin JD, et al: Electrocardiogram changes and therapeutic desipramine and 2-hydroxy-desipramine concentrations in elderly depressives. Br J Psychiatry 148:676–679, 1986

Lai AA, Levy RH, Cutler RE: Time course of interaction between carbamazepine and clonazepam in normal man. Clin Pharmacol Ther 24:316–323, 1978

Lazarus LW, Groves L, Gierl B, et al: Efficacy of phenelzine in geriatric depression. Biol Psychiatry 21:699–701, 1986

Lemberger L, Bergstrom RF, Wolen RL, et al: Fluoxetine: clinical pharmacology and physiologic disposition. J Clin Psychiatry 46:14–19, 1985

Lemberger L, Rowe H, Bosomworth JC, et al: The effect of fluoxetine on the pharmacokinetics and psychomotor responses of diazepam. Clin Pharmacol Ther 43:412–419, 1988

Levine A: Buspirone and agitation in head injury. Brain Injury 2:165–167, 1988

Levine S, Napoliello MJ: A study of buspirone coprescribed with histamine H_2-receptor antagonists in anxious outpatients. Int Clin Psychopharmacol 3:83–86, 1988

Lieberman JA, Cooper TB, Suckow RF, et al: Tricyclic antidepressant and metabolite levels in chronic renal failure. Clin Pharmacol Ther 37:301–307, 1985

Lieberman JA, Kane JM, Johns CA: Clozapine: guidelines for clinical management. J Clin Psychiatry 50:329–338, 1989

Lin SC, Hsu T, Fredrickson PA, et al: Yohimbine- and tranylcypromine-induced postural hypotension (letter). Am J Psychiatry 144:119, 1987

Lingam VR, Lazarus LW, Groves L, et al: Methylphenidate in treating poststroke depression. J Clin Psychiatry 49:151–153, 1988

Lipinski JF, Mallya G, Zimmerman P, et al: Fluoxetine-induced akathisia: clinical and theoretical implications. J Clin Psychiatry 50:339–342, 1989

Lippman SB, Manshadi MS, Gultekin A: Lithium in a patient with renal failure on hemodialysis. J Clin Psychiatry 45:444, 1984

Lose G, Jorgensen L, Thunedborg P: Doxepin in the treatment of female detrusor overactivity: a randomized double-blind crossover study. J Urol 142:1024–1026, 1989

Lowry MR, Dunner FJ: Seizures during tricyclic therapy. Am J Psychiatry 137:1461–1462, 1980

Macfarlane JG, Jalali S, Grace EM: Trimipramine in rheumatoid arthritis: a randomized double-blind trial in relieving pain and joint tenderness. Curr Med Res Opin 10:89–93, 1986

Manoach M, Netz H, Varon D, et al: The effect of tricyclic antidepressants on ventricular fibrillation and collateral blood supply following acute coronary occlusion. Heart Vessels 2:36–40, 1986

Manoach M, Varon D, Neuman M, et al: Reduction of infarct size following acute coronary occlusion by augmenting collateral blood supply induced by infusion of tricyclic antidepressants. Heart Vessels 3:80–83, 1987

Manoach M, Varon D, Neuman M, et al: The cardio-protective features of tricyclic antidepressants. Gen Pharmacol 20:269–275, 1989

Matson AM, Thurlow AC: Hypotension and neurological sequelae following intramuscular midazolam (letter). Anaesthesia 43:896, 1988

Mattes JA: Clozapine for refractory schizophrenia: an open study of 14 patients treated up to 2 years. J Clin Psychiatry 50:389–391, 1989

Max MB, Culnane M, Schafer SC, et al: Amitriptyline relieves diabetic neuropathy pain in patients with normal or depressed mood. Neurology 37:589–596, 1987

May T, Rambeck B: Serum concentrations of valproic acid: influence of dose and comedication. Ther Drug Monit 7:387–390, 1985

McCue RE, Georgotas A, Suckow RF, et al: 10-Hydroxynortriptyline and treatment effects in elderly depressed patients. J Neuropsychiatry 1:176–180, 1989a

McCue RE, Georgotas A, Nagachandran N, et al: Plasma levels of nortriptyline and 10-hydroxynortriptyline and treatment-related electrocardiographic changes in the elderly depressed. J Psychiatr Res 23:73–79, 1989b

McElroy SL, Pope HG (eds): The Use of Anticonvulsants in Psychiatry: Recent Advances. Clifton, NJ, Oxford Health Care Inc., 1988

McElroy SL, Keck PE, Pope HG, et al: Valproate in psychiatric disorders: literature review and clinical guidelines. J Clin Psychiatry 50 (suppl 3):23–29, 1989

McGrath PJ, Stewart JW, Quitkin FM: A possible L-deprenyl induced hypertensive reaction. J Clin Psychopharmacol 9:310–311, 1989

Mellstrom B, Bertilsson L, Sawe J, et al: E- and Z-10-hydroxylation of nortriptyline: relationship to polymorphic debrisoquine hydroxylation. Clin Pharmacol Ther 30:189–193, 1981

Meltzer HY, Fleming R: Effect of buspirone on prolactin and growth hormone secretion in laboratory rodents and man. J Clin Psychiatry 43:76–79, 1982

Mendoza R, Djenderedjian AH, Adams J, et al: Midazolam in acute psychotic patients with hyperarousal. J Clin Psychiatry 48:291–292, 1987

Merikangas JR, Merikangas KR: Calcium channel blockers in MAOI-induced hypertensive crisis (abstract). Psychopharmacology 96 (suppl):229, 1988

Michaels I, Serrings M, Shier N, et al: Anesthesia for cardiac surgery in patients receiving monoamine oxidase inhibitors. Anesth Analg 63:1041–1044, 1984

Miller ME, Perry CJ, Siris SG: Psychosis in association with combined cimetidine and imipramine treatment. Psychosomatics 28:217–219, 1987

Molitor JA, Gammans RE, Carroll CM, et al: Effect of buspirone on mixed function oxidase in rats (abstract). Fed Proc 44:1257, 1985

Morrow JI, Routledge PA: Poisoning by anticonvulsants. Adverse Drug React Acute Poisoning Rev 8:97–109, 1989

Naber D, Leppig M, Grohmann R, et al: Efficacy and adverse effects of clozapine on schizophrenia and tardive dyskinesia—a retrospective study of 387 patients. Psychopharmacology 99:S73–S76, 1989

Navis GJ, deJong PE, deZeeuw D: Volume homeostasis, angiotensin converting enzyme inhibition, and lithium therapy. Am J Med 86:621, 1989

Nelson JC, Jatlow PI, Bock J, et al: Major adverse reactions during desipramine treatment: relationship to drug plasma concentrations, concomitant antipsychotic treatment and patient characteristics. Arch Gen Psychiatry 39:1055–1061, 1982

Nelson JC, Atillasoy E, Mazure C: Hydroxydesipramine in the elderly. J Clin Psychopharmacol 8:428–433, 1988a

Nelson JC, Mazure C, Jatlow PI: Antidepressant activity of 2-hydroxydesipramine. Clin Pharmacol Ther 44:283–288, 1988b

Nordin C, Bertilsson L, Siwers B: Clinical and biochemical effects during treatment of depression with nortriptyline: the role of 10-hydroxynortriptyline. Clin Pharmacol Ther 42:10–19, 1987

Noveske FG, Hahn KR, Flynn RJ: Possible toxicity of combined fluoxetine and lithium (letter to the editor). Am J Psychiatry 146:1515, 1989

Ostergaard K, Dupont E: Clozapine treatment of drug induced psychotic symptoms in late stages of Parkinson's disease (letter). Acta Neurol Scand 78:349–350, 1988

Palmer H: Potentiation of pethidine (letter). Br Med J 2:944, 1960

Parvin R, Milo R, Klein C, et al: Amitriptyline for intractable hiccup (letter). Am J Gastroenterol 83:1007–1008, 1988

Patterson JF: Triazolam syndrome in the elderly. South Med J 80:1425–1426, 1987a

Patterson J: Metoclopramide therapy of MAOI orthostatic hypotension (letter). J Clin Psychopharmacol 7:112–113, 1987b

Peck AW, Stern WC, Watkinson C: Incidence of seizures during treatment with tricyclic antidepressant drugs and bupropion. J Clin Psychiatry 44:197–201, 1983

Perucca E, Garratt A, Hebdige S, et al: Water intoxication in epileptic patients receiving carbamazepine. J Neurol Neurosurg Psychiatry 41:713–718, 1978

Physician's Desk Reference for Nonprescription Drugs, 11th Edition. Oradell, NJ, Medical Economics, 1990

Pieri L: Preclinical pharmacology of midazolam. Br J Clin Pharmacol 16 (suppl 1):17S–27S, 1983

Pisani F, Fazio A, Oteri G, et al: Sodium valproate and valpromide: differential interactions with carbamazepine in epileptic patients. Epilepsia 27:548–552, 1986

Pohl R, Balon R, Berchou R, et al: Allergy to tartrazine in antidepressants. Am J Psychiatry 144:237–238, 1987

Pollock BG, Perel JM, Stiller RL, et al: Comparative cardiotoxicity and pharmacokinetics of nortriptyline and its isomeric 10-hydroxymetabolites in unanesthetized swine (abstract). Fed Proc 46:1305, 1987

Pollack M, Rosenbaum J: Management of antidepressant-induced side effects: a practical guide for the clinician. J Clin Psychiatry 48:3–8, 1987

Port FK, Kroll PD, Rosenzweig J: Lithium therapy during maintenance hemodialysis. Psychosomatics 20:130–131, 1979

Preskorn SH, Othmer SC: Evaluation of bupropion hydrochloride: the first of a new class of atypical antidepressants. Pharmacotherapy 4:20–34, 1984

Price LH, Charney DS, Heninger GR: Effects of tranylcypromine treatment on neuroendocrine, behavioral, and autonomic responses to tryptophan in depressed patients. Life Sci 37:809–818, 1983

Price WA, Bielefeld M: Buspirone-induced mania. J Clin Psychopharmacol 9:150–151, 1989

Price W, Giannini RJ: Neurotoxicity caused by lithium-verapamil synergism. J Clin Pharmacol 26:717–719, 1986

Prien RF, Gelenberg AJ: Alternatives to lithium for preventive treatment of bipolar disorder. Am J Psychiatry 146:840–848, 1989

Pulik M, Lida H: Interaction lithium-inhibiteurs de l'enzyme de conversion. (letter). La Presse Medicale 17:755, 1988

Puzynski S, Klosiewicz L: Valproic acid amide in the treatment of affective and schizoaffective disorders. J Affective Disord 6:115–121, 1984

Realmuto GM, August GJ, Garfinkel BD: Clinical effect of buspirone in autistic children. J Clin Psychopharmacol 9:122–125, 1989

Redenbaugh JE, Sato S, Penry JK, et al: Sodium valproate: pharmacokinetics and effectiveness in treating intractable seizures. Neurology 30:1–6, 1980

Reed SM, Wise MG, Timmerman I: Choreoathetosis: a sign of lithium toxicity. Journal of Neuropsychiatry 1:57–60, 1989

Regan WM, Margolin RA, Mathew RJ: Cardiac arrhythmia following rapid imipramine withdrawal. Biol Psychiatry 25:482–484, 1989

Rickels K, Freeman E, Sondheimer S: Buspirone in treatment of premenstrual syndrome. Lancet 1:777, 1989

Risby ED, Risch SC, Stoudemire A: Mood disorders, in Clinical Psychiatry for Medical Students. Edited by Stoudemire A. Philadelphia, PA, JB Lippincott, 1990, pp 157–198

Ritchie EC, Bridenbaugh RH, Jabbari B: Acute generalized myoclonus following buspirone administration. J Clin Psychiatry 6:242–243, 1988

Rivers N, Horner B: Possible lethal reaction between Nardil and dextromethorphan (letter to the editor). Can Med Assoc J 103:85, 1970

Roberts HE, Dean RC, Stoudemire A: Clozapine treatment of psychosis in Parkinson's disease. Journal of Neuropsychiatry 1:190–192, 1989

Robinson D, Cooper TB, Howard D, et al: Amitriptyline and hydroxylated metabolite plasma levels in depressed outpatients. J Clin Psychopharmacol 5:83–88, 1985

Robinson D, Napoliello MJ, Schenk J: The safety and usefulness of buspirone as an anxiolytic drug in elderly versus young patients. Clin Ther 10:740–746, 1988

Robinson DS, Alms DR, Shrotriya RC, et al: Serotonergic anxiolytics and treatment of depression. Psychopathology 22 (suppl 1):27–36, 1989

Rochel M, Ehrenthal W: Haematological side effects of valproic acid, in Chronic Toxicity of Antiepileptic Drugs. Edited by Oxley J, Janz D, Meinardi H. New York, Raven, 1983, pp 101–104

Roose SP, Glassman AH, Giardina EGV, et al: Cardiovascular effects of imipramine and bupropion in depressed patients with congestive heart failure. J Clin Psychopharmacol 7:247–251, 1987

Roose SP, Glassman AH, Dalack GW: Depression, heart disease, and tricyclic antidepressants. J Clin Psychiatry 50 (suppl):12–16, 1989

Rudorfer MV, Potter WZ: Combined fluoxetine and tricyclic antidepressants. Am J Psychiatry 146:562–564, 1989

Salama AA, Shafey M: A case of severe lithium toxicity induced by combined fluoxetine and lithium carbonate (letter). Am J Psychiatry 146:278, 1989

Salmeron S, Brenot F, Rain B, et al: Maprotiline and pulmonary alveolitis (letter). Ann Intern Med 109:758–759, 1988

Samiy AH, Rosnick PB: Early identification of renal problems in patients receiving chronic lithium treatment. Am J Psychiatry 144:670–672, 1987

Satel SL, Nelson JCN: Stimulants in the treatment of depression: a critical overview. J Clin Psychiatry 50:241–249, 1989

Scheffner D, Konig S, Rauterberg-Rutland I, et al: Fatal liver failure in 16 children with valproate therapy. Epilepsia 29:530–542, 1988

Schenker S, Bergstrom RF, Wolen RL, et al: Fluoxetine disposition and elimination in cirrhosis. Clin Pharmacol Ther 44:353–359, 1988

Schneider LS, Cooper TB, Staples FR, et al: Prediction of individual dosage of nortriptyline in depressed elderly outpatients. J Clin Psychopharmacol 7:311–314, 1987

Schneider LS, Cooper TB, Severson JA, et al: Electrocardiographic changes with nortriptyline and 10-hydroxynortriptyline in elderly depressed outpatients. J Clin Psychopharmacol 8:402–408, 1988

Schou M: Lithium prophylaxis: myths and realities. Am J Psychiatry 146:573–576, 1989

Schou M, Vestergaard P: Use of propranolol during lithium treatment: an enquiry and a suggestion. Pharmacopsychiatry 20:131, 1987

Schou M, Vestergaard P: Prospective studies on a lithium cohort, 2: renal function, water and electrolyte metabolism. Acta Psychiatr Scand 78:427–433, 1988

Secor JW, Schenker S: Drug metabolism in patients with liver disease. Adv Intern Med 32:379–406, 1987

Sellers EM, Bendayan R: Pharmacokinetics of psychotropic drugs in selected patient populations, in Psychopharmacology: The Third Generation of Progress. Edited by Meltzer HY. New York, Raven, 1987, pp 1397–1406

Series F, Cormier Y, LaForge J: Changes in day and night time oxygenation with protriptyline in patients with chronic obstructive lung disease. Thorax 44:275–279, 1989

Sethna M, Solomon G, Cedarbaum J, et al: Successful treatment of massive carbamazepine overdose. Epilepsia 30:71–73, 1989

Shukla S, Mukherjee S, Decina P: Lithium in the treatment of bipolar disorders associated with epilepsy: an open study. J Clin Psychopharmacol 8:201–204, 1988

Sides CA: Hypertension during anaesthesia with monoamine oxidase inhibitors. Anaesthesia 42:633–635, 1987

Simonds AK, Parker RA, Branthwaite MA: Effects of protriptyline on sleep related disturbances of breathing in restrictive chest wall disease. Thorax 41:586–590, 1986

Simonson M: Controlling MAO inhibitor hypotension. Am J Psychiatry 120:1118–1119, 1964

Simpson GM, Singh H: Buspirone and dyskinesia (letter). J Clin Psychiatry 49:503, 1988

Specht U, Boenigk HE, Wolf P: Discontinuation of clonazepam after long-term treatment. Epilepsia 30:458–463, 1989

Stack CG, Rogers P, Linter SPK: Monoamine oxidase inhibitors and anaesthesia. Br J Anaesth 60:222–227, 1988

Stark P, Hardison CD: A review of multicenter controlled studies of fluoxetine vs. imipramine and placebo in outpatients with major depressive disorder. J Clin Psychiatry 46:53–58, 1985

Stark P, Fuller RW, Wong DT: The pharmacologic profile of fluoxetine. J Clin Psychiatry 46:7–13, 1985

Steiner W, Fontaine R: Toxic reaction following the combined administration of fluoxetine and L-tryptophan: five case reports. Biol Psychiatry 21:1067–1071, 1986

Stephens WP, Espir MLE, Tattersall RB, et al: Water intoxication due to carbamazepine. Br Med J 1:754–755, 1977

Sternbach H: Danger of MAOI therapy after fluoxitine withdrawal. Lancet 2:850–851, 1988

Stoudemire A, Atkinson P: Use of cyclic antidepressants in patients with cardiac conduction disturbances. Gen Hosp Psychiatry 10:389–397, 1988

Stoudemire A, Clayton L: Successful use of clozapine in a patient with a history of neuroleptic malignant syndrome. Journal of Neuropsychiatry 1:303–305, 1989

Stoudemire A, Fogel BS: Psychopharmacology in the medically ill, in Principles of Medical Psychiatry. Edited by Stoudemire A, Fogel BS. Orlando, FL, Grune & Stratton, 1987, pp 79–112

Stoudemire A, Moran MG, Fogel BS: Psychotropic drug use in the medically ill: Part I. Psychosomatics 31:377–391, 1990

Stoudemire A, Moran MG, Fogel BS: Psychotropic drug use in the medically ill: Part II. Psychosomatics (in press)

Sussman N: Treatment of anxiety with buspirone. Psychiatric Annals 17:114–117, 1987

Taylor DC: Alarming reaction to pethidine in patients on phenelzine. Lancet 2:410–412, 1962

Tiller JWG, Dakis JA, Shaw JM: Short-term buspirone treatment in disinhibition with dementia. Lancet 2:510, 1988

Trimble MR: Nonmonoamine oxidase inhibitor antidepressants and epilepsy: a review. Epilepsia 19:241–250, 1978

Tuomisto J, Smith DF: Effects of tranylcypromine enantiomers on monoamine uptake and release and imipramine binding. J Neural Transm 65:135–145, 1986

Van Sweden B: Rebound antidepressant cardiac arrhythmia. Biol Psychiatry 24:360–369, 1988

Van Sweden B, Van Moffaert M: Valproate as psychotropic agent. Acta Psychiatr Scand 72:315–317, 1985

Vaughan DA: Interaction of fluoxetine with tricyclic antidepressants (letter to the editor). Am J Psychiatry 145:1478, 1988

Vendsborg PB: Lithium and glucose tolerance in manic-melancholic patients. Acta Psychiatr Scand 59:306–316, 1979

Verbeeck RK: Glucuronidation and disposition of drug glucuronides in patients with renal failure. Drug Metab Dispos 10:87–89, 1982

Vieweg WVR, Yank GR, Row WT, et al: Increase in white blood cell count and serum sodium level following the addition of lithium to carbamazepine treatment among three chronically psychotic male patients with disturbed affective states. Psychiatr Q 58:213–217, 1986–87

Vieweg WVR, Godleski LS: Carbamazepine and hyponatremia. Am J Psychiatry 145:1323–1324, 1988

Vieweg WVR, Glick JL, Herring S, et al: Absence of carbamazepine-induced hyponatremia among patients also given lithium. Am J Psychiatry 144:943–947, 1987

Vincent HH, Weimar W, Schalekamp MADH: Effect of cyclosporine in fractional excretion of lithium and potassium in kidney transplant recipients (abstract). Kidney Int 31:1048, 1987

Weber JJ: Seizure activity associated with fluoxetine therapy. Clin Pharm 8:296–298, 1989

Wells DG, Bjorksten AR: Monoamine oxidase inhibitors revisited. Can J Anaesth 36:64–74, 1989

Wenger TL, Stern WC: The cardiovascular profile of bupropion. J Clin Psychiatry 44:176–182, 1983

Wenger TL, Bustrack JA, Cohn JB: Comparison of the electrocardiographic effects of amitriptyline and bupropion (abstract). Clin Pharmacol Ther 31:280, 1982

Wenger TL, Cohn JB, Bustrack J: Comparison of the effects of bupropion and amitriptyline on cardiac conduction in depressed patients. J Clin Psychiatry 44:174–175, 1983

White MG, Fetner CD: Treatment of the syndrome of inappropriate secretion of antidiuretic hormone with lithium carbonate. N Engl J Med 292:390–392, 1975

White PF, Vasconez LO, Mathes SA, et al: Comparison of midazolam and diazepam for sedation during plastic surgery. Plast Reconstr Surg 81:703–710, 1988

Wibell L: The serum level and urinary excretion of beta 2-microglobulin in health and renal disease. Pathol Biol (Paris) 26:295–301, 1978

Williams RL, Mamelok RD: Hepatic disease and drug pharmacokinetics. Clin Pharmacokinet 5:528–547, 1980

Wong KC: Preoperative discontinuation of monoamine oxidase inhibitor therapy: an old wives tale? Seminars in Anesthesia 5:145–148, 1986

Wong T, Tiessen E: Seizure in gradual clonazepam withdrawal. Psychiatr J Univ Ottawa 14:484, 1989

Wood IK, Parmelee DX, Foreman JW: Lithium-induced nephrotic syndrome. Am J Psychiatry 146:84–87, 1989

Woods SW, Tesar GE, Murray GB, et al: Psychostimulant treatment of depressive disorders secondary to medical illness. J Clin Psychiatry 47:12–15, 1986

Wyant M, Diamond BI, O'Neal E, et al: The use of midazolam in acutely agitated psychiatric patients. Psychopharmacol Bull 26:126–129, 1990

Yassa R, Iskandar H, Nastase C, et al: Carbamazepine and hyponatremia in patients with affective disorder. Am J Psychiatry 145:339–342, 1988

Yatham LN, Barry S, Dinan TG: Serotonin receptors, buspirone, and premenstrual syndrome. Lancet 1:1447–1448, 1989

Young RC, Alexopoulos GS, Shamoian CA, et al: Plasma 10-hydroxy-nortriptyline in elderly depressed patients. Clin Pharmacol Ther 35:540–544, 1984a

Young RC, Alexopoulos GS, Shamoian CA, et al: Heart failure associated with high plasma 10-hydroxynortriptyline levels. Am J Psychiatry 141:432–433, 1984b

Young RC, Alexopoulos GS, Shamoian CA, et al: Plasma 10-hydroxy-nortriptyline and ECG changes in elderly depressed patients. Am J Psychiatry 142:866–868, 1985

Youssef MS, Wilkinson PA: Epidural fentanyl and monoamine oxidase inhibitors. Anaesthesia 43:210–212, 1988

Ziegler DK, Hurwitz A, Hassanein RS, et al: Migraine prophylaxis: a comparison of propranolol and amitriptyline. Arch Neurol 44:486–489, 1987

Zung WWK: Review of placebo-controlled trials with bupropion. J Clin Psychiatry 44:104–114, 1983

Chapter 3

Anesthetic Management of the High-Risk Medical Patient Receiving Electroconvulsive Therapy

Gundy B. Knos, M.D.
Yung-Fong Sung, M.D.

In December 1989, the American Psychiatric Association issued practice guidelines for the use of electroconvulsive therapy (ECT) and characterized the procedure as "safe and very effective for certain severe mental illnesses" ("APA issues practice guidelines for ECT" 1990). Nonetheless, practitioners should be aware that the cardiovascular and autonomic changes that can occur during ECT may be profound in some patients. This chapter is meant to acquaint the reader with the physiological changes associated with ECT and to serve as a guide in the application of ECT to the psychiatric treatment of the medically frail patient. In this chapter, we will assume that an anesthesiologist or anesthetist is present for the procedure, and that the psychiatrist will collaborate with the person administering anesthesia to manage risks associated with the procedure.

PHYSIOLOGICAL EFFECTS OF ECT

The physiological response to electrically induced convulsions determines the risks of ECT in medically ill patients. Figure 3-1 illustrates the sequence of physiological changes that occur during and after ECT. ECT has profound effects on the hypothalamus, the pituitary, and the thyroid glands, and, most importantly (from the point of view of an anesthesiologist or anesthetist), on the adrenal cortex and medulla (Pitts 1982; Selvin 1987).

Endocrine Response to ECT

After ECT stimulus, there is an immediate increase in adrenocorticotropic hormone (ACTH) levels followed by a later increase in serum cortisol and glucagon. Glucose-mediated insulin secretion may be inhibited. These effects appear to have little clinical consequence except in persons with severe diabetes, in whom they may cause potentially dangerous hyperglycemia (Selvin 1987). There have been some reports of improvement of diabetic status in some patients with recent-onset diabetes or in those with non-insulin-dependent diabetes (Fakhri et al. 1980). With these variable effects of ECT on blood glucose levels in diabetic patients, it is reasonable to monitor blood glucose closely during a treatment series and, it is suggested, for as long as 3 weeks after the end of treatment (Finestone and Weiner 1984).

Cardiovascular Response to ECT

Of far greater importance to the health and well-being of the medically frail ECT patient is the dramatic increase in levels of circulating catecholamines. Catecholamines are largely released from the adrenal medulla, with a smaller contribution from the sympathetic nerve endings themselves (Selvin 1987). The first autonomic event observed after stimulus is an increase in parasympathetic tone (Selvin 1987). Bradycardia and even asystole may be observed (Gaines and Rees 1986). This parasympathetically mediated sinoatrial node inhibition in the heart may cause ectopic foci to appear, resulting in premature ventricular contractions (PVCs) and ventricular escape beats. The increased vagal tone may produce hypotension and bradycardia.

In 10–15 seconds, the parasympathetic manifestations are replaced by the signs of sympathetic stimulation, as plasma epinephrine may

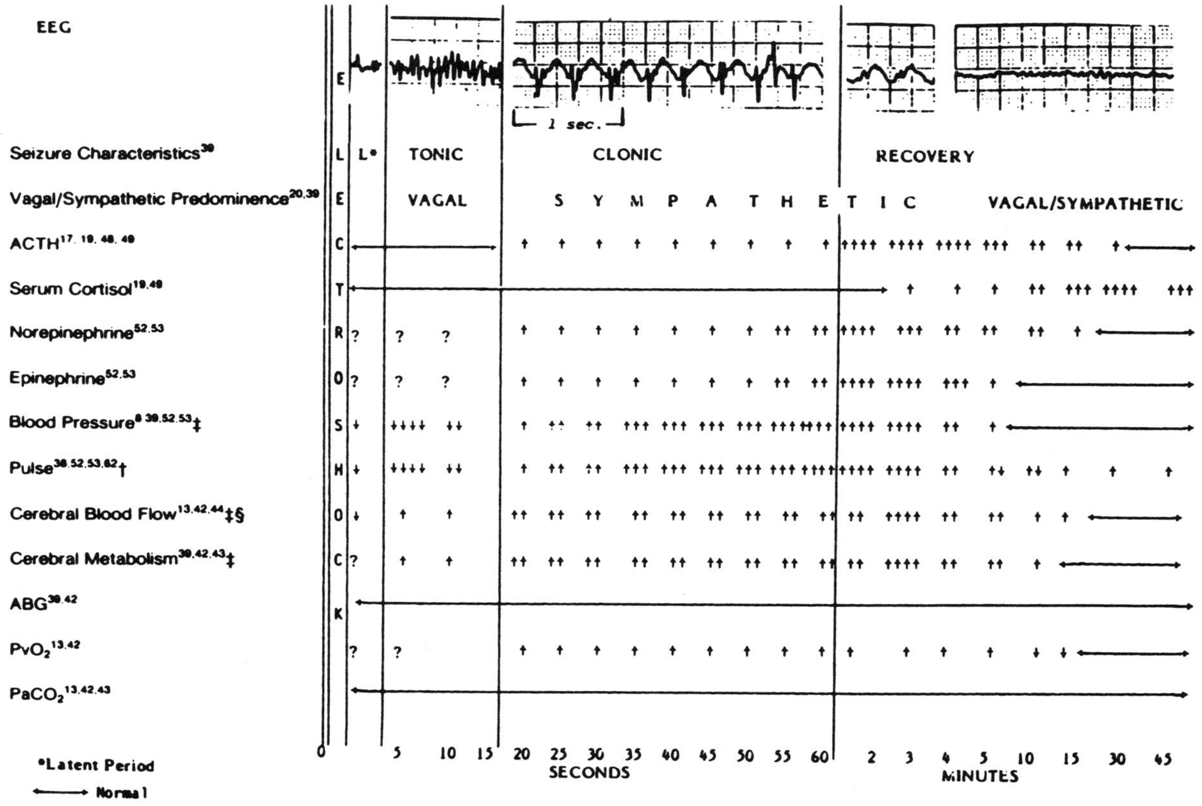

EEG

SEIZURE CHARACTERISTICS

	EEG	TONIC	CLONIC	RECOVERY
	L* L	VAGAL	SYMPATHETIC	VAGAL/SYMPATHETIC

Vagal/Sympathetic Predominance[20,39]

Seizure Characteristics[30]

ACTH[17,18,48,49]

Serum Cortisol[18,49]

Norepinephrine[52,53]

Epinephrine[52,53]

Blood Pressure[38,52,53,62] ‡

Pulse[38,52,53,62] †

Cerebral Blood Flow[13,42,44] ‡§

Cerebral Metabolism[39,42,43] ‡

ABG[39,42]

PvO2[13,42]

PaCO2[13,42,43]

*Latent Period
→ Normal

SECONDS: 0 5 10 15 20 25 30 35 40 45 50 55 60
MINUTES: 2 3 4 5 10 15 30 45

1 sec.

Figure 3-1. Diagram of physiological events related to ECT (modified). Reprinted with permission from Selvin BL: Electroconvulsive therapy—1987. Anesthesiology 67:367–385, 1987.

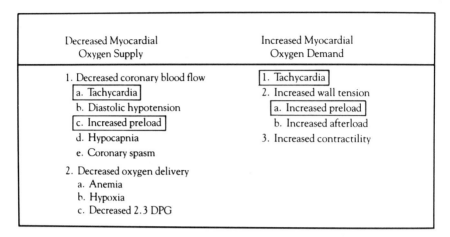

Decreased Myocardial Oxygen Supply	Increased Myocardial Oxygen Demand

1. Decreased coronary blood flow
  a. Tachycardia
  b. Diastolic hypotension
  c. Increased preload
  d. Hypocapnia
  e. Coronary spasm
2. Decreased oxygen delivery
  a. Anemia
  b. Hypoxia
  c. Decreased 2.3 DPG
	1. Tachycardia
	2. Increased wall tension
	  a. Increased preload
	  b. Increased afterload
	3. Increased contractility

Figure 3-2. Detrimental changes in the myocardial oxygen balance. Factors in boxes affect both myocardial oxygen supply and myocardial oxygen demand and are therefore doubly detrimental to the patient's health. DPG = diphosphoglycerate. Reprinted with permission from Kaplan J: Anesthesia for patients with coronary artery disease (monograph, Audio Rounds for Anesthesiologists). Ossining, NY, Cortlandt Group, 1982, pp 1–6.

increase to 15 times normal levels and plasma norepinephrine may reach 3 times normal levels. Heart rate and blood pressure may soar, and cardiac dysrhythmias may occur in response to the arrhythmogenic effects of the catecholamine surge (Gaines and Rees 1986; Selvin 1987). These changes, along with the increase in muscular tone and activity, may produce an increase in myocardial oxygen consumption. Myocardial ischemia and even infarction may result (Gaines and Rees 1986). Tachycardia is a well-known detrimental factor in myocardial oxygen balance. It increases myocardial oxygen demand at the same time that it decreases myocardial oxygen supply due to reduced time in diastole when most of coronary blood flow occurs (Figure 3-2). Pharmacologic interventions for high-risk patients focus on attenuating these autonomic changes and their secondary effects.

Cerebrovascular Response to ECT

The cerebrovascular system is also affected by ECT. As the electrical stimulus occurs, there is a concurrent brief period of cerebrovascular constriction. This is followed by a 1.5- to 7-fold increase in cerebral blood flow from baseline, due to increased systemic arterial pressure and in response to the increase in cerebral oxygen consumption by the actively seizing cells. As a result, a dramatic but transient increase in intracranial pressure occurs, which may have profound detrimental effects in patients with cranial arteriovenous malformations, intracranial mass lesions, or increased intracranial pressure for any reason (Gaines and Rees 1986).

Intraocular and Intragastric Pressure Responses to ECT

Intraocular pressure has been reported to increase transiently with seizure onset. This increase begins with the sudden hypertension associated with ECT and lasts for about 5 minutes after the seizure has ended. The intraocular pressure may increase to 30 mmHg (Epstein et al. 1975). In chronic open-angle glaucoma, this is usually of no clinical consequence (Nathan et al. 1986; Weiner and Coffey 1987). More serious ophthalmic risk may occur with ECT in patients with acute narrow-angle glaucoma (Sibony 1985). Consequently, before undergoing ECT, the glaucoma in these patients should be well controlled. As discussed later, some of the medications used in controlling glaucoma may have interesting interactions with anesthetic drugs.

Intragastric pressure is also increased with seizure onset (Hurwitz 1974). The rise in intragastric pressure may lead to problems with regurgitation and pulmonary aspiration of gastric contents in patients with symptomatic hiatal hernias who have a tendency to reflux when ventilated with a mask and Ambu bag. Aspiration pneumonitis is a dreaded complication that carries a mortality rate of 28% (Bynum and Pierce 1976). If a history of reflux is obtained from the patient, especially if it occurs when the patient lies flat or with an empty stomach, oral administration of histamine (H2) receptor antagonists such as cimetidine or ranitidine should be strongly considered in the evening and morning before ECT. Oral metoclopramide (to facilitate gastric emptying) may be needed and should be given 60 minutes before ECT. Preoxygenation with endotracheal intubation and cricoid pressure prior to electrical stimulus may have to be considered in patients with severe symptoms to provide a physical barrier, in the form of the endotracheal tube balloon, to tracheal trespass of gastric contents. It is also imperative to have a suction apparatus ready if regurgitation should unexpectedly occur.

CONTRAINDICATIONS TO ECT

The list of contraindications to ECT is based on data that have shown many times that the contraindicating condition combined with ECT may often produce a poor outcome or even death. Certain conditions, however, may justify proceeding with ECT despite the presence of these contraindications. Management of patients under these circumstances is dealt with later in the chapter. In this section, discussion will focus on the physiological change in each condition and how it may relate adversely to ECT.

"Absolute" Contraindications to ECT

Intracranial mass lesions.   The presence of an intracranial space-occupying lesion (with or without increases in intracranial pressure) is universally considered to be an absolute contraindication to ECT (Scalafani 1988; Selvin 1987). This concern arises from the dynamics of intracranial pressure and volume (Figure 3-3). Initially, the pressure volume curve is flat and horizontal, representing a phase of high compliance. This is followed by an intermediate area of transition. The steep, nearly vertical terminal portion of the curve represents the area of low compliance. The initial stable portion represents a time of central nervous system compensation. An increase in volume of one of the intracranial components (e.g., brain mass increased by a tumor) is compensated for by a decrease in another intracranial component (e.g., cerebrospinal fluid). Such a patient can have a normal or nearly normal intracranial pressure, with no neurological changes, and still be at the limit of his or her compensatory mechanisms (Donegan 1983b). Consequently, even a small increase in intracranial volume such as occurs with increased cerebral blood flow to the brain during ECT can cause the emergence of abnormal neurological signs due to changes in cerebral cellular permeability, vascular tone, and increased edema around the brain tumor, causing sudden tremendous increases in intracranial pressure (Kalinowski et al. 1982; Selvin 1987).

ECT has been performed safely in some patients with brain tumors (Maltbie et al. 1980). These patients, generally, were neurologically stable before their treatment, with no signs of increased intracranial pressure. Usually these patients had small, asymptomatic tumors such as meningiomas (Alexopoulos et al. 1989; Fried and Mann 1988; Greenberg et al. 1988). However, a good result cannot be presumed when these criteria are present, because some patients who appeared neu-

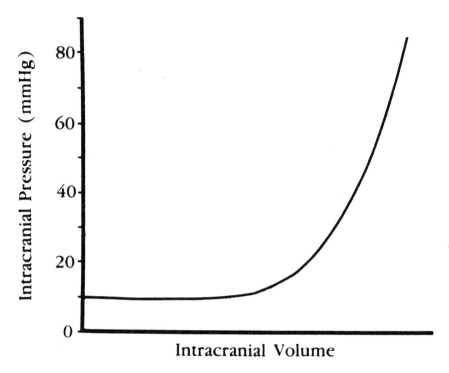

Figure 3-3. Intracranial pressure–volume curve illustrating rapid loss of intracranial compliance with small increases in intracranial volume after exhaustion of compensatory mechanisms. Reprinted with permission from Donegan 1983b. Copyright Little, Brown, 1983.

rologically stable with apparently normal intracranial pressure had poor post-ECT results with permanent neurological deterioration (Dressler and Folk 1975; Gassell 1960; Kalinowski et al. 1982; Karliner 1978; Maltbie et al. 1980; Shapiro and Goldberg 1957). A 74% overall morbidity is reported in patients with brain tumors who receive ECT, including a 1-month mortality rate of 28% (Maltbie et al. 1980). It is still a valid conclusion that a space-occupying intracranial lesion is a strong contraindication to ECT.

Cerebrovascular infarct. A recent cerebrovascular accident has been considered an absolute contraindication to ECT (Scalafani 1988). It has been reported that ECT in patients within 6 weeks of an infarct may increase the risk for further neurological deterioration (Anderson and Kissane 1977). In patients with a recent cerebrovascular accident, vascular integrity may be compromised and a potential for further adverse neuropathological changes exists (Adams and Victor 1977; Anderson and Kissane 1977); however, the risk is minimized once healing has occurred (Hsiao et al. 1987). It is also conceivable that ECT could dislodge a second embolus in patients with a history of cerebrovascular embolism due to blood pressure surges (Alexopoulos et al. 1989). However, ECT has been successfully performed in a patient with a cerebral infarct of 4 days duration (Gassell 1960) and in four patients within 1 month of a stroke (Murray et al. 1986). Many practitioners feel that ECT can be administered safely 1 month or later after a cerebrovascular accident (Hsiao et al. 1987; Murray et al. 1986).

Intracranial aneurysms and cerebrovascular malformations. These have been considered absolute contraindications to ECT. However, ECT has been successfully performed in these circumstances (Drop et al. 1988; Greenberg et al. 1986), but tight control of blood pressure should be exercised to prevent increased aneurysmal wall stress, which is thought to be related to increased mean arterial pressure or pulse pressure (Peerless 1983). When considering ECT in this setting, the practitioner must be aware that the situation is analogous to that of driving down the highway in a car with a bulging tire. One can never be sure at what speed (blood pressure) the tire (aneurysm) will blow out.

Recent myocardial infarction (MI). This is considered a strong contraindication to ECT. Several reports have shown that patients who have recently had MIs have an increased risk of reinfarction with surgical stress or ECT (Goldman et al. 1977; Rao et al. 1983; Steen et al. 1978). In addition, mortality rates can exceed 50% should reinfarction occur. When the previous MI is 0–3 and 4–6 months old, perioperative reinfarction occurs in 36% and 16% of patients, respectively. After 6 months, the rate for reinfarction in patients with a previous MI returns to the baseline rate of 7%. The risk of reinfarction with subsequent high mortality can be decreased to 6% or less in surgical patients with recent MIs by preoperative optimization of the patient's status, aggressive invasive monitoring of the hemodynamic parameters, and prompt treatment of any hemodynamic aberrations (Rao et al. 1983). ECT has been performed successfully in a few patients 2–3 weeks after an MI, although ischemic changes have been reported on the ECG during treatment (Dec et al. 1985; Kerr et al. 1982; Regestein and Reich 1985; Solomon 1979). A patient in our institution had a successful series of ECT treatments within 1 month of her MI. During her treatments, she had episodes of multifocal PVCs and one episode of a 4- to 5-beat run of ventricular tachycardia requiring 100 mg iv (2 mg/kg) of lidocaine during the recovery phase of ECT. No S-T segment depression was noted.

After MI, 6–8 weeks are required for infarcted myocardium to heal, i.e., for scar tissue replacement of the infarcted area to occur. Early complications of MI include an increased incidence of cardiac arrhythmias, particularly ventricular fibrillation. Extensive tissue necrosis may lead to congestive heart failure. A major consideration in the care of these patients is the fact that infarct size can vary with time. Ischemic areas around the infarcted tissue may depend on collateral blood flow, which may vary with changes in myocardial oxygen supply and demand. Therefore, factors that increase the work of the heart may increase the size of the infarct (Pasternak et al. 1987). As was discussed previously, catecholamine release with ECT stimulus has considerable adverse effects on myocardial oxygen supply and demand. ECT in a patient with recent MI may cause potentially fatal extension of the infarct. As stated earlier in this chapter, there is evidence that this risk may be decreased by tight hemodynamic control (Rao et al. 1983). These methods will be discussed later in the chapter in the section "Management of Specific Medical Problems During ECT."

Unstable aortic aneurysm. Unstable aortic aneurysms have been considered absolute contraindications to ECT. The rationale for this concern relates to the problems of increased blood pressure during ECT, producing increased intramural pressure on the weakened aortic wall. ECT has been successfully performed in patients with abdominal aortic aneurysms (Pomeranze et al. 1968; Wolford 1957). However, it is well known that the mortality rate in patients with unrepaired unstable aortic aneurysms is 80% or more in 5 years (Figure 3-4) (Estes 1950) and the surgical mortality of abdominal aortic aneurysm repair is 1.4–3.9%. Therefore, thought should be given to surgical repair of the aneurysm before ECT (Youngberg 1988). Each case should be decided individually, among the attending psychiatrist, anesthesiologist, and vascular surgeon, as to whether the patient's depression is so severe as to make it unlikely for him or her to survive the stress of surgery versus the chance for aneurysmal rupture during ECT. If the decision is made to proceed with ECT before aneurysmectomy, the patient, family, and all others concerned should be aware that the circumstances are not ideal and that there is an increased risk of an acute disastrous event during the ECT. Aneurysmal rupture carries a mortality rate of up to 50% even if the patient is managed aggressively

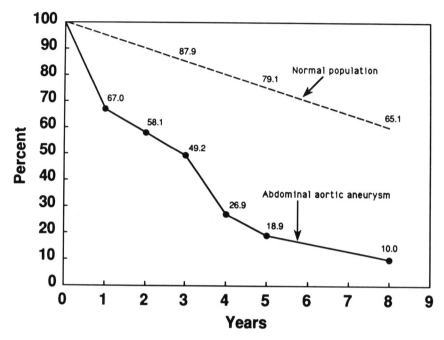

Figure 3-4.   Survival rates for traced patients who had abdominal aortic aneurysm compared with survival rates of the normal population aged 65 years. Modified from Estes JE Jr: Abdominal aortic aneurysm; a study of 102 cases. Circulation 2:258–264, 1950. By permission of the American Heart Association, Inc.

and quickly brought to the operating room (Darling and Brewster 1980; Hiatt et al. 1984). Also, it should be considered that patients with peripheral vascular-occlusive disease or abdominal aortic aneurysms also have a high incidence (30–60%) of occult coronary atherosclerotic heart disease (Youngberg 1988).

Pheochromocytoma and hypertension.   The presence of a pheochromocytoma is considered an absolute contraindication to ECT (Drake and Ebaugh 1956; Scalafani 1988; Selvin 1987). This position is understandable considering the dramatic catecholamine surges that occur during ECT and the concern that in the presence of a catecholamine-secreting tumor, the response could be a pressor crisis. Patients who present with paroxysmal hypertension should be tested for the presence of a pheochromocytoma (Drop and Welch 1989) because up to 0.1% of patients with hypertension have this tumor (Landsberg and Young 1987).

Surgical excision of the pheochromocytoma should precede ECT (Drop and Welch 1989; Selvin 1987). However, ECT has been successfully performed in the presence of an unsuspected pheochromocytoma (Carr and Woods 1985; Simon and Evans 1986), but this is a situation that few knowledgeable physicians would enjoy.

Blood pressure in patients with intrinsic systemic arterial hypertension should be under the best possible control before ECT. This may be complicated by the patient's anxiety causing a high catecholamine state despite "adequate" medical control. Studies have shown that patients with diastolic blood pressures greater than 110 mmHg show greater hemodynamic instability during anesthesia and that patients with untreated or poorly controlled hypertension are at greater risk for episodes of myocardial ischemia associated with either hypertension or hypotension (Goldman and Caldera 1979). Medications for coronary artery disease and hypertension (with the possible exception of diuretics) should be continued as usual. In fact, withholding beta-blocking agents could precipitate ischemic episodes, particularly under the stress of ECT (Scalafani 1988). Exceptions to this rule are the rauwolfia alkaloids, which produce their antihypertensive effects by intraneuronal catecholamine and 5-hydroxytryptophan depletion. Serious consequences of ECT in patients taking these alkaloids include prolonged apnea, profound hypotension, cardiac dysrhythmias, and death (Foster and Gayle 1955). Therefore, these medications should be discontinued 2 weeks before ECT, and another antihypertensive medication should be substituted, if necessary (Scalafani 1988).

Monoamine oxidase inhibitor therapy. Monoamine oxidase inhibitors (MAOIs) have been a traditional concern for anesthesiologists before any surgical procedure. These drugs act by blocking the oxidative deamination of catecholamines. The possibility exists for an intensified sympathetic response with hypertension, hypotension, hyperreflexia with convulsions, and hyperpyrexia (Drop and Welch 1989; Scalafani 1988; Selvin 1987). Central nervous system depressants, such as the barbiturates, may be potentiated, producing increased sleep time and sedation (Gaines and Rees 1986). Also, phenelzine sulfate (Nardil) has been reported to reversibly reduce serum pseudocholinesterase activity, causing paralysis for up to an hour after a dose of succinylcholine in patients on this drug (Bodley et al. 1969).

Traditionally, it has been recommended to discontinue MAOIs for 10–14 days before ECT. In some severely depressed patients, this may not be advisable. Recent studies have shown that a 2-week washout period may not be necessary, because no increase in ventricular ectopies or change in blood pressure responses were seen in the presence or absence of MAOI withdrawal (El-Ganzouri et al. 1985; Freese 1985; Remick et al. 1987). However, cardiac arrest has occurred after both modified and unmodified ECT in patients taking MAOIs (Marks 1984), and a recent informal survey of 60 board-certified anesthesiologists revealed that only 8 (13.3%) would administer an elective anesthetic to a patient on an MAOI, and then only with invasive blood pressure monitoring (Gevirtz 1989). Although this traditional stance may be shown to be overly conservative in future well-controlled studies, most anesthesiologists (including us) will be reluctant to proceed with elective ECT in a patient on an MAOI considering that there are numerous other antidepressant medications available. Why add to a patient's anesthetic risk merely to save 2 weeks? On the other hand, if ECT becomes necessary as an urgent treatment of last resort, as in an actively suicidal patient on an MAOI, then it may be necessary to accept what may only be theoretical increased risk and proceed with ECT. Doubtless, this issue may be a source of contention between psychiatrists and anesthesiologists for some time to come.

Summary.   Each patient who has a condition thought to be an absolute contraindication for ECT must be considered on an individual basis. The patient could be dying (wasting away with dehydration and lack of nourishment) due to catatonic depression. The patient could be actively suicidal with multiple daily attempts at self-destruction. If the condition that contraindicates ECT is surgically correctable, but the patient is at higher risk for mortality from the surgical procedure in the depressed state, or if ECT seems to be the only alternative to imminent death from depression in a surgically noncorrectable condition, it may be necessary to proceed with ECT. However, these cases must be carefully considered, and this must be a joint decision among the attending psychiatrist, anesthesiologist, surgeon and/or cardiologist, and, especially, the patient and family. All parties involved must be fully aware that there is a higher risk involved in proceeding with ECT under the circumstances, but that the only other likely alternative to ECT is the patient's death from depression. Documentation regarding the decision made, alternative possibilities with their probable outcomes, the persons involved in the decision-making process, and the seriousness of the patient's condition must be charted. The patient's physical condition must be optimized, and stringent care must be applied during the ECT procedure and in the recovery period.

Relative Contraindications to ECT

A great diversity of opinion exists as to what constitutes a relative contraindication to ECT. Frequently mentioned medical conditions in this category are angina pectoris, congestive heart failure, presence of cardiac pacemakers, glaucoma, retinal detachment, severe osteoporosis, major bone fractures, and severe acute and chronic pulmonary disease (Gaines and Rees 1986; Hurwitz 1974). However, ECT has been successfully performed in all these circumstances; a guide to the specific management of patients with some of these problems will be addressed in the section "Management of Specific Medical Problems During ECT."

CONSIDERATIONS IN SOME TYPES OF PATIENTS REFERRED FOR ECT

Elderly Depressed Patients

Elderly depressed patients referred for ECT are often frail and suffer from cardiovascular and pulmonary diseases. These patients may be malnourished and dehydrated, and chronic diseases may be in poor control due to lack of compliance with prescribed medications or diets. Often these persons have poor dentition, osteoporosis, and arthritis. If psychotic or catatonic features are present, it may be impossible to obtain a good medical history from the patient.

Patients on Tricyclic Antidepressants

Patients referred for ECT may be on tricyclic antidepressants (TCAs), which block the uptake of norepinephrine and/or of serotonin or dopamine into presynaptic nerve terminals. This has the effect of increasing central and peripheral adrenergic tone (Janowsky et al. 1981). TCAs may augment the effects of barbiturates used before ECT stimulus, causing increased sleep time and sedation (Gaines and Rees 1986). TCAs may also have anticholinergic effects. Therapeutic doses of TCAs have been associated with dysrhythmias and tachycardia, and there may be an increased response to direct sympathomimetics used to treat hypotension. Hyperthermia, hypertensive crises, and death have been reported in association with TCAs (Gaines and Rees 1986). The arrhythmogenic effects of epinephrine released during ECT could be potentiated by the presence of a TCA. Systemic adaptations in response to chronic TCA therapy may explain a lack of adverse responses of some patients during ECT, but patients on TCAs for less than 1 month may not be adapted and therefore may be at higher risk (Selvin 1987). A prolonged drug-free period is probably not necessary and might even be ill-advised in some patients (Azar and Lear 1984; Gaines and Rees 1986; Weiner and Coffey 1987). However, if there is no reason for TCA therapy during a course of ECT, they probably should be discontinued (Drop and Welch 1989).

Patients on Lithium

Lithium therapy in combination with barbiturates has been reported to prolong recovery time when serum lithium levels are above the therapeutic range. The action of muscle relaxants has been shown to be prolonged in patients on lithium therapy, which may contribute to prolonged inability of the patient to ventilate after relaxation for ECT (Gaines and Rees 1986). Lithium has been reported to decrease the therapeutic response to ECT (Gaines and Rees 1986; Weiner and Coffey 1987) and in combination with ECT may induce neurotoxicity and delirium (Drop and Welch 1989). Therefore, lithium probably should be discontinued before beginning ECT (Selvin 1987).

PRE-ECT ASSESSMENT

The attending physician, whether psychiatrist or anesthesiologist, may be the first physician to critically examine the general medical condition of patients referred for ECT. These patients may not have received consistent care from a primary physician due to their disinterest in their own health secondary to their depression. Further, medical "clearance" of psychiatric patients often leaves gaps. Therefore, neither the psychiatrist nor the anesthesiologist should assume that all medical problems were addressed in the routine examination received by the patient on admission to the hospital.

History

The physician consulted to assess a psychiatric patient referred for ECT should approach the patient as he or she would approach any patient before surgery. If possible, a history should be obtained from the patient or the patient's family regarding cardiovascular status, exercise tolerance, pulmonary status, gastric reflux, hypertension, diabetes, allergies, and any other pertinent medical factors, such as endocrine problems or family history suggesting malignant hyperthermia or pseudocholinesterase deficiency.

Obtaining a medical history may be difficult, as these patients may be catatonic and incapable of providing any personal information. They may be psychotically anxious as a result of their illness and may be terrified of undergoing "shock treatments." Family members, if available, may have little information to offer. Old medical charts should be carefully examined, and specialists should be consulted for any doubts regarding the patient's condition. The current medical chart should be examined for stability of the patient's vital signs.

Physical Examination

The patient's airway should be examined carefully, especially with regard to dentition. Due to long-standing depression, these patients may have disregarded their dental hygiene, resulting in loose and broken teeth. Neck range of motion should be established, especially in arthritic patients, because neck and jaw mobility may be extremely restricted or there may be instability of the first cervical vertebra on the second cervical vertebra leading to difficult airway management (Kallos and Smith 1989). The neck should be examined for a thyroid goiter. Because hyperthyroidism may be associated with depression, signs of hyperthyroidism, such as exophthalmos, fine tremor, palpitations, and muscle weakness, should be noted (Cassem 1987).

Careful auscultation of the heart and lungs should be performed. Cardiac murmurs and gallops, inspiratory and expiratory wheezes, jugular venous distension, and dependent edema should be noted. Signs of orthopnea can be elicited in patients suspected of having congestive heart failure by placing them in a supine position for 30 minutes. Frequent inspirations during normal conversation, pursed lips, barrel chest, and use of accessory muscles during resting ventilation are signs of significant pulmonary disease. If pulmonary disease is suspected, an impromptu test of a patient's pulmonary reserve could consist of a brisk walk down the hospital hall or the ability to ascend a flight of hospital stairs. Abnormalities should be followed up by consultation with the appropriate specialist and objective tests as indicated (see below).

The patient's hydration status should be examined carefully, especially in catatonic patients who are taking very little food or liquids by mouth. Skin turgor, neck vein distension, lying and standing (if possible) pulses and blood pressures, and appearance of mucus membranes should be assessed. A dehydrated patient should be adequately rehydrated with oral or, if necessary, intravenous fluids before undergoing ECT.

Objective Tests

Laboratory values such as the hematocrit and sodium levels may give additional clues to hydration status. A high hematocrit may indicate severe dehydration. Weekly measurement of electrolyte levels is important in patients treated with diuretics for hypertension or with digitalis for arrhythmias. There is also a correlation between low potassium levels and the incidence of PVCs (Rao et al. 1974). Low potassium levels in patients on digitalis have been associated with emergence of digitalis-toxic arrhythmias. The possibility of digitalis toxicity should be entertained in any patient on digoxin with premature ventricular beats, atrial tachycardia with variable atrioventricular (AV) block, or a heart rate of less than 50 beats/minute due to AV block (Braunwald 1987). Patients on digitalis should have a minimum potassium level of 3.5 mg/dl (Curling et al. 1984). Hypokalemia and digitalis toxicity should be corrected before initiating ECT.

Patients referred for ECT should have a recent ECG, chest X ray, and, if indicated, cervical spine films (particularly in arthritic patients). In patients with unstable blood pressures, studies should be done to rule out intracranial neoplasms or aneurysms, thyroid dysfunction, and pheochromocytoma. These patients should be prepared with the same care given any surgical patient.

A cardiologist should be consulted to evaluate cardiovascular status and to optimize medication regimens in patients with moderate to severe angina, unstable angina, history of multiple or recent MI, poorly controlled hypertension, valvular heart disease, or chronic congestive heart failure. In patients with more than mild stable angina well-controlled on medication, pretreatment evaluation with echocardiography and/or coronary angiography may be indicated (McPherson and

Lipsey 1988). Coronary artery disease and ability to handle cardiac stress can be evaluated with a stress-test ECG. In catatonic patients or patients unable to perform the exercise stress test, a dipyridamole-thallium myocardial perfusion scan will disclose areas of ischemia as well as areas of old infarction. In patients with congestive heart failure, a gaited pool study, chest radiograph, and arterial blood gas may be indicated to assess myocardial function (Drop and Welch 1989). Echocardiography and/or cardiac catheterization may be necessary to assess the severity of certain critical heart valve lesions such as aortic stenosis. The frequency and severity of cardiac dysrhythmias noted on pretreatment ECG or suggested by history (e.g., Stokes-Adams attacks) may require evaluation with Holter monitoring for 24–48 hours (Adams and Martin 1987).

In the patient suspected of pulmonary disease, room-air arterial blood gas analysis and clinical spirometry are the optimal tests for evaluation of pulmonary reserve before ECT (Gal 1986). A single spirometric study will provide critical information, such as the forced vital capacity (FVC), the forced expiratory volume at 1 second (FEV_1), the FEV_1-to-FVC ratio, maximal voluntary ventilation (MVV), and forced expiratory flow at 25–75% of the vital capacity (FEF_{25-75}). Values that indicate increased risk for morbidity and mortality due to pulmonary disease are shown below.

FVC < 50% predicted
FEV_1 < 50% predicted or < 2.0 liter
FEV_1/FVC < 50%
MVV < 50% predicted or < 50 liters/minute
FEF_{25-75} < 50% predicted

Any patient who does not surpass these criteria should be evaluated and optimized by an expert in pulmonary medicine (Boysen 1988).

PREOPERATIVE ORDERS

Patients should have nothing by mouth for 6–8 hours before ECT. Cimetidine (300 mg) or ranitidine (150 mg) po may be given at bedtime and on the morning of ECT to increase gastric fluid pH and decrease the risk of aspiration pneumonitis in patients who will undergo positive pressure ventilation by mask. However, patients with bronchial asthma may develop bronchoconstriction on administration of these H2-receptor blocking agents (Stoelting 1986). Therefore, the decision to give these medications must be made on an individual basis.

Glycopyrrolate (0.2 mg im) or atropine (0.4 mg im) 30–45 minutes before ECT is often ordered by the psychiatrist to attenuate the initial bradycardia seen after the ECT stimulus and to decrease airway secretions (Selvin 1987). Whether pretreatment with anticholinergic agents is necessary before ECT treatment is a controversial issue (Gaines and Rees 1986).

All usual medications, such as antihypertensive agents, cardiac medications, bronchodilators, thyroid medications, etc., should be continued as usual on the morning of ECT, with small sips of water. Exceptions include diuretics such as furosemide or hydrochlorothiazide. The insensible fluid loss associated with 8 hours of no oral intake ("npo past midnight") produces a deficit of more than a liter in a 70-kg patient at 2 ml/kg per hour (Giesecke and Egbert 1986).

Insulin-dependent diabetic patients, particularly those with brittle diabetes, should be evaluated in consultation with an endocrinologist. Pretreatment management may require glucose and insulin drips through the "npo" period. Certainly, when any diabetic patient presents for ECT, a pretreatment glucose level must be checked. These patients should also be scheduled early in the day so that there is minimal disturbance of their insulin or medication regimens (Natof 1985). Evening doses of NPH insulin with peak effects 11 hours later may need to be withheld before treatment. In our center, morning doses of regular insulin are withheld until after treatment when the patient demonstrates the ability to eat and drink with no nausea or vomiting. In caring for patients on oral antihyperglycemic agents such as the sulfonylureas (e.g., acetohexamide, chlorpropamide), the practitioner should be aware that these agents often have long durations of action (12–60 hours) and that the hypoglycemic effects of these agents can be severe and profound (Foster 1987). The decision about how to administer these medications in the treatment period may require expert consultation. Remember, glucose is the primary energy substrate of the brain, and, in the short run, hypoglycemia is far more dangerous than hyperglycemia (Foster and Rubenstein 1987).

In patients on chronic steroid therapy, persistent hypotension has been reported during perioperative stress in the absence of steroid supplements (Knudsen et al. 1981). This has led to the practice of giving supplementary steroids (e.g., 100–300 mg of hydrocortisone phosphate per 70 kg body weight) to steroid-dependent patients, or any patient who has received steroids within 1 year. The rationale is that steroid supplementation is a low-risk procedure and the potential risk of no steroid supplementation may be higher (Roizen 1986). Because we have established that ECT is a stressful procedure, and until we have better data, our practice is to give steroid supplements to these patients before ECT treatment.

MONITORING DURING ECT

The ECT patient should be monitored just as closely as any other patient undergoing a surgical procedure under either regional or general anesthesia—and perhaps even more closely due to the potentially dramatic hemodynamic changes. An ECG, blood pressure cuff, and precordial stethoscope are considered necessities, along with oxygen and an Ambu bag for ventilation. A pulse oximeter and peripheral nerve stimulator are innovations that may further enhance patient safety. (Pulse oximetry is a relatively inexpensive intraoperative monitor that is now considered a standard in anesthesia practice).

The area where ECT is performed should be equipped with suction, intubation equipment, defibrillator, and cardiac resuscitative medications (Scalafani 1988). The ECT machine itself should be inspected, calibrated, and maintained on a regular basis by qualified biomedical technicians (Kendell 1981).

Patients with a tendency to rapid oxygen desaturation, such as obese patients or patients with severe pulmonary disease and/or cardiac disease, should be given 100% oxygen by mask for a few minutes before induction with intravenous anesthetics. If the patient objects excessively to the mask, ventilation with 100% oxygen should commence immediately as loss of consciousness occurs (Selvin 1987).

Particular attention must be paid to the ECG before, during, and after the treatment, and it may be advisable to run a pre-ECT ECG rhythm strip for purposes of comparison in any patient who has any risk factors for coronary artery disease. Clinicians who regularly perform anesthesia for ECT can be amazed at the high incidence of arrhythmias, marked tachycardia, and S-T segment changes, which are often noticed with a little close observation of the ECG. Due to the wide range of dysrhythmias and treatment courses available, in-depth discussion of this topic is beyond the scope of this chapter. Generally, dysrhythmias that will require treatment are those that produce significant hemodynamic instability (e.g., hypotension) or those that have a potential for deteriorating into malignant dysrhythmias, such as ventricular tachycardia. ECG changes suggestive of myocardial ischemia should also be managed aggressively. The decision of how and when to treat such ECG changes is at the discretion of the attending anesthesiologist. Intravenous lidocaine pretreatment has been shown to be effective in preventing arrhythmias during ECT; however, it also has been shown to suppress or shorten the seizure activity in a dose-related manner (Selvin 1987).

INTRAVENOUS ANESTHETIC-INDUCTION AGENTS USED IN ECT

Intravenous anesthetic agents are usually given before induction of ECT to provide amnesia during the shock in case a "missed" or "incomplete" seizure occurs. Regardless of the presence or absence of an anesthetic agent, retrograde amnesia occurs after a successful electrically induced seizure (Selvin 1987). Ideally, the anesthetic agents used during ECT should have rapid onset with short duration of action and rapid return to consciousness after ECT. They should not shorten the seizure time since treatment efficacy is related to total seizure time (Selvin 1987). Short-acting barbiturates (methohexital and thiopental) have been the intravenous agents most commonly used. Large doses of intravenous anesthetic agents, such as the barbiturates, have been shown to have no beneficial effect in controlling hypertension and tachycardia during ECT (Gravenstein et al. 1965) and will actually shorten seizure time (Lunn et al. 1981). This should come as no surprise, since these agents are in the same general pharmaceutical class as medications used to treat seizure disorders. With lighter anesthesia, it has been shown that seizure time may be longer due to a lower seizure threshold, and fewer treatments may be necessary (Maletzky 1978).

Tables 3-1 and 3-2 provide a comparison of various intravenous agents used in ECT.

Barbiturates

Methohexital has been touted as the intravenous anesthetic agent of choice for ECT due to alleged reduction in the incidence of arrhythmias and other ECG abnormalities in ECT patients as compared with thiopental and other agents such as thiamylal and diazepam (Gerring and Shields 1982; Pitts 1982; Pitts et al. 1965; Rich et al. 1969; Woodruff et al. 1969). However, due to variations in methodology, protocols, and techniques, it is difficult to draw a definitive conclusion as to the

Table 3-1. Comparison of intravenous induction agents used in electroconvulsive therapy

	Methohexital	Thiopental	Diazepam	Propofol	Etomidate	Ketamine
Pain	Yes	No	Yes	Yes	Yes	No
Phlebitis	Rare	Rare	Yes	No	Yes	No
Onset (seconds)	30	30	120	<60	30	30
Duration (minutes after single dose)	5–10	10–15	15 minutes to 3 hours	4–8	3	5–10
Emergence	Smooth	Smooth	Smooth	Smooth	Smooth	Stormy
Respiratory effects	Transitory respiratory depression	Transitory respiratory depression	Mild respiratory depression	Transitory respiratory depression	Transitory respiratory depression	Minimal; reflexes intact
Hemodynamic effects	Mild CV depression	Mild CV depression; increased HR	Hypotension	Hypotension; CV depression	None	Increased HR and BP
Effect on seizure threshold	Increased; however, may activate seizure foci	Increased; also increased incidence of ECG abnormalities	Increased; 60% incidence of ECG abnormalities	Increased	May activate seizure foci; use with caution in patients with focal epilepsy	No change
Other effects	Muscle tremors; hiccups; excessive salivation as compared with thiopental	Decreased cerebral blood flow and intracranial pressure may cause bronchospasm	May have prolonged effects in elderly	Involuntary muscle movement; coughing, hiccups	Involuntary muscle movement; increased muscle tone	Increased intracranial cerebral blood flow; hallucinations

Note. CV = cardiovascular. HR = heart rate. BP = blood pressure.
Source. Data from Cockshott 1985; Fragen and Avram 1989; Lebowitz et al. 1982; Reves 1986; Selvin 1987; Stoelting 1987c; Sung 1988a.

Table 3-2. Comparison of pharmacokinetic parameters of anesthetic-induction agents

	Methohexital	Thiopental	Diazepam	Propofol	Etomidate	Ketamine
Protein binding (%)	73	83.4	98	95–98	77	12
Alpha distribution half-life	5.6 minutes	2.5–8.5 minutes	30–60 minutes	1.8–8.3 minutes	2.5 minutes	20–40 minutes
Beta elimination half-life	3.9 hours	5–12 hours	20–50 hours	30–90 minutes	3–5 hours	2–4 hours
Clearance (ml/kg per minute)	10.9	3.4	0.2–0.5	30–60	17.9	20
Active metabolites	No	No	Yes	No	No	Yes

Source. Data from Cockshott 1985; Fragen and Avram 1989; Lebowitz et al. 1982; Reves 1986; Selvin 1987; Stoelting 1987c; Sung 1988a.

superiority of methohexital with regard to cardiovascular stability (Selvin 1987).

Disadvantages of methohexital appear to be a greater incidence of hiccup, pain on injection, muscle twitching, and salivation, as compared with thiopental (Gaines and Rees 1986; Greenan et al. 1983). Thiopental has a somewhat longer duration of action than methohexital, which may be a disadvantage (Scalafani 1988).

Thiamylal has been used in ECT since the early 1960s but may be associated with more sympathetic arrhythmias, a higher incidence of S-T segment depression in ECG, and more severe vagal arrhythmias even in the presence of atropine (Pitts 1982).

Benzodiazepines

Although it is known to raise seizure threshold and has a relatively long duration of action, diazepam (5–10 mg iv) has been used for ECT induction in some centers. It has been associated with a 60% incidence of ECG abnormalities that may be multiple and persistent, compared to a 19% incidence with methohexital (Allen et al. 1980; Pitts 1982; Selvin 1987). A longer induction period and delayed recovery have been reported (McCleave and Blakemore 1975). Therefore, use of diazepam in ECT should be restricted to patients in whom barbiturates are contraindicated. Midazolam, a new short-acting benzodiazepine, will probably have effects on seizure threshold and possibly on incidence of ECG abnormalities similar to diazepam, although there are no reports in the literature on midazolam in ECT. Midazolam (1–2 mg iv) has been used in our facility to stop ECT seizures of excessive length. When using midazolam, one should recall that it is three to four times more potent than diazepam and it may have profound effects on hypoxic ventilatory response. Midazolam should be titrated carefully because respiratory arrest may occur with larger doses, especially in patients with chronic obstructive pulmonary disease and/or in patients who have received narcotics. Patients who have received midazolam should be carefully monitored for adequate ventilation and stable vital signs until they are fully alert (Kastrup 1988).

Diisopropylphenol and Other Agents

Propofol (diisopropylphenol; Diprivan) was developed by ICI Pharmaceutical Clinical Research Laboratory. Investigators were searching for an ideal intravenous agent that would produce rapid, smooth induction of anesthesia and would be rapidly metabolized. Propofol was developed for use as both an induction and a maintenance agent and allows speedy recovery as soon as it is stopped.

Propofol was first used clinically by Kay and Rolly in 1977 in Cremophor EL form. Because of allergic reactions, it was reformulated into an oil-based emulsion 5–6 years later.

Propofol is about 2–2.5 times more potent than thiopental and has been reported to produce a rapid, smooth induction of anesthesia with more rapid recovery than thiopental when used as maintenance anesthesia for short procedures (Sung et al. 1988a). Similar to thiopental, propofol causes unawareness and amnesia during anesthesia maintenance in combination with nitrous oxide (Sung et al. 1990a, 1990b). Also similar to thiopental, propofol does not cause venous sequelae (Sung et al. 1988b); however, both will cause apnea during induction.

There is a statistically significant heart rate increase during the first 3 minutes of induction of anesthesia with thiopental. In contrast, there is no significant change in heart rate when using propofol for induction. Also, there is a significant decrease in mean arterial pressure when propofol is used, but not when thiopental is used. Therefore, propofol may have an advantage over thiopental as an intravenous anesthetic for some patients undergoing ECT.

Recent reports comparing propofol and methohexital as induction agents for ECT show that propofol tends to produce shorter electroconvulsions, both grossly and electrically (Dwyer et al. 1988; Simpson et al. 1988). For this reason, some authorities do not recommend its use in ECT (R. Weiner, 1990, personal communication).

Alfentanil can be used as a supplement to propofol, to decrease dosage of the latter for ECT. Use of propofol and alfentanil in combination may lengthen ECT-induced seizures as compared with using propofol alone. Further clinical study of this drug combination seems clearly warranted.

Etomidate compared with methohexital in ECT has been shown to have increased involuntary muscle movement, increased muscular tone, and prolonged recovery time (O'Carroll et al. 1977). Cardiovascular effects of etomidate during ECT have not been reported (Selvin 1987).

There have been no reports of disordered thinking after ECT with ketamine induction (Selvin 1987); however, if ECT is not successful, one must question the wisdom of using a drug that can produce hallucinations in a psychiatric patient. Also, ketamine is a very potent dilator of the cerebral vasculature, which can cause a marked increase in intracranial pressure in patients with both normal and elevated intracranial pressure (Donegan 1983a). Combining this drug with a treatment known to increase intracranial pressure may be unwise.

Short-Acting Narcotic Induction Agents

Recently, we have introduced the short-acting narcotic alfentanil in 300- to 700-μg intravenous doses for ECT induction. It has allowed us to decrease the barbiturate induction dose by 50%. Our experience shows that this has permitted a significant reduction of the electrical stimulus with no adverse effect on seizure time or recovery of consciousness. The reduced electrical stimulus could confer increased cardiovascular stability (Anton et al. 1977). The only ill effect associated with this use was increased complaints of nausea, which was effectively resolved with small doses of droperidol (0.625 mg iv) given 5 minutes before ECT induction.

MUSCLE RELAXANTS USED IN ECT

Depolarizing Muscle Relaxants

Succinylcholine, a short-acting intravenous depolarizing muscle relaxant, is an inherent part of the "modified" ECT technique. Since its introduction in ECT, it has markedly decreased the incidence of associated fractures (Selvin 1987). It is used in doses of 0.5–1.5 mg/kg. At lower doses, tonic-clonic motor activity is discernible. At higher doses, most motor activity ceases and seizure duration can be monitored by EEG. Higher doses also may be necessary if endotracheal intubation is indicated, as in the patient with moderate to severe reflux or in the obese patient with a difficult mask airway and a tendency to rapid oxygen desaturation. A depressed patient well into her pregnancy, with associated decreased gastric motility, slow stomach emptying, and increased risk of gastric reflux, could fall in this category (Cheek and Gutsche 1987). The clinician should be aware, before deciding to intubate a patient, that intubation itself is extremely stimulating, with marked tachycardia and hypertension occurring due to increases in circulating norepinephrine (Derbyshire et al. 1983). Dysrhythmias are occasionally associated with severe hypertension (Fox et al. 1977), and adding further insult in the form of a catecholamine-releasing ECT stimulus may prove too much for a frail patient. These considerations must be weighed in the decision of whether to intubate.

The presence of certain medical conditions is considered a serious contraindication to the use of succinylcholine. These conditions include denervation injuries, such as paraplegia or amyotrophic lateral sclerosis, in which severe hyperkalemia and cardiac arrest may occur. Patients with a family or personal history of malignant hyperpyrexia should not be exposed to succinylcholine for fear of precipitating a malignant hyperpyrexia crisis with its associated significant mortality rate. Patients with a contraindication to succinylcholine can undergo ECT with one of the short-acting nondepolarizing muscle relaxants.

Succinylcholine may also be contraindicated in a patient with a family or personal history suggestive of abnormal pseudocholinesterase. This is an inherited disorder that may be tested by determination of the dibucaine number. Dibucaine inhibits normal plasma pseudocholinesterase by about 80%. Abnormal plasma cholinesterase may be inhibited only 20% by dibucaine (Miller and Savarese 1986). An abnormal dibucaine number may predict a prolonged response (hours) to succinylcholine. Such patients have been successfully handled during ECT with atracurium relaxation and edrophonium reversal (Hickey et al. 1987; Stack et al. 1988). An additional note of caution is necessary with regard to the use of succinylcholine. Medications that the patient may be taking concurrently with ECT may inhibit the action of pseudocholinesterase. These drugs include echothiophate, an eyedrop used in the treatment of glaucoma that can inhibit pseudocholinesterase activity 15–40%; phenelzine, an MAOI; and cytotoxic drugs such as cyclophosphamide (Miller 1981). Preferably in these patients, one of the nondepolarizing muscle-relaxants should be used instead of succinylcholine, as outlined below. If succinylcholine must be used, before the first ECT treatment and after barbiturate administration, it can be titrated in small doses while the patient is monitored with a peripheral nerve stimulator to determine sensitivity to the drug.

Succinylcholine administration has been associated with subsequent muscle pains, with an incidence of 0.2–89% (Brodsky et al. 1979), although only a 2% incidence has been reported in ambulatory patients given modified ECT (Kerr et al. 1982). Because some of our patients have complained of muscle pain, we routinely use 3 mg iv of d-tubocurarine 3 minutes before succinylcholine administration to attenuate the myalgic pain (Waters and Mapleson 1971). Also, elevations of intraocular pressure and intragastric pressure may be decreased or eliminated (Miller 1972)—a beneficial effect in a patient ventilated by Ambu bag and mask who will have his or her intraocular pressure increased by the ECT treatment itself. If a defasciculating dose of *d*-tubocurarine is chosen, the succinylcholine dose should be increased by 30–50% to offset the effect of *d*-tubocurarine on receptor sensitivity to succinylcholine (Miller 1972).

Nondepolarizing Muscle Relaxants

There are reports in the literature of the use of nondepolarizing muscle relaxants in ECT. There is one report of administration of ECT using thiopental and gallamine without apparent adverse effects (Brunton and Free 1983). In our facility, we have used atracurium in two patients for ECT when succinylcholine was contraindicated (one patient with a family history of pseudocholinesterase deficiency, another with neuroleptic malignant syndrome). The dosages used were 0.25–0.4 mg/kg, given with the induction dose of thiopental. (The lower dose was used in the patient with neuroleptic malignant syndrome due to extreme muscle wasting.) A nerve stimulator was used, and shock was withheld until muscle twitch was suppressed 90%. After ECT, the patients were immediately reversed with neostigmine (0.06 mg/kg) and glycopyrrolate (0.2 mg per 1.0 mg of neostigmine iv). No adverse effects, cardiovascular or otherwise, were noted in either patient. There are reports in the literature of similar doses of atracurium being used during ECT in patients with pseudocholinesterase deficiency (Hickey et al. 1987; Stack et al. 1988).

MANAGEMENT OF SPECIFIC MEDICAL PROBLEMS DURING ECT

Intracranial Mass Lesions

As discussed in the section on absolute contraindications, ECT in the presence of an intracranial mass lesion with associated symptoms, such as headache, neurological signs, and possible obstruction of flow of cerebrospinal fluid with increased intracranial pressure, has a high incidence of morbidity and mortality. If excision of a symptomatic brain tumor or relief of intracranial pressure by surgical means is not possible and ECT is the only hope for life-threatening depression, all persons involved must be fully aware of the high incidence of death and neurological deterioration in this situation. Stringent efforts to

decrease intracranial pressure to as close to normal as possible are
necessary before, during, and after ECT. Pharmacologic maneuvers to
decrease intracranial hypertension before each treatment may require
the intervention of a neurologist. Steroids such as dexamethasone (1.5
mg four times a day before and after ECT) may be indicated to reduce
perifocal edema around malignant brain tumors (Dressler and Folk
1975; Gutin 1977; Maltbie et al. 1980). Mannitol (0.25–0.50 mg/kg)
can be infused 30 minutes before the ECT treatment to decrease brain
volume by increasing plasma osmolality, which moves water from the
brain into the intravascular space. Mannitol's action begins within 10–
15 minutes and its effects last about 2 hours (Newfield 1987). Furosemide (0.15–1 mg/kg) can also decrease brain volume by effecting a
systemic diuresis and decreasing brain cerebrospinal fluid production
(Cottrell et al. 1977).

Hyperventilation before ECT induction can decrease brain volume
due to decreased cerebral blood flow from cerebrovascular vasoconstriction. The effects of hyperventilation are almost immediate. This
vasoconstriction in response to hypocapnia may counteract the 1.5- to
7-fold increase in cerebral blood flow that occurs during ECT (Gaines
and Rees 1986). However, the effectiveness of this measure may be
compromised by impaired responses to CO_2 by diseased vessels around
the brain tumor. Also, an arterial CO_2 less than 30 mmHg due to
excessive hyperventilation may impair brain oxygenation because of
severe restriction of cerebral blood flow (Newfield 1987). The patient
should be placed in a 15°–20° head-up tilt with the head in the midline
position to keep jugular venous drainage open. Coughing and straining,
which cause venous hypertension, should be avoided.

The small barbiturate doses used in induction of anesthesia during
ECT may help decrease intracranial pressure (Bruce 1983; Donegan
1983a). Glucose-free crystalloid solutions should be used, because there
is evidence that should brain ischemia occur, it may be exacerbated
in the presence of increased blood glucose (Pulsinelli et al. 1983).

Blood pressure should be controlled during ECT, because blood
vessels in and around the tumor may be fragile and prone to rupture.
Sublingual nifedipine has been shown to be effective in preventing
severe blood pressure increases during and after ECT (Kalayam and
Alexopoulos 1989). Nitroprusside infusion, esmolol, or labetalol may
be necessary to maintain rigorous blood pressure control. Use of these
medications is described in a later section of the chapter, "Recent
Myocardial Infarction and Unstable Angina." After ECT, these patients
should be observed for a fairly long time to ensure that their mental
status is quite stable. Any sudden deterioration in mental status may

indicate hemorrhage in the area of the tumor, which may require emergency surgical decompression.

Patients who have had surgical excision of their brain tumor can probably safely undergo ECT 3 months later. Consecutive CT scans have shown that the postoperative changes of brain surgery are stabilized in about 3 months (Jefferies et al. 1980). Before that time, post-surgical intracranial bleeding, due to the increased cerebral blood flow and pressure changes during ECT, can occur (Husum et al. 1983). ECT has been successfully administered to a patient 4 months after surgical excision of an intracranial meningioma (Hsiao and Evans 1984).

Cerebrovascular Infarction

Patients can safely undergo ECT 4–6 weeks after a cerebrovascular infarction (Alexopoulos et al. 1989; Anderson and Kissane 1977). If ECT must be performed within 1 month of the infarction, the methods outlined below for stabilizing blood pressure changes during ECT in patients with a recent MI should be followed to avoid further insult. Also, sublingual nifedipine may help prevent severe blood pressure increases after ECT (Kalayam and Alexopoulos 1989).

Intracranial Aneurysms and Cerebrovascular Malformations

The primary consideration for safely performing ECT in a patient with an unclipped cerebral arterial malformation is tight blood pressure control during ECT (Drop and Welch 1989). The main anesthetic goal during the ECT procedure should be avoiding increased stress on the aneurysmal wall. The principles of management are similar to those for patients with unstable aortic aneurysms, outlined below. An increase in the mean arterial pressure or a fall in the intracranial pressure (as with hyperventilation) will increase the transmural pressure, the wall stress, and the risk of aneurysm rupture (Peerless 1983). Consequently, maneuvers to decrease intracranial pressure in these patients (as opposed to patients with intracranial mass lesions) should not be pursued (Colley 1983). Intravenous propranolol and hydralazine, oral timolol, and nitroprusside infusions have all been used to moderate blood pressure increases in these patients (Drop et al. 1988; Husum et al. 1983).

Recent Myocardial Infarction and Unstable Angina

As discussed previously, ECT patients with a recent MI should be handled with extreme caution. A crash cart with a charged functional defibrillator should be ready. Lidocaine (200 mg) should be ready in a syringe at the patient's bedside. An arterial line should be strongly considered to aid in meticulous blood pressure control for the first one or two treatments until the patient's response to ECT is determined. ECT monitoring with a modified V5 lead for myocardial ischemia is essential. A pre-ECT ECG recording is advisable for comparison to ECG changes noted post-ECT.

A nitroglycerine infusion is strongly advised in this setting. Nitroglycerine is an organic nitrate that causes relaxation of smooth muscles in venous (primarily) and arterial walls, including coronary vessels, leading to favorable redistribution of coronary blood flow to ischemic areas. It can also be used to treat brief hypertensive episodes during ECT. Nitroglycerine has the advantage of a rapid onset of action and short half-life with easy titratability in infusion form. It is prepared by diluting 50 mg into 250 ml of 5% dextrose in water to yield 200 μg/ml. The infusion should be started at about 10 μg/minute and should be titrated to the patient's blood pressure response. It may be initiated before or after application of the electrical stimulus (Abrams and Roberts 1983). Rapid adjustments in the infusion rate may be necessary, and up to 400 μg/minute may be required to maintain blood pressure control (Drop and Welch 1989). The rate of the infusion is tapered as the seizure and hypertension subside. Nitroglycerine may produce a reflex tachycardia in response to a decrease in blood pressure (Waller et al. 1979). Nitroglycerine 2% ointment applied 45 minutes before treatment has been reported to be effective in moderating ECT-related hypertension (Lee et al. 1985).

Nitroprusside, a nonselective vasodilator, can dramatically control blood pressure during ECT. A nitroprusside infusion is made by mixing 50 mg into 250 ml or 500 ml of 5% dextrose in water. The resulting concentrations are 200 μg/ml or 100 μg/ml, respectively. Infusion has a rapid effect on blood pressure and should be titrated cautiously, starting with an initial dose of 0.5 μg/kg per minute (Drop and Welch 1989). Nitroprusside may produce considerable reflex tachycardia, which, as discussed previously, may have significant detrimental effects on myocardial oxygen supply and demand. It also should be used with caution in patients with potential myocardial ischemia because it has been reported to produce "intracoronary steal" or shunting of blood away from ischemic myocardium by dilation of coronary vessels to non-ischemic myocardium (Waller et al. 1979). Also, sodium nitroprusside has been associated with persistent hypotension after ECT (Ciraulo et al. 1978).

Due to cardiovascular changes that occur during ECT, beta-blocking agents, such as propranolol (0.5–4.0 mg iv), have been used to decrease hypertension and incidence of ventricular arrhythmias (Husum et al. 1983; Selvin 1987). However, cardiac arrest has been reported after propranolol (0.5–1.0 mg) given before ECT (Decina et al. 1984). The duration of action of propranolol may last too long for the brief hemodynamic disturbance caused by ECT. Recently, two new short-acting beta-blocking agents, esmolol and labetalol, have been shown to be effective in controlling the cardiovascular responses during ECT (Hay 1989; Knos et al. 1990). Esmolol, in a bolus of 1 mg/kg followed by an infusion of 500 μg/kg per minute or 24 mg/minute, has been shown to provide greater hemodynamic stability during ECT (Black et al. 1989; Klein et al. 1988; Kovac et al. 1988). Labetalol (5 mg) given intravenously before ECT induction has also been effective in controlling heart rate and blood pressure during ECT (Knos et al. 1990; Stoudemire et al., in press).

Lidocaine pretreatment is effective in attenuating or preventing ventricular arrhythmias; however, it causes a dose-related suppression of seizure activity (Selvin 1987). After seizure induction, lidocaine (2 mg/kg) or procainamide may be necessary for treatment of ventricular arrhythmias (Hood and Mecca 1983).

It should be remembered that preoxygenation and ventilation are paramount in preventing ventricular arrhythmias. In nonoxygenated cardiac patients, ventricular arrhythmias may be as high as 75% (McKenna et al. 1970). Finally, there is a report of ECT-induced changes in the ECG mimicking MI, without any changes in cardiac isoenzymes or thallium-201 scan that would indicate that an actual MI had occurred (Gould et al. 1983).

Chronic Congestive Heart Failure

Patients with a history of congestive heart failure should be evaluated by a cardiologist before undergoing ECT. Optimal control of heart failure should be achieved by proper adjustments of the patient's medications, such as digitalis, diuretics, calcium channel blockers, and vasodilators. ECT may cause decompensation and pulmonary edema in the patient with compromised cardiac function due to the increase in myocardial work. Control of the hypertensive response via the pharmacologic mechanisms listed in the preceding sections will help reduce this risk (Drop and Welch 1989). Beta-blocking agents should be used cautiously in these patients as they may precipitate cardiac failure due to their negative inotropic effects (Stoelting 1987a). Intravenous fluids should be given sparingly, and myocardial depressant drugs such as methohexital should be titrated to the minimal doses that provide anesthesia (Drop and Welch 1989).

Pacemakers

Pacemakers present special problems for the clinician who performs ECT; however, ECT has been successfully performed in such patients (Abiuso et al. 1978; Gibson et al. 1973; Pitts 1982). Animal studies have shown that an electrical stimulus to the head does not influence pacemaker function, probably due to the high electrical resistance of body tissues (Youmans et al. 1969). However, if the pacemaker's lead insulation is broken, or when a low-resistance pathway is created to the heart by improperly grounded electrical devices, an ECT stimulus could cause pacemaker dysfunction (Drop and Welch 1989).

Before performing ECT in a patient with a pacemaker, the type of pacemaker should be determined. The patient, a family member, or the patient's cardiologist should have the information. If these sources are not helpful, the hospital where the pacemaker was placed will have the information in the patient's medical record. The ventricular-inhibited pacemaker is the most common type in use today. Certain considerations apply in the treatment of patients with this pacemaker type. The ECT device and the ECG monitor should be properly grounded. Intact insulation of the pacemaker leads should be confirmed with a chest X ray. Adequate doses of succinylcholine should be used to prevent seizure-induced muscle potentials of sufficient magnitude to inhibit the pacemaker. Three minutes before using succinylcholine, an intravenous dose of d-tubocurarine should be administered (3 mg/70 kg body weight) to minimize succinylcholine-induced muscle defasciculations, which may in themselves shut off the pacemaker. Patients with pacemakers should not be excessively hyperventilated because potassium influx into the myocardial cells will decrease the resting membrane potential beyond normal and produce noncapture of the pacemaker's impulse, and a higher current will be required to depolarize the myocardium. The nonreprogrammable ventricular-inhibited pacemaker may be converted to an asynchronous mode by placing the magnet over the pulse generator. Asynchronous activity eliminates possible interference of pacemaker function by ECT stimulus, and the asynchronous mode may avoid ECT-induced severe bradycardia (Drop and Welch 1989; Selvin 1987).

A greater number of patients now receive programmable pacemakers. A magnet should not be used in this type of pacemaker as the combination of the magnet and ECT stimulus could reprogram the pacemaker into an unknown rhythm, or no rhythm. A cardiologist should be consulted to advise management of patients with this type of pacemaker. Consider preparing an external transthoracic pacer in case it is needed during treatment in these patients.

Unstable Aortic Aneurysm

Successful ECT in a patient with an unstable aortic aneurysm depends on careful control of blood pressure and heart rate (Pomerantz et al. 1968). The means to achieve this cardiovascular stability are similar to those outlined for the patient with unstable cardiac disease, with special emphasis on control of blood pressure. In a patient with possible imminent aneurysmal rupture, ECT should not be performed without a large-bore IV (16 gauge or larger). Because a patient tends to respond similarly to each ECT, the first couple of treatments should be performed in the vicinity of a prepared operating room with several units of blood readily available. Serious consideration should be given to an arterial line and nitroprusside infusion for tight blood pressure control. After the patient's response pattern and treatment mode have been determined, these excessive precautions with exception of the large-bore IV may no longer be necessary.

Pheochromocytoma

If ECT must be performed in the presence of a known pheochromocytoma (pheo), an endocrinologist must be consulted to stabilize the patient's condition as much as possible before starting ECT. Patients with untreated pheos are at risk for cerebrovascular hemorrhage, heart failure, dysrhythmias, or MI due to severe hypertensive crises.

Alpha-methyltyrosine, an agent that inhibits the tyrosine hydroxylase enzyme that is the rate-limiting step in catecholamine synthesis, may be instituted to reduce catecholamine synthesis. These patients are also started on a regimen of phenoxybenzamine, a long-acting alpha-blocking agent, in 10-mg doses tid, which is increased incrementally until the blood pressure is controlled. After alpha-blockade is established, beta-blocking agents are added. Dehydration and plasma volume reduction occur in these patients due to their severe hypertension and renal compensation. They must be hydrated very carefully because life-threatening hypotension can occur in response to anesthetic-induction agents (Graf and Rosenbaum 1989). For the first treatments, an arterial line monitor should be established with a nitroprusside infusion for tight blood pressure control. Phentolamine, a short-acting alpha-antagonist, may also be used in 2- to 5-mg boluses to aid in blood pressure control. Esmolol infusions (discussed earlier) can be used for control of heart rate (Graf and Rosenbaum 1989).

Pulmonary Disease

Patients with severe pulmonary disease should have their respiratory function maximized before ECT. This may require evaluation and regulation of medications by a consulting pulmonologist. Several studies have shown that preoperative treatment of patients with pulmonary disease decreases perioperative respiratory complications (Brown 1986). Currently, spirometry and arterial blood gas analysis seem to be the most reliable and cost-effective means of evaluating pulmonary risk (Boysen 1988).

Reversible airway obstruction and wheezing may require treatment with corticosteroids such as hydrocortisone in a 1- to 3-mg/kg dose. Selective beta$_2$-agonist agents such as albuterol and terbutaline will treat bronchospasm with fewer undesirable side effects such as the tachyarrhythmias seen with agents with more beta$_1$ effects (such as isoproterenol). Albuterol can be given orally, but the treatment of choice is two or three puffs of aerosolized albuterol before start of the ECT treatment to minimize airway reactivity. Patients with severe bronchospasm may require treatment with infusions of aminophylline, a water-soluble salt of theophylline. Before starting ECT, aminophylline therapy should be adjusted to obtain serum blood levels in the therapeutic range of 10–20 μg/ml. A loading dose of 5.6 mg/kg is recommended, followed by an infusion of 0.5–0.9 mg/kg per hour to maintain therapeutic levels. Anticholinergic agents such as atropine and glycopyrrolate may be useful in some patients, particularly those with chronic obstructive pulmonary disease (COPD) with a reactive component. Administration of these drugs via aerosol may avoid some of the undesirable cardiovascular and central nervous system effects. However, these drugs are less effective than the beta$_2$-adrenergic agonists, and they actually play a minor role in the treatment of pulmonary disease (Hirshman 1988).

H2 receptor antagonists, such as cimetidine and ranitidine, may precipitate bronchospasm due to their inhibition of H2 receptor–mediated bronchodilation (Stoelting 1987b). The benefits of using these drugs to increase gastric pH to avoid aspiration pneumonia should be weighed against the severity of the patient's reactive airway disease (Hirshman 1988). Ranitidine may have a milder effect on airway reactivity than cimetidine (Kastrup 1988).

Short-acting narcotic agents should be used sparingly in patients with severe pulmonary disease, due to their depressant effect on respiration. As stated previously, midazolam should be used cautiously in these patients due to its adverse effect on respiratory drive. Thiopental has been shown to have no increased incidence of bronchospasm in nonintubated patients compared with patients receiving regional anesthesia (Schnider and Papper 1961), and its use during ECT induction probably is quite safe in these patients in the absence of intubation. If beta-antagonist drugs are needed to control heart rate in a patient with mild bronchospastic disease during ECT, beta$_1$-selective drugs, such as metoprolol, atenolol, or esmolol, should be used to avoid bronchospasm induced by beta-blockade. In patients with severe bronchospastic disease, any beta-blocking agents are probably contraindicated, and their use should be weighed against the severity of the patient's cardiac disease (Merin 1986).

COMPLICATIONS OF ECT

Morbidity

The complication rate in ECT has been cited to be 1 in 1,700 treatments (Frederiksen and D'Elia 1978). Before the introduction of modified ECT with short-acting muscle relaxants, the most common complication was fracture of thoracic vertebrae and/or long bones (Scalafani 1988). Today, the most common complaint by patients undergoing ECT relates to memory disturbances after treatment (Hood and Mecca 1983). This appears to be worsened by bipolar electrode placement (Squire and Slater 1978). Skin burns, lacerations of the tongue and oral mucosa, and tooth and eye damage have all been described in situations where vigilance by attending personnel has been lax (Scalafani 1988; Selvin 1987). Headaches, muscle aches, and anxiety following treatment are common complaints. In our institution, where small doses (300–700 μg) of alfentanil are used with decreased barbiturate doses for anesthesia induction, nausea has been a problem, without small preinduction doses (0.625 mg) of intravenous droperidol. All things considered, these complications are rather minor considering the improvement (often dramatic) that can be seen in a patient's depressive symptoms after a course of ECT.

Mortality

The mortality from ECT is considered rare (Scalafani 1988; Selvin 1987). Four large studies in the last 15 years reported no deaths directly attributable to ECT (Rich and Smith 1981). Current mortality is quoted as 0.03%, or 3 per 10,000 treated patients, or 0.0045% of individual treatments (Fink 1979). Four deaths in 2,594 patients were reported in a 1984 study from the United Kingdom (Marks 1984). A study of ECT in the United States cites an incidence of 0.2 deaths per 10,000 treatments (Kramer 1985). Certainly, these statistics compare favorably to the most recent statistics citing anesthesia mortality in hospitalized surgical patients as 0.9 deaths per 10,000 cases (Keenan and Boyan 1985). However, before we congratulate ourselves, it should be remembered that these statistics include those patients undergoing major surgery and high-risk procedures. To compare patients undergoing ECT, a relatively "minor" procedure, with a group containing patients undergoing abdominal aortic aneurysm repair, or coronary artery bypass surgery, is not quite fair. Rather, we should demand that ECT mortality approach that of ambulatory patients undergoing minor procedures, which was recently quoted as 0.0016 deaths per 10,000 cases (Green and Taylor 1984).

The most frequent cause of death during ECT is due to the cardiovascular system, in the form of arrhythmias, MI, congestive heart failure, and cardiac arrest. These complications often occur during the recovery period of ECT (Alexopoulos et al. 1984; Gerring and Shields 1982; Weiner 1979). Cardiac arrhythmias and myocardial ischemia are not uncommon complications during ECT, with an incidence varying between 8 and 80%, with the higher incidence seen in cardiac patients (Alexopoulos et al. 1984; Gerring and Shields 1982; Kitamura and Page 1984; Pitts 1982). During the active convulsing phase of ECT, sinus and ventricular tachycardias and PVCs (often multifocal, bigeminy, or trigeminy) are common arrhythmias (Selvin 1987). This may be related to the arrhythmogenic effects of the elevated circulating catecholamines. The incidence and severity of complications appear to be increased in patients who are hypoxic or hypercapnic, or who have respiratory acidosis. Elderly hypertensive patients who have cardiovascular disease and/or are taking digitalis or undergoing antiarrhythmic or diuretic therapy have a higher incidence of complications (Gerring and Shields 1982; Kraus and Remick 1982; Weiner 1979). Patients tend to exhibit the same arrhythmia after each treatment (Selvin 1987).

The best course of action to follow in treating medically frail patients with ECT is to monitor heart rhythm, blood pressure, and oxygenation throughout the treatment until the patient is well awake and stable. (Return to awake status usually requires 30–45 minutes of observation after ECT treatment is finished.) A crash cart with full resuscitative supplies and defibrillator should be readily available. Lidocaine (2 mg/cc) should be ready in a syringe and at the patient's bedside, and a person trained in advanced cardiac life support (ACLS) should be available within seconds of the ECT area.

CONCLUSION

ECT is reemerging as a viable treatment modality for refractive depression. As the population ages, with increased incidence of serious disease and depression, the clinician performing ECT will be required to treat these severely depressed patients regardless of their increased risk. Meticulous preparation and care of the patient before, during, and after ECT will reduce these risks significantly.

REFERENCES

Abiuso P, Dunkelman R, Proper M: Electroconvulsive therapy in patients with pacemakers. JAMA 240:2459–2460, 1978

Abrams JJ, Roberts J: First American conference on nitroglycerine therapy. Am J Med 74:1–66, 1983

Adams RD, Martin JB: Faintness, syncope, and seizures, in Harrison's Principles of Internal Medicine. Edited by Braunwald E, Isselbacher KJ, Petersdorf RG, et al. New York, McGraw-Hill, 1987, pp 64–70

Adams RD, Victor M: Principles of Neurology. New York, McGraw-Hill, 1977

Alexopoulos GS, Shamoian CJ, Lucas J, et al: Medical problems of geriatric patients and younger controls during electroconvulsive therapy. J Am Geriatr Soc 32:651–654, 1984

Alexopoulos GS, Young RC, Abrams RC: ECT in the high-risk geriatric patient. Convulsive Therapy 5:75–87, 1989

Allen RE, Pitts SN, Summers WK: Drug modification of ECT: methohexital and diazepam: II. Biol Psychiatry 15:257–264, 1980

Anderson WD, Kissane JM: Pathology. St. Louis, MO, CV Mosby, 1977

Anton AH, Uy DS, Redderson CL: Autonomic blockade and the cardiovascular and catecholamine response to electroshock. Anesth Analg 56:46–54, 1977

APA issues practice guidelines for ECT, calls it 'safe.' AMA News, Jan 12, 1990, p 6

Azar I, Lear E: Cardiovascular effects of electroconvulsive therapy in patients taking tricyclic antidepressants. Anesth Analg 63:1139, 1984

Black HA, Howie MB, Martin DJ, et al: Attenuation of electroconvulsive (ECT) autonomic hyperactivity by esmolol. Anesth Analg 68:S1–S321, 1989

Bodley PO, Halwax K, Potts L: Low serum pseudocholinesterase levels complicating treatment with phenalzine. Br Med J 3:510–512, 1969

Boysen PG: Pulmonary function testing, in Current Practice in Anesthesiology. Edited by Rogers MC. Toronto, BC Decker, 1988, pp 9–11

Braunwald E: Heart failure, in Harrison's Principles of Internal Medicine. Edited by Braunwald E, Isselbacher KJ, Petersdorf RG, et al. New York, McGraw-Hill, 1987, pp 905–916

Brodsky JB, Brock-Unte JG, Samuels SI: Pancuronium pretreatment and post-succinylcholine myalgias. Anesthesiology 51:259, 1979

Brown M: Assessment and treatment of the patient with hypoxemia (lecture 132), in 1986 Annual Refresher Course Lectures, American Society for Anesthesiologists. American Society for Anesthesiologists, 1986, pp 1–6

Bruce DA: Head trauma: management, in Handbook of Neuroanesthesia: Clinical and Physiologic Essentials. Edited by Newfield P, Cottrell JE. Boston, MA, Little, Brown, 1983, pp 283–301

Brunton CR, Free CW: ECT without suxamethonium. Anaesth Intensive Care 11:177–178, 1983

Bynum LJ, Pierce AK: Pulmonary aspiration of gastric contents. Am Rev Respir Dis 114:1129–1136, 1976

Carr ME, Woods JW: ECT in a patient with unsuspected phaeochromocytoma. South Med J 78:613–615, 1985

Cassem EH: Approach to the patient with mental and emotional complaints, in Harrison's Principles of Internal Medicine. Edited by Braunwald E, Isselbacher KJ, Petersdorf RG, et al. New York, McGraw-Hill, 1987, pp 60–64

Cheek TG, Gutsche BB: Maternal physiologic alterations during pregnancy, in

Anesthesia for Obstetrics, 2nd Edition. Edited by Shnider SM, Levinson G. Baltimore, MD, Williams & Wilkins, 1987, pp 3–13

Ciraulo D, Lind L, Salzman C, et al: Sodium nitroprusside treatment of ECT-induced blood pressure elevations. Am J Psychiatry 135:1105–1106, 1978

Cockshott ID: Propofol (DIPRIVAN') pharmacokinetics and metabolism—an overview. Postgrad Med J 61 (suppl 3):45–50, 1985

Colley PS: Anesthesia in intracranial aneurysms, in Handbook of Neuroanesthesia: Clinical and Physiological Essentials. Edited by Newfield P, Cottrell JE. Boston, MA, Little, Brown, 1983, pp 183–206

Cottrell JE, Robustelli A, Post K, et al: Furosemide- and mannitol-induced changes in intracranial pressure and serum osmolarity and electrolytes. Anesthesiology 47:28–30, 1977

Curling PE, Duke PG, Levy JH, et al: Management of the postoperative cardiac patient, in Clinical Essays of the Heart, Vol 3. Edited by Hurst JW. New York, McGraw-Hill, 1984, pp 257–286

Darling RC, Brewster DC: Elective treatment of abdominal aortic aneurysms. World J Surg 4:661–667, 1980

Dec DW, Stern TA, Welch C: The effect of electroconvulsive therapy on serial electrocardiograms and serum cardiac enzyme values. JAMA 253:2525–2529, 1985

Decina P, Malitz S, Sackeim A, et al: Cardiac arrest during ECT modified by beta-adrenergic blockade. Am J Psychiatry 141:298–300, 1984

Derbyshire DR, Chmielewski A, Fell D, et al: Plasma catecholamine responses to tracheal intubation. Br J Anaesth 55:855–860, 1983

Donegan J: Effect of anesthesia on cerebral physiology and metabolism, in Handbook of Neuroanesthesia: Clinical and Physiologic Essentials. Edited by Newfield P, Cottrell J. Boston, MA, Little, Brown, 1983a, pp 16–27

Donegan J: Physiology and metabolism of the brain and spinal cord, in Handbook of Neuroanesthesia: Clinical and Physiologic Essentials. Edited by Newfield P, Cottrell J. Boston, MA, Little, Brown, 1983b, pp 3–15

Drake FR, Ebaugh FG: Pheochromocytoma and electroconvulsive therapy. Am J Psychol 113:295–301, 1956

Dressler DM, Folk J: The treatment of depression with ECT in the presence of brain tumor. Am J Psychiatry 132:1320–1321, 1975

Drop LJ, Welch CA: Anesthesia for electroconvulsive therapy in patients with major cardiovascular risk factors. Convulsive Therapy 5:88–101, 1989

Drop LJ, Bouckoms AJ, Welch CA: Arterial hypertension and multiple cerebral aneurysms in a patient treated with electroconvulsive therapy. J Clin Psychiatry 49:280–282, 1988

Dwyer R, McCaughey W, Lavery J, et al: Comparison of propofol and methohexitone as anaesthetic agents for electroconvulsive therapy. Anaesthesia 43:459–462, 1988

El-Ganzouri AR, Ivankovich AD, Braverman B, et al: Monoamine oxidase inhibitors: should they be discontinued preoperatively? Anesth Analg 64:592–596, 1985

Epstein HM, Fagman W, Bruce DL, et al: Intraocular pressure changes during anesthesia for electroshock therapy. Anesth Analg 54:479–481, 1975

Estes JE Jr: Abdominal aortic aneurysm; a study of 102 cases. Circulation 2:258–264, 1950

Fakhri O, Fadhli A, Rawi R: Effect of electroconvulsive therapy on diabetes mellitus. Lancet 2:775–777, 1980

Finestone DH, Weiner RD: Effects of ECT on diabetes mellitus. Acta Psychiatr Scand 70:321–326, 1984

Fink M: Convulsive Therapy: Theory and Practice. New York, Raven, 1979

Foster DW: Diabetes mellitus, in Harrison's Principles of Internal Medicine. Edited by Braunwald E, Isselbacher KJ, Petersdorf RG, et al. New York, McGraw-Hill, 1987, pp 1778–1797

Foster DW, Rubenstein AH: Hypoglycemia, insulinoma, and other hormone-secreting tumors of the pancreas, in Harrison's Principles of Internal Medicine. Edited by Braunwald E, Isselbacher KJ, Petersdorf RG, et al. New York, McGraw-Hill, 1987, pp 1800–1807

Foster MW Jr, Gayle RF Jr: Dangers in combining reserpine with electroconvulsive therapy. JAMA 154:257–260, 1955

Fox EJ, Sklar GS, Hill CH, et al: Complications related to the pressor response to endotracheal intubation. Anesthesiology 47:524–525, 1977

Fragen RJ, Avram MJ: Nonopioid intravenous anesthetics, in Clinical Anesthesia. Edited by Barash P, Cullen BF, Stoelting RK. Philadelphia, PA, JB Lippincott, 1989, pp 227–253

Frederiksen S, D'Elia G: Electroconvulsive therapy in Sweden. Br J Psychiatry 134:283–287, 1978

Freese KJ: Can patients safely undergo ECT while receiving monoamine oxidase inhibitors? Convulsive Therapy 1:190–194, 1985

Fried D, Mann JJ: Electroconvulsive therapy of a patient with known intracranial tumor. Biol Psychiatry 23:176–180, 1988

Gaines GY, Rees DI: Electroconvulsive therapy and anesthetic considerations. Anesth Analg 65:1345–1356, 1986

Gal TJ: Pulmonary function testing, in Anesthesia, 2nd Edition, Vol 3. Edited by Miller RD. New York, Churchill Livingstone, 1986, pp 2053–2075

Gassell MM: Deterioration after electroconvulsive therapy in patients with intracranial meningioma. Arch Gen Psychiatry 3:504–506, 1960

Gerring JP, Shields HM: The identification and management of patients with a high risk for cardiac arrhythmias during modified ECT. J Clin Psychiatry 43:140–143, 1982

Gevirtz C: Anesthesia and monoamine oxidase inhibitors (letter). JAMA 261:3407, 1989

Gibson TC, Leaman DM, Devors J, et al: Pacemaker function in relation to electroconvulsive therapy. Chest 63:1025–1027, 1973

Giesecke Jr AH, Egbert LD: Perioperative fluid therapy—crystalloids, in Anesthesia, 2nd Edition, Vol 2. Edited by Miller RD. New York, Churchill Livingstone, 1986, pp 1313–1328

Goldman L, Caldera DL: Risks of general anesthesia and elective operation in the hypertensive patient. Anesthesiology 50:285–292, 1979

Goldman L, Caldera DL, Nussbaum SR, et al: Multifactorial index of cardiac risk in non-cardiac surgical procedures. N Engl J Med 297:845–850, 1977

Gould L, Gopalaswamy C, Chandy F, et al: Electroconvulsive therapy-induced ECG changes simulating a myocardial infarction. Arch Intern Med 143:1786–1787, 1983

Graf G, Rosenbaum S: Anesthesia and the endocrine system, in Clinical Anesthesia. Edited by Barash P, Cullen BF, Stoelting RK. Philadelphia, PA, JB Lippincott, 1989, pp 1185–1214

Gravenstein JS, Anton AH, Wiener SM, et al: Catecholamine and cardiovascular response to electro-convulsive therapy in man. Br J Anaesth 37:833–839, 1965

Green RA, Taylor TH: An analysis of anesthesia medical liability claims in the United Kingdom 1977–1982. Int Anesthesiol Clin 22:73–90, 1984

Greenan J, DeWar M, Jones CJ: Intravenous glycopyrrolate and atropine at induction of anesthesia: a comparison. J R Soc Med 76:369–371, 1983

Greenberg LB, Anand A, Roque CT, et al: Electroconvulsive Therapy and cerebral venous angioma. Convulsive Therapy 2:197–202, 1986

Greenberg LB, Mofson R, Fink M: Prospective electroconvulsive therapy in a delusional depressed patient with a frontal meningioma. Br J Psychiatry 153:105–107, 1988

Gutin PH: Corticosteroid therapy in patients with brain tumors. National Cancer Institute Monograph 46:151–156, 1977

Hay DP: Electroconvulsive Therapy in the medically ill elderly. Convulsive Therapy 5:8–16, 1989

Hiatt JCG, Barker WF, Machleder HL, et al: Determinants of failure in the treatment of ruptured abdominal aortic aneurysm. Arch Surg 119:1264–1268, 1984

Hickey DR, O'Connor JP, Donati F: Comparison of atracurium and succinylcholine for electroconvulsive therapy in a patient with atypical plasma cholinesterase. Can J Anaesth 34:280–283, 1987

Hirshman CA: Perioperative management of the patient with asthma (lecture 264), in 1988 Annual Refresher Course Lectures, American Society of Anesthesiologists, 1988, pp 1–7

Hood DD, Mecca RS: Failure to initiate electroconvulsive seizures in a patient pretreated with lidocaine. Anesthesiology 58:379–381, 1983

Hsiao JK, Evans DL: ECT in a depressed patient after craniotomy. Am J Psychiatry 141:442–444, 1984

Hsiao JK, Messenheimer JA, Evans DL: ECT and neurological disorders. Convulsive Therapy 3:121–136, 1987

Hurwitz TD: Electroconvulsive therapy: a review. Compr Psychiatry 15:303–314, 1974

Husum B, Vester-Andersen T, Buchmann G, et al: Electroconvulsive therapy and intracranial aneurysm. Anaesthesia 38:1205–1207, 1983

Janowsky EC, Risch SC, Janowsky DS: Psychotropic agents, in Drug Interactions in Anesthesia. Edited by Smith NT, Miller RD, Corbascio AN. Philadelphia, PA, Lea and Febiger, 1981, pp 177–195

Jefferies BF, Kishore PRS, Singh KS, et al: Postoperative computed tomographic changes in the brain. Radiology 135:751–753, 1980

Kalayam B, Alexopoulos GS: Nifedipine in the treatment of blood pressure rise after ECT. Convulsive Therapy 5:110–113, 1989

Kalinowsky LB, Hippius H, Klein HE (eds): Biological Treatments in Psychiatry. New York, Grune & Stratton, 1982, pp 255–260

Kallos T, Smith TC: Anesthesia and orthopedic surgery, in Clinical Anesthesia. Edited by Barash P, Cullen BF, Stoelting RK. Philadelphia, PA, JB Lippincott, 1989, pp 1163–1184

Kaplan J: Anesthesia for patients with coronary artery disease (monograph, Audio Rounds for Anesthesiologists). Ossining, NY, Cortlandt Group, 1982, pp 1–6

Karliner W: ECT for patients with CNS disease. Psychosomatics 19:781–783, 1978

Kastrup EK (ed): Drug Facts and Comparisons. St. Louis, JB Lippincott, 1988

Kay B, Rolly G: A new intravenous induction agent. Acta Anaesthesiol Belg 28:303–316, 1977

Kendell RE: The present status of electroconvulsive therapy. Br J Psychiatry 139:265–283, 1981

Kennan RL, Boyan CP: Cardiac arrest due to anesthesia: a study of incidence and causes. JAMA 253:2373–2377, 1985

Kerr RA, McGraith JJ, O'Kearney RT, et al: ECT: misconceptions and attitudes. Aust N Z J Psychiatry 16:43–49, 1982

Kitamura T, Page AJF: Electrocardiographic changes following electroconvulsive therapy. Eur Arch Psychiatry Neurol Sci 234:147–148, 1984

Klein M, Martin D, Soloff P, et al: Comparison of the effect of nitroglycerin and esmolol on the cardiovascular response to ECT. Anesthesiology 69:A41, 1988

Knos GB, Sung YF, Stoudemire A, et al: Use of labetalol to control cardiovascular responses to electroconvulsive therapy. Anesth Analg 70:S210, 1990

Knudsen L, Christiansen LA, Lorentzen JE: Hypotension during and after operation in glucocorticoid-treated patients. Br J Anaesth 53:295–301, 1981

Kovac AL, Unruh GK, Goto H, et al: Evaluation of esmolol infusion in controlling increases of heart rate and blood pressure during electroconvulsive therapy. Anesthesiology 69:A895, 1988

Kramer BA: Use of ECT in California, 1977–1983. Am J Psychiatry 142:1190–1192, 1985

Kraus R, Remick R: Diazoxide in the management of severe hypertension after electroconvulsive therapy. Am J Psychiatry 139:504–505, 1982

Landsberg L, Young JB: Pheochromocytoma, in Harrison's Principles of Internal Medicine. Edited by Braunwald E, Isselbacher KJ, Petersdorf RG, et al. New York, McGraw-Hill, 1987, pp 1775–1778

Lebowitz P, Newberg L, Gillette M: Clinical Anesthesia Procedures of the Massachusetts General Hospital. Edited by Lebowitz P, Newberg L, Gillette M. Boston, MA, Little, Brown, 1982

Lee JT, Erbguth PH, Stevens WC, et al: Modification of electroconvulsive therapy induced hypertension with nitroglycerin ointment. Anesthesiology 62:793–796, 1985

Lunn RJ, Savageau MM, Beatty WW, et al: Anesthetics and electroconvulsive therapy seizure duration: implications for therapy from a rat model. Biol Psychiatry 16:1163–1175, 1981

Maletzky BM: Seizure duration and clinical effect in electroconvulsive therapy. Compr Psychiatry 19:541–550, 1978

Maltbie AA, Wingfield MS, Volow MR, et al: Electroconvulsive therapy in the presence of brain tumor: case reports and evaluation of risks. J Nerv Ment Dis 168:400–405, 1980

Marks RJ: Electroconvulsive therapy; physiological and anaesthetic considerations. Can Anaesthetists Soc J 31:541–548, 1984

McCleave DJ, Blakemore WB: Anaesthesia for electroconvulsive therapy. Anaesth Intensive Care 3:250–256, 1975

McKenna G, Engle RP, Brooks H, et al: Cardiac arrhythmias during electroshock therapy: significance, prevention and treatment. Am J Psychiatry 127:530–533, 1970

McPherson RW, Lipsey JR: Electroconvulsive therapy, in Current Practice in Anesthesiology. Edited by Rogers MC. Toronto, BC Decker, 1988, pp 212–217

Merin RG: Pharmacology of the autonomic nervous system, in Anesthesia, 2nd Edition, Vol 2. Edited by Miller RD. New York, Churchill Livingstone, 1986, pp 945–982

Miller RD: The advantages of giving *d*-tubocurarine before succinylcholine. Anesthesiology 37:568–569, 1972

Miller RD: Neuromuscular blocking agents, in Drug Interactions in Anesthesia. Edited by Smith NT, Miller RD, Corbascio AN. Philadelphia, PA, Lea and Febiger, 1981, pp 249–269

Miller RD, Savarese JJ: Pharmacology of muscle relaxants and their antagonists, in Anesthesia, 2nd Edition, Vol 2. Edited by Miller RD. New York, Churchill Livingston, 1986, pp 889–943

Murray GB, Shea V, Conn DK: Electroconvulsive therapy for post stroke depression. J Clin Psychiatry 47:258–260, 1986

Nathan RS, Dowling R, Peters JL, et al: ECT and glaucoma. Convulsive Therapy 2:132–133, 1986

Natof HE: Complications, in Anesthesia for Ambulatory Surgery. Edited by Wetchler BV. Philadelphia, PA, JB Lippincott, 1985, pp 321–356

Newfield P: Anesthetic considerations in patients with increased intracranial pressure (lecture 176), in 1987 Annual Refresher Course Lectures, American Society of Anesthesiologists, 1987, pp 1–7

O'Carroll TM, Blogg CE, Hoinville ES, et al: Etomidate in electroconvulsive therapy. Anaesthesia 32:868–872, 1977

Pasternak RC, Braunwald E, Alpert JS: Acute myocardial infarction, in Harrison's Principles of Internal Medicine. Edited by Braunwald E, Isselbacher KJ, Petersdorf RG. New York, McGraw-Hill, 1987, pp 190–993

Peerless SJ: Intracranial aneurysms: neurosurgery, in Handbook of Neuroanesthesia: Clinical and Physiologic Essentials. Edited by Newfield P, Cottrell JE. Boston, MA, Little, Brown, 1983, pp 173–183

Pitts FN: Medical physiology of ECT, in Electroconvulsive Therapy: Biological Foundations and Clinical Applications. Edited by Abrams R, Essman WB. New York, Spectrum Publications, 1982, pp 57–89

Pitts FN, Desmarais GN, Stewart W, et al: Induction of anesthesia with methohexital and thiopental in electroconvulsive therapy. N Engl J Med 273:353–360, 1965

Pomeranze J, Karliner W, Triebel WA, et al: Electroshock in the presence of serious organic disease: depression and aortic aneurysm. Geriatrics 23:122–124, 1968

Pulsinelli WA, Levy DE, Sigsbee B, et al: Increased damage after ischemic stroke in patients with hyperglycemia with or without established diabetes mellitus. Am J Med 74:540–544, 1983

Rao G, Ford WB, Zikria EA, et al: Prevention of arrhythmias after direct myocardial revascularization surgery. Vascular Surgery 8:82–89, 1974

Rao TLK, Jacobs KH, El-Etr AA: Reinfarction following anesthesia in patients with myocardial infarction. Anesthesiology 59:499–505, 1983

Regestein QR, Reich PR: Electroconvulsive therapy in patients at high risk for physical complications. Convulsive Therapy 1:101–114, 1985

Remick RA, Jewesson P, Ford RWJ: Monoamine oxidase inhibitors in general anesthesia: a reevaluation. Convulsive Therapy 3:196–203, 1987

Reves JG: Comparative pharmacology of intravenous anesthetic induction drugs. Review Course Lecture, 60th Congress, International Anesthesia Research Society, 1986

Rich CL, Smith NT: Anaesthesia for electroconvulsive therapy: a psychiatric viewpoint. Can Anaesthetists Soc J 28:153–157, 1981

Rich CL, Woodruff RA, Cadoret R, et al: Electrotherapy: the effects of atropine on EKG. Diseases of the Nervous System 30:622–626, 1969

Roizen MF: Anesthetic implications of concurrent diseases, in Anesthesia, 2nd Edition, Vol 1. Edited by Miller RD. New York, Churchill Livingston, 1986, pp 255–357

Scalafani SG: The patient for electroconvulsive therapy. Anesthesiology News, Feb 1988, pp 9–18

Selvin BL: Electroconvulsive therapy—1987. Anesthesiology 67:367–385, 1987

Shapiro MF, Goldberg HH: Electroconvulsive therapy in patients with structural disease of the central nervous system. Am J Med Sci 233:186–195, 1957

Shnider SM, Papper EM: Anesthesia for the asthmatic patient. Anesthesiology 22:886–892, 1961

Sibony PA: ECT risks in glaucoma. Convulsive Therapy 1:283–287, 1985

Simon JS, Evans D: Phaeochromocytoma, depression and ECT. Convulsive Therapy 2:296–298, 1986

Simpson KH, Halsall PJ, Carr CME, et al: Propofol reduces seizure duration in patients having anaesthesia for electroconvulsive therapy. Br J Anaesth 61:343–344, 1988

Solomon JG: Electroconvulsive therapy: an overview. Va Med 106:180–188, 1979

Squire LR, Slater PC: Bilateral and unilateral ECT: effects on verbal and nonverbal memory. Am J Psychiatry 135:1316–1360, 1978

Stack CG, Abernethy MH, Thacker M: Atracurium for ECT in plasma cholinesterase deficiency. Br J Anaesth 60:244–245, 1988

Steen PA, Tinker JH, Tarhan S: Myocardial reinfarction after anesthesia and surgery. JAMA 239:2566–2570, 1978

Stoelting RK: Psychological preparation and preoperative medication, in Anesthesia, 2nd Edition, Vol 1. Edited by Miller RD. New York, Churchill Livingstone, 1986, pp 381–397

Stoelting RK: Alpha and beta-adrenergic receptor antagonists, in Pharmacology and Physiology in Anesthetic Practice. Philadelphia, PA, JB Lippincott, 1987a, pp 280–293

Stoelting RK: Histamine and histamine receptor antagonists, in Pharmacology and Physiology in Anesthetic Practice. Philadelphia, PA, JB Lippincott, 1987b, pp 373–384

Stoelting RK: Pharmacology, Section I, in Pharmacology and Physiology in Anesthetic Practice. Philadelphia, PA, JB Lippincott, 1987c, pp 69–147

Stoudemire A, Knos G, Gladson M, et al: Labetalol in the control of cardiovascular responses to electroconvulsive therapy in high risk depressed medical patients. J Clin Psychiatry (in press)

Sung YF, Freniere S, Tillette T, et al: Comparison of propofol and thiopental anesthesia in outpatient surgery: speed of recovery. Anesthesiology 69(3A): A562, 1988a

Sung YF, Weinstein MS, Biddle MR: Comparison of Diprivan (propofol) and thiopental as intravenous induction agents: cardiovascular effects, respiratory change, recovery, and postoperative venous sequelae. Seminars in Anesthesia 7 (suppl 1):52–56, 1988b

Sung YF, Tillette T, Freniere S, et al: Retrograde amnesia, anterograde amnesia and impaired recall by using either thiopentone or propofol as induction and maintenance anaesthetic agents, in Memory and Awareness in Anaesthesia. Edited by Bonke B, Fitch W, Millar K. Swets and Zeitlinger Publishers, 1990a, pp 175–179

Sung YF, Reiss N, Tillette T, et al: The differential cost of anesthesia and recovery with propofol, nitrous oxide anesthesia versus thiopental-isoflurane-nitrous oxide (abstract). Anesth Analg 70:S396, 1990b

Waller JL, Kaplan JA, Jones EL: Anesthesia for coronary revascularization, in Cardiac Anesthesia. Edited by Kaplan JA. New York, Grune & Stratton, 1979, pp 241–280

Waters DJ, Mapleson WW: Suxamethonium pains: hypothesis and observation. Anaesthesia 26:127–141, 1971

Weiner RD: The psychiatric use of electrically-induced seizures. Am J Psychiatry 136:1507–1517, 1979

Weiner RD, Coffey CE: Electroconvulsive therapy in the medically ill, in Principles of Medical Psychiatry. Edited by Stoudemire A, Fogel BS. New York, Grune & Stratton, 1987, pp 113–134

Wolford JA: Electroshock therapy and aortic aneurysm. Am J Psychiatry 113:656, 1957

Woodruff RA, Pitts FN, Craig A: Electrotherapy: the effects of barbiturate anesthesia, succinylcholine and preoxygenation on EKG. Diseases of the Nervous System 30:180–185, 1969

Youmans CR, Bourianoff G, Allensworth DC, et al: Electroshock therapy and cardiac pacemakers. Am J Surg 118:931–937, 1969

Youngberg JA: Perioperative management of the patient having vascular surgery (lecture 132), in 1988 Annual Refresher Course Lectures, American Society of Anesthesiologists. American Society of Anesthesiologists, 1988, pp 1–7

Chapter 4

Special Technical Considerations in Laboratory Testing for Illicit Drugs

Robert M. Swift, M.D., Ph.D.
William Griffiths, Ph.D.
Paul Camara, M.S.

In the last decade, the use of illicit psychoactive drugs has become commonplace. Based on data obtained by the 1988 National Household Survey of Drug Abuse, it is estimated that 72.4 million Americans aged 12 years or older (37% of the population) have used an illicit psychoactive drug at least once in their lifetime. Although the prevalence of current use of illicit drugs appears to have declined over the last decade, 14.5 million Americans (7% of the population) were estimated to have used at least one illicit psychoactive substance in the month before the survey (NIDA 1989). Illicit drug use is even more prevalent among psychiatric and medical patients. Up to 50% of psychiatric admissions involve use of psychoactive substances (Crowley et al. 1974; Hall et al. 1977).

The use of illicit psychoactive substances has significant implications for the diagnosis and treatment of patients with medical and psychiatric disorders. Because even sporadic or recreational use of illicit drugs may have deleterious medical, psychiatric, or social consequences, it is important for physicians to have knowledge of drug use.

Unfortunately, most patients are reluctant to report and often deny the use of illicit drugs.

The testing of body fluids for illicit substances has become an increasingly common procedure in diagnosis and treatment of medical and psychiatric patients. Abnormal results on blood or urine toxicological testing provide important confirmatory evidence of illicit substance abuse. The proper use of drug testing in diagnostic and treatment protocols requires that the clinician have knowledge and skills about the capabilities and limitations of the procedures, about the interpretation of results, and about how the results are to be used in the diagnosis and treatment of an individual patient. A variety of confounding issues are introduced by use and interpretation of toxicological testing and include legal and ethical as well as technical and clinical considerations (Department of Health and Human Services 1986; Finkle 1987; MacKenzie et al. 1987; Schwartz 1988). This chapter reviews the application of blood and urine toxicological testing in the evaluation and treatment of patients with illicit prescription or street drug use.

GENERAL CONSIDERATIONS

Toxicological analysis of body fluids for illicit substances is a complex process with multiple clinical, legal, and technical ramifications. In deciding to test a patient for drugs or medication, the clinician must first consider the objectives of the testing procedures. Are the data obtained from the analysis for illicit drugs to be used for drug-abuse screening, for diagnosis, for compliance determinations, for treatment, or for legal and forensic issues? The proper choice of sample collection protocols, choice of analytical methods, and proper interpretation of the data depend to a large extent on the ultimate use of the data. For example, if the results are to be used for forensic or legal purposes, strict protocols and documentation procedures may be required.

The analysis proper is composed of sequential stages, each of which is important to the ultimate interpretation of the data (Table 4-1). These include 1) sample collection, 2) sample storage and transport, 3) sample analysis methodology and accuracy, 4) interpretation of reported data, and 5) use of data. Improper procedures at any stage of the sequence may render data inaccurate or uninterpretable; unfortunately, this occurs commonly (Hansen et al. 1985).

In deciding on methodology, the clinician should always consider three technical questions:

1. How accurate are the procedures?
2. How fast can the data be produced?
3. How much do the procedures cost?

USE OF THE DATA

Although use of the data is the final stage of toxicological testing, several important considerations are required on the part of the clinician before initiating the testing process. First, the toxicological analysis for illicit drugs must always occur within a clinical context. Indications for testing, the specific procedures, and potential treatment plans dependent on results should be established before drug testing. Second, the intention to test should be discussed with the patient, including the purpose and indications for testing, the manner and schedule of sample collection, and how the results are to be used. This essentially constitutes obtaining informed consent. The plan should include a method of providing the test results to the patient and a discussion of other parties who may have access to the information and should specify what therapeutic actions are to be taken in light of the results of the laboratory data. In addition, the clinician should always consider the possible consequences resulting from erroneous data because false-positive and false-negative results may occur. Confronting patients with inaccurate data has been shown to result in a breakdown of trust between patient and clinician and in poor outcome of substance-abuse treatment (Harford and Kleber 1978; Swift et al. 1988; Trellis et al. 1975).

Table 4-1.   Sequential stages of drug testing

1. Sample collection—type of body fluid and method of collection

2. Sample storage and transport

3. Laboratory testing: methodology and accuracy of sample analysis

4. Interpretation of test results

5. Use of test results (medical and legal considerations)

THE SAMPLE

Sample Type

The decision whether to obtain blood or urine for analysis depends on several factors. Certain drugs are preferentially distributed in one body fluid, such as amphetamines and opiates in urine and alcohol in blood. Blood sampling may provide both quantitative and qualitative information about a drug, whereas urine analysis provides only qualitative information. Plasma levels may be especially important in the assessment of overdose or of prescription-drug intoxication and dependence. Blood sampling is more invasive and requires personnel with specific training in phlebotomy, whereas urine testing requires less technical skill. The required amount of specimen to be obtained should be known in advance so as to eliminate results reported as "QNS" (quantity not sufficient).

Sample Collection Procedures

Sample collection procedures, although a frequently ignored aspect of toxicological analysis, are important for reliable analysis of samples and for interpretation of results. The process of sample collection must be designed to ensure the integrity and stability of the analytes and the dignity and confidentiality of the patient. Factors to be considered include type of sample to be obtained (blood, urine, or both), amount of sample (volume needed), timing of sample collection, frequency of sample collection, and observation of the collection process. If the data may be used in any legal proceeding, then it is essential that the samples be collected and handled in a way that is acceptable in the courtroom. This may include documentation that the subject being tested has consented to (and understands the ramifications of) the process.

Considerable controversy exists over the legal ramifications of the drug screening process and the need for informed consent. At present, the issue is unresolved, as proposals for widespread screening of federal employees are involved in litigation. In most states, information contained in a medical record may be obtained by law enforcement agencies, insurance companies, and other parties. The best policy for the clinician is to perform screening in the context of a treatment plan negotiated with the patient, with the patient's informed consent. However, this is not always possible in the case of the delirious, psychotic, or incompetent patient. In that case, the clinician must utilize whatever procedures are necessary as part of a diagnostic workup, but be aware that any data obtained become part of the medical record. In the case of children or adolescents, it is important to negotiate a treatment plan with the patient or guardian and decide on how the information is to be used before testing.

Timing and frequency of collection should be determined by the uses of the data. If samples are to be used for assessing treatment compliance or for drug-abuse screening, samples should be obtained on a random basis, as soon as possible after announcement of the intention to perform testing. Frequency of testing should be determined according to the half-life of the drug to be tested, resources available for testing, and the expected frequency of drug use. One admitted cocaine abuser was never detected because the employer always announced the intention to test 7–10 days before sample collection.

The specimen must be acquired in a way that obviates the possibility of substitution or tampering by the subject and must then be put in a labeled tamper-evident container. Urine samples should be obtained under direct observation, with the observer being of the same sex as the patient. Samples should be collected in a confidential manner, preferably in a private area. Nevertheless, some patients are extremely adept in substituting or adulterating samples, particularly urine. A small rubber tube taped to the penis that leads to a urine-filled rubber bulb in a pocket can produce a stream of urine that appears naturally produced. A useful method to identify some instances of adulteration or substitution is to check the sample pH and temperature at the time of collection. However, patients have been known to preheat substituted urine in a microwave prior to collection. Table 4-2 depicts several common methods used for adulterating urine samples.

Sample Storage and Transport

After collection, samples should be placed in proper containers or tubes containing any required additives and centrifuged, frozen, or refrigerated as necessary. They should be analyzed within an appropriate time frame to prevent deterioration of the sample. At this point, a chain of custody form must be created. This form will then accompany the specimen on its trail to the testing laboratory (and perhaps beyond) and serves as a written description and documentation of its itinerary. It also serves to identify all those who have had the specimen in their possession. The steps taken to maintain the accurate identity and in-

Table 4-2.   Common methods used in adulterating urine samples

Method	Effect
Addition of diluent or excessive consumption of liquids	Dilution of analyte beyond sensitivity of assay
Addition of acidic or alkaline material (e.g., soap, vinegar)	Changes pH of sample, affecting extractability in certain methods
Addition of benzalkonium chloride (i.e., Visine eyedrops)	False-negative cannabinoid results
Vinegar ingestion	Decreased methadone concentration in urine
Ingestion of poppy seeds	Justifies positive test for opioids in urine
Ingestion of decongestants	Justifies positive test for amphetamine in urine
Submission of someone else's urine for analysis	May be drug free depending on the integrity of the donor

tegrity of the specimen are of paramount importance in all cases of testing for illicit drugs. The written documentation of these steps will be less important in cases not likely to involve forensic or legal applications.

LABORATORY ANALYSIS

The accuracy of the actual analysis of the specimen depends on the technique or combination of techniques employed and the training, experience, and competence of the laboratory staff. When examining accuracy of drug assay procedures, one must consider both qualitative and quantitative accuracy. Careful consideration must be given to the process of acquiring and handling the specimen before and during the analysis, and to the treatment and reporting of the data afterward. The analytical process itself will have a greater or lesser degree of inaccuracy associated with it depending on the techniques and equipment chosen. The potential for random error (as opposed to expected variability) is greater in the pre- and postanalytical operations. In a well-run laboratory, the inaccuracy will be known and characterized and should be carefully controlled.

Sample Verification

The first step in the laboratory analysis is to perform *verification operations* on the sample. These may include visual inspection, pH and osmolality determinations, or even determination of normal urine or blood components. There are numerous legendary and factual methods of doctoring samples in a way that can cause interferences with drug analysis techniques. The most common schemes include diluting the sample, substituting some other fluid or someone else's blood or urine, or adding adulterants that affect the pH (e.g., surfactant, vinegar, lye). It must be noted, however, that as hard as we may try to protect the sample, new ways of tampering will always appear. Recently, a method for producing false-negative cannabinoid results using Visine eyedrops was described (Pearson et al. 1989). This technique affected cannabinoid results with both the Abbott TDx and the Syva EMIT systems.

In the analysis of specimens, laboratories use a two-tiered approach. An initial, inexpensive screening method is used to analyze all samples. Subsequently, only those samples that are positive for an illicit substance on initial screening are subjected to a second analysis, usually (but not always) by a different analytic method. Only those samples that are determined to be positive by the second method as well are reported to the clinician as positive. A wide variety of methodologies are available for use and may vary considerably between laboratories (Table 4-3).

Chromatographic and *immunochemical* techniques are the two most widely used for testing for illicit drugs. Applications of both types have been made very successfully to screening, confirmation, and quantification. Typically, the testing process begins with screening, followed by a confirmation of positive results by an alternative method and, if necessary, quantification. Methods should be chosen such that

---

Table 4-3. Commonly used techniques for sample analysis

●**Immunochemical**
   Fluorescein polarization immunoassay (FPIA)
   Enzyme-multiplied immunoassay test (EMIT)
   Radioimmunoassay (RIA)

●**Chromatographic**
   Thin-layer chromatography (TLC)
   Gas chromatography/mass spectrometry (GC/MS)

the screening process is accomplished quickly and inexpensively. Automated immunochemical methods lend themselves very well to this step.

Depending on the patient population, only a fraction of the screened samples will need confirmation and quantification. Thus, the more laborious and expensive techniques should be relegated to these tasks. All the immunochemical methods discussed below can be used to detect the most popular drugs of abuse in urine.

Immunochemical methods. All immunochemical methods for illicit-drug screening are based on the recognition of the three-dimensional structure of a drug by an antibody. These are typically monoclonal antibodies developed for a molecule whose structure is representative of a given target drug family. Beyond this, the methods differ considerably in the mode of detection of the antigen-antibody complex. It is important to note that, in all immunochemical techniques, the limits for the sensitivity of the test are dictated not only by the detection mechanism, but also by the cross-reactivity of the antibody for the drug of interest. Because the antibody does not "see" all members of a drug family equally, the concentrations needed to achieve an equivalent analytical response will sometimes be considerably different for closely related substances. It is very important for the testing laboratory to be well informed in this area and to educate the users of the analytical data as to their true interpretation.

Fluorescence polarization immunoassay (FPIA), originally developed for the quantitative determination of therapeutic drug concentrations, has also become a very popular tool for qualitative and semiquantitative analysis for drugs of abuse in urine. It is the method of analysis used in the Abbott TDx and ADx analyzers. With this method, urine is mixed with a solution of monoclonal antibody specific for the drug of interest, and with fluorescein-labeled drug. The unlabeled drug in the patient's urine competes with the labeled drug in the reagent for a limited number of binding sites on the antibody. The greater the concentration of the drug in the patient's urine, the less the labeled drug in the reagent will bind to the antibody, and vice versa.

When excited by plane-polarized light, fluorescein will emit fluorescence with a degree of polarization inversely related to its rotation (i.e., the faster it rotates, the lesser the degree of polarization). Thus, the greater the concentration of drug in the patient's urine, the less the fluorescein-labeled drug will bind to the antibody. Unbound antibody has increased rotation, and therefore decreased polarization. By measuring the degree of polarization of the mixture, we can therefore assess the concentration of drug in the patient's urine (the lesser the polarization, the greater the concentration of drug). Using the instrumental configurations described above, the technique is accurate, very precise, and extremely easy to use and to teach. The stability of the stored standard curve (at least 1 month) is a great advantage that may be somewhat offset, however, by the price of the reagents. This method works well both as a screening technique and as a confirmatory method if the screening is performed by a nonimmunochemical method.

Enzyme-multiplied immunoassay test (EMIT) was the first nonisotopic immunochemical technique to gain wide acceptance in the clinical laboratory as a tool for *quantifying* serum drug concentrations. It is now used by many as the method of choice for urinary drug screening. With this technique, urine is mixed with reagent containing antibody to the drug of interest. Given the excess of antibody, all drug in the patient's urine is bound. The same drug, but labeled with an enzyme, is then added to the mixture. This drug takes up binding sites on the remaining antibody. In this process, the enzymatic activity of the label is altered either by an actual change in its conformation or by steric hindrance. Unbound drug-enzyme complex sees no effect in its activity. Thus, the greater the concentration of drug in the patient's urine, the fewer binding sites left available for the drug-enzyme complex, and the greater the enzymatic activity of the solution. When a substrate is added and a chromophore formed, the resulting absorbance of the solution is directly proportional to the concentration of the drug in the patient's urine. This method is adaptable to a number of automated systems (e.g., Hitachi 700 series, Roche Cobas MIRA) and thus can be used in a random-access mode. Stability of a stored standard curve is, at best, 1–2 weeks, but any cost incurred by running extra standards is usually compensated for by a reagent price that is typically lower than that of FPIA reagents. Like FPIA, EMIT is also useful for screening and confirmation.

Radioimmunoassay (RIA), originally developed by Berson and Yalow (1968) as a technique for the quantification of insulin, has found broad application in many disciplines in the clinical laboratory. The Roche Abuscreen is still used in many labs as a urine screening technique for drugs of abuse. Rather than using an enzyme or fluorophore, RIA methods use a radioactive isotope (usually a gamma emitter such as ^{125}I), and detection is accomplished in a gamma counter. The patient's urine is mixed with antibody to the drug of interest and with isotopic-labeled drug. The drug in the urine competes with the labeled drug for binding sites on the antibody. After an appropriate incubation period, the bound isotope is separated from the unbound fraction. If the bound fraction is counted, the counts will bear a direct relationship to the concentration of drug in the patient's urine. If the unbound fraction is counted, the counts and the drug concentration in the urine will be inversely related. This technique is very sensitive and is not difficult to perform, although the incubation times are considerably longer than those for EMIT and FPIA. The reagents are relatively inexpensive, but the problems associated with regulation of the isotopes and disposal of the waste make this an ill-advised choice for screening. It can, however, be very useful as a confirmatory method.

Chromatographic methods.   The basis for all chromatographic analysis is that separation of analytes in a mixture is possible based on their physicochemical characteristics. As with other analytical techniques, "positives" in chromatography are only presumptive until confirmed by another method. Gas chromatography/mass spectrometry (GC/MS), as described below, incorporates the confirmation test in its detection step. Chromatographic methods, although able to resolve specific members within a given drug family and to do so relatively inexpensively (after an initial capital outlay), nevertheless are more labor-intensive and time-consuming. Consequently, with the exception of the Toxi-Lab thin-layer chromatography system, they are usually reserved for use as confirmatory procedures.

Thin-layer chromatography (TLC) takes place on silica gel bonded to a solid support (usually a glass plate). Initially, the urine is extracted (liquid/liquid, or solid phase) to remove interferents and to concentrate the analytes of interest. The dried product is then redissolved (usually in methanol) and applied, via a capillary pipette, to the thin-layer plate. After the samples have dried, the plate is placed in a developing tank containing enough developing solvent to cover the lower 10 mm of the plate. The developing solvent migrates up the plate by capillary action, causing a migration of the drugs contained in the patient's urine. Through an interaction of the physicochemical properties of the silica, the solvent, and each drug in the urine sample, the drugs are resolved from each other as the process continues. At certain points up the plate, various constituents in the sample will stop migrating, whereas others will continue. After development of the plate is complete, it is removed from the developing tank and left to dry. After drying, the drugs are detected either by ultraviolet light for naturally fluorescing drugs, or by spraying or dipping the plate with some appropriate color-developing reagent. This technique is not as sensitive as the immunochemical methods or GC/MS but sensitivity can be enhanced for certain drugs by including an acid hydrolysis step before the extraction to cleave glucuronide conjugates, releasing the unconjugated drug into the urine.

TLC is an inexpensive, sensitive, and relatively simple chromatographic method for use in urinary drug screening. Instrumentation (densitometers, automated applicators) has been introduced to enhance its use, but this is certainly not required. A laboratory may provide a very effective drug screening service without these additions. Historically, the turnaround time for TLC (3–4 hours) has always been greater than that of the immunochemical methods, but the trade-off is increased specificity (individual drugs rather than drug families), and significantly less expense.

Gas chromatography/mass spectrometry (GC/MS) gives the analytical laboratory the ability to identify unknowns completely and specifically. This very accurate and sensitive technique can be used to irrefutably confirm a presumptively positive result generated by another method. Considered by many to be the gold standard in drug screening, it is required for National Institute on Drug Abuse (NIDA) certification and it is considered "fully defensible" in court when used as a confirmatory test to TLC or one of the immunochemical methods (Hoyt et al. 1987).

As in TLC, a preliminary extraction (usually liquid/liquid) of the sample is always necessary to eliminate interferences and to increase the concentration of the extracted analytes. Subsequently, chemical derivitization is employed to increase the volatility of a drug or metabolite (e.g., molecules with phenolic, carboxylic acid, amine, or hydroxyl functionalities) or to decrease it (e.g., amphetamines) and, in many cases, to improve chromatographic resolution and to give a more distinctive mass spectrum to similar low-molecular-weight compounds.

After extraction and derivitization, the sample is ready to be analyzed. A very small volume of sample (1 or 2 µl) is injected into the GC column, which resolves, to a greater or lesser degree, the components in the mixture. A small amount of the column effluent is then fed directly into the ionization chamber of the mass spectrometer, which produces neutral and ionic fragments of each resolved drug. These fragments can be directly related back to the parent compound. The charged species are then accelerated, separated by mass, and measured by a detector. The mass spectrum for any given analyte has characteristic, well-defined peaks that include those produced from ionic fragments, and those produced from the whole species (the molecular ion). Using a computerized data library, the analyst can then proceed to identify the compound. This information, coupled with the retention data from the chromatographic analysis, typically provides a result that is unambiguous.

GC/MS can be used qualitatively and quantitatively for either serum or urine analysis. Its importance in the drug screening process is its lack of ambiguity. The data usually cannot reasonably be refuted. Also, along with confirming the presence of commonly abused drugs, GC/MS can be used to detect the newer "designer" drugs provided the computer library has their standard mass spectra. This is important in cases of overdose when the causative agent is not immediately apparent or cannot be detected by the less inclusive immunochemical or chromatographic techniques. Although GC/MS is a premier method in the toxicology laboratory, its expense and need for a high level of technical expertise prevent its use from being widespread.

Other methods.   Certain abused substances can be detected through specific screens, but require suspicion of abuse, as these screens are not normally utilized. For example, abuse of phenolphthalein-containing laxatives can be best detected through colorimetric analysis of a stool specimen. Diuretic abuse may be best determined through analysis of urine electrolytes.

CHOOSING AN ANALYTIC METHODOLOGY

In comparing different analytic methodologies for the detection of illicit drugs, it must be kept in mind that there are inverse relationships between accuracy and cost and between speed and accuracy. In an acute psychiatric emergency such as a drug ingestion, speed of analysis is paramount and accuracy and sensitivity can be sacrificed. A rapid screening method such as an automated EMIT assay may produce results in as little as 15 minutes, which can be confirmed later. However, the ability to perform rapid analyses may depend on the presence of trained personnel and automated equipment, which are expensive.

In an outpatient mental health or drug-abuse treatment setting, time may not be so important a factor as sensitivity and accuracy of results. Turnaround time for TLC or GC/MS (3–4 hours) has always been greater than that for the immunochemical methods, but the trade-off is increased specificity in identifying individual drugs rather than drug families. When toxicological analyses are used for screening many individuals or a single individual on several occasions, cost considerations become important.

CHOOSING A LABORATORY

Laboratories have been shown to vary considerably in their accuracy of analysis (Hansen et al. 1985), so it is important to be aware of the quality control of the laboratory being used. The federal government has recently instituted certification procedures for laboratories engaged in drug testing of federal employees (Department of Health and Human Services 1987). This so-called NIDA standard is so stringent and the methodology so expensive that only a few large laboratories have become certified. However, the NIDA certification will probably eventually become the de facto standard for all laboratory analyses of illicit drugs.

Although few laboratories achieve the "NIDA standard," most laboratories utilize quality-control procedures to determine reliability and reproducibility of their analyses. The clinician should inquire about quality-control procedures and, on request, be provided with a laboratory's false-positive and false-negative report rate. Some large users of analytic services submit known samples to laboratories on a regular basis, so as to assess quality control for themselves. If possible, the clinician should also perform reliability studies by periodically submitting test samples of known composition for laboratory analyses. Another method of checking reliability is to divide samples into two or more aliquots and submit each for a separate analysis. Any discrepancies need to be brought to the attention of the laboratory director, who should be open to discussing possible sources of error.

The clinical laboratory business can be quite lucrative and is very competitive. In most locations there are often several laboratories, both large and small, that compete for the clinician's business, and that are often willing to be quite accommodating to retain business. When a clinician does have a choice of laboratories, several factors should determine the decision of which laboratory to use. These may include cost of analyses, location of the laboratory, timeliness of reporting, and accuracy of reporting. The clinician should have a "contact" at the laboratory to whom questions and problems can be addressed. Some clinicians, especially those who are hospital-based, may have limited input into the choice of a laboratory for analyses of patient specimens. Nevertheless, the clinician should lobby hard with administrators for an adequate analytical laboratory as it is important to good patient care.

INTERPRETATION OF TESTING RESULTS

Aspects of analytical accuracy include sensitivity and specificity. The sensitivity of a technique designed to detect and/or quantify an illicit drug is usually stated in terms of the minimum concentration of the drug in a sample that can be distinguished from zero concentration with a defined certainty, usually 95%, when the method is operated under optimum conditions. However, most laboratories do not report drug concentrations, but rather report results only as a "positive" or "negative." With most methods, particularly the immunologic methods, it is common to set an arbitrary cutoff concentration somewhat higher than the highest likely sensitivity limits and define any result lower than the cutoff as negative, or "none detected" (Table 4-4).

It is important to the user of the data to know what the analytical sensitivity means in terms of the timing and quantity of the drug ingested. This requires some knowledge of the peak sample (urine or blood) concentrations reached at various doses as well as the in vivo drug half-life. It is useful to know whether the drug use has occurred as a single event or on a chronic basis, as blood levels of drug are higher and therefore detectable longer with repeated dosing, especially for drugs with long half-lives such as cannabinoids and phenobarbital. For "well-behaved" drugs such as ethanol and barbiturates, knowledge of two or three sequential timed serum concentrations can yield a reasonable deduction as to the original dose. At the other extreme are drugs such as THC or anabolic steroids. These have such a long half-life that, particularly in a habitual user, there is little relationship between blood concentration and dose, and even less relationship between blood concentration and time of ingestion.

Specificity in drug testing usually is defined as the ability of an analytic method to distinguish among different chemical compounds and is critically important to the interpretation of results. Analytic methods designed for rapid screening, such as EMIT, have poor specificity and may not discriminate compounds with related chemical properties. For example, the ingestion of poppy seed bagels has been reported to give a false-positive result for opioids, and use of decongestants may yield a false-positive result for amphetamines. Some methods for benzodiazepines may yield false-negatives for the triazolobenzodiazepines such as alprazolam because these drugs are different chemically from other benzodiazepines. The specificity of analysis can be greatly increased through use of an alternative chemical analytic

Table 4-4. Cutoff* (threshold) concentrations and detection times for popular drugs of abuse in urine

Drug	Immunoassay		Chromatography		Length of Detection[†]
	FPIA	EMIT	TLC	GC/MS	
Amphetamines	300	300	500	10	1–2 days
Barbiturates	300	400		5	2–14 days
Benzodiazepines	300	800	500	5	2–14 days
Benzoylecgonine	300	300	2000	5	2–4 days
Cannabinoids	25	20 or 100	25	1	48 hours to 8 weeks
Methadone	500	500	5500	10	7 days
Opiates	200	300	500	5	2–5 days
Phencyclidine	75	75	500	5	48 hours to 8 weeks

Note. Concentrations are given in ng/ml. FPIA = fluorescein polarization immunoassay, TDx/ADx, Abbott Laboratories; cutoff can be user adjusted. EMIT = enzyme-multiplied immunoassay test, Syva Co. TLC = Thin-layer chromatography. GC/MS = gas chromatography/mass spectrometry.

Cutoff is a term applied to an arbitrary concentration, set by the laboratory or the manufacturer, above which the test is positive and below which it is negative. It is used interchangeably with *threshold*. It is usually not the lower limit of sensitivity of an assay. In this table, the concentration shown for the immunoassay is the cutoff, but the concentration shown for the chromatographic technique is the sensitivity.

[†]*Length of detection* denotes outer time boundary that evidence of the drug can be detected by laboratory testing after use by the patient.

Table 4-5. Definition of drug test outcomes

	Reality	
Result	Drug taken	Drug not taken
Test positive	True positive	False positive
Test negative	False negative	True negative

method for confirmation of positive results. For example, a laboratory may use EMIT or FPIA for initial screening and TLC or GC/MS for confirmation. The clinician should *never* rely on positive results that have not been confirmed through use of an alternative method.

Thus, a positive drug test (assuming accuracy) is a demonstration of probable use of the drug, although the time of usage and dosage cannot be determined. A negative test is evidence of the absence of use only in the context of the analytical sensitivity of the test, and within a time frame that is dependent on the pharmacology. When quantitative analytical methods are employed, some correlation can be made between drug concentration and likely acute physiologic effect, but only in the case of those drugs with a demonstrated concentration-effect relationship (i.e., barbiturates but not steroids). Drug-analysis results in themselves can never yield a diagnosis of psychoactive substance dependence. Table 4-5 shows possible outcomes of laboratory analysis and the interpretations that the clinician must consider.

SUMMARY

Properly utilized, toxicological analysis of illicit drugs can provide important information for the clinician treating medical and psychiatric patients. However, the testing should be performed in the context of a well-developed treatment plan and the testing results always correlated with the clinical state.

REFERENCES

Berson SA, Yalow RS: General principles of radioimmunoassay. Clin Chim Acta 22:51–69, 1968

Crowley TJ, Chesluk D, Dilts S, et al: Drug and alcohol abuse among psychiatric admissions. Arch Gen Psychiatry 30:13–20, 1974

Department of Health and Human Services: Urine testing for drugs of abuse (NIDA Research Monograph 73). Edited by Hawks RL, Chiang CN. Washington, DC, U.S. Government Printing Office, 1986

Department of Health and Human Services: Scientific and technical guidelines for federal drug testing programs: standards for certification of laboratories engaged in urine drug testing for federal agencies: notice of proposed guidelines. Federal Register 52(157):30638–30652, 1987

Finkle BS: Drug analysis technology: overview and state of the art. Clin Chem 33(11):13B–18B, 1987

Hansen HJ, Caudill SP, Boone DJ: Crisis in drug testing: results of CDC blind study. JAMA 253:2382–2387, 1985

Hall RCW, Popkin NK, DeVaul R, et al: The effect of unrecognized drug abuse on diagnosis and therapeutic outcome. Am J Drug Alcohol Abuse 4:455–465, 1977

Harford RJ, Kleber HD: Comparative validity of random-interval and fixed-interval urinalysis schedules. Arch Gen Psychiatry 35:356–359, 1978

Hoyt DW, Finnigan RE, Nee T, et al: Drug testing in the workplace—are methods legally defensible? JAMA 258:504–509, 1987

MacKenzie RG, Cheng M, Haftel AJ: The clinical utility and evaluation of drug screening techniques. Pediatr Clin North Am 34:423–436, 1987

NIDA: National Household Survey of Drug Abuse. Science 245:1192, 1989

Pearson SD, Ash KO, Urry FM: Mechanism of false negative urine cannabinoid immunoassay screens by Visine eyedrops. Clin Chem 35:1163(A), 1989

Schwartz RH: Urine testing in the detection of drugs of abuse. Arch Intern Med 148:2407–2412, 1988

Swift RM, DePetrillo PB, Camara P, et al: False positive urine screen for quinine from tonic water. Addict Behav 14:213–215, 1988

Trellis ES, Smith FF, Alston DC, et al: The pitfalls of urine surveillance: the role of research in evaluation and remedy. Addict Behav 1:83–88, 1975

Chapter 5

Advances in EEG-Based Diagnostic Technologies

M. Eileen McNamara, M.D.

Electrodiagnostics are becoming an increasingly important part of psychiatry. In line with the medicalization of their field in recent years, psychiatrists have employed a variety of EEG-based technologies in an effort to improve diagnostic specificity. Ironically, the large number of studies that employ EEG technology in the psychiatric literature stands in marked contrast to the paucity of EEG training most psychiatrists receive during their residency training. Psychiatrists need the ability to assess critically the often contradictory research that abounds in the literature, including the sometimes exuberant claims of manufacturers of EEG-based diagnostic apparatuses.

Understanding the sensitivity and specificity of any diagnostic test is mandatory for its proper use. Before considering the meaning of EEG reports, the critical reviewer should be aware of the great variability in EEG interpretation among encephalographers with various training. For example, Williams et al. (1985) provided 100 encephalographers with the same EEG samples and found significant differences of interpretation that were influenced by respondent characteristics such as EEG board certification, age, and experience.

The competence of the EEG technician is also crucial. Artifacts in EEGs can be indistinguishable from true brain activity, and it is the technician, not the encephalographer, who is present at the time of recording. A record produced by a poorly trained or inattentive technician may be invalid no matter how great the skill of the encephalographer who later reads it.

The growth of the use of surgery for epilepsy, guided by the use of depth electrodes, has greatly increased our understanding of the meaning of EEG signals recorded from the scalp. For example, while focal slow, sharp, or spike activity is almost always abnormal, the area of the brain that is later proved abnormal at surgery or depth electrode study may be quite different from the localization suggested by scalp EEG. Depth electrodes have shown that some discharges project along neuronal pathways from deep structures to more distant superficial cortical reflections, or across the corpus callosum and subcortical structures to the contralateral hemisphere. Thus, the EEG may falsely localize and at times even falsely lateralize. Sammaritano et al. (1987) reported on three patients whose seizures were shown by depth electrodes to originate on the side opposite to that indicated by scalp and sphenoidal recording (1987). Unilateral tumors or ictal foci can commonly present with bilateral findings on EEG (Hughes and Zak 1987). In a review of 106 patients studied by both scalp and depth electrodes for refractory seizures, Spencer et al. (1988) reported that the accuracy of localization by scalp ictal EEG for lobe of onset was scarcely better than chance, at 21–38%, and only 46–49% for side of seizure onset. These studies place serious constraints on research that attempts to discriminate right versus left temporal lobe epilepsy in terms of psychiatric characteristics or to define areas of brain injury in populations of patients based on EEG alone.

Even with special techniques, a routine EEG may not detect a seizure focus. Patients with frontal lobe seizures, in particular, may have a normal EEG even during an ictus. Williamson et al. (1985) reported that 7 of 10 patients with frontal lobe seizures had no appreciable scalp EEG changes other than artifact during some seizures; these seizures could only be confirmed with depth electrodes. Since frontal lobe seizures are often bizarre, repetitive, extremely frequent, and without postictal lethargy, they are often mistakenly thought to be functional. Eight of Williamson's 10 patients, in fact, had been previously diagnosed as hysteric.

EEG PATTERNS IN SPECIFIC SITUATIONS

Seizures

The detection of seizures is the most common reason for an EEG. Although EEG is the most sensitive test for this disorder, the clinician must be aware of several important limitations.

For an ictal focus to be detectable by EEG, the electrical discharge must be accessible to the recording electrode. Because the routine EEG is recorded from the scalp, small and deep foci from the insula, amygdala, and mesial and basal frontal and temporal lobes can easily escape detection. Unfortunately, these limbic areas are the most likely to cause seizures with psychiatric symptomatology. In a comparison of depth versus scalp electrodes, Lieb et al. (1976) reported that 68% of ictal discharges from deep gray matter did not reach the surface. Further, 14% of clinical seizures and 82% of auras, confirmed as ictal by depth electrodes, had no evidence of surface seizure activity.

An ictal focus, moreover, must be active to be detected. Between discharges, the EEG may be normal. Because routine EEG only samples for 25–45 minutes, during the daytime, it is easy to miss a true ictal focus. It has been estimated that one or two of every three EEGs in a true epileptic patient may be normal (Desai et al. 1988). Thus, a normal EEG does not rule out a seizure disorder. Three or more serial EEGs may be necessary to find an interictal focus.

A further example of this that is of particular interest to psychiatry is the phenomenon of "forced normalization" of the EEG. In 1958, Landolt observed that occasionally a previously abnormal EEG spontaneously normalized, accompanied by the development of psychosis in the epileptic patient. Paradoxically, when the EEG improved, the patient deteriorated. Whereas in the original cases of Landolt the EEG changes were spontaneous, Pakalnis et al. (1987) reported that the same phenomenon could occur when seizure control was achieved by the introduction of effective antiepileptic drugs. Pakalnis presented a convincing argument that the psychosis was not the effect of medications, structural injury, etc., by showing the clear temporal relation of the seizures, seizure control, normalization of the EEG, and the development of psychosis. Without such careful history, the clinician might well be tempted to think that the pristine condition of the EEG indicated that seizures had nothing to do with the patient's psychosis.

Provocative maneuvers and special electrodes. Several maneuvers are used to increase the yield of abnormalities on EEG and facilitate the diagnosis of seizures (Table 5-1). Sleep deprivation is the most common, as both fatigue and stage 2 sleep are thought to greatly increase the yield of focal abnormalities. Veldhuizen et al. (1983) reported, however, that sleep deprivation may not be necessary. He investigated 69 patients from whom a routine EEG, a secobarbital-induced sleep record, and an EEG following 24 hours of sleep deprivation were obtained in random order. The study confirmed the marked activating effects of light sleep on the EEG, but found no evidence of

Table 5-1.   Maneuvers to increase the yield of abnormal EEGs

Technique	Advantages	Disadvantages
24-hour sleep deprivation	Produces natural sleep; activates seizure foci	May cause convulsions; inconvenient
Barbiturate-induced sleep	Increases yield of interictal abnormalities	May cause drug-induced EEG artifact
Nasopharyngeal leads	Aids in localization of foci	Many artifacts
Sphenoidal leads	May help specify "nonspecific" abnormalities	Many artifacts
Anterior temporal (T1 and T2) leads	May detect abnormalities not seen on surface EEG	Muscle artifact
Intensive inpatient monitoring	Prolonged recording time, increasing detection if interictal activity is infrequent and increasing likelihood of recording a seizure	High cost; inconvenient
Ambulatory cassette EEG	Prolonged recording time; recording in natural setting	Lower cost than inpatient EEG, but still expensive; many artifacts, so that highly specialized interpretive skills are needed

an overall increase in discharge rate after sleep deprivation in either the waking state or in various sleep stages. In other words, it did matter that the patient slept during EEG, by natural or pharmacological means, but sleep deprivation itself did not appear to increase abnormalities. Since sleep deprivation is inconvenient and carries the small but real risk of inducing grand mal seizures even in patients who have never had them, sleep alone, even if induced by barbiturates, may be as satisfactory.

Another maneuver to increase the yield of focal abnormalities is the use of additional electrodes to record from a broader cortical surface than in the standard "10-20" system of electrode placements. The most common of these additional electrodes are the nasopharyngeal, which are inserted in the nose to rest against the posterior pharyngeal wall and detect discharges from the mesial and basal temporal structures, particularly from the uncus and anterior part of the hippocampal gyrus. Somewhat more invasive are sphenoidal electrodes, which are thin wires inserted through the skin at the angle of the jaw to pass below the zygomatic arch to rest near the foramen ovale and enhance recording from the anterior and mesiobasal portions of the temporal lobe.

Nasopharyngeal and sphenoidal electrodes can be quite valuable for the detection of deep, mesial foci and the clarification of scalp EEG findings. Extreme caution, however, must be used in interpreting results from these specialized electrodes, and they should only be used by experienced encephalographers, for if a discharge is only seen at the invasive electrodes and not on the surface, there is always the possibility that the discharge is an artifact. Because these electrodes are deep and not visible during recording and are not glued in place like other electrodes, they are quite susceptible to motion artifact, which can at times appear very similar to a seizure discharge.

Silverman (1960) reported that additional surface electrodes placed slightly lateral and superior to the outer canthus of each eye (T1 and T2) were as sensitive as nasopharyngeal electrodes in the detection of temporal abnormalities. These scalp electrodes are far simpler and safer than more invasive electrodes and can be directly observed by the technician for artifact. Nowack et al. (1988) reported that the use of these anterior temporal electrodes added further diagnostic information in 18.8% of 624 EEGs.

Sperling and Engel (1985) performed a prospective study to compare the usefulness of ear, anterior temporal (T1 and T2), and nasopharyngeal electrodes for recognizing temporal lobe foci. Pathological discharges seen in nasopharyngeal electrodes were invariably seen also in ear and anterior temporal electrodes as well, and the authors concluded that the routine use of nasopharyngeal electrodes added no further benefit. T1 and T2 electrodes themselves, however, are no less immune from artifact than other placements (Bromfield et al. 1989) and are best used in a judicious integration with other findings.

Relationship of seizures to EEG abnormalities.   There is no single finding on EEG that is pathognomonic for seizures, with the possible exception of the distinct 3-Hz generalized spike and wave of absence seizures (petit mal). The most common epilepsy in adults—complex partial seizures, previously known as temporal lobe epilepsy—however, has no simple EEG correlate. A frank seizure discharge is rarely captured on routine EEG; only interictal abnormalities are usually found. These take the form of focal slow, sharp, or spike, or spike and wave activity. Focal abnormalities are found in various abnormal brain conditions, however, only one of which is a seizure disorder. Focal slow activity may be the only surface manifestation of a deep seizure discharge. On the other hand, focal slow activity can also signify a tumor, cortical contusion, or stroke. Focal sharp activity and, even more so, focal spike activity indicate increased brain irritability and are more likely to indicate a seizure focus, but these too can be associated with conditions other than a seizure discharge. It has been estimated that one-third to two-thirds of focally abnormal EEGs are found in patients who do not have seizures. Although "interictal" discharges should alert the physician to the possibility of seizures or the other abnormal brain conditions noted above, frank spike activity occurs in 0.4% of otherwise healthy populations, 3.5% of family members of epileptic patients, and 2.2% of patients suffering from cerebral disease without seizures (Gastaut and Tassinari 1975). Focal sharp and dysrhythmic activity is even more common in patients who have no clinical evidence of seizures, although such patients might arguably have a lower seizure threshold. A patient with focal slow, sharp, or spike activity on EEG does not necessarily have seizures.

On the other hand, as noted above, a focal slow, sharp, or spike focus may be the only surface manifestation of a deep-occurring seizure discharge. Given this, the meaning of the term *interictal* or *epileptiform* becomes somewhat obscure, for it is only by depth electrodes that one can reliably say whether a discharge is interictal or actually ictal itself. Siebelink et al. (1988) performed neuropsychological testing under EEG monitoring on children who had partial seizures with frequent interictal discharges. The children's performance was impaired on subtests of short-term memory during periods of epileptiform activity, strongly suggesting that the "interictal" discharges may actually have represented very focal ictal discharges that were confined to limbic structures. In a related study, Bridgman et al. (1989) performed neuropsychological testing with depth electrodes in two patients. Seizures that were confined to the left hippocampus showed no surface alteration of the EEG, no impairment of speech, and no alteration of consciousness and caused no subjective sensation in the patient, but did impair memory. In short, these exquisitely focal seizures were undetectable by the patient, the observer, and routine EEG, but nonetheless caused functional impairment.

Bridgers (1987) reported that 3.4% of psychiatric patients had epileptiform abnormalities on routine EEG. Epileptiform abnormalities were more common in patients younger than age 25, and in older patients on multiple psychotropics. Diagnoses of anorexia nervosa, explosive behavior in adolescence, and barbiturate abuse were also associated with an increased finding of epileptiform abnormalities. Bridgers contended that when patients who had a diagnosis of epilepsy

Table 5-2.   Causes of altered mental status detectable by EEG

Cause	EEG finding
Delirium	Diffuse slowing
Nonconvulsive status epilepticus	Runs of spikes and waves
Postictal states	Diffuse or focal slowing
Stroke (embolic, cortical)	Focal slowing, with or without spikes or sharp waves
Herpes encephalitis	Temporal lobe slow and sharp activity
Encephalitis (other causes)	Diffuse slowing with or without sharp waves or spikes
Benzodiazepine or barbiturate abuse	Excess frontal beta activity
Lithium encephalopathy	Diffuse slowing with paroxysmal bursts of delta activity

on the requisition were excluded, the incidence of epileptiform abnormalities, 2.6%, was no higher than that of a general population reported by Zivin and Ajmone-Marsan (1968). Because the criteria used by the referring psychiatrists for making a diagnosis of epilepsy are not reported, the meaning of this latter conclusion is somewhat uncertain.

Altered Mental Status

EEG is an excellent and underutilized tool in the evaluation of altered mental status. The differential diagnosis of changes in level of alertness is quite broad, and the EEG can suggest many diagnostic possibilities (Table 5-2).

Delirium is an important cause of change in mental status. In clinical practice, delirium is often confused with depression and types of primary psychiatric illness, or with simple apathy. The clinical symptoms can be subtle or florid, adding to the diagnostic uncertainty. Here the EEG is of great utility. All deliriums are accompanied by EEG slowing. The converse is not true: not every patient with diffuse slowing will be delirious. Still, if a clinician suspects delirium in the patient and wishes to confirm the diagnosis, an EEG is mandatory.

Of particular interest to psychiatrists is the report by Hauser et al. (1989) of delirium induced by benzodiazepine withdrawal in patients with partial seizure disorders. Features of this withdrawal syndrome included catatonic behavior, auditory hallucinations, and agitation accompanied by mild to moderate slowing of the EEG. The authors suggested that the absence of epileptiform abnormalities on EEG argued against an ictal cause of the behavior and suggested that the phenomenon of "forced normalization" might underlie the syndrome. Abrupt discontinuation of benzodiazepines is a well-known precipitant of convulsions in epileptic patients, however, and the authors left unaddressed the possibility of partial status epilepticus without scalp EEG reflection. Their first case, in particular, in which the patient exhibited bizarre stereotyped behavior after benzodiazepine discontinuation, strongly suggests frontal lobe seizures.

Nonconvulsive status epilepticus is another cause of altered mental status that can be clinically indistinguishable from delirium, and it may be either of the absence, spike-wave stupor, or partial complex type (Tomson et al. 1986). An EEG, interpreted with knowledge of its limitations, is the only way to make this diagnosis. Nonconvulsive status can occur not only in patients with known epilepsy, but can also be the first or only manifestation of seizures in some patients. Lee (1985) described new-onset ictal confusion in late life. He reported a series of 11 patients, aged 42–76 years, without prior history of seizures or petit mal who developed acute prolonged confusion with prominent behavioral disturbances. Many of the patients were considered "hysterical" and were admitted to the psychiatric service. Subsequent EEGs demonstrated runs of 1- to 2.5-Hz generalized spike-wave and polyspike activity.

A related condition is the finding of *periodic lateralized epileptiform discharges* (PLEDs), biphasic or polyphasic, usually 100- to 200-msec medium-amplitude complexes of predominantly negative spikes or sharp waves and a slow wave, with a quasi-periodic repetition rate of 1–2 seconds and a wide distribution. PLEDs are almost always associated with an obtunded mental status. PLEDs can be seen with both metabolic and structural disturbances such as stroke and may respond to anticonvulsants (Kuroiwa and Celesia 1980). Terzano et al. (1986) reported a series of seven elderly patients who had recurring confusional episodes with prominent psychiatric symptoms, including depression and hallucinations, associated with PLEDs; episodes cleared with intravenous diazepam. A similar series of cases was reported by Drury et al. (1985), who described four patients with abrupt onset of psychosis and periodic, diffuse sharp waves on EEG.

Some *strokes* will present chiefly as altered mental status and a paucity of other findings, particularly right hemisphere and posterior strokes. The EEG will be focally abnormal, in many cases several days before the stroke can be visualized on computed tomography (CT).

Herpes encephalitis is another notorious cause of altered mental status. In this disorder, the EEG is often focally abnormal several days before there are findings on CT or physical examination. Because herpes has a predilection for the temporal lobes, patients present with confusion, agitation, disorientation, and fever, but no paralysis, and are frequently initially diagnosed as suffering from a primary psychiatric illness. I have seen at least two such patients admitted to psychiatric hospitals. Delay in diagnosis for even a day has significant implications for ultimate morbidity and mortality, since the condition is treatable with antiviral agents. Therefore, all patients with an unexplained acute change in mental status should have an EEG.

Drug Use

The EEG can at times give a clue regarding unexpected drug use. Use of benzodiazepines, barbiturates, and other sedatives can be associated with abundant beta activity on the EEG. Acute intoxication can produce a diffusely slow record. (Although it sounds contradictory, an EEG record can be "fast and slow" from superimposed beta and theta or delta rhythms.) Sedative and alcohol withdrawal can produce a diffusely sharp and irritable record. Chronic alcoholic patients often have a low-voltage and flat-appearing EEG. While none of these changes are specific, their presence can be a hint to the physician to pursue a substance-related diagnosis.

The EEG can also be useful as an index of the degree of metabolic encephalopathy induced by psychotropics. For example, apathy and slowness can be symptoms of depression but may alternatively be side effects of the psychotropics prescribed for depression. A new finding of generalized slowing on an EEG is a strong argument for cognitive slowing induced by such psychotropics.

Lithium is among the psychotropics with the most pronounced effects on the EEG. Experienced encephalographers can often correctly guess even before reading the requisition that a patient is receiving lithium. Struve (1987) reviewed a large series of EEGs obtained on psychiatric patients and reported that 39.4% of patients receiving lithium, most in the therapeutic range, had abnormal generalized slowing combined with high-voltage paroxysmal bursts of diffuse delta activity. Clinically, these patients were sometimes mildly lethargic and slowed. In comparison, the incidence of such changes in other groups ranged from a low of only 0.9% of patients on minor tranquilizers to 10.3% of patients treated with haloperidol. More than half, 69.6%, of the

Table 5-3. EEG and dementia

Type of dementia	Usual EEG findings
Alzheimer's disease	Early: normal or mild slowing Later: diffuse slowing
Multi-infarct (large-vessel cortical strokes)	Focal or multifocal slowing
Multi-infarct (lacunar strokes)	Normal
Creutzfeldt-Jakob disease	Early: normal Later: repetitive, synchronous, bilateral sharp waves
Normal-pressure hydrocephalus	Normal (in most cases), or diffuse or focal delta

lithium-treated patients had also at some point had an EEG while not on lithium. All of these EEGs were without the EEG abnormalities observed during lithium therapy. While the implications for such EEG findings have not been fully explored, the presence of such dramatic changes on the EEG should alert the clinician to examine the patient for the well-described cognitive impairments associated with lithium therapy. However, since most lithium-treated patients without neurologic symptoms or signs are not referred for EEG, reported case series may overestimate the occurrence of EEG abnormalities in lithium-treated patients.

Dementia

The EEG can be useful in the evaluation of dementia (Table 5-3), but in many early cases where the diagnosis is most difficult, the EEG is normal. Thus, a normal EEG does not rule out dementia. In early Alzheimer's disease the EEG is often normal or shows some slowing of the alpha rhythm. Such slowing of the alpha rhythm can also be found in normal aging, however, and therefore does not aid in differential diagnosis. As Alzheimer's disease progresses and dementia becomes more severe, generalized slowing becomes evident. For these more severe cases, the degree of slowing has been reported to correlate with the degree of neuropsychological impairment (Kaszniak et al. 1979).

In multi-infarct dementia, background alpha activity is generally better preserved than in Alzheimer's disease, and focal slowing is more common. Multi-infarct dementia consists of two major categories, dementia from small-vessel lacunar disease (etat lacunaire), and that resulting from large-vessel strokes. Because lacunae are deep and remote from the surface, a patient may have significant dementia from lacunar infarcts without a change in EEG (Muller and Schartz 1978). Large-vessel strokes, on the other hand, are more likely to present with focal slowing, particularly if they involve cortex. For reasons that are uncertain, however, the EEG occasionally normalizes about 6 months after a stroke even when a large infarct persists on CT.

EEG is particularly helpful in the diagnosis of Creutzfeldt-Jakob disease. Although in early stages the EEG can be normal, as in other dementias, eventually distinctive repetitive, synchronous, and bilateral sharp waves appear, distinguishing Creutzfeldt-Jakob disease from other degenerative dementias. These waves can be seen occasionally in hepatic failure and other metabolic disturbances (Busse 1983), but almost never in Alzheimer's. About 10% of patients with Alzheimer's disease display the myoclonic jerks that are typical of Creutzfeldt-Jakob disease; the EEG has special usefulness in assessing demented patients with myoclonus.

SPECIALIZED EEG TECHNIQUES

Topographic EEG Mapping

The popularity of topographic EEG mapping has far exceeded its documented scientific validity. In computer-assisted quantitative EEG, the EEG is analyzed into frequency spectra, and selected frequencies are displayed as a color-coded map over a graphic of the brain surface. Although the pictures the computer generates are attractive and appear to be interpretable by individuals not skilled in interpreting EEGs, they are deceptively fraught with risk of error. While mapping has been hailed by some as a simpler way to use EEG, it is in fact far more difficult. The chief problem is that the most sophisticated computer program is not able to discriminate reliably between artifact and genuine brain activity. Mapping requires the input of both a sophisticated encephalographer and a trained technician to screen data prior to processing. Otherwise, to borrow a phrase from computing, "garbage in, garbage out."

In addition to the problems of correctly entering EEG data, there remain numerous difficulties with the various computer programs that process the raw data (Nuwer 1988). Programs commonly reject epileptic spikes, which usually occur singly, as artifact, and likewise reject PLEDs and frontal intermittent rhythmic delta activity (FIRDA) (Hooshmand et al. 1989). Statistical programs for spectral analysis, spatial and temporal resolution, and statistical rejection of artifact can introduce further errors. Moreover, the lack of standards for recording procedures such as location and number of electrodes, epoch length for analysis, and artifact rejection criteria makes comparisons between studies difficult (Nuwer 1989).

The American Academy of Neurology recently took a very strong stand concerning EEG brain mapping, worth quoting at some length:

> The clinical application of EEG brain mapping is still very limited. Most scientific reports on these techniques have demonstrated research applications rather than clinical usefulness. Among the clinical reports, few have been prospectively verified or reproduced. . . .
>
> On the basis of the present medical literature, their sensitivity and specificity fail to substantiate a role for these tests in the clinical diagnostic evaluation of individual patients for possible tumors, multiple sclerosis, minor head trauma, dyslexia, attention deficit disorder, schizophrenia, depression, alcoholism or drug use. . . .
>
> **Executive Summary.** EEG brain mapping is of limited usefulness in clinical neurology. The tests are best used by physicians highly skilled in EEG, in conjunction with analysis of the concurrent polygraph EEG. (American Academy of Neurology, Therapeutics and Technology Assessment Subcommittee 1989, pp. 1100–1101)

The crucial point of this opinion is the distinction between the research and clinical applications of topographic mapping. The science of computer-based EEG analysis, although making significant strides over the past decade, and holding great promise, is still in its infancy and is not yet ready for general clinical application. Further, the power of any tool rests not only in its design but also in the skill of its user. A Porsche, while an elegant and sophisticated machine, will not travel very far when operated by someone who cannot pass his driver's test. If you are willing to be a passenger on a high-speed trip, you had better be sure of the qualifications of the driver.

At the moment, the proper use of topographic mapping requires, as the Academy of Neurology pointed out, a skilled encephalographer familiar with all the caveats of its proper use. The marketing of topographic mapping equipment to the general psychiatric community before its basic principles of design, statistical software, and interpretation are fully tested and standardized is a true scandal. The clinician who bases a diagnostic judgment on topographic mapping alone, done by an unqualified practitioner, may end up in a scientifically indefensible position, and at risk for an adverse result from litigation if the consequences of the decision are untoward.

There are as yet no specific clinical situations for which topographic mapping is a practical diagnostic method. If an abnormality seen on mapping is also seen on routine EEG, then mapping is superfluous. If an abnormality is noted on mapping, but not on other diagnostic techniques, then its significance is still under debate and therefore of questionable clinical utility. Statements such as "routine EEG *may* (italics mine) still be a sensible first choice..." (Garber et al. 1989) that suggest that topographic mapping might be a reasonable alternative to routine EEG, are premature, to say the least.

Duffy (1989), currently the leading scientific developer of topographic mapping, agrees with these reservations, but still finds that topographic mapping may be a valuable clinical tool when used correctly: "In our view, qNP [quantified neurophysiology] studies should never be 'diagnostic.' They provide information that contributes to a diagnosis, along with other available clinical information." He does not support the exaggerated claims made by some manufacturers and proponents and stresses the need for sophisticated knowledge of EEG, scrupulous technique, a normative data base, and consistent standards of practice.

The difficulty of collecting a normative data base, which sounds like a straightforward issue, is illustrated by Kohrman et al. (1989), who examined the differences in alpha power between the resting and the cognitive test states in a group of normal subjects. He found that there could be marked changes in the alpha frequency band, from 2.5 to 7 standard deviations, in an individual subject under the two conditions, and that such changes were reproducible over time. Because of the large variability among subjects, however, differences averaged out, and when analyzed as a group, no changes between the two conditions could be demonstrated. Niedermeyer et al. (1989), using routine EEG, have also noted significant intersubject variability in alpha response to mental activation and suggest that what may be activating to one person may not be as activating for another. Subtracting serial 7s, for example, is far harder for some people than for others.

In related work, Shagass et al. (1988) have suggested that mood state may also affect EEG reactivity. In a study comparing medicated and unmedicated depressive patients with control subjects, unmedicated depressive patients showed more reactivity with higher amplitude and more wave asymmetry with eyes closed and higher frequency with eyes open. Shagass has suggested that these findings may reflect a lower-than-normal level of activation in depressive patients, which would seem consistent with the common clinical observations of psychomotor retardation, slowed cognition, and pseudodementia in depressive patients.

Brain mapping appears most sensitive for the detection of low-amplitude slow activity that is difficult to detect by eye. Care needs to be taken, however, to reject sources of low-frequency artifact (Lee and Buchsbaum 1987) such as respiration, slow eye movements, electrode motion, or problems due to montage design (Hughes and Miller 1988; Nuwer and Jordan 1987). Jerrett and Corsak (1988) compared findings on routine EEG, brain mapping, and neuroimaging (CT and/or magnetic resonance imaging [MRI]) in 100 patients. They reported that abnormal EEG maps corresponded to all lesions detected on abnormal CT and/or MRI, whereas normal routine EEG failed to detect the abnormalities in 11% (6 of 54) of abnormal maps. Overall, of the patients with abnormal maps of EEG slowing, 30% had either sole or better localization by topographic mapping than with routine EEG, and there were no false localizing abnormalities.

Oken et al. (1989), however, produced contradictory results in their analysis of the sensitivity and specificity of EEG frequency analysis in patients with focal abnormalities on both EEG and CT or MRI. They reported that 2 of 20 patients with focal lesions had normal computerized EEG studies, a result that appears in direct opposition to that of Jerrett and Corsak (although the lesions, subjects, and techniques may not have been identical). Oken et al. suggest that computerized EEG may fail to detect abnormalities that can be seen on routine EEG because of computer averaging of episodic slowing, obscuration of asymmetries by bilateral slowing, or the failure to screen out drowsiness or other artifact before computer analysis. Although false-negative studies could have been minimized by changing evaluation parameters, the cost would have been an increase in the false-positive rate. Since obvious focal lesions were missed, the authors questioned the utility of computerized EEG to detect more subtle lesions.

Conflicting reports, like these and others, are likely due to differences in both the equipment and the test parameters used and also to differences in the encephalographers. Fundamental debates among experts regarding parameters of proper use indicate that mapping is not ready for use by those less than expert.

Despite these cautionary notes, few would deny that Duffy and his colleagues have initiated a quantum leap in EEG sophistication and usefulness. I have no doubt that some day all EEGs will be analyzed by computerized technology, and that this will lead to a vast improvement in standardization and utility of the EEG. A technique that can analyze and document rapidly evolving brain activity by the millisecond, and do this over hours and days of investigation, will likely be far more powerful than single-photon emission computer tomography (SPECT) or positron-emission tomography (PET) in increasing our understanding of the neurophysiology and functional anatomy of cognition.

The evolution of computerized EEG can be viewed somewhat like the evolution of computers themselves. The science is still largely in the research and development stage, and arguments about the best procedures should not be viewed as ultimate judgments about the technology itself. Still, while computers have reached the stage where technologically unsophisticated users can have them in their homes, computerized EEG is still at a point where its use should be reserved for experts.

EVOKED POTENTIALS

Evoked potentials (EPs) are an electrodiagnostic tool related to EEG. In this procedure, volleys of repetitive stimuli are used to evoke electrical changes, or potentials, in the EEG. Routine EEG also contains patterns that occur in response to external stimuli, such as photic driving and the K complex of sleep. Most reactive changes, however, have a low signal-to-noise ratio and are too small to be clearly seen on routine EEG. To be noted by the human eye, responses must have an amplitude that stands out against background activity. With EPs, an attempt is made to get around this limitation by presenting hundreds of stimuli and computer averaging the responses so that background EEG activity unrelated to the stimulus will cancel out. The responses to physiologically simple stimuli—visual, sensory, and auditory—are relatively stable across states of alertness, drowsiness, and sleep, maximizing the yield.

An EP is a computer-generated, irregular line that represents the changes in EEG power over time in response to a stimulus. Peaks are named for their positive (P) or negative (N) polarity and for their approximate latency after the presentation of the stimulus. The early portions of the waveform are thought to be related to reception of the sensory information in primary cortical sensory areas, whereas the later components are thought to arise from more complex cognitive processing of the stimulus such as occurs in association and multimodal cortex and limbic structures. The first positive deflection in the cortical auditory evoked responses, for example, P1, arises from the primary auditory cortex. The first negative deflection, N1, is thought to arise from the lateral surface of the superior temporal gyrus or the supratemporal plane, P2 from the temporal lobe cortical structure, P3 from limbic structures, and so forth. Noting delays or attenuation of expected components in the EP helps to determine the site of the lesion.

EPs are particularly useful in the evaluation of hysteria. Documentation of the expected response to stimuli is a strong argument in support of a diagnosis of hysterical blindness, deafness, or numbness. Although major EP waves are present, patients with conversion reactions may have minor changes in amplitudes, which might be related to attentional or physiological factors (Gordon et al. 1986). Another common clinical problem is the patient with vague and fleeting sensory symptoms and a normal neurological examination, in whom the diagnosis of either conversion disorder or multiple sclerosis can be entertained. Visual EPs are exquisitely sensitive to the presence of multiple sclerosis and can often noninvasively detect the patient with demyelinating disorder.

While EPs are most sensitive and reliable in determining sensory disturbance, researchers have tried to explore their utility in other disorders. Because the "long-latency" components of the EP appear to arise in part from limbic and association cortex, other disorders that involve these structures are potentially demonstrable by EP. Stefanatos et al. (1989), for example, reported abnormal auditory EPs in developmental dysphasia and have suggested that this disorder is associated with defects of higher-level sensory encoding preceding the cognitive and linguistic processing of speech.

Some caution should be employed in the interpretation of long-latency EP results. This field of study is still relatively young, and methods are largely unstandardized, making comparisons difficult between studies. Investigators differ widely in electrode placement; electrode number, which can vary from 1 to 32; testing conditions; and stimulus parameters. Moreover, there is not yet universal consensus on the criteria for and significance of normal and abnormal long-latency EP results.

The P300

A reduced P300 component of the cortical event–related potential in schizophrenic patients has been reported most consistently. The P300, or P3 wave, is a large positive wave that peaks at approximately 350 msec after the stimulus, which is recorded over the midparietal area but may arise from the hippocampus, amygdala, and associated structures (Pritchard 1986). The P300 is a particular long-latency component that arises in response to infrequent, or novel, "oddball" events in the repetitive stimuli. For example, if the subject has been hearing a series of low tones, an unexpected high-pitched tone may elicit the P300 response. Production of the P300 is enhanced if, in response to the oddball event, the patient is required to do some cognitive processing such as counting or reacting. A reduction in P300 amplitude is thought to be related to emotional unresponsiveness or attentional impairments (Romani et al. 1987; Roth et al. 1980).

The decrease in P300 amplitude seen in schizophrenia has been reported by some, but not all, investigators to be unrelated to medications (Blackwood et al. 1987), duration of illness, or patient compliance (Morstyn 1983). Latencies to P300 are reported as normal by most investigators, suggesting that the reductions of P300 amplitude are not the result of abnormal processing before P300 (Pritchard 1986). Investigations of dementing processes such as Huntington's, Parkinson's, and Alzheimer's diseases generally, but not invariably, show P300 waves of normal amplitude but prolonged latencies (Hansch et al. 1982; Polich et al. 1986; Rosenberg et al. 1985).

P300 amplitude reductions are not specific for schizophrenia, however, and are also reported in a variety of neuropsychiatric disorders including some cases of dementia (Pfefferbaum et al. 1980), psychotic depression (Roth et al. 1980), autism (Courchesne et al. 1984), borderline personality disorder, and depression (Kutcher et al. 1987), as well as traumatic brain injury and stroke (Gummow et al. 1986).

As noted, investigators have varied widely in the parameters used to evoke P300. Duncan et al. (1987) compared the relative effects of modality, (visual versus auditory) and probability (frequency of occurrence of the novel stimulus) on P300 in schizophrenic and normal patients. They found that P300 amplitude was reduced in schizophrenic patients only for low-probability auditory stimuli, and that in contrast to other reports P300 latency was also prolonged. A marked increase in amplitude of P300 was also associated with successful pharmacologic treatment of schizophrenia. Wagner et al. (1989) also failed to find

P300 abnormalities in schizophrenic patients when visual, rather than auditory, stimuli were used. These studies underline the crucial need to standardize procedures in the investigation of psychiatric patients.

Several authors have pointed out that determination of P300 latency and amplitude in abnormal patient populations can be difficult and at times arbitrary (Michalewski et al. 1986; Rodin et al. 1989). P300 is not a unitary event but rather part of a late positive complex of several components (Sutton and Ruchkin 1984), and deciding which of several peaks at various latencies is P300 can at times be problematic. Also as yet unstandardized is the establishment of the extent of variability of the P300 latency in normal subjects. Investigators can vary widely in what is accepted as a normal range for P300, and hence in what is considered a prolonged latency. Rosenberg et al. (1985) used a standard error of 26 msec, whereas Pfefferbaum et al. (1980) used a standard error of 51 msec. A normal P300 latency may well vary by the modality and complexity of the task assigned, methods for defining P300, sample size, age, and intelligence of the controls (Rosenberg et al. 1985). This may explain why some studies have not been reproducible.

Brain Electrical Activity Mapping

Some investigators have merged the techniques of EPs and topographic EEG mapping to better display and analyze the spatiotemporal evolution of the components of the EP. Duffy et al. (1979) have been the leading proponents of brain electrical activity mapping (BEAM), which displays computer-extracted changes in EEG spectral power over time in response to visual and auditory stimuli, mapped to a video display of the brain. The caveats of topographic mapping and EPs all apply to BEAM, necessitating that this technique should only be used by experienced encephalographers.

Faux et al. (1987), of Duffy's group, have reported that the topographic mapping of the middle latency auditory EP, P200, is abnormal in schizophrenia, with a right-deviated positive maximum and deficient activity in the left temporal lobe. Faux et al. reported that the altered topography of P200 correctly classified 73% of schizophrenic patients and 78% of control subjects. Because P200 is generated from different temporal lobe structures than P300, this would provide supportive evidence of left temporal abnormalities in schizophrenia.

MAGNETOENCEPHALOGRAPHY

As will be remembered from physics, electrical currents produce magnetic fields. The magnetic fields generated by brain electrical activity can be detected by a device somewhat fancifully called a SQUID, for superconducting quantum interference device. By extrapolating backward from the known spatial resolution of the magnetic field, researchers attempt to better define the spatial resolution of the electrical source. Magnetoencephalography (MEEG) is particularly helpful for defining electrical currents in regions of the brain that are usually not well seen on regular EEG, such as the depths of gyri (Reeve et al. 1989). MEEG is a promising new technique to detect and localize ictal foci by noninvasive means. It has also been used in conjunction with EEG and electrocorticography to define the origins of the EP response (Sutherling et al. 1988). Reite et al. (1989) have used MEEG to identify differences in anatomic location, rather than latency or amplitude, in the origins of auditory N100 evoked responses in schizophrenic patients. If reproducible, this may indicate differences in auditory processing in this patient group.

The necessary equipment for MEEG is large and cumbersome and can only cover a small portion of the brain at any one time. MEEG remains in the research and development stage, and further developments in localization methods are needed before it can be applied clinically. It does appear, however, that MEEG will be an excellent tool for the definition of the small, deep ictal foci that are of particular interest in psychiatry (Rose et al. 1987; Sutherling and Barth 1989).

DIPOLE LOCALIZATION METHOD

Dipole localization method (DLM) is a computer-assisted mathematical method based on electrical field theory, similar to localization methods currently used by electrocardiographers. Localization of EEG foci is based on volume conduction models, and scalp voltages are translated backward to infer the deep intracranial source of the discharges. Usually, the high resistivity of the skull, approximately 80 times that of the brain, impairs transmission of recordable signals from deep midline structures. Smith et al. (1985) reported that deep foci generated from a known source via depth electrodes could be accurately localized by scalp electrodes using DLM. With further development,

DLM may be another useful technique for the detection of small epileptic foci in psychiatric patients.

Dipole methods have also been employed to determine the origins of the components of EPs (Scherg and Von Crammon 1985).

AMBULATORY CASSETTE EEG

As previously noted, prolonged EEG monitoring, particularly through sleep, can significantly increase detection of epileptiform abnormalities. Although closed-circuit, inpatient EEG monitoring (CCEEG) is unquestionably the "gold standard" of prolonged recording, it is cumbersome, expensive, and of limited availability. Ambulatory cassette EEG (A/EEG) is a procedure intermediate between routine and inpatient CCEEG, with several advantages that make it of particular utility for psychiatric patients.

Similar to a Holter monitor, the A/EEG records 8 channels of brain or heart activity on a cassette tape that is later played back on a monitor. The recording equipment is the size of a purse, considerably reduced from a desk-sized regular EEG machine, and is entirely portable. Two recorders can be easily worn to increase the number of EEG channels to 16. Patients can be recorded at home, or without transfer from their present place of treatment such as a psychiatric unit. During the course of the recording, patients or observers are asked to complete a diary of any paroxysmal events. The recorder contains a clock and an event button, so that symptoms can be correlated with EEG or ECG changes when the tape is reviewed. Individual recordings last 24 hours, but recording can be continued indefinitely by daily changes of the tape and batteries, and regluing of the electrodes.

Although 8-channel A/EEG uses fewer channels than regular EEG or CCEEG, its sensitivity compares favorably to these more traditional modalities. In adults, most focal interictal abnormalities are anterior, and generalized ictal abnormalities are usually most prominent in the anterior regions as well. Most A/EEG montages exploit this fact by concentrating channels in the anterior regions of the scalp while sacrificing coverage of the occiput. Leroy and Ebersole (1983) and Ebersole and Bridgers (1985) have reported that the frontotemporal montage most commonly used in A/EEG detects 74–100% of interictal epileptiform events. Bridgers and Ebersole (1985) obtained A/EEG before intensive monitoring in 33 patients referred to an epilepsy center. They reported that A/EEG found 83% of the epileptiform abnormalities later

Table 5-4.   Ambulatory EEG findings in 100 patients with "funny spells"

Feature	Number of patients
Symptomatic events	55
Associated with seizures	3
Associated with cardiac arrhythmia	3
Associated with drowsiness	12
Cardiac arrhythmias	8
Disturbed nocturnal sleep	30
Daytime naps	41

Source. Data from McNamara ME, Nordin NL, Shriner RL, et al: Quantification of sleep in episodic alterations of consciousness: daytime sleepiness in patients with funny spells (abstract). Presented at the North Eastern regional sleep meeting, White Plains, NY, March 31, 1989.

determined by CCEEG, at considerable cost savings. A/EEG was also 2.5 times more likely than routine EEG to yield evidence in support of epilepsy. Bridgers (1988) also reported that 11% of psychiatric patients had interictal epileptiform abnormalities on A/EEG, compared to 0.5% of headache patients (Bridgers et al. 1989), and that A/EEG could be used to clarify the nature of suspicious clinical episodes in selected patients.

Although the workup of generalized convulsions is fairly straightforward, the diagnosis and treatment of the patient with more subtle episodic symptoms such as alterations in consciousness, sensation, or behavior is a more difficult and more common problem in clinical practice. While the bulk of the literature has focused on the discrimination of epileptic from nonepileptic events, the differential diagnosis of paroxysmal symptoms includes not only seizures, but also cardiac events, metabolic disturbance with delirium, and drowsiness with microsleeps. The ability of A/EEG to monitor EEG, ECG, and sleep architecture simultaneously for prolonged periods in a cost-effective manner makes it ideally suited to investigate these patients.

McNamara et al. (1989) reviewed 100 A/EEGs of patients who were referred for the investigation of "funny spells" (Table 5-4). Symptomatic events were reported by 55 of the patients during the course of recording. Of these, only 3 corresponded with episodes of A/EEG seizure activity, a percentage consistent with that reported by Bridgers for psychiatric patients (1988). Unexpected cardiac arrhythmias were seen in 8 patients, and in 3 of these patients, symptoms correlated with the cardiac arrythmia. In 12 of the patients, symptoms correlated with periods of drowsiness as defined by the appearance of generalized theta activity of mixed frequency, absence and/or disappearance of alpha activity, and the emergence of slow roving eye movements. These patients also had evidence of either hypersomnia or fragmented and diminished nocturnal sleep, which suggested that their episodic symptoms were related to hypnagogic phenomena and drowsiness. As a group, the patients with episodic symptoms had a high incidence of sleep disturbance, with 30% showing significant abnormalities of nocturnal sleep. These included markedly fragmented sleep with numerous arousals in 21%, hypersomnia with total sleep time more than 10 hours in 5%, and alpha-delta patterns in 4%.

Also interesting was the observation that 41 of the 100 patients took naps at some point in the recording (McNamara et al. 1989), a figure that is far higher than the 15–20% reported by Broughton et al. (1988) in a study of normal subjects by A/EEG. These data suggest that sleep disorders and drowsiness, rather than seizures, may be a more important and somewhat neglected cause of episodic symptoms. Traditional, inpatient polysomnography has inherent limitations for the study of hypersomnia. Sleep laboratories are rarely staffed for 24-hour studies, and the patient is by definition not in her or his natural environment, which causes observational artifact. The A/EEG technique, recording a full 24 hours in the patient's natural environment, is likely to give more definitive evidence regarding hypersomnia. Its ability to record naps and other daytime sleep episodes is particularly relevant when studying psychiatric aspects of medical illnesses that may shift or disrupt the sleep-wake cycle.

A number of services have sprung up offering A/EEG, but the clinician should check their qualifications carefully before ordering. Such services vary considerably in their expertise. In many, the tape is reviewed by a technician only, who then sends paper printouts to a local physician for review. This entirely omits the power of the A/EEG to detect abnormalities by sound, rather than visual image. Accuracy is entirely dependent on the ability of the technician to select abnormalities, and the expertise of the local physician to read tapes that appear quite different from regular EEG. Diagnostic yield may be considerably improved when tapes are read directly by trained encephalographers.

CONCLUSION

A/EEG, computerized EEG topography, long-latency EPs, and the other advanced EEG-based technologies that have been discussed here are powerful, promising tools for neuropsychiatry. To use them cor-

Table 5-5.   EEG in psychiatry: key points

1. A normal EEG does not rule out a seizure disorder.
2. A patient with focal slow, sharp, or spike activity on EEG does not necessarily have seizures.
3. All deliriums are accompanied by EEG slowing in comparison with the patient's baseline.
4. All patients with an unexplained acute change in mental status should have an EEG.
5. A normal EEG does not rule out dementia.
6. Brain mapping is not easier than regular EEG, it is harder.

rectly, it is crucial that the physician understands their specificity, sensitivity, and limitations (Table 5-5). When used correctly, such tests offer exciting opportunities to better define the pathophysiology of psychiatric illness.

REFERENCES

American Academy of Neurology, Therapeutics and Technology Assessment Subcommittee: Assessment: EEG brain mapping. Neurology 39:1100–1101, 1989

Blackwood DH, Whalley LJ, Christie JE, et al: Changes in auditory P3 event-related potential in schizophrenia and depression. Br J Psychiatry 150:154–160, 1987

Bridgers SL: Epileptiform abnormalities discovered on electroencephalographic screening of psychiatric patients. Arch Neurol 44:312–316, 1987

Bridgers SL: Ambulatory cassette electroencephalography of psychiatric patients. Arch Neurol 45:71–74, 1988

Bridgers SL, Ebersole JS: The clinical utility of ambulatory cassette EEG. Neurology 35:166–173, 1985

Bridgers SL, Wade PB, Ebersole JS: Estimating the importance of epileptiform abnormalities discovered on cassette electroencephalographic monitoring. Arch Neurol 46:1077–1079, 1989

Bridgman PA, Malamut MA, Sperling MD, et al: Memory during subclinical hippocampal seizures. Neurology 39:853–856, 1989

Bromfield E, Sato S, McBurney J, et al: Letter to the editor. Clin Electroencephalogr 20:VII–VIII, 1989

Broughton R, Dunham W, Newman J, et al: Ambulatory 24-hour sleep wake monitoring in narcolepsy-cataplexy compared to matched controls. Electroencephalogr Clin Neurophysiol 70:473–481, 1988

Busse EW: Electroencephalography, in Alzheimer's Disease. Edited by Reisberg B. New York, Free Press, 1983, pp 231–236

Courchesne E, Kilman BA, Galambos R, et al: Autism: processing of novel auditory information assessed by event-related brain potentials. Electroencephalogr Clin Neurophysiol 59:238–248, 1984

Desai B, Whitman S, Bouffard DA: The role of the EEG in epilepsy of long duration. Epilepsia 29:601–606, 1988

Drury I, Klass DW, Westmoreland BF, et al: An acute syndrome with psychiatric symptoms and EEG abnormalities. Neurology 35:911–914, 1985

Duffy FH: Clinical value of topographic mapping and quantified neurophysiology. Arch Neurol 46:1133–1134, 1989

Duffy FH, Burchfiel JL, Lombroso CT: Brain electrical activity mapping (BEAM): a method for extending the clinical utility of EEG and evoked potential data. Ann Neurol 5:309–321, 1979

Duncan CC, Perlstein WM, Morihisa JM: The P300 metric in schizophrenia: effects of probability and modality. Electroencephalogr Clin Neurophysiol [Suppl] 40:670–674, 1987

Ebersole JS, Bridgers SL: Direct comparison of 3- and 8-channel ambulatory cassette EEG with intensive inpatient monitoring. Neurology 35:846–854, 1985

Faux SF, Shenton ME, McCarley RW, et al: P200 topographic alterations in schizophrenia: evidence for left temporal-centroparietal region deficits. Electroencephalogr Clin Neurophysiol [Suppl] 40:681–687, 1987

Garber HJ, Weilburg JB, Duffy FH, et al: Clinical use of topographic brain electrical activity mapping in psychiatry. J Clin Psychiatry 50:205–211, 1989

Gastaut H, Tassinari CA: Epilepsies, in Handbook of EEG and Clinical Neurophysiology, Vol 13. Edited by Remond A. Amsterdam, Elsevier, 1975

Gordon E, Kraiuhin C, Kelly P, et al: A neurophysiological study of somatization disorder. Compr Psychiatry 27:295–301, 1986

Gummow LJ, Dustman RE, Keaney RP: Cerebrovascular accident alters P300 event-related potential characteristics. Electroencephalogr Clin Neurophysiol 63:128–137, 1986

Hansch EC, Syndulko K, Cohen SN, et al: Cognition in Parkinson's disease: an event-related potential perspective. Ann Neurol 11:599–607, 1982

Hauser P, Devinsky O, De Bellis M, et al: Benzodiazepine withdrawal delirium with catatonic features: occurrence in patients with partial seizure disorders. Arch Neurol 46:696–699, 1989

Hooshmand H, Beckner E, Radfar F: Technical and clinical aspects of topographic brain mapping. Clin Electroencephalogr 20:235–247, 1989

Hughes JR, Miller JK: Eye movements on brain maps. Clin Electroencephalogr 19:210–213, 1988

Hughes JR, Zak SM: EEG and clinical changes in patients with slowly growing brain tumors. Arch Neurol 44:540–543, 1987

Jerrett SA, Corsak J: Clinical utility of topographic EEG brain mapping. Clin Electroencephalogr 19:134–143, 1988

Kaszniak AW, Garron DC, Fox JH, et al: Cerebral atrophy, EEG slowing, age, education and cognitive functioning in suspected dementia. Neurology 29:1273–1279, 1979

Kohrman MH, Sugioka C, Huttenlocher PR, et al: Inter- versus intra-subject variance in topographic mapping of the electroencephalogram. Clin Electroencephalogr 20:248–253, 1989

Kuroiwa Y, Celesia GC: Clinical significance of periodic EEG patterns. Arch Neurol 37:1359–1361, 1980

Kutcher SP, Blackwood DH, St. Clair D, et al: Auditory P300 in borderline personality disorder and schizophrenia. Arch Gen Psychiatry 44:645–650, 1987

Landolt H: Serial electroencephalographic investigations during psychotic episodes in epileptic patients and during schizophrenic attacks, in Lectures on Epilepsy. Edited by de Haas L. New York, Elsevier, 1958

Lee SI: Nonconvulsive status epilepticus: ictal confusion in late life. Arch Neurol 42:778–781, 1985

Lee S, Buchsbaum MS: Topographic mapping of EEG artifacts. Clin Electroencephalogr 18:61–67, 1987

Leroy RF, Ebersole JS: An evaluation of ambulatory, cassette EEG monitoring, I: montage design. Neurology 33:1–7, 1983

Lieb JP, Walsh GO, Babb TL, et al: A comparison of EEG seizure patterns recorded with surface and depth electrodes in patients with temporal lobe epilepsy. Epilepsia 17:137–160, 1976

McNamara ME, Nordin NL, Shriner RL, et al: Quantification of sleep in episodic alterations of consciousness: daytime sleepiness in patients with funny spells (abstract). Presented at the North Eastern regional sleep meeting, White Plains, NY, March 31, 1989

Michalewski HJ, Prasher DK, Starr A: Latency variability and temporal interrelationships of the auditory event-related potentials (N1, P2, N2, and P3) in normal subjects. Electroencephalogr Clin Neurophysiol 65:59–71, 1986

Morstyn R, Duffy FH, McCarley RW: Altered P300 topography in schizophrenia. Arch Gen Psychiatry 40:729–734, 1983

Muller HF, Schartz G: Electroencephalograms and autopsy findings in geropsychiatry. J Gerontol 33:504–513, 1978

Niedermeyer E, Krauss GL, Peyser CF: The electro-encephalogram and mental activation. Clin Electroencephalogr 20:215–227, 1989

Nowack WJ, Janati A, Metzer WS, et al: The anterior temporal electrode in the EEG of the adult. Clin Electroencephalogr 19:199–204, 1988

Nuwer MR: Quantitative EEG, 1: techniques and problems of frequency analysis and topographic mapping. J Clin Neurophysiol 5:1–43, 1988

Nuwer MR: Uses and abuses of brain mapping. Arch Neurol 46:1134–1136, 1989

Nuwer MR, Jordan SE: The centrifugal effect and other spatial artifacts of topographic EEG mapping. J Clin Neurophysiol 4:321–326, 1987

Oken BS, Chiappa KH, Salinsky M: Computerized EEG frequency analysis: sensitivity and specificity in patients with focal lesions. Neurology 39:1281–1287, 1989

Pakalnis A, Drake ME, Kuruvilla J, et al: Forced normalization: acute psychosis after seizure control in seven patients. Arch Neurol 44:289–292, 1987

Pfefferbaum A, Horvath TB, Roth WT, et al: Auditory brain stem and cortical evoked potentials in schizophrenia. Biol Psychiatry 15:209–223, 1980

Polich J, Ehlers CL, Otis S, et al: P300 latency reflects the degree of cognitive decline in dementing illness. Electroencephalogr Clin Neurophysiol 63:138–144, 1986

Pritchard WS: Cognitive event-related potentials in schizophrenics. Psychol Bull 100:43–66, 1986

Reeve A, Rose DF, Weinberger DR: Magnetoencephalography: applications in psychiatry. Arch Gen Psychiatry 46:573–576, 1989

Reite M, Teale P, Goldstein L, et al: Late auditory magnetic sources may differ in the left hemisphere of schizophrenic patients: a preliminary report. Arch Gen Psychiatry 46:565–572, 1989

Rodin E, Khabbazeh Z, Twitty G, et al: The cognitive evoked potential in epilepsy patients. Clin Electroencephalogr 20:176–182, 1989

Romani A, Merello S, Gozzoli L, et al: P300 and CT scans in patients with chronic schizophrenia. Br J Psychiatry 151:506–513, 1987

Rose DF, Sato S, Smith PD, et al: Localization of magnetic interictal discharges in temporal lobe epilepsy. Ann Neurol 22:348–354, 1987

Rosenberg C, Nudleman K, Starr A: Cognitive evoked potentials (P300) in early Huntington's disease. Arch Neurol 42:984–987, 1985

Roth WT, Pfefferbaum A, Horvath TB, et al: P3 reduction in auditory evoked potentials of schizophrenics. Electroencephalogr Clin Neurophysiol 49:497–505, 1980

Sammaritano M, de Lobiniere A, Andermann F, et al: False lateralization by surface EEG of seizure onset in patients with temporal lobe epilepsy and gross focal cerebral lesions. Ann Neurol 21:361–369, 1987

Scherg M, Von Crammon D: Two bilateral sources of the late AEP as identified by a spatio-temporal dipole model. Electroencephalogr Clin Neurophysiol 62:32–44, 1985

Shagass C, Roemer RA, Josiassen RC: Some quantitative EEG findings in unmedicated and medicated major depressives. Neuropsychobiology 19:169–175, 1988

Siebelink BM, Bakker DJ, Binnie CD, et al: Psychological effects of subclinical epileptiform EEG discharges in children, II: general intelligence tests. Epilepsy Research 2:117–121, 1988

Silverman DA: The anterior temporal electrode and the ten-twenty system. Electroencephalogr Clin Neurophysiol 12:735–737, 1960

Smith DB, Sidman RD, Flanigin H, et al: A reliable method for localizing deep intracranial sources of the EEG. Neurology 35:1702–1707, 1985

Spencer SS, Williamson PD, Bridgers SL, et al: Reliability and accuracy of localization by scalp ictal EEG. Neurology 35:1567–1575, 1988

Sperling MR, Engel J: Electroencephalographic recording from the temporal lobes: a comparison of ear, anterior temporal, and nasopharyngeal electrodes. Ann Neurol 17:510–513, 1985

Stefanatos GA, Green GGR, Ratcliff GG: Neurophysiological evidence of auditory channel anomalies in developmental dysphasia. Arch Neurol 46:871–875, 1989

Struve FA: Lithium-specific pathological electro-encephalographic changes: a successful replication of earlier investigative results. Clin Electroencephalogr 18:46–53, 1987

Sutherling WW, Barth DS: Neocortical propagation in temporal lobe spike foci on magnetoencephalography and electroencephalography. Ann Neurol 25:373–381, 1989

Sutherling WW, Crandall PH, Darcey TM, et al: The magnetic and electrical fields agree with intracranial localizations of somatosensory cortex. Neurology 38:1705–1714, 1988

Sutton S, Ruchkin DS: The late positive complex: advances and new problems. Ann NY Acad Sci 423:1–21, 1984

Terzano MG, Parrino L, Mazzucchi A, et al: Confusional states with periodic lateralized epileptiform discharges (PLEDS): a peculiar epileptic syndrome in the elderly. Epilepsia 27:446–457, 1986

Tomson T, Svanborg E, Wedlund JE: Nonconvulsive status epilepticus: high incidence of complex partial status. Epilepsia 27:276–285, 1986

Veldhuizen R, Binnie CD, Beintema DJ: The effect of sleep deprivation on the EEG in epilepsy. Electroencephalogr Clin Neurophysiol 55:505–512, 1983

Wagner M, Kurtz G, Engel RR: Normal P300 in acute schizophrenics during a continuous performance test. Biol Psychiatry 6:792–795, 1989

Williams GW, Luders HO, Brickner A, et al: Interobserver variability in EEG interpretation. Neurology 35:1714–1719, 1985

Williamson PD, Spencer DD, Spencer SS, et al: Complex seizures of frontal lobe origin. Ann Neurol 18:497–504, 1985

Zivin L, Ajmone-Marsan C: Incidence and prognostic significance of epileptiform activity in the EEG of nonepileptic subjects. Brain 91:751–777, 1968

Section II

Specific Syndromes and Disease Categories

Chapter 6

Psychiatric Aspects of Hematologic Disorders

Elisabeth J. Shakin, M.D.
Troy L. Thompson II, M.D.

In this chapter, we focus on hematologic disorders that affect people of various ages. Hemophilia, sickle cell disease, and thalassemia affect both children and young adults. We present hemophilia as a model for understanding the psychiatric aspects of other chronic hematologic disorders of childhood. Porphyria, vitamin B_{12} deficiency, folate deficiency, and the hyperviscosity syndrome are primarily diseases of adults; we present their clinical presentations, laboratory diagnosis, and treatment. Finally, we present two unusual hematologic problems with which psychiatrists should be familiar: psychogenic purpura (auto-erythrocyte sensitization) and anticoagulant malingering. We do not discuss hematologic malignancies in this chapter because the psychiatric issues in hematologic oncology are discussed elsewhere (Lesko et al. 1987). As the laboratory analysis and interpretation of clinical symptoms may be quite complicated in some of these disorders, the psychiatrist may need to work with other medical specialists, for example, hematologists, neurologists, and clinical pathologists.

The authors acknowledge the advice of David Agle, M.D., Samir Ballas, M.D., Margaret Hilgartner, M.D., Sandor Shapiro, M.D., and Mrs. Joan Tannebaum, and the technical assistance of Judith Ferko in the preparation of this chapter.

Table 6-1.   Components of psychosocial and educational programs for children with hemophilia and their families

- General counseling or guidance at time of diagnosis
- Groups such as self-help and support groups for parents
- Education for families about the disease itself, available services, encouragement of socialization, and prevention of isolation
- Marital counseling, including stress reduction
- Child care counseling, including appropriate interventions and level of protection versus overprotection
- Social services
- Liaison to schools and employers
- Adolescent counseling, including dating, sexual activity, education, and vocational planning
- HIV counseling, including sexual activity and information for spouses
- Psychiatric referral for psychotherapy, medications, pain management, and other treatments

Source.   Adapted from Handford and Mayes 1989; Simon 1989.

HEMOPHILIA

In the United States, hemophilia affects at least 25,000 males. Hemophilia A and B may account for up to 65% of patients with inherited coagulation disorders. Hemophilia A, or classic hemophilia, is caused by deficiency in the clotting activity of factor VIII. It is more common than hemophilia B, or Christmas disease, which is caused by a deficiency of the clotting activity of factor IX. The two cannot be distinguished clinically.

Since 1976, federal legislation has stipulated that hemophilia treatment center eligibility must include the provision of mental health services as part of a comprehensive multidisciplinary program, and that mental health services for hemophilia patients should include psychosocial support, financial counseling, and vocational programs (Table 6-1). Ideally, comprehensive programs should promote normal psychosocial development and prevent the development of major psychiatric disorders (primary prevention), should identify and intervene at early presentations of emotional dysfunction (secondary prevention), and should provide specific treatment for established psychiatric disorders to prevent complications (Agle 1984; Agle and Heine, in press). Recent evidence suggests that younger hemophilia patients (ages 18–24 years) generally function better emotionally than their older counterparts (over age 35 years) who did not have the benefit of comprehensive care, including mental health interventions, during their childhood and teenage years (Hernandez et al. 1989).

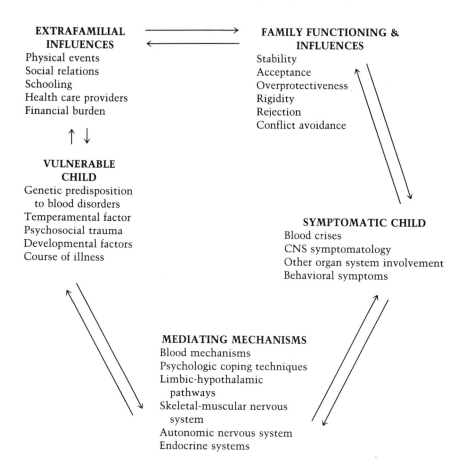

Figure 6-1. Open systems model for approaching patients with a blood disorder. Reprinted with permission from Mattsson A, Kim SP: Blood disorders. Psychiatr Clin North Am 5:345–356, 1982.

Hemophilia is a chronic, life-threatening disorder. An open-systems model helps conceptualize the psychosocial impact of this illness on children and their families (Figure 6-1). A hemophilia patient often feels socially isolated, stigmatized, and defective. The patient's lifestyle and age-related life goals are virtually always interrupted or disrupted by the disease (Magrab 1985; Mattsson 1984; Mattsson and Kim 1982). (See also Chapter 14 for generic issues affecting families of medically ill children.)

Reports of "spontaneous" bleeding following increased stress, anxiety, and even presumptively positive emotional situations (e.g., school vacations) support the potential contribution of psychological factors to exacerbations of hemophilia. These reports are generally anecdotal, and the effect of stress on bleeding episodes has not been rigorously demonstrated. The pathophysiological mechanisms of this phenomenon are not yet known (Agle 1964; Agle and Heine, in press; Browne et al. 1960; Mattsson and Gross 1966a). Furthermore, even when patients have comparable disease severity, the use of antihemophilic factor infusions can vary considerably (Handford et al. 1980). Hypnosis and psychotherapy have been used to decrease anxiety and have generally resulted in decreased bleeding (Lucas 1975) and in decreased blood product usage (Handford et al. 1980; LaBaw 1975; LeBaron and Zeltzer 1984; Lichstein and Eakin 1985; Lucas 1965; Swirsky-Sacchetti and Margolis 1986).

Disease-Related Complications

Hemophilia is inherited through a recessive X-linked gene and is transmitted from asymptomatic carrier mothers to their children. Therefore, daughters of carrier mothers have a 50% chance of becoming carriers, whereas sons have a 50% chance of inheriting the disease. In patients with no family history of the disease, a spontaneous mutation in the mother is thought to have occurred (Hilgartner et al. 1985; Mattsson and Kim 1982).

With mild factor deficiencies, excessive bleeding is only expected with surgery, dental extractions, or major trauma. With severe deficiencies, recurrent hemorrhages occur spontaneously or with minor trauma. Patients with severe deficiencies have less than 1% of either factor VIII or IX. These patients usually suffer repeated episodes of acute pain from bleeding into their large joints and muscles. Moreover, hemarthrosis often results in arthritis, producing chronic pain. The acute pain of bleeding episodes may respond to factor replacement. Treatment of chronic pain may include behavioral approaches, transcutaneous electrical nerve stimulators (TENS), analgesics, orthopedic rehabilitation, and possibly joint reconstruction (Choiniere and Melzack 1987; Holdredge and Cotta 1989; Roche et al. 1985; Varni 1981). When bleeding occurs into pharyngeal soft tissue or the central nervous system (CNS), emergency interventions may be necessary for the life-threatening complications of respiratory compromise or increased intracranial pressure. Before the era of factor replacement, crippling ar-

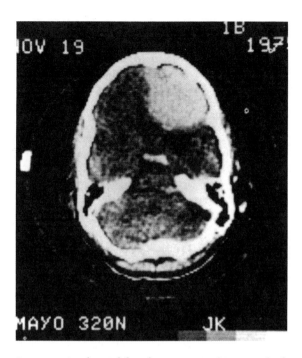

Figure 6-2. Computerized axial head tomogram (CT scan) of a 19-year-old male with factor VIII deficiency, showing a large right frontal hematoma. There was a right frontal skull fracture, and at surgery, the hematoma was found to be epidural in location. Reprinted with permission from Gilchrist GS, Piepgras DG: Neurologic complications in hemophilia, in Progress in Pediatric Hematology and Oncology, Vol 1: Hemophilia in Children. Edited by Hilgartner M, Pochedly C. Littleton, MA, PSG, 1976, pp 79–97. Copyright 1976, PSG Publishing Company.

thritis and early death, often secondary to CNS hemorrhage, were common with hemophilia (Figure 6-2). Primarily as a result of factor replacement therapy, the mean age of death for patients with hemophilia increased to 30.7 years in 1974 from 19.6 years in 1968 (S. Dietrich, 1979, personal communication to Hilgartner et al. 1985). Currently, in human immunodeficiency virus (HIV)–seronegative hemophilia patients, a normal life span can be expected (S. Shapiro, 1990, personal communication).

Additional complications may result from blood component therapy. Some patients develop an antibody or an inhibitor to the transfused factor. The presence of an inhibitor complicates treatment because infused factor concentrates are rapidly consumed (Hilgartner 1980; Hilgartner et al. 1985). Before 1985, exposure to pooled blood products often led to increased risk of exposure to hepatitis and HIV. However, these risks are almost nil with current screening methods for factor VIII. A new generation of factor IX products probably will be equally safe (S. Shapiro, 1990, personal communication).

Family Adaptation to Hemophilia

Early education and psychosocial support are crucial in preventing or lessening maladaptive coping in patients with hemophilia and their families. The early age at onset of hemophilia and the current emphasis on home care make family interventions especially important. Families experience stress at all stages of the disease, but stress may be greatest at the time of diagnosis (Reis et al. 1982). Mothers often have been criticized for becoming overprotective of their hemophiliac sons; they are afraid that their sons will fall, thereby causing an episode of bleeding. Each mother needs to learn more about the disease so that she will allow her child to explore his environment without incurring undue trauma. She will thus also lessen her guilt about having given birth to a hemophiliac son. Despite what is often an intense emotional situation, most mothers are able to remain calm and competent during events requiring home administration of blood products. On the other hand, fathers more often report feeling left out and helpless during such bleeding episodes. Although fathers may be present less often during clinic visits, they should be encouraged to remain involved as male role models for their sons and as emotional supports for their families (Meijer 1980–81; Salk et al. 1972). Despite education, however, a certain amount of fear, anxiety, and anticipatory grief over the child's disability and possible early death from disease complications is to be expected (Agle and Mattsson 1968). After the death of a child with hemophilia, the need for support to the surviving family should be assessed, and services should be made available when deemed necessary.

In some dysfunctional families, parents may reject or neglect the hemophiliac child because of their own limitations or because of rigid, dysfunctional relationships. Hemophiliac children may serve as scapegoats or as a way to avoid other marital conflicts (Mattsson 1984; Mattsson and Kim 1982). In extreme situations, breakup of the marriage resulted from the birth of a hemophiliac child (Salk et al. 1972).

Male siblings should be given time to ventilate their concerns about their hemophiliac brother(s) and should neither be neglected nor burdened with the responsibility of achieving what an impaired brother could not accomplish, either because of his physical limitations or because of his premature death from acquired immunodeficiency syndrome (AIDS). Female siblings should discuss and hopefully learn to integrate their potential carrier status with future choices about childbearing (Agle 1964; Handford and Mayes 1989; Mattsson 1984; Mattsson and Gross 1966a; Mattsson et al. 1971). Finally, the attention given to the child with hemophilia may divert parental attention away from the needs of siblings of both sexes.

Families also may be affected by financial limitations associated with the disease and by the need to live near treatment facilities. Although New York City and Rochester, New York, are exceptions, in most cities Medicaid, Social Security Insurance, and Crippled Children's Services will only reimburse parents for blood factor replacement given in emergency room settings, not for factor given at home (Hilgartner et al. 1985). The disease may affect choice of family size, choice of job based on its location or schedule, the numbers of hours worked by parents, whether both parents work outside the home, etc. Finally, insurance discrimination may create an additional financial obstacle for families with hemophiliac members (Handford and Mayes 1989), especially with the advent of AIDS.

Special Issues for Children With Hemophilia

Bleeding episodes that require transfusion often occur by age 4 years. Young children do not understand their illness or the rationale for treatment and may be especially frightened by immobilization with orthotic devices, separation from their families because of hospitalizations, and pain from the disease and medical treatments. In response, some children may deny pain to avoid transfusions (Holdredge and Cotta 1989). As hemophiliac children grow older, they are able to understand more about the disease and hopefully can learn to report trauma earlier, thereby allowing prompt home intervention with factor replacement.

Home treatment has significantly decreased morbidity and decreased the number of necessary absences from school. Older children should be taught that pain is not a punishment for their real or imagined misdeeds, a common illness-associated fantasy. Older children also are able to participate more in their home treatment.

Most hemophiliac children do not differ from the general population of children on psychometric measures (Steinhausen 1976), and some actually perform slightly better intellectually, possibly because of more parental attention and a shift from physical to intellectual pursuits due to their physical vulnerability (Agle and Mattsson 1970; Handford et al. 1986; Hilgartner et al. 1985; Mattsson and Gross 1966a). The incidence and prevalence rates of major psychopathology in hemophiliac children are not yet known, and as a result, rates of psychopathology in this population cannot be compared with rates in other pediatric populations.

Special Issues for Teenagers With Hemophilia

Teenagers have the difficult task of trying to integrate the normal developmental tasks of adolescence with a realistic sense of vulnerability from their disease. Their ability to work, earn a living, and perform sexually are important in the development of their masculinity and self-esteem. Fears, sometimes unrealistic, regarding these issues are not uncommon.

Although most hemophiliac teenagers are able to cope fairly well, extreme passivity and dependency on the one hand and extreme risk-taking on the other hand have been reported as examples of poor coping. Poor coping in the adolescent with hemophilia has been related to how well the child's mother has been able to master her emotional reactions to his illness, including her sense of guilt (Mattsson and Gross 1966b). In the risk-taker, daredevil acts are often thought to be a counterphobic response: the patient is denying his extreme fear of hurting himself by placing himself in situations in which he is likely to be hurt (Agle 1964; Handford and Mayes 1989; Mattsson 1984; Mattsson and Gross 1966a; Mattsson et al. 1971).

Specific Psychiatric Issues

Several warning signs that should prompt formal medical and psychiatric evaluation for hemophiliac patients of any age include over- or underutilization of factor transfusions; bleeding that is excessive considering the patient's blood level of factor VIII or IX; behavioral problems, psychiatric symptoms, or medical illness in family members; inappropriate use of drugs, alcohol, or analgesics; and sudden changes in the use of medical resources (Simon 1984). For example, patients with equally severe disease tend to use similar amounts of factor products over a month; a marked deviation from usual amounts should prompt further investigation. In addition, the patient who gives himself excessive factor transfusions for a single bleeding episode or whose use of factor products markedly changes over time should be evaluated for his understanding of appropriate treatment and for anxiety that could be interfering with his ability to stop transfusions after an appropriate amount of factor product.

For patients with hemophilia who develop major psychiatric disorders, the full spectrum of interventions from outpatient individual therapy or family therapy to psychiatric hospitalization should be considered. For example, group therapy with parents of hemophiliac children often is a useful mode of education and a forum for ventilation of emotional concerns (Mattsson and Agle 1972). Although antidepressant and antipsychotic medications are not contraindicated, recommended dosages may need to be decreased in patients with impaired renal or hepatic function. The clinician must be aware, however, that sedation, possibly leading to falls, may result from the use of these medications in conjunction with analgesic medications for pain control (Jonas 1977, 1989). The monoamine oxidase inhibitors (MAOIs) should be reserved for exceptional situations because they can potentially cause hypertensive crises with dietary indiscretions or in combination with narcotics. Such crises are associated with increased risks of intracranial hemorrhage in patients with bleeding disorders (Handford and Mayes 1989).

Analgesics and benzodiazepines are not necessarily associated with drug dependency and addiction in patients with hemophilia (Brunner et al. 1982). Patients at increased risk for drug abuse tend to be older and to have had more psychiatric hospitalizations and more suicide attempts by overdose. Those who do abuse drugs tend to be polysubstance abusers (Jonas 1989). A complete history of drugs obtained from all sources, including over-the-counter medications and street drugs, should be obtained as part of any consultation to prevent or manage withdrawal states.

Finally, a change in a hemophiliac patient's mental status should precipitate a neurologic workup for CNS hemorrhage and/or CNS complications of AIDS. Of hemophiliac patients with intracranial hemorrhage, 50% have no known history of head trauma. Although intracranial hemorrhage is an infrequent event, the current mortality rate from intracranial hemorrhage is about 30% among hemophiliac patients (Gilchrist et al. 1989). If death does not occur, residual neurologic complications may include seizures, cognitive impairment, aphasia, and hydrocephalus (Handford and Mayes 1989; Mattsson and Kim 1982). Neuropsychiatric evaluation may assist in differentiating early organic mental syndromes from functional psychiatric disorders and in quantifying cognitive impairments. A computed tomography (CT) scan or magnetic resonance imaging (MRI) scan of the brain may provide a definitive diagnosis. However, conventional skull X rays may detect linear fractures missed on CT scans (Gilchrist et al. 1989).

Other Issues Related to AIDS

About 70–90% of patients with moderate and severe hemophilia A and about 30–50% of those with moderate and severe hemophilia B who regularly used blood products before 1985 are now thought to be HIV seropositive (S. Shapiro, 1990, personal communication). Of those patients with severe deficiencies of factor VIII, 6% now have AIDS in addition to their hemophilia, and it is estimated that the large majority of HIV-seropositive hemophiliac patients will probably develop AIDS (Jason et al. 1989). Therefore, increased morbidity and mortality from opportunistic infections and the CNS complications of AIDS can be anticipated in many of these individuals (Agle 1989; Levine 1985). (See Chapter 7 for details on psychiatric aspects of HIV infection.)

Although most families of hemophiliac patients are coping well with the realistic fear of developing AIDS, some families have significant difficulties carrying out their day-to-day responsibilities and experiencing pleasure. Parents must cope with increased anxiety and social problems because not only does their child have hemophilia, he has also tested seropositive for HIV. This situation may increase overprotection by the parents and, secondarily, increase the child's dependency, rebellion, or problems with self-esteem, especially among adolescents. In addition, patients with hemophilia who are frightened of AIDS are at increased risk for hypochondriasis and medical noncompliance. The patient's emotional stability is further threatened by his awareness of his increased vulnerability and the social ostracism associated with HIV seropositivity (Agle 1989; Agle et al. 1987; Mayes et al. 1988).

Sexual counseling is now an additional responsibility for the mental health team in hemophilia treatment centers. While some patients with hemophilia who are HIV-positive have chosen abstinence, either as a result of altruism or because of preexisting difficulties with sexual intimacy, other patients continue to engage in risky behaviors that may transmit the virus to others. Engaging in risky behaviors may relate to multiple factors, including denial, a wish not to be further stigmatized and not to feel defective, decreased ability to process information (e.g., AIDS dementia), lack of concern for the welfare of others, anger that they contracted AIDS, a "retaliatory" wish to transmit it to others, and cultural biases or sexual preferences regarding condom use (Agle 1989; Levine 1984). Recently, the Executive Board of Hemophilia Region II Centers (New York, New Jersey, and Puerto Rico) recommended that staff breach confidentiality with HIV-positive hemophiliac patients to inform their sexual partners of their risk status (Simon 1989).

The already complex staff-patient relationship for hemophiliac patients and their families may be further stressed by the staff's guilt over having prescribed HIV-infected products, staff discomfort in confronting sexual issues, and staff concerns about contracting the virus themselves. The patients' anger and fear about having been given infected products are only intensified by the inability to seek treatment elsewhere and lead to mistrust in the staff who had reassured them about the safety of blood products. The tasks of the consulting psychiatrist now include not only evaluating patients with hemophilia and their families, but also working with staff and physicians concerning several AIDS-related issues, including HIV-related distress and psychiatric complications, safe-sex counseling, terminal illness, and death (Agle 1989; Faulstick 1987).

SICKLE CELL DISEASE

Sickle cell disease refers to the gamut of conditions that result from having sickle hemoglobin (e.g., sickle cell anemia, sickle cell–hemoglobin C, sickle cell–beta-thalassemia). These conditions are also referred to as the sickle cell syndromes. The World Health Organization has estimated that sickle cell anemia (SCA) is responsible for the deaths of at least 80,000 children worldwide each year (Huntsman 1985). The significant morbidity and early mortality of SCA result in a multitude of psychosocial problems for patients with SCA and their families. Because of its wide prevalence, our discussion will focus on SCA; the issues discussed are common to all of the sickle cell diseases.

The lay population is often unaware of the distinction between sickle cell trait and sickle cell anemia. The gene for sickle cell hemoglobin must be inherited from both parents to produce sickle cell anemia; the carrier state (sickle cell trait) results when the gene is inherited from one parent (Huntsman 1985). Sickle cell carriers who mistakenly think they have SCA often experience unnecessary anxiety and impaired self-esteem and may make unwarranted decisions regarding life-style, marriage, and reproduction (Whitten and Nishiura 1985). Physicians may wish to ask about this misconception in siblings of sickle cell patients. More widespread public education regarding the difference between sickle cell trait and SCA is important for families who are unaware of the distinction and its implications and who may benefit from genetic counseling.

SCA is characterized by anemia and its sequelae, painful or vaso-occlusive crises, and organ damage. *Aplastic crises* result from reduced erythropoietic activity of the marrow which may follow infections; shortened red cell survival caused by increased red cell fragility can make these crises life threatening, especially if the hemoglobin drops precipitously. *Vaso-occlusive crises* result from the obstruction of vasculature by the sickled cells. Patients with SCA have sickled red cells at all times, but have enough normal red cells for blood to flow. Under certain conditions, including dehydration, infection, low temperature, other physical stressors, and possibly anxiety, the proportion of sickled cells increases, leading to vascular occlusion. For most crises, however, the exact cause cannot be determined. Organs normally supplied by the occluded vasculature undergo ischemia and necrosis. Pain and organ damage result. The lungs, kidneys, bones, CNS, and the penis (possibly leading to priapism) are some of the possible sites of organ damage.

The management of patients of all ages with SCA includes hydration, broad-spectrum antibiotic treatment for infections, analgesics and behavioral techniques for pain management, and transfusions for aplastic crises or severe anemia secondary to increased hemolysis. Problems seen within the first year of life include dactylitis (painful and swollen hands and feet) and increased susceptibility to infections (Powars 1975; Whitten and Nishiura 1985).

Older children with SCA may be unable to concentrate their urine, causing isosthenuria; as a result, they often drink large amounts of fluid, sometimes resulting in bed-wetting. Enuresis has been reported in as many as 45% of 8- to 11-year-olds with SCA (Hurtig and White 1986). Damage to the CNS from cerebrovascular accidents may be associated with intellectual impairment. Damage to the retina may result in progressive loss of sight; this loss occurs in children with SCA who are less than 10 years old (Mattsson and Kim 1982), but is more common in patients with hemoglobin sickle cell (sickle cell–hemoglobin C) disease (Ballas et al. 1982). In addition, physicians should be alert to the possibility of growth retardation and delayed puberty in children with SCA. However, one prospective cohort study did not find significant differences in physical growth in children with SCA (Kramer et al. 1978).

Functioning of SCA Patients

Although most children with SCA have no impairments in intelligence, about 5% do suffer cerebrovascular accidents that lead to decreased intellectual function (Whitten and Nishiura 1985). Intellectually impaired patients with SCA often have accompanying motor and sensory dysfunction (Powars 1975). In addition to cerebrovascular events, other factors may play a role in poor academic achievement in patients with SCA; these include socioeconomic factors, family dynamics, physical limitations such as increased fatigue, and absences from school. However, even in children matched for age, race, sex, and socioeconomic status, children with SCA have impaired reading and spelling skills (Fowler et al. 1988). Visuomotor and attentional deficits were greater in older children with SCA; however, the physical severity of their SCA did not correlate with their achievement scores or neuropsychological functioning.

Chronic microvascular insults without gross cerebrovascular accidents may result in subtle neurological deficits, thereby contributing to decreased school performance. In addition, the incidence of crossdominance is increased in children with sickle cell disease (Leavell and Ford 1983). These findings are important since standard IQ tests (e.g., Wechsler Intelligence Scale for Children) do not show significant differences between children with SCA and their siblings without SCA (Chodorkoff and Whitten 1963). The greater sensitivity of MRI over CT may help provide an explanation for SCA-related intellectual problems.

Psychosocial Issues in Children With SCA and Their Families

Many issues of families and children coping with SCA are generic to chronic illness and have already been addressed in the discussion of hemophilia. Stress from SCA can result from the diagnosis, the treatment, and the individual family's response (Whitten and Nishiura 1985). In contrast to hemophilia, most patients with SCA are managed by private physicians; therefore, comprehensive care, including specialized psychosocial support and education, often is not available or offered. Overall, however, when studies have controlled for age, race, and socioeconomic status, children with SCA do not differ from healthy children on measures of social and personal adjustment (Kumar et al. 1976; Lemanek et al. 1986). In one study that used several self-report measures of anxiety and depression, physically healthy siblings of children with SCA were more vulnerable to depression than their brother or sister with SCA, especially if the affected child or the affected child's mother had increased psychological distress (Treiber et al. 1987). Therefore, awareness of psychosocial distress in one family member may serve to alert the clinician to the possibility of distress in other family members.

Children may fear that they will be abandoned during hospitalizations. Their sense of control over their disease and developing self-esteem also are threatened by the unpredictable course of sickle cell crises (Whitten and Fischhoff 1974). Growth retardation, delayed puberty, and the inability to compete physically with their peers may lead to children with SCA being teased by their peers and treated as if they were much younger (Whitten and Fischhoff 1974; Whitten and Nishiura 1985). To foster adaptive emotional coping mechanisms, emotional concerns should be discussed both between and during crises, and the patient should return to the appropriate level of independence when crises have subsided.

Specific Psychosocial Issues in Adolescents With SCA

Adolescents with SCA are generally less satisfied with the appearance of their bodies and more withdrawn socially and have more symptoms of depression than adolescents without SCA (Morgan and Jackson 1986). Drug dependency, acting out, anxiety, and hypochondriasis have been observed in adolescents with SCA. Other adolescents with SCA do not regress but can be described as more mature and may have more adaptive coping skills than age-matched adolescents without SCA; in some cases, a form of compensatory pseudomaturity may develop (Hurtig and White 1986; Williams et al. 1983).

Specific Psychosocial Issues in Adults With SCA

Leavell and Ford (1983) did not demonstrate a specific personality type or psychiatric diagnosis in 16 adult patients with sickle cell disease. However, 2 patients had passive-aggressive traits and 1 patient was sociopathic. Their study population ranged in intelligence from 2 patients diagnosed as mentally retarded to 4 patients who obtained a college education. Increased numbers of environmental stressors were correlated positively with the subsequent development of sickle cell symptoms. In addition, as patients with sickle cell disease approach the age with which they associate death from their illness, they may become anxious, depressed, and preoccupied with death (Whitten and Fischhoff 1974).

Larger studies may yield more accurate prevalence rates for specific psychiatric disorders in the sickle cell population. The perception on the part of hospital staff members that these patients have more psychosocial problems than other medically ill populations may relate to the small percentage of SCA patients with more severe disease who are repeatedly hospitalized. This population accounts for about 6% of patients with sickle cell syndromes at our medical center in Philadelphia (S. Ballas, 1990, personal communication). Frequently hospitalized patients may be more manipulative and may be more at risk for problems with pain control and drug addiction, thereby further contributing to this misconception.

Pain Management in SCA

Painful sickle cell episodes may be severe enough to warrant the use of narcotics and hospitalization. At other times, crises can be managed at home with only aspirin or without medication (Whitten and Nishiura 1985). The severity of sickle cell disease and the clinical course of painful episodes cannot be reliably predicted (Benjamin 1989). Painful crises that do not have clear precipitants may include several specific signs and symptoms in children, such as fever, joint involvement, loss of bowel sounds, and abdominal rebound tenderness. In adults, however, less than 50% of such crises are associated with localized findings, and pain is often less well localized (Powars 1975). In younger children, pain often can be managed with the use of adjunctive measures alone, including local application of heat, increased ingestion of fluids, whirlpool treatments on the affected area, and emotional support (Powars 1975; Whitten and Fischhoff 1974).

Despite their pain, patients with SCA generally are encouraged to maintain as normal a life-style as possible. As a result, behavioral manifestations of pain may be deceiving. For example, if patients in acute pain are relatively stoic, their pain may be perceived as not severe;

however, if they cry and "carry on," staff members may believe they are acting immaturely or overdramatizing to procure narcotics (Whitten and Nishiura 1985). Staff members may inappropriately withhold or underprescribe narcotics in either of these circumstances. Staff members' fears of inducing iatrogenic addiction also may lead to inadequate treatment of pain (Benjamin 1989).

The question of malingering is often raised for patients with SCA. Despite this question, no objective means exists to distinguish malingering from a true crisis. In general, if any doubt exists, patients with SCA should be treated as if they were experiencing a true crisis. For example, rather than reflecting drug-seeking behavior, requests for specific drugs may reflect patients' desire to avoid drugs that they associate with drug abuse (e.g., morphine and methadone) and may reflect their past knowledge of which drug is most effective and has the fewest side effects for them. Routine dosages of analgesics are useful in reducing pain in 80% of patients with SCA (Benjamin 1989).

Some patients with SCA may be managed by clinicians who are overly concerned or preoccupied with iatrogenic addiction, have inadequate knowledge about pain and its management, and mistrust the patient's motives for requesting analgesics. Clinicians can avoid several common errors in treating pain in SCA patients. First, when patients are discharged from the emergency room or hospital, they should not be given the same dosage of oral medication that they were receiving parenterally. If so, they often will either return or seek help elsewhere because the equianalgesic dose of an oral narcotic is significantly higher than the parenteral dose. As a result, patients with SCA have been known to visit several emergency rooms in one night to achieve relief from pain. Second, patients should not be given prescriptions for narcotic analgesics to treat pain that might occur between visits. Occasionally, in patients known to have frequent crises, a limited supply of narcotic analgesics may be given to avoid repeated emergency room visits and to compensate for clinics that are not open 7 days a week. Third, patients who are aware of their caretakers' negative feelings about narcotic analgesics may avoid treatment until pain becomes unbearable. At this point, patients in acute pain may become acutely agitated and may escalate their behavior to procure medications for pain control. If clinicians teach patients about pain management and convey a supportive attitude, this phenomenon may decrease. Finally, although problems of physical addiction may occasionally result from the frequent use of narcotics for chronic pain management, drug abuse and dependence need not be consequences of the management of sickle cell disease (Benjamin 1989).

A combination of narcotic analgesics and non-narcotic drugs can have an additive or synergistic effect that facilitates pain management. Narcotics act on the CNS, whereas non-narcotics, such as acetaminophen and the nonsteroidal anti-inflammatory drugs act primarily on the peripheral nervous system, closer to the site that is generating pain. Ongoing education about the assessment and the management of pain is crucial if a rational approach is to be instituted for the treatment of patients with SCA. For a more detailed discussion of the rationale behind the following suggestions for pain management, see Benjamin (1989) and Goldberg et al. (1987).

1. A full history of the pain should include the following information: quality, intensity, location, precipitants (if any), prior episodes, duration of episodes, hospitalizations, and psychological factors contributing to the pain or exacerbated by it.
2. Treatment of the pain should occur early in the assessment to reduce secondary psychological and physical debilitation.
3. Start with aspirin or a nonsteroidal anti-inflammatory drug. Add a mild narcotic analgesic if pain remains uncontrolled. If pain becomes more severe or the above means are ineffective, switch to a stronger opiate (e.g., hydromorphone, morphine, or meperidine).
4. Combinations of drugs may reduce side effects. For example, hydroxyzine in combination with a narcotic may reduce nausea and vomiting while potentiating analgesia. Bowel regimens to prevent narcotic-induced constipation should be routine. The physician should be aware that narcotics (and also phenothiazines) may lower the seizure threshold (Mattsson and Kim 1982); patients with known past seizures or cerebrovascular accidents may need anticonvulsant coverage.
5. The starting dose is based on the patient's prior analgesic requirements, if any, and can be quite variable (e.g., 75 mg meperidine im in a patient who has never received narcotics). Medications should be dosed at frequent intervals at first (e.g., every 2 hours as needed) and then changed to an around-the-clock regimen. This regimen helps maintain plasma levels and avoids undermedicating patients. Undermedication commonly occurs when patients finally fall asleep with the first sign of relief from severe pain and then awake in extreme pain because medications were withheld while

they were sleeping. The role of continuous patient-controlled analgesia is still somewhat controversial in these patients.
6. Analgesic drug dosages should be tapered slowly. Routes of administration and dosage intervals should remain constant if at all possible.
7. Consider adjunctive measures to help decrease anxiety and improve pain control, e.g., thermal biofeedback, relaxation, and self-hypnosis (Cozzi et al. 1987; Thomas et al. 1984).
8. Consider adjunctive analgesics such as tricyclic antidepressants.

THALASSEMIA

Compared with the large number of people with thalassemia in Greece and Italy, thalassemia is relatively uncommon (1 in 40,000 live births) in the United States. In 1979, only 1,000 people had thalassemia in the United States. Most people with thalassemia are clustered in Chicago, San Francisco, and the Northeast. However, the incidence of thalassemia is expected to rise in the United States as a result of ongoing immigration from the Far East and Southeast Asia (Hilgartner et al. 1985). Thalassemia, like hemophilia, requires ongoing dependency on blood products and on the medical community. Similarly, psychosocial issues affecting people with thalassemia relate to their ability to cope with an inherited chronic childhood illness. However, the clinical course of thalassemia is quite different from hemophilia and typically results in a somewhat different set of psychological issues for these patients.

Disease-Related Issues in Patients With Thalassemia

Thalassemia is inherited via an autosomal recessive mode. Therefore, thalassemia must be transmitted by both parents to produce an affected child. If both parents are heterozygous for the affected gene, a male or female child has a 25% chance of being homozygous for the gene (severely affected), a 50% chance of being heterozygous (the carrier state), and a 25% chance of being born without the gene. The disease results from the inability to synthesize sufficiently either the alpha-, beta-, gamma-, and/or delta-globin chains of hemoglobin. For example, beta-thalassemia refers to the insufficient synthesis of beta-globin chains of hemoglobin in people who are homozygous for that specific gene. The beta variant is the most common type of thalassemia and is also called beta-thalassemia major, Mediterranean anemia, or Cooley's anemia.

Clinical symptoms in thalassemia result from intramedullary hemolysis and ineffective erythropoiesis. Beta-thalassemia typically presents within the first year of life with progressive anemia, irritability, poor appetite, and failure to thrive. In attempting to correct for this anemia, the body increases production of red blood cells in the bone marrow, liver, spleen, and lymph nodes. Increased bone marrow production may cause a distorted cranium, abnormal facial features, and fractures in long bones. Hypersplenism often leads to further destruction of blood components, and the resulting anemia may cause further decreased tissue oxygenation.

Repeated transfusions and splenectomy are the primary treatments for thalassemia. Maintaining an adequate hemoglobin level helps to prevent the development of facial distortion, but despite therapy, death typically occurs prematurely from recurrent infections following splenectomy and/or from cardiac failure. Multiple transfusions often lead to iron overload, which may result in discolored skin, cirrhosis, and multiple cardiac abnormalities, including arrhythmias, pericarditis, and heart failure. Iron overload also may cause endocrine dysfunction, including hypothyroidism, diabetes, hypoparathyroidism and hypocalcemia, and/or delayed growth and sexual development. Iron chelation with deferoxamine mesylate (Desferal) can retard the effects of iron overload and is available intravenously or via a subcutaneous infusion pump (Hilgartner et al. 1985). In addition to iron overload, multiple transfusions increase the risk of hepatitis, HIV exposure, AIDS, and the development of antibodies against multiple blood components, which may produce transfusion reactions (Pochedly 1986). Fortunately, the risk of exposure to hepatitis and HIV has been considerably reduced with current screening practices. Bone marrow transplantation is the most recent advance in the treatment of patients with thalassemia. Gene therapy remains at the investigational level.

As a result of the medical complications of thalassemia and its treatment, clinicians might expect a spectrum of associated organic mental syndromes. However, these syndromes have not been well documented in the literature, possibly because of the relatively small number of experts in this field, the small number of patients with the disorder in this country, and the earlier death of these patients, especially before the introduction of deferoxamine mesylate in the 1970s.

Depressed verbal IQs have been noted in some children with thalassemia, and it is unclear whether this phenomenon is secondary to cerebral effects of anemia or whether cognitive impairment may be a result of cerebral iron deposition (Sherman et al. 1985). Psychiatric symptoms also might result from hypothyroidism or other types of endocrine dysfunction in these patients. Psychiatric syndromes resulting from endocrine dysfunction are discussed in more detail by O'Shanick and colleagues (1987).

Psychosocial Issues of Patients With Thalassemia and Their Families

Patients with thalassemia and their families perceive day-to-day emotional stress as their second major concern, outranked only by their concern with financial burdens imposed by the disease. Complaints about the lack of convenient routine medical care for this condition are also commonplace (Giordano 1985; Hilgartner et al. 1985). The emotional stresses that these families experience may be caused by many uncertainties, including concerns about new treatment outcomes, unpredictable life expectancies for affected children, and possible genetic transmission to future offspring. Families at risk for the disease often are eager to be screened once they are made aware of the possible genetic consequences of the carrier state (Rowley et al. 1985). Prenatal diagnosis using amniocentesis and fetoscopy is available but is associated with increased risk of fetal morbidity and mortality. The majority of families with affected children appear to resolve their uncertainties by choosing not to conceive any more children (Hilgartner et al. 1985). It is unclear what impact the advent of chorionic villi sampling and percutaneous umbilical blood sampling will have on such decision making.

Communication and cooperation among family members are important sources of support within these families. For example, concern about depression in a wife or mother, which is fairly common because of guilty feelings for having transmitted the disease, will optimally lead to increased support from the family and sometimes to an outside referral for psychotherapy or formal support. As with the initial reports on hemophilia, there has been little documented research about how fathers of thalassemic children typically cope with having transmitted the disease. However, studies have described depression, anxiety, and issues of impaired self-esteem and body image in affected children (Hilgartner et al. 1985; Mattsson and Kim 1982). As with hemophilia, extreme passivity and unrealistic levels of denial have been described in some thalassemic adolescents (Becker et al. 1980). Finally, there is one report of a family case study linking bipolar affective disorder and thalassemia minor (Joffe et al. 1986).

PORPHYRIAS

The porphyrias are a heterogeneous group of inherited disorders of the synthesis of the heme portion of hemoglobin. The porphyrins are intermediate metabolites in the synthesis pathway (Figure 6-3) that leads to heme formation by the addition of iron to protoporphyrin IX. Deficiencies of the associated enzymes or partial blocks in this pathway lead to the accumulation of porphyrins and their precursors. Despite this, total heme production remains normal.

Although porphyrins can be synthesized in virtually all cells, in the porphyrias, abnormal porphyrins are synthesized in the liver and bone marrow. The site of synthesis is used in the diagnostic nomenclature to subdivide the porphyrias into the erythropoietic, hepatic, and erythrohepatic porphyrias (Table 6-2). Of the multiple types of porphyrias, only three of the four hepatic porphyrias have been associated with neuropsychiatric findings: acute intermittent porphyria, hereditary coproporphyria, and variegate porphyria. The term *latent porphyria* is used to describe patients who have biochemical abnormalities but no clinical symptoms (Goldberg et al. 1983; Meyer 1980; Robinson 1977); this condition explains why patients may not have a positive family history even though genetic transmission is autosomal dominant (Lishman 1987a).

Clinical Presentations

Clinically, the hepatic porphyrias are characterized by acute, life-threatening attacks that typically include abdominal pain and a variety of neuropsychiatric symptoms. Such attacks do not occur in the other porphyrias. Alcohol, various medications, pregnancy, menstruation, infections, and decreased calorie intake (e.g., dieting or fasting) can precipitate attacks in acute intermittent porphyria, hereditary coproporphyria, and variegate porphyria. Barbiturates, griseofulvin, and the sulfonamides are the most commonly cited medication precipitants (Table 6-3) (Jefferson and Marshall 1981a; Meyer 1980; Robinson 1977).

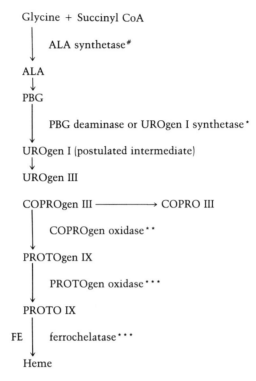

Figure 6-3. Synthesis of porphyrins in acute intermittent porphyria (AIP), hereditary coproporphyria (HCP), and variegate porphyria (VP). # = site of action for hematin and glucose. * = site of deficiency in AIP. ** = site of deficiency in HCP. *** = possible sites of deficiency in VP. Colorless compounds: ALA = delta-aminolevulinic acid. PBG = porphobilinogen. UROgen = uroporphyrinogen. COPROgen = coproporphyrinogen. PROTOgen = protoporphyrinogen. Colored compounds: COPRO = coproporphyrin. PROTO = protoporphyrin. Adapted from Meyer 1980, p. 496; Robinson 1977, p. 154.

In many instances, attacks are not preceded by identifiable emotional distress or stressful events (Ackner et al. 1962). Attacks of porphyria may resolve completely, may result in long-standing psychiatric or neurologic disability, or may end in death (Goldberg et al. 1983; Lishman 1987a).

In acute intermittent porphyria, abdominal pain is usually the first symptom and may be accompanied by headaches, persistent constipation, vomiting, fever, postural hypotension, hypertension, tachycardia, urinary retention, and increased sweating (Lishman 1987a; Meyer

Table 6-2. The porphyrias

- **Erythropoietic porphyria**
  Congenital erythropoietic porphyria

- **Hepatic porphyria**
  Acute intermittent porphyria*
  Hereditary coproporphyria*
  Variegate porphyria*
  Porphyria cutanea tarda

- **Erythrohepatic porphyria**
  Protoporphyria

*Porphyrias with neuropsychiatric manifestations.

1980). Neurologic manifestations typically occur late in the disease and may include peripheral neuropathy (usually motor), sensory changes (e.g., hypesthesia, paresthesia, and painful extremities), paralysis (sometimes including respiratory paralysis), cranial nerve dysfunction (e.g., optic nerve atrophy, ophthalmoplegia, and dysphagia), and other CNS involvement (e.g., seizures, dementia, delirium, and coma) (Jefferson and Marshall 1981a; Meyer 1980). Respiratory compromise and bulbar paralysis may lead to death. The above neuropsychiatric and gastrointestinal symptoms often confuse the clinician and may lead to mistaken diagnoses, frequently including intestinal obstruction, appendicitis, pancreatitis, renal colic, poliomyelitis, Guillain-Barré syndrome, or hypertensive encephalopathy (Jefferson and Marshall 1981a; Lishman 1987a).

Psychiatric disturbances are present in 30–70% of patients with acute intermittent porphyria. Psychiatric disturbances may be among the initial symptoms or may be the sole presenting complaint (Ackner et al. 1962; Jefferson and Marshall 1981a; Meyer 1980; Tishler et al. 1985). Psychotic symptoms are usually a late manifestation of acute intermittent porphyria (Jefferson and Marshall 1981a). In 1945, Roth proposed that porphyria occurred much more frequently in patients with severe neurosis or personality disorders. Neurotic and hysterical features in these patients also were described by other authors (Copeman 1891; Jefferson and Marshall 1981a). However, other researchers have disputed these claims, stating that clinical evidence for premorbid personality abnormalities is lacking (Wetterberg and Osterberg 1969). Other investigators argue that earlier observations of psychiatric symptomatology were actually accounted for by episodic manifestations of the disease itself (Ackner et al. 1962). Other researchers postulate that

Table 6-3. Psychotropic drug use in porphyrias with neuropsychiatric manifestations

Safe (do not precipitate attacks of porphyria)	Unsafe (may precipitate attacks of porphyria)
Analgesics	Alcohol
Dihydrocodeine	Anticonvulsants
Morphine, other opiates (meperidine)	Carbamazepine
Antihistamines	Phenytoin, other hydantoins
Diphenhydramine	Antidepressants
Antihypertensives	Amitriptyline
Propranolol	Imipramine
Reserpine	Barbiturates
Antipsychotics	Often still used with Amytal
Chlorpromazine	interviews, electroconvulsive
Promazine	therapy, and laparotomy
Trifluoperazine	Benzodiazepines
	Chlordiazepoxide
	Nitrazepam
	Oxazepam
	Hormones
	Contraceptives
	Estrogens
	Other steroids
Miscellaneous	Miscellaneous
Atropine	Amphetamines
Diazepam for seizures	Cocaine
Nitrous oxide	Dichloralphenazone
	("Welldorm")
	Meprobamate
	Methyldopa
	Pentazocine

Source. Adapted from Eilenberg and Scobie 1960; Goldberg et al. 1983; Lishman 1987a; Meyer 1980; Robinson 1977; Wells and Duncan 1980.

psychiatric symptoms between episodes may result from both the stress of having a chronic episodic illness and possibly from having unnecessary surgery and psychiatric hospitalization as a result of misdiagnosis (Cashman 1961; Whittaker and Whitehead 1956). Acute intermittent porphyria has been misdiagnosed as schizoaffective disorder, hysteria, schizophrenia (with catatonia, paranoia, and auditory hallucinations), depressive disorder, anxiety, and atypical psychosis (Jefferson and Marshall 1981a; Lishman 1987a; Tishler et al. 1985).

Neuropsychiatric attacks are indistinguishable in acute intermittent porphyria, hereditary coproporphyria, and variegate porphyria. Acute intermittent porphyria is distinguished from the other porphyrias by the absence of photodermatitis. Hereditary coproporphyria presents with photosensitivity in one-third of patients. In variegate porphyria, skin involvement is even more common and may present simultaneously with neuropsychiatric symptoms. Skin involvement may include abrasions and blisters after minimal trauma, secondary infections of skin lesions, hyperpigmentation, and hypertrichosis (in women).

Laboratory Findings in Acute Intermittent Porphyria, Hereditary Coproporphyria, and Variegate Porphyria

Laboratory abnormalities in acute intermittent porphyria may include leukocytosis, transient normochromic normocytic anemia, and hyponatremia (secondary to vomiting or inappropriate secretion of antidiuretic hormone). Increased catecholamine excretion may be responsible for hypertension and tachycardia when they are present. Other abnormalities in acute attacks may include increased thyroxine levels without hyperthyroidism, hypercholesterolemia, hypomagnesemia, and abnormal glucose tolerance tests. Routine liver function tests can be normal (Meyer 1980) or show elevations of the transaminases and bilirubin (Goldberg et al. 1983).

While the EEG is usually abnormal, it may sometimes be normal even during acute attacks; therefore, serial EEGs during attacks may be more useful than isolated recordings to confirm the organic nature of symptoms (Ackner et al. 1962; Lishman 1987a). Neuropsychological testing also may reveal significant cognitive abnormalities, suggesting some organicity, or may confirm dementia (Tishler et al. 1985).

Laboratory testing should include specimens of urine and feces. The Watson-Schwartz or Hoesch test can be used as a qualitative measure of porphobilinogen in the urine during an acute attack. Either of these tests should be the first step in screening patients in an acute attack. These tests reflect elevated delta-aminolevulinic acid (ALA) and porphobilinogen (PBG) in the urine but do not distinguish between acute intermittent porphyria, hereditary coproporphyria, and variegate porphyria during acute attacks. In acute intermittent porphyria, elevated PBGs present in fresh urine are colorless. However, when the urine of an acute intermittent porphyria patient is left standing, exposed to sunlight, acidified, or heated, it darkens (turns pink to red to black) as uroporphyrins and coproporphyrins are formed (Figure 6-3 and Table 6-4). False-positive test results may occur in lead poisoning, alcohol ingestion, and iron-deficiency anemia because excretion of circulating porphyrins increases in these conditions (Goldberg et al. 1983).

Table 6-4.   Characteristics of porphyrias causing neuropsychiatric symptoms

	Acute intermittent porphyria	Hereditary coproporphyria	Variegate porphyria
Enzyme deficiency	PBG deaminase or UROgen I synthetase	COPROgen oxidase	PROTOgen oxidase or ferrochelatase
Photodermatitis	No	Infrequent	Yes
Laboratory tests			
Erythrocyte levels			
Protoporphyrins	Normal	Normal	Normal
Coproporphyrins	Normal	Sometimes increased in attacks	Normal
Urine			
ALA	Very high in acute attacks	Raised only in acute attacks	Raised in acute attacks
PBG	Very high in acute attacks	Raised only in acute attacks	Raised in acute attacks
Uroporphyrin	Usually raised	Sometimes raised in acute attacks	Sometimes raised
Coproporphyrin	Sometimes raised	Usually raised, always raised in acute attacks	Sometimes raised
Feces			
Porphyrin	Normal	Sometimes raised, especially if photo-sensitivity present	Very high in acute attacks
Protoporphyrin	Sometimes raised	Raised or normal	Very high
Coproporphyrin	Sometimes raised	Very high	Raised

Note.   PBG = porphobilinogen. UROgen = uroporphyrinogen. COPROgen = coproporphyrinogen. PROTOgen = protoporphyrinogen. ALA = aminolevulinic acid.

False-positive test results also have been reported in patients on phenothiazines (Reio and Wetterberg 1969).

False-negative results may be obtained with the Watson-Schwartz test not only in latent porphyria but also in some affected patients with acute intermittent porphyria who are between acute attacks, in whom urinary excretion of PBG and ALA may be normal or only mildly elevated during remissions (Jefferson and Marshall 1981a; Lishman 1987a; Meyer 1980). If the Watson-Schwartz or Hoesch test is negative, ALA and PBG in the urine should be quantitatively measured; such tests use chromatographic techniques. In acute intermittent porphyria, hereditary coproporphyria, and variegate porphyria, the absolute levels of ALA and PBG do not correlate with the severity or even the presence of neuropsychiatric symptoms (Ackner et al. 1962; Meyer 1980). If ALA and PBG are measured as normal, however, decreased enzymatic activity of uroporphyrinogen I synthetase in lymphocytes, erythrocytes, or skin fibroblasts can be measured and will confirm the diagnosis of acute intermittent porphyria (Meyer 1980; Tishler et al. 1985).

Hereditary coproporphyria is characterized by significant elevations of coproporphyrin III in feces and urine (Table 6-4). In hereditary coproporphyria, the Watson-Schwartz and Hoesch tests will be positive during acute attacks because ALA and PBG excretion is increased in the urine. These levels return to normal with remission. Leukocytes and cultured skin fibroblasts show partial deficiencies of coproporphyrinogen oxidase (Goldberg et al. 1983; Meyer 1980).

In contrast, in variegate porphyria, ALA and PBG may remain elevated in the urine between attacks, so the Watson-Schwartz or Hoesch test may remain positive. In patients with variegate porphyria who have only skin symptoms or who are in remission, the levels of ALA, PBG, and the porphyrins in the urine will be normal or increased. Significant elevations of protoporphyrin and coproporphyrin when clinical symptoms are minimal should suggest the possible diagnosis of variegate porphyria. In contrast to hereditary coproporphyria, in variegate porphyria, fecal elevations of protoporphyrins are greater than the elevations of coproporphyrins (Goldberg et al. 1983; Meyer 1980). Decreased enzyme activity is not routinely measured.

Treatment of Acute Intermittent Porphyria, Hereditary Coproporphyria, and Variegate Porphyria

Patients should be taught to avoid known precipitants and should be given genetic counseling. Early diagnosis and increased awareness about porphyria may prevent unnecessary surgery because of misdiagnosis and may prevent inappropriate psychiatric hospitalization. Patients with dermatologic manifestations should wear protective clothing and avoid direct sunlight (Meyer 1980).

Acute attacks can sometimes be aborted by using intravenous glucose. If neuropsychiatric symptoms do not abate, hematin may be used. Hematin and glucose not only may abate acute attacks, but also reduce the overproduction of porphyrins and their precursors. In laboratory animals, they suppress the induction of hepatic ALA synthetase (Figure 6-3), thereby preventing the accumulation of heme precursors. Analgesics (e.g., meperidine, dihydrocodeine, morphine) are used to manage severe abdominal pain. Other supportive measures include the correction of fluid and electrolyte abnormalities, the use of beta-blockers for hypertension and tachycardia, and respiratory support in severe cases.

Psychiatric manifestations may be treated safely with a variety of psychotropic medications (Table 6-3). Barbiturates may be inadvertently given to psychiatric patients who have undiagnosed or misdiagnosed porphyria, most commonly when they are either undergoing electroconvulsive therapy (Mann 1961) or during barbiturate interviews for conversion symptoms (Hirsch and Dunsworth 1955); acute attacks of porphyria leading to death may result under such circumstances. The role of nonbarbiturate hypnotic agents (e.g., propofol) that induce and maintain anesthesia has not been determined in these patients.

VITAMIN B_{12} DEFICIENCY

Vitamin B_{12} Metabolism

Vitamin B_{12} is present in meat, fish, dairy products, and legumes, which are contaminated by bacteria that synthesize the vitamin. It is released from other proteins in the stomach and then bound to intrinsic factor, a glycoprotein produced by stomach parietal cells. The resultant complex is absorbed in the ileum and then bound to transcobalamins (transport proteins in the serum) which are responsible for vitamin B_{12} distribution. Although transcobalamin II binds most of the newly absorbed vitamin B_{12}, in the circulation, the majority of vitamin B_{12} is bound to transcobalamin I because clearance of vitamin B_{12} is relatively faster from transcobalamin II compared with its clearance from transcobalamin I. There is a small percentage of vitamin B_{12} that is bound to transcobalamin III. Body stores (2–5 mg in adult males) are primarily in the liver

Table 6-5. Most frequent causes of vitamin B$_{12}$ deficiency

Decreased ingestion
- Decreased food intake (e.g., starvation)
- Strict vegetarianism

Decreased absorption
- Decreased intrinsic factor
  Pernicious anemia (most common cause)
  Gastrectomy
  Congenital absence of intrinsic factor
- Ileal defects
  Sprue
  Regional enteritis
  Post-surgery, involving the ileum
  Malignancy, involving the ileum
- Increased competition for vitamin B$_{12}$
  Fish tapeworm
  Overgrowth of intestinal flora-blind loops
- Drugs that interfere with absorption, e.g., *p*-amino salicylic acid, neomycin, and colchicine

Impaired utilization
- Abnormal or deficient binding proteins

Note. Vitamin B$_{12}$ deficiency state = <80 pg/ml serum; normal state = 175–725 pg/ml serum.
Source. Adapted from Babior and Bunn 1980; Gross 1987.

and are far greater than daily requirements of the vitamin (approximately 2.5 µg). As a result, in a previously healthy and well-nourished individual, deficiency states may take years to develop (Cooper and Rosenblatt 1987; Hillman 1980; Jefferson and Marshall 1981b). Common causes of vitamin B$_{12}$ deficiency are outlined in Table 6-5.

Methylcobalamin and adenosylcobalamin are the major active forms of vitamin B$_{12}$ in the body. Because methylcobalamin donates a methyl group as a cofactor in the conversion of homocysteine to methionine, serum elevations of homocysteine might be expected in vitamin B$_{12}$ deficiency. Methylcobalamin itself is also generated by the transfer of a methyl group from methyltetrahydrofolic acid, the inactive form of folate, leaving tetrahydrofolate, the active form of folate. As a result, in states of methylcobalamin deficiency, folate is only available in its inactive form, which results in a functional folate deficiency. Since tetrahydrofolate is needed for purine and pyrimidine synthesis, in tetrahydrofolate deficiency, DNA synthesis is impaired. This type of impairment of DNA synthesis is thought to account for the anemia seen in vitamin B$_{12}$ deficiency. Adenosylcobalamin, the second active form of vitamin B$_{12}$, is used in lipid and carbohydrate metabolism. Deficiency of adenosylcobalamin is thought to impair myelin synthesis, thereby resulting in neurologic symptoms. As adenosylcobalamin is needed in the isomerization of methylmalonyl–coenzyme A (CoA) to succinyl-CoA, elevation of methylmalonic acid would be expected in states of vitamin B_{12} deficiency (Carmel 1983; Chanarin 1987; Hillman 1980).

Clinical Manifestations of Vitamin B_{12} Deficiency

Neurologic manifestations of vitamin B_{12} deficiency may include symmetrical peripheral neuropathy, myelopathy (subacute combined degeneration), and encephalopathy. For instance, paresthesias, impaired vibration sense, decreased deep tendon reflexes, and moderate or severe impairments of intellectual function were present in over 55% of the 42 patients studied by Roos (1978). Visual impairment may occasionally present as the initial manifestation of vitamin B_{12} deficiency, and even in patients without clinical evidence of visual impairments, visual-evoked potentials may be abnormal. For a more detailed discussion of the neurological manifestations of vitamin B_{12} deficiency, see Adams and Victor (1985).

Hematologic abnormalities caused by vitamin B_{12} deficiency may be seen in virtually all cell lines: normochromic macrocytic anemia, ineffective erythropoiesis and consequent hemolysis, neutrophil hypersegmentation, leukopenia, and thrombocytopenia (Gross 1987). However, in some instances of vitamin B_{12} deficiency, the peripheral blood and bone marrow may be normal. The megaloblastosis normally seen in vitamin B_{12} deficiency can be masked by superimposed iron deficiency or folate supplementation (Jefferson and Marshall 1981b). Therefore, psychiatric symptoms resulting from vitamin B_{12} deficiency can occur without any neurologic or hematologic abnormalities being manifest (Reynolds 1976a; Strachan and Henderson 1965; Zucker et al. 1981). In addition to hematologic and neurologic symptoms, vitamin B_{12} deficiency also can affect other organ systems. For example, gastrointestinal symptoms may include glossitis, anorexia, abdominal pain, weight loss, constipation, and diarrhea. Cardiovascular and respiratory problems can include congestive heart failure, chest pain, palpitations, and dyspnea (Jefferson and Marshall 1981b).

Psychiatric Presentations of Vitamin B_{12} Deficiency

Vitamin B_{12} deficiency may not only be a cause of psychiatric symptoms, but may also result from inadequate nutrition in chronic psychiatric patients (Elsborg et al. 1979; Lishman 1987b; Zucker et al. 1981). Psychiatric presentations of vitamin B_{12} deficiency have ranged from mild depression to full-blown psychosis (Roos 1978). Depression, mania, paranoid states, dementia, and other confusional states have been described as a result of vitamin B_{12} deficiency and were reported as early as 1849 by Addison (Addison 1849; Zucker et al. 1981). However, many of these reports came from psychiatric populations in which the psychiatric symptoms did not always respond to vitamin B_{12} therapy (Carney and Sheffield 1970; Edwin et al. 1965; James et al. 1986; Shulman 1967a). Furthermore, depression improved before treatment with vitamin B_{12}, i.e., after patients had been informed of their diagnosis and reassured about the outcome of treatment (Shulman 1967b).

The incidence of psychiatric symptoms in vitamin B_{12} deficient–patients ranges from 4 to 16% for psychotic symptoms to as high as 75% for less dramatic presentations (Jefferson 1977; Jefferson and Marshall 1981b). Suicide attempts have been reported in up to 20% of some vitamin B_{12}–deficient populations (Roos and Willanger 1977). Initial complaints are often vague and lead to misdiagnosis. Jefferson (1977) reported one such case: a man who presented with poor appetite, weight loss, crying spells, depression, progressive numbness of the extremities, impotence, and numbness of his testicles. Although his symptoms were initially thought to be psychogenic, they disappeared after parenteral vitamin B_{12} administration.

The potential benefits of screening psychiatric patients for vitamin B_{12} deficiency have been debated by many researchers (Geagea and Ananth 1975; Jefferson and Marshall 1981b; Phillips and Kahaner 1988; Shulman 1967c). Early diagnosis and treatment are clearly important to prevent irreversible neurologic symptoms (Hart and McCurdy 1971). However, it seems logical to restrict screening to those patients at highest risk for deficiency: elderly patients, postgastrectomy patients, patients with evidence of cognitive impairment, patients with neurological symptoms, and patients with the characteristic anemia. An aggressive diagnostic workup is probably appropriate in such cases of suspected vitamin B_{12} deficiency.

Laboratory Diagnosis of Vitamin B_{12} Deficiency

The level of vitamin B_{12} (cobalamin) is currently measured by a radioisotope-dilution method. However, up to 20% of patients with a vitamin B_{12} deficiency are evaluated as having normal serum levels by this procedure because both active cobalamin and inactive cobalamin analogues are measured by the commercial binding proteins (Kolhouse et al. 1978). This finding is particularly true among patients without anemia. If pure intrinsic factor was used as the binding protein, only true cobalamins would be measured and the problem of false-normal serum vitamin B_{12} levels in states of vitamin B_{12} deficiency would be eliminated (Cooper and Whitehead 1978). Serum vitamin B_{12} levels also can be normal in patients who have recently received parenteral vitamin B_{12}, although these patients' total body stores of vitamin B_{12} may still be low (Jefferson and Marshall 1981b).

If serum vitamin B_{12} levels are low or low normal, then the clinician should consider more sensitive tests. Elevations of methylmalonic acid and total homocysteine in the serum occur early in vitamin B_{12} deficiency, often before hematologic evidence of vitamin B_{12} deficiency. Furthermore, the test remains positive within 24 hours of vitamin B_{12} administration so that even if treatment has been initiated, a definitive diagnosis can be made. Treatment is usually lifelong. However, these tests are costly, and therefore, not yet performed routinely. Elevated urinary methylmalonic acid or homocysteine has been measured in vitamin B_{12} deficiency states for a long time, but these tests are more cumbersome than the serum tests and are, therefore, no longer used (Carmel 1983; Lindenbaum et al. 1988). The most specific indicators of vitamin B_{12} deficiency include the following tests: serum elevations of methylmalonic acid and homocysteine, methylmalonic aciduria, lack of clinical response to adequate doses of folate in cases where only folate was inappropriately given to correct a presumed deficiency, and reticulocytosis in response to sufficient doses of vitamin B_{12} (Edwin et al. 1965; Gross 1987; Hillman 1980).

The cerebrospinal fluid–serum ratio of vitamin B_{12} is usually 0.05. Low cerebrospinal fluid vitamin B_{12} levels with normal serum levels have been reported in a variety of psychiatric conditions, including dementia, organic mood disorder, and postpartum depression (Van Tiggelen et al. 1983). Low levels in the presence of normal serum levels have also been reported in patients on anticonvulsants (Frenkel et al. 1971, 1973). However, the clinical relevance of cerebrospinal fluid vitamin B_{12} levels still is unclear.

An abnormal Schilling test (quantitative test of absorption with radiolabeled vitamin B_{12}) and gastric achlorhydria after histamine stimulation will make the diagnosis of pernicious anemia. (Pernicious anemia should be distinguished from other causes of vitamin B_{12} deficiency.) During the Schilling test, a parenteral flushing dose of nonradioactive vitamin B_{12} is given 2 hours after giving radioactive vitamin B_{12} orally. Vitamin B_{12} absorption is assayed by studying urinary excretion of the radioactive vitamin. This test leads to increased urinary excretion of the radioactive vitamin B_{12}. Therefore, the Schilling test will be inaccurate in the presence of impaired renal function and incomplete urine collection (Katz 1985). In the second part of the test, intrinsic factor is given with the radioactive vitamin B_{12}, which is followed again by the flushing dose of nonradioactive vitamin B_{12}. The second test should show normal excretion of the radioactive vitamin B_{12} if the vitamin B_{12} deficiency was secondary to pernicious anemia (i.e., impaired absorption).

The administration of parenteral cobalamin in the Schilling test is therapeutic and, therefore, may subsequently interfere with making the diagnosis of vitamin B_{12} deficiency (Carmel 1983; Katz, 1985). Low serum vitamin B_{12} levels have been reported in patients with senile and presenile dementia (Abalan and Delile 1985). Normal Schilling tests have been reported in elderly patients with dementia with abnormal vitamin B_{12} absorption (Burns and Jacoby 1988) and in elderly patients with low serum vitamin B_{12} levels and no pernicious anemia (Rao 1988).

EEG abnormalities are common (48–64%) in patients with vitamin B_{12} deficiency, but are not diagnostically significant. These abnormalities are thought to be related to a defect in cerebral metabolism and tend to reverse with treatment of the deficiency (Evans et al. 1983; Roos and Willanger 1977; Walton et al. 1954).

Treatment of Vitamin B_{12} Deficiency

Treatment is aimed at inducing remission and replenishing stores of vitamin B_{12}. Commercial preparations of vitamin B_{12} (cyanocobalamin and hydroxocobalamin) must be converted to an active form by the body before they can be used. Parenteral vitamin B_{12} (1,000 μg im) is given daily over the first 1–2 weeks, and every week thereafter until the anemia is corrected and then monthly, usually for the remainder of the patient's life. Patients with neurologic symptoms may require biweekly therapy for the first 6 months (Gross 1987).

Within 24 hours after vitamin B_{12} therapy is initiated, patients often report an improved sense of well-being (Gross 1987; Katz 1985). Full recovery of neuropsychiatric symptoms and signs may require months and does not always occur. Although folate may partly reverse hematologic abnormalities, in vitamin B_{12}–deficient patients, it may either exacerbate, precipitate, or not change neurologic symptoms. Hematologic abnormalities typically reverse with treatment of the vitamin deficiency. Within 2 weeks, megaloblastosis is corrected, reticulo-cytes increase, and the hematocrit normalizes. The reversal of such abnormalities is identical in folate and vitamin B_{12} deficiencies (Gross 1987; Hillman 1980).

FOLATE DEFICIENCY

Folate Metabolism

The reduced form of pteroylmonoglutamic acid (folate) is tetra-hydrofolate. It is used in amino acid metabolism and is a coenzyme in the synthesis of methionine, norepinephrine, serotonin, and DNA. Impaired neurohormonal synthesis may explain the psychiatric manifestations reported with folate deficiency (Thornton and Thornton 1978). Impaired DNA synthesis secondary to folate deficiency results in megaloblastic transformation (Gross 1987).

Folate is abundant in leafy green vegetables, liver, and yeast. Dietary requirements (50 µg per day) do not lead to large stores of folate (5–10 mg is stored in the liver), and as a result, stores can be depleted within months (Jefferson and Marshall 1981b). The major causes of folate deficiency are outlined in Table 6-6. Alcohol and anticonvulsants particularly should be noted as common causes of secondary folate deficiency (Hunter et al. 1967).

Clinical Manifestations of Folate Deficiency

Folate and vitamin B_{12} deficiencies may cause similar hematologic signs and symptoms, and both folate and vitamin B_{12} deficiency can occur in the absence of anemia or bone marrow changes (Strachan and Henderson 1967). However, the spectrum of neuropsychiatric illness due to folate deficiency is somewhat different from vitamin B_{12} deficiency. Peripheral neuropathy (Shorvon et al. 1980) and subacute combined degeneration (Botez et al. 1977; Manzoor and Runcie 1976) can be present but are far less frequent findings of folate deficiency. Folate deficiency can occur in up to 30% of psychiatric inpatients (Reynolds 1976b; Thornton and Thornton 1978) and has been reported most frequently in those inpatients with depression, organic mental syndromes, and epilepsy (Carney 1967; Reynolds et al. 1970). Folate deficiency has been reported in up to 20% of geriatric admissions. The incidence is even greater in geriatric patients with psychiatric symptoms (Reynolds 1976b).

Table 6-6. Major causes of folate deficiency

- Decreased ingestion of folate (most common)
  Alcoholism
  Poverty
  Advanced age
  Overcooking food

- Decreased absorption
  Malabsorption syndromes—sprue, Crohn's disease
  Blind loops
  Drugs—phenytoin, ethanol, barbiturates

- Impaired utilization
  Folate antagonists—pyrimethamine, methotrexate, triamterene, pentamidine,
    trimethoprim
  Enzyme deficiency
  Vitamin B_{12} deficiency
  Scurvy
  Alcoholism

- Increased requirements
  Pregnancy
  Infancy
  Malignancy
  Increased hematopoiesis (hemolytic anemia)

Note. Folate deficiency state = <3 mg/ml serum, <140 mg/ml red blood cell level; normal state
= >6 mg/ml serum, >160 mg/ml red blood cell level.
Source. Adapted from Babior and Bunn 1980; Gross 1987; Jefferson and Marshall 1981b.

Mood disorders were the most common neuropsychiatric finding associated with folate deficiency in general hospital inpatients (Shorvon et al. 1980). The relationship of depression (or other neuropsychiatric symptoms) and folate deficiency may be complex and often relates to several factors. First, chronic depression may lead to inadequate intake of folate. Second, depression may be a secondary result of disturbances in CNS serotonin and catecholamine metabolism, resulting from folate deficiency (Reynolds et al. 1970). Third, the fatigue associated with folate deficiency may mimic or worsen a depression (Botez et al. 1977). Finally, folate deficiency may be unrelated to depression that has developed because of other factors (Reynolds 1976b).

Organic mental disorders that have been associated with folate deficiency include dementia, mental retardation (Reynolds 1976b; Strachan and Henderson 1967), organic delusional states resembling schizophrenia (Freeman et al. 1975; Reynolds 1967a), and nonspecific cognitive deficits (Feigenbaum et al. 1988). Botez et al. (1977) have reported impaired memory and concentration and minor abnormalities on CT scans of folate-deficient patients. Reports regarding the reversibility of cognitive impairments are mixed because organic mental syndromes associated with folate deficiency respond to treatment with folate (Lishman 1987b).

Laboratory Diagnosis of Folate Deficiency

Serum folate levels are usually determined by microbiologic techniques. Serum folate levels must be obtained concurrently with vitamin B_{12} levels because clinical symptoms may be indistinguishable in the two deficiency states. Because folate levels can be falsely elevated with recent dietary intake and because over 95% of the folate in the blood is in red blood cells, red blood cell folate levels are a more accurate reflection of the status of folate stores (Gross 1987). Because red blood cell folate levels take longer than serum levels to return to normal, if folate was administered before the serum folate level was obtained, a red blood cell folate level might be a way to make the definitive diagnosis of folate deficiency. This is not yet performed routinely. It is not clear whether radioisotope techniques of folate measurement will be associated with a high percentage of falsely elevated folate levels as has been noted with these techniques in the measurement of vitamin B_{12}. In addition, elevated levels of homocysteine have been associated with folate deficiency, but such tests are not yet performed routinely (Carmel 1983; Freeman et al. 1975; Lindenbaum et al. 1988).

Mechanisms involved in the production of cerebrospinal fluid are known to concentrate folate, so that cerebrospinal fluid folate levels may more accurately reflect CNS stores. The cerebrospinal fluid–serum folate ratio ranges from 2.5 to 4.0. There are mixed reports on whether cerebrospinal fluid levels are lowered in patients on anticonvulsants. In general, the clinical relevance of cerebrospinal fluid folate levels remains unclear (Reynolds et al. 1972; Weckman and Lehtovaara 1969; Wells and Casey 1967).

Treatment of Folate Deficiency

Most patients with folate deficiency require daily folic acid (1–5 mg orally) for 4–5 weeks to replenish their stores. Occasionally, lifetime therapy or initial doses of up to 30 mg per day have been required (Botez et al. 1977; Gross 1987).

Although folate may improve the mental state of patients with seizure disorders, it has worsened their seizures in some cases (Reynolds 1967b). More recent investigators have questioned the validity of these early findings, and in most folate-deficient epileptic patients who are given folate supplementation, seizure frequency does not increase (Lishman 1987b). Consultation with a neurologist and/or a hematologist may be helpful when compiling a history of treatment decisions in particular instances. For example, this may help clinicians to decide whether to give folate to the patient with a history of seizures who is maintained on phenytoin and who shows a mild macrocytosis and mild sensory impairments.

Mood, confusion, and psychosis usually improve within weeks of therapy initiation with folate and are followed over several months by neurologic improvements (Manzoor and Runcie 1976). Elevations in mood and improvements in concentration, drive, self-confidence, and sociability have been noted by Reynolds (1967b) when folate is given; however, severe mood swings and aggressive behavior also have been noted. Psychiatric inpatients with depression, schizophrenia, and organic delusional disorders who were treated with folate were discharged earlier and in better condition than those who were not treated with folate (Carney and Sheffield 1970). Despite such reports of improvements in psychiatric symptoms with folate therapy, a causal link between folate deficiency and the subsequent development of neuropsychiatric symptoms remains unclear (Gross 1987).

HYPERVISCOSITY SYNDROME

The hyperviscosity syndrome (HVS) may result from a variety of hematologic conditions and on occasion may have psychiatric manifestations. In adults, HVS is most often caused by elevated serum immunoglobulins (as in multiple myeloma and Waldenstrom's macroglobulinemia), by elevated blood counts (as in polycythemia and leukemia), and by decreased blood cell deformability (as in sickle cell disease) (Fahey et al. 1965; Forconi et al. 1987; Mueller et al. 1983). HVS is usually characterized by the clinical syndrome of retinopathy, a bleeding diathesis, a variety of ischemic neurological symptoms, and hypervolemia with cardiac failure (Bergsagel 1983a; Crawford et al. 1985; Euler et al. 1985; Stern et al. 1985). It also can result in renal insufficiency.

The psychiatrist must consider HVS as a cause of delirium or, less commonly, dementia, especially in the above-mentioned conditions.

HVS patients may complain of slowed thinking, fatigue, headaches, and visual disturbances. A thorough mental status examination with serial reassessments of cognitive function is important in the ongoing evaluation of patients susceptible to HVS (Bergsagel 1983b; Silberfarb and Bates 1983).

Serum viscosity (relative to distilled water) in HVS usually is greater than 4 (normal is less than 1.8) when circulatory and hemostatic disturbances become evident (Bergsagel 1983c). Rouleaux formation on the blood smear may indicate that HVS may be present. If HVS is suspected, whole-blood viscosity should be measured because severe cognitive impairments can occur with only mild elevations in serum viscosity (Mueller et al. 1983). EEG abnormalities have been reported with HVS-related dementia and with neuropsychiatric symptoms secondary to partial complex seizures. In some cases, cognitive changes and neurologic disturbances have been reversible if serum viscosity is reduced by treatment of HVS. Specific treatment of the HVS is, of course, dependent on the underlying condition; for example, hydration, chemotherapy, and plasmapheresis may be instituted when appropriate (Crawford et al. 1985; Euler et al. 1985; Mueller et al. 1983; Stern et al. 1985).

PSYCHOGENIC PURPURA (AUTOERYTHROCYTE SENSITIZATION)

Although the phenomenon of psychogenic purpura is unusual, the clinician should be aware of its existence. Gardner and Diamond (1955) were the first to describe the syndrome, which is characterized by the appearance of repeated crops of painful bruises, often having an inflammatory component. Similar bruises often can be reproduced by the intracutaneous injection of autologous blood, suggesting that they result from autoerythrocyte sensitization. Despite this phenomenon, antierythrocyte antibodies have not been confirmed in published reports. In addition, unlike other bleeding disorders, no known hemostatic defect exists in psychogenic purpura. There also is no evidence of immunologic, renal, or infectious processes that might explain this phenomenon.

Bruises sometimes may be induced by hypnotic suggestion in susceptible patients, implying that psychophysiologic factors may play a role in their pathogenesis (Sorensen et al. 1985). Patients with psychogenic purpura are typically females with multiple systemic complaints;

bruises are often preceded by a reported history of trauma. However, in the absence of trauma, emotional distress in some individuals can precipitate these lesions. These patients sometimes have been characterized as having hysterical and masochistic character traits, as having difficulty modulating their own hostility, and, commonly, as having secondary depression and anxiety. There often is a history of sexual trauma and intrapsychic conflicts (Agle et al. 1967; Mattsson and Agle 1979; Ratnoff and Agle 1968; Sorenson et al. 1985).

The syndrome is not generally thought to be a factitious disorder or the result of malingering. However, several case reports have described the factitious production of similar lesions. In most patients the voluntary production of such lesions cannot be proven. However, it is more evident that severe emotional stressors are present in almost all such patients.

Patients with psychogenic purpura have been treated with psychotherapy, biofeedback, and psychotropic medications (antidepressants, antihistamines, hormones, and steroids). Other patients have received reassurance alone. No one therapeutic modality or agent has been proven to be more effective than any of the other approaches. In fact, in a 2-year follow-up, some patients did not have a recurrence of bruises (Mattsson and Agle 1979; Sorensen et al. 1985).

ANTICOAGULANT MALINGERING

Voluntary ingestion of the coumarin derivatives may result in a multitude of hemorrhagic complaints (Agle et al. 1970; Stafne and Moe 1951). Labeling these patients as "malingerers" is probably incorrect because there is no evidence for secondary gain. They should be more correctly considered to have a factitious disorder with physical symptoms.

The diagnosis of anticoagulant malingering should be considered in the presence of unexplained hemorrhagic complaints and a prolonged prothrombin time. The diagnosis can be confirmed by detection of the anticoagulants in the patient's plasma, i.e., a significant warfarin (Coumadin) level in a patient who does not acknowledge taking warfarin. The prothrombin time may remain elevated for up to 3 days after warfarin ingestion, and therefore, in these patients, a warfarin level may not be detectable. Persistent clotting abnormalities should prompt an extensive diagnostic workup for other causes of abnormal clotting.

Deficiencies of factors II, VII, VIII, and IX are easily corrected with the parenteral administration of vitamin K_1.

Patients with anticoagulant malingering have been described as having histrionic and masochistic personality traits, like patients with psychogenic purpura. In contrast, however, many patients have sadistic impulses or fantasies of inducing bleeding in others. Their past history often includes violent descriptions of bleeding problems in themselves and/or in family members. These patients are sometimes knowledgeable about side effects of anticoagulants and typically have access to them through their jobs or from prescriptions given to family members or the patients themselves. The primary physician should take responsibility for making the diagnosis known to the patient and for correcting the bleeding problem. Appropriate evaluation and treatment planning should include psychiatric consultation and possibly psychiatric hospitalization to prevent patients from harming themselves or others. Psychotropic medications should be used whenever indicated (Agle et al. 1970).

The prognosis is variable. Some patients gain insight and are able to control their self-destructive behavior. Two reported patients who remained in psychotherapy did not have further bleeding. One patient who refused psychotherapy showed some improvement in self-destructive behavior following confrontation with the diagnosis and continued medical management. Coordinated follow-up between the patient's physician and psychiatrist is considered the preferred treatment at this time (Agle et al. 1970).

CONCLUSION

In this chapter, we have discussed the psychiatric aspects of several hematologic disorders. Consulting psychiatrists may encounter many of these conditions, either on general hospital units or in routine office practice. An understanding of the clinical course and an awareness of the most common psychiatric presenting problems associated with these disorders is important to avoid unnecessary psychiatric hospitalizations and to direct the most appropriate medical, surgical, and psychiatric interventions.

REFERENCES

Abalan F, Delile JM: B_{12} deficiency in presenile dementia (letter to the editor). Biol Psychiatry 20:1251, 1985

Ackner B, Cooper JE, Gray CH: Acute porphyria: a neuropsychiatric and biochemical study. J Psychosom Res 6:1–24, 1962

Adams RD, Victor M: The neurologic manifestations of vitamin B_{12} deficiency, in Principles of Neurology. New York, McGraw-Hill, 1985, pp 773–776

Addison T: Anemia: disease of the suprarenal capsules. London Medical Gazette 8:517–518, 1849

Agle DP: Psychiatric studies of patients with hemophilia and related states. Arch Intern Med 114:76–82, 1964

Agle DP: Hemophilia—psychological factors and comprehensive management. Scandinavian Journal of Haematology 33 (suppl 40):55–63, 1984

Agle DP: The hemophiliac population and HIV infection. Presented at the American Psychosomatic Society meeting, San Francisco, CA, March, 1989

Agle DP, Heine P: The psychosocial dimensions of the Hemophilia Treatment Center Project (brochure). The Hemophilia Treatment Center History Project, co-sponsored by the Office of Maternal and Child Health, U.S. Public Health Department and the National Hemophilia Foundation, in press.

Agle DP, Mattsson A: Psychiatric and social care of patients with hereditary hemorrhagic disease. Modern Treatment 5:111–124, 1968

Agle DP, Mattsson A: Psychiatric factors in hemophilia: methods of parental adaptation. Bibliotheca Haematologica 34:89–94, 1970

Agle DP, Ratnoff OD, Wasman M: Studies in autoerythrocyte sensitization: the induction of purpuric lesions by hypnotic suggestion. Psychosom Med 29:491–503, 1967

Agle DP, Ratnoff OD, Spring GK: The anticoagulant malingerer: psychiatric studies of three patients. Ann Intern Med 73:67–72, 1970

Agle D, Gluck H, Pierce GF: The risk of AIDS: psychological impact on the hemophilic population. Gen Hosp Psychiatry 9:11–17, 1987

Babior BM, Bunn HF: Megaloblastic anemias, in Harrison's Principles of Internal Medicine. Edited by Isselbacher KJ, Adams RD, Braunwald E. New York, McGraw-Hill, 1980, pp 1518–1525

Ballas SK, Lewis CN, Noone AM, et al: Clinical, hematological and biochemical features of Hb SC disease. Am J Hematol 13:37–51, 1982

Becker RD, Cividalli G, Cividalli NJ: Psychological considerations in the management of patients with thalassemia major, 1: reactions to chronic illness in childhood and adolescence: a report of a case. The Arts in Psychotherapy 7:165–195, 1980

Benjamin LJ: Pain in sickle cell disease, in Current Therapy of Pain. Edited by Foley KM, Payne RM. Toronto, BC Decker, 1989, pp 90–104

Bergsagel D: Macroglobulinemia, in Hematology, 3rd Edition. Edited by Williams WJ, Beutler E, Ersler AJ. New York, McGraw-Hill, 1983a, pp 1104–1109

Bergsagel D: Plasma cell myeloma, in Hematology, 3rd Edition. Edited by Williams WJ, Beutler E, Ersler AJ. New York, McGraw-Hill, 1983b, pp 1078–1104

Bergsagel D: Plasma cell neoplasms—general considerations, in Hematology, 3rd Edition. Edited by Williams WJ, Beutler E, Ersler AJ. New York, McGraw-Hill, 1983c, pp 1067–1078

Botez MI, Fontaine F, Botez T: Folate-responsive neurological and mental disorders: report of 16 cases. Eur Neurol 16:240–246, 1977

Browne WJ, Mally MA, Kane RP: Psychosocial aspects of hemophilia: study of 28 children and their families. Am J Orthopsychiatry 30:730–740, 1960

Brunner RL, Schapera NE, Gruppa RA: Pain, psychosocial adjustment and drug use: their interactions in hemophilia (abstract). Psychosom Med 44:120, 1982

Burns A, Jacoby R: Vitamin B_{12} deficiency in demented patients. J Am Geriatr Soc 36:85–86, 1988

Carmel R: Clinical and laboratory features of the diagnosis of megaloblastic anemia, in Nutrition in Hematology. Edited by Lindenbaum J. New York, Churchill Livingstone, 1983, pp 1–31

Carney MWP: Serum folate values in 423 psychiatric patients. Br Med J 4:512–516, 1967

Carney MWP, Sheffield BF: Associations of subnormal serum folate and vitamin B_{12} values and effects of replacement therapy. J Nerv Ment Dis 150:404–412, 1970

Cashman MD: Psychiatric aspects of acute porphyria. Lancet 1:115–116, 1961

Chanarin I: Megaloblastic anemia, cobalamin, and folate. J Clin Pathol 40:978–984, 1987

Chodorkoff J, Whitten CF: Intellectual status of children with sickle cell anemia. J Pediatr 63:29–35, 1963

Choiniere M, Melzack R: Acute and chronic pain in hemophilia. Pain 31:317–331, 1987

Cooper BA, Rosenblatt DS: Inherited defects of vitamin B_{12} metabolism. Annu Rev Nutr 7:291–320, 1987

Cooper BA, Whitehead VM: Evidence that some patients with pernicious anemia are not recognized by radiodilution assay for cobalamin in serum. N Engl J Med 299:816–818, 1978

Copeman SM: In proceedings of the pathological society of London. Lancet 1:196–197, 1891

Cozzi L, Tyron WW, Sedlacek K: The effectiveness of biofeedback-assisted relaxation in modifying sickle cell crises. Biofeedback and Self-Regulation 12:51–61, 1987

Crawford J, Cox EB, Cohen HS: Evaluation of hyperviscosity in monoclonal gammopathies. Am J Med 79:13–22, 1985

Edwin E, Holten K, Norum KR: Vitamin B_{12} hypovitaminosis in mental diseases. Acta Med Scand 177:689–699, 1965

Eilenberg MD, Scobie BA: Prolonged neuropsychiatric disability and cardiomyopathy in acute intermittent porphyria. Br Med J 1:858–860, 1960

Elsborg L, Hansen T, Rafaelsen OJ: Vitamin B_{12} concentrations in psychiatric patients. Acta Psychiatr Scand 59:145–152, 1979

Euler HH, Schmitz N, Loeffler H: Plasmapheresis in paraproteinemia. Blut 50:321–330, 1985

Evans DL, Edelson GA, Golden RN: Organic psychosis without anemia or spinal cord symptoms in patients with vitamin B_{12} deficiency. Am J Psychiatry 140:218–221, 1983

Fahey JL, Barth WF, Solomon A: Serum hyperviscosity syndrome. JAMA 192:464–467, 1965

Faulstick ME: Psychiatric aspects of AIDS. Am J Psychiatry 144:551–556, 1987

Feigenbaum LZ, Lee D, Ho J: Routine assessment of folate levels in geriatric assessment for dementia (letter to the editor). J Am Geriatr Soc 36:755, 1988

Forconi S, Pieragalli D, Guerrini M: Primary and secondary blood hyperviscosity syndromes, and syndromes associated with blood hyperviscosity. Drugs 33 (suppl 2):19–26, 1987

Fowler MG, Whitt JK, Lallinger RR: Neuropsychologic and academic functioning of children with sickle cell anemia. J Dev Behav Pediatr 9:213–220, 1988

Freeman JM, Finkelstein JD, Mudd SH: Folate-responsive homocystinuria and "schizophrenia." N Engl J Med 292:491–496, 1975

Frenkel EP, McCall MS, White JD: An isotopic measurement of vitamin B_{12} in cerebrospinal fluid. Am J Clin Pathol 55:58–64, 1971

Frenkel EP, McCall MS, Sheehan RG: Cerebrospinal fluid folate, and vitamin B_{12} in anticonvulsant-induced megaloblastosis. J Lab Clin Med 81:105–115, 1973

Gardner FH, Diamond LK: Autoerythrocyte sensitization: a form of purpura producing painful bruising following autosensitization to red cells in certain women. Blood 10:675–690, 1955

Geagea K, Ananth J: Response of a psychiatric patient to vitamin B_{12} therapy. Diseases of the Nervous System 36:343–344, 1975

Gilchrist GS, Piepgras DG: Neurologic complications in hemophilia, in Progress in Pediatric Hematology and Oncology, Vol 1: Hemophilia in Children. Edited by Hilgartner M, Pochedly C. Littleton, MA, PSG, 1976, pp 79–97

Gilchrist GS, Piepgras DG, Roskos RR: Neurologic complications in hemophilia, in Hemophilia in the Child and Adult. Edited by Hilgartner M, Pochedly C. New York, Raven, 1989, pp 45–68

Giordano V: Psychosocial impacts on a thalassemic patient's life. Ann NY Acad Sci 445:324–326, 1985

Goldberg A, Moore MR, McColl KEL: Porphyrin metabolism and the porphyrias, in Oxford Textbook of Medicine, Vol 1. Edited by Weatherall DJ, Ledingham JGG, Warrell DA. New York, Oxford University Press, 1983, pp 9.81–9.89

Goldberg RJ, Sokol MS, Cullen LO: Acute pain management, in Principles of Medical Psychiatry. Edited by Stoudemire A, Fogel BS. Orlando, FL, Grune & Stratton, 1987, pp 365–388

Gross LS: Neuropsychiatric aspects of vitamin deficiency states, in Textbook of Neuropsychiatry. Edited by Hales RE, Yudofsky SC. Washington, DC, American Psychiatric Press, 1987, pp 327–338

Handford HA, Mayes SD: The basis of psychosocial programs in hemophilia, in Hemophilia in the Child and Adult. Edited by Hilgartner M, Pochedly C. New York, Raven, 1989, pp 195–212

Handford HA, Charney D, Ackerman L: Effect of psychiatric intervention on use of antihemophilic factor concentrate. Am J Psychiatry 137:1254–1256, 1980

Handford HA, Mayes SD, Bixler EO: Personality traits of hemophilic boys. J Dev Behav Pediatr 4:224–229, 1986

Hart RJ, McCurdy PR: Psychosis in vitamin B_{12} deficiency. Arch Intern Med 128:596–597, 1971

Hernandez J, Gray D, Lineberger HP: Social and economic indicators of well-being among hemophiliacs over a 5 year period. Gen Hosp Psychiatry 11:241–247, 1989

Hilgartner MW: Comprehensive care for hemophilia (U.S. Department of Health, Education, and Welfare Publ No 79-5129). Washington, DC, U.S. Government Printing Office, 1980

Hilgartner MW, Aledort L, Giardina PJV: Thalassemia and hemophilia, in Issues in the Care of Children With Chronic Illness. Edited by Hobbs N, Perrin JM. San Francisco, CA, Jossey-Bass, 1985, pp 299–323

Hillman RS: Vitamin B_{12}, folic acid, and the treatment of megaloblastic anemias, in The Pharmacologic Basis of Therapeutics. Edited by Gilman AG, Goodman LS, Gilman A. New York, Macmillan, 1980, pp 1331–1346

Hirsch S, Dunsworth FA: An interesting case of porphyria. Am J Psychiatry 111:703, 1955

Holdredge SA, Cotta S: Physical therapy and rehabilitation in the care of the adult and child with hemophilia, in Hemophilia in the Child and Adult. Edited by Hilgartner M, Pochedly C. New York, Raven, 1989, pp 235–262

Hunter R, Jones M, Jones TG: Serum B_{12} and folate concentrations in mental patients. Br J Psychiatry 113:1291–1295, 1967

Huntsman RG: Hemoglobinopathies. Medicine North America 29:3998–4008, 1985

Hurtig AL, White LS: Psychosocial adjustment in children and adolescents with sickle cell disease. J Pediatr Psychol 11:411–427, 1986

James SP, Golden RN, Sack DA: Single case study: vitamin B_{12} deficiency and the dexamethasone suppression test. J Nerv Ment Dis 174:560–561, 1986

Jason L, Lui K-J, Ragni MV, et al: Risk of developing AIDS in HIV-infected cohorts of hemophilic and homosexual men. JAMA 261:725–727, 1989

Jefferson JW: The case of the numb testicles. Diseases of the Nervous System 38:749–751, 1977

Jefferson JW, Marshall JR: Metabolic disorders, in Neuropsychiatric Features of Medical Disorders. New York, Plenum, 1981a, pp 201–206

Jefferson JW, Marshall JR: Vitamin disorders, in Neuropsychiatric Features of Medical Disorders. New York, Plenum, 1981b, pp 231–257

Joffe RT, Horvath Z, Tarvydas I: Bipolar affective disorder and thalassemia minor (letter to the editor). Am J Psychiatry 143:7, 1986

Jonas DL: Psychiatric aspects of hemophilia. Mt Sinai J Med 44:457–463, 1977

Jonas DL: Drug abuse in hemophilia, in Hemophilia in the Child and Adult. Edited by Hilgartner M, Pochedly C. New York, Raven, 1989, pp 227–233

Katz M: Megaloblastic anemia. Medicine North America 29:3966–3979, 1985

Kolhouse JF, Kondo H, Allen NC: Cobalamin analogues are present in human plasma and can mask cobalamin deficiency because current radioisotope dilution assays are not specific for true cobalamin. N Engl J Med 299:785–792, 1978

Kramer MS, Rooks Y, Pearson HA: Growth and development in children with sickle cell trait. N Engl J Med 299:686–689, 1978

Kumar S, Powars D, Allen J: Anxiety, self-concept, and personal and social adjustments in children with sickle cell anemia. J Pediatr 88:859–863, 1976

Labaw WL: Autohypnosis in hemophilia. Haematologica 9:103–110, 1975

Leavell SR, Ford CV: Psychopathology in patients with sickle cell disease. Psychosomatics 24:24–37, 1983

LeBaron S, Zeltzer LK: Research on hypnosis in hemophilia—preliminary success and problems: a brief communication. Int J Clin Exp Hypn 32:290–295, 1984

Lemanek KL, Moore SL, Gresham FM: Psychological adjustment of children with sickle cell anemia. J Pediatr Psychol 11:397–409, 1986

Lesko LM, Massie MJ, Holland JC: Oncology, in Principles of Medical Psychiatry. Edited by Stoudemire A, Fogel BS. Orlando, FL, Grune & Stratton, 1987, pp 495–520

Levine PH: The acquired immunodeficiency syndrome in persons with hemophilia. Ann Intern Med 103:723–726, 1985

Levine SB: Introduction to the sexual consequences of hemophilia. Scandinavian Journal of Haematology 33 (suppl 40):75–82, 1984

Lichstein KL, Eakin TL: Progressive versus self-control relaxation to reduce spontaneous bleeding in hemophiliacs. J Behav Med 8:149–162, 1985

Lindenbaum J, Healton EB, Savage DG, et al: Neuropsychiatric disorders caused by cobalamin deficiency in the absence of anemia or macrocystosis. N Engl J Med 318:1720–1728, 1988

Lishman WA: Endocrine diseases and metabolic disorders, in Organic Psychiatry: The Psychological Consequences of Cerebral Disorders. Oxford, Blackwell Scientific, 1987a, pp 428–485

Lishman WA: Vitamin deficiencies, in Organic Psychiatry: The Psychological Consequences of Cerebral Disorder. Oxford, Blackwell Scientific, 1987b, pp 501–507

Lucas ON: Dental extractions in the hemophiliac: control of emotional factors by hypnosis. Am J Clin Hypn 7:301–307, 1965

Lucas ON: The use of hypnosis in hemophilia dental care. Ann NY Acad Sci 240:263–266, 1975

Magrab PR: Psychosocial development of chronically ill children, in Issues in the Care of Children With Chronic Illness. Edited by Hobbs N, Perrin JM. San Francisco, CA, Jossey-Bass, 1985, pp 698–716

Mann J: Acute porphyria provoked by barbiturates given with electroshock therapy. Am J Psychiatry 118:509–511, 1961

Manzoor M, Runcie J: Folate-responsive neuropathy: report of 10 cases. Br Med J 1:1176–1178, 1976

Mattsson A: Hemophilia and the family: life-long challenges and adaption. Scandinavian Journal of Haematology 33 (suppl 40):65–74, 1984

Mattsson A, Agle D: Group therapy with parents of hemophiliacs: therapeutic process and observations on parental adaption to chronic illness in children. J Am Acad Child Adolesc Psychiatry 11:558–571, 1972

Mattsson A, Agle DP: Psychophysiologic aspects of adolescence: hemic disorders. Adolesc Psychiatry 7:269–280, 1979

Mattsson A, Gross S: Adaptational and defensive behavior in young hemophiliacs and their parents. Am J Psychiatry 122:1349–1356, 1966a

Mattsson A, Gross S: Social and behavioral studies on hemophilic children and their families. J Pediatr 68:952–964, 1966b

Mattsson A, Kim SP: Blood disorders. Psychiatr Clin North Am 5:345–356, 1982

Mattsson A, Gross S, Hall TW: Psychoendocrine study of adaptation in young hemophiliacs. Psychosom Med 33:215–225, 1971

Mayes SD, Handford HA, Kowalski C: Parent attitudes and child personality traits in hemophilia: a six-year longitudinal study. Int J Psychiatry Med 18:339–355, 1988

Meijer A: Psychiatric problems of hemophilic boys and their families. Int J Psychiatry Med 10:163–172, 1980–81

Meyer UA: Porphyrias, in Harrison's Principles of Internal Medicine. Edited by Isselbacher KJ, Adams RD, Braunwald E. New York, McGraw-Hill, 1980, pp 494–500

Morgan SA, Jackson J: Psychological and social concomitants of sickle cell anemia in adolescents. J Pediatr Psychol 11:429–440, 1986

Mueller J, Hotson JR, Langston JW: Hyperviscosity-induced dementia. Neurology (NY) 33:101–103, 1983

O'Shanick GJ, Gardner DF, Kornstein SG: Endocrine disorders, in Principles of Medical Psychiatry. Edited by Stoudemire A, Fogel BS. Orlando, FL, Grune & Stratton, 1987, pp 641–658

Phillips SL, Kahaner KP: An unusual presentation of vitamin B_{12} deficiency (letter to the editor). Am J Psychiatry 145:529, 1988

Pochedly C: Key questions on chronic blood transfusions in children. Resident and Staff Physician 32:65–68, 1986

Powars DR: Natural history of sickle cell disease—the first ten years. Semin Hematol 12:267–285, 1975

Rao MG: Low serum B_{12} level and normal Schilling's test. J Am Geriatr Soc 36:649–650, 1988

Ratnoff OD, Agle DP: Psychogenic purpura: a re-evaluation of the syndrome of autoerythrocyte sensitization. Medicine 47:475–500, 1968

Reio L, Wetterberg L: False porphobilinogen reactions in the urine of mental patients. JAMA 207:148–150, 1969

Reis E, Linhart R, Lazerson J: Using a standard form to collect psychosocial data about hemophilia patients. Health Soc Work 7:206–214, 1982

Reynolds EH: Schizophrenia-like psychoses of epilepsy and disturbances of folate and vitamin B_{12} metabolism induced by anticonvulsant drugs. Br J Psychiatry 113:911–919, 1967a

Reynolds EH: Effects of folic acid on the mental state and fit-frequency of drug-treated epileptic patients. Lancet 1:1086–1088, 1967b

Reynolds EH: The neurology of vitamin B_{12} deficiency. Lancet 2:832–833, 1976a

Reynolds EH: Neurologic aspects of folate and vitamin B_{12} metabolism. Clinics in Hematology 5:661–696, 1976b

Reynolds EH, Preece JM, Bailey J: Folate deficiency in depressive illness. Br J Psychiatry 117:287–292, 1970

Reynolds EH, Gallagher BB, Mattson RH, et al: Relationship between serum and cerebrospinal fluid folate. Nature 240:155–157, 1972

Robinson SH: Hypochromic anemias, II: heme metabolism and the porphyrias, in Hematology. Edited by Beck WS. Cambridge, MA, MIT Press, 1977, pp 153–164

Roche PA, Gijsbers K, Belch JJF: Modification of haemophiliac haemorrhage pain by transcutaneous electrical nerve stimulation. Pain 21:43–48, 1985

Roos D: Neurological complications in patients with impaired vitamin B_{12} absorption following partial gastrectomy. Acta Neurol Scand [Suppl] 69:4–77, 1978

Roos D, Willanger R: Various degrees of dementia in a selected group of gastrectomized patients with low serum B_{12}. Acta Neurol Scand 55:363–376, 1977

Roth N: The neuropsychiatric aspects of porphyria. Psychosom Med 7:291–301, 1945

Rowley PT, Loader S, Walden ME: Toward providing parents the option of avoiding the birth of the first child with Cooley's anemia: response to hemoglobinopathy screening and counseling during pregnancy. Ann NY Acad Sci 445:408–416, 1985

Salk L, Hilgartner MW, Granich B: The psychosocial impact of hemophilia on the patient and his family. Soc Sci Med 6:491–505, 1972

Sherman M, Koch D, Giardina P: Thalassemic children's understanding of illness: a study of cognitive and emotional factors. Ann NY Acad Sci 445:327–336, 1985

Shorvon SD, Carney MWP, Chanarin I: The neuropsychiatry of megaloblastic anemia. Br Med J 281:1036–1038, 1980

Shulman R: Vitamin B_{12} deficiency and psychiatric illness. Br J Psychiatry 113:252–256, 1967a

Shulman R: Psychiatric aspects of pernicious anemia: a prospective controlled investigation. Br Med J 3:266–270, 1967b

Shulman R: A survey of vitamin B_{12} deficiency in an elderly psychiatric population. Br J Psychiatry 113:241–251, 1967c

Silberfarb PM, Bates GM: Psychiatric complications of multiple myeloma. Am J Psychiatry 140:788–789, 1983

Simon R: Hemophilia and the family system. Psychosomatics 25:845–849, 1984

Simon RM: The family and hemophilia, in Hemophilia in the Child and Adult. Edited by Hilgartner M, Pochedly C. New York, Raven, 1989, pp 213–226

Sorensen RU, Newman AJ, Gordon EM: Psychogenic purpura in adolescent patients. Clin Pediatr 24:700–704, 1985

Stafne WA, Moe AE: Hypoprothrombinemia due to Dicumarol in a malingerer: a case report. Ann Intern Med 35:910–911, 1951

Steinhausen H: Hemophilia: a psychological study in chronic disease in juveniles. J Psychosom Res 20:461–467, 1976

Stern TA, Purcell JJ, Murray GB: Complex partial seizures associated with Waldenstrom's macroglobulinemia. Psychosomatics 26:890–892, 1985

Strachan RW, Henderson JG: Psychiatric syndromes due to avitaminosis B_{12} with normal blood and marrow. Q J Med 34:303–317, 1965

Strachan RW, Henderson JG: Dementia and folate deficiency. Q J Med 36:189–204, 1967

Swirsky-Sacchetti T, Margolis CG: The effects of a comprehensive self-hypnosis training program on the use of factor VIII in severe hemophilia. Int J Clin Exp Hypn 34:71–83, 1986

Thomas JE, Koshy M, Patterson L: Management of pain in sickle cell disease using biofeedback therapy: a preliminary study. Biofeedback and Self-Regulation 9:413–420, 1984

Thornton WE, Thornton BP: Folic acid, mental function and dietary habits. J Clin Psychiatry 39:315–322, 1978

Tishler PV, Woodward B, O'Connor J: High prevalence of intermittent acute porphyria in a psychiatric patient population. Am J Psychiatry 142:1430–1436, 1985

Treiber F, Mabe PA, Wilson G: Psychological adjustment of sickle cell children and their siblings. Children's Health Care 16:82–88, 1987

Van Tiggelen CJM, Peperkamp JPC, Tertoolen JFW: Vitamin B_{12} levels of cerebrospinal fluid in patients with organic mental disorder. Journal of Orthomolecular Psychiatry 12:305–311, 1983

Varni JW: Self-regulation techniques in the management of chronic arthritic pain in hemophilia. Behavior Therapy 12:185–194, 1981

Walton JN, Kiloh LG, Osselton JW: The electroencephalogram in pernicious anemia and subacute combined degeneration of the cord. Electroencephalogr Clin Neurophysiol 6:45–64, 1954

Weckman N, Lehtovaara R: Folic acid and anticonvulsants. Lancet 1:207–208, 1969

Wells CE, Duncan GW: Other neurologic disorders important for the psychiatrist, in Neurology for Psychiatrists. Philadelphia, PA, FA Davis, 1980, pp 203–204

Wells DG, Casey HJ: Lactobacillus casei CSF folate activity. Br Med J 3:834–836, 1967

Wetterberg L, Osterberg E: Acute intermittent porphyria: a psychometric study of twenty-five patients. J Psychosom Res 13:91–93, 1969

Whittaker SRF, Whitehead TP: Acute and latent porphyria. Lancet 1:547–551, 1956

Whitten CF, Fischhoff J: Psychosocial effects of sickle cell disease. Arch Intern Med 133:681–689, 1974

Whitten CF, Nishiura EN: Sickle cell anemia, in Issues in the Care of Children

With Chronic Illness. Edited by Hobbs N, Perrin JM. San Francisco, CA, Jossey-Bass, 1985, pp 236–260

Williams I, Earles AN, Pack B: Psychological considerations in sickle cell disease. Nurs Clin North Am 18:215–229, 1983

Zucker DK, Livingston RL, Nakra R: B_{12} deficiency and psychiatric disorders: case report and literature review. Biol Psychiatry 16:197–205, 1981

Chapter 7

Human Immunodeficiency Virus and Other Infectious Disorders Affecting the Central Nervous System

Paul Summergrad, M.D.
Randy S. Glassman, M.D.

Infectious diseases represent an important source of neuropsychiatric disturbances. A wide variety of viruses, bacteria, fungi, and parasites can infect the central nervous system (CNS), contributing greatly to human suffering. For many patients, agitation, confusion, or lethargy may accompany the early stages of CNS infection and may bring patients to psychiatric attention. Non-CNS infections can also have psychiatric complications; for example, elderly patients with mild, stable dementias can become delirious after developing a urinary tract infection, pneumonia, or dehydration associated with fever. While a truly comprehensive discussion on the neuropsychiatric impact of infectious diseases would include these disorders, in this chapter we limit the focus to four disorders that may directly involve the CNS—three of unquestioned infectious etiology: human immunodeficiency virus (HIV) infection, syphilis, and Lyme disease—and one of presumed infectious etiology: the chronic fatigue syndrome. These disorders are likely to bring patients to psychiatric attention or may be areas of intense concern for patients seen by psychiatrists for other reasons. In the sections below, we review the epidemiology, pathogenesis, clinical description, diagnosis, and treatment of these four disorders and discuss clinical dilemmas in the care of patients who suffer from them.

HUMAN IMMUNODEFICIENCY VIRUS INFECTION

Infection with HIV, the causative agent of acquired immunodeficiency syndrome (AIDS), represents one of the major public health problems of this era. The expanding burden and changing demography of HIV infection, its association with a wide variety of other infectious diseases, its pleomorphic presentation, and the high frequency of neuropsychiatric illness associated with it make detailed knowledge of HIV infection essential for all psychiatrists.

AIDS was first described in 1981 after outbreaks of a heretofore rare infectious disorder, Pneumocystis carinii pneumonia, and a previously rare vascular tumor, Kaposi's sarcoma, in young homosexual men in New York and California (Friedman-Kien et al. 1981; Gottlieb et al. 1981; Masur et al. 1981; Siegal et al. 1981). While initial reports focused on these and other symptoms of immune compromise, it rapidly became clear that patients with AIDS frequently developed neuropsychiatric illness (Nurnberg et al. 1984; Snider et al. 1983). This illness burden was generally distributed in four areas: 1) psychiatric disturbances, particularly depression, but also affective and schizophreniform psychoses probably directly related to effects of the virus on the CNS; 2) a chronic dementing disorder, variously called AIDS or HIV encephalopathy or the AIDS dementia complex, also related to the direct CNS effects of the virus; 3) a large number of other opportunistic infections and malignancies of the CNS associated with significant neuropsychiatric symptoms; and 4) psychological reactions to the risk or actuality of HIV infection and its sequelae: AIDS-related complex (ARC) and AIDS itself (Faulstich 1987; Forstein 1984; Navia et al. 1986a).

In this section, we focus on the neuropsychiatric consequences of HIV infection, primarily the AIDS dementia complex, and other psychiatric syndromes directly related to HIV infection. We review other opportunistic CNS infections, especially as they may confound the evaluation and management of patients with HIV infection. Psychological reactions to HIV infection are noted in passing because these reactions have been covered extensively elsewhere (Holland and Tross

1985; Forstein 1984). Finally, we review issues related to serologic testing, psychopharmacologic management of HIV infection, and emerging medical-psychiatric dilemmas in the care of patients with HIV-related illness.

Epidemiology

Approximately 1–2 million Americans are believed to be infected with HIV (Rubin 1988). As of September 1990, 152,126 persons have been diagnosed as having AIDS, usually on the basis of infections or malignancies indicative of significant immune compromise (Centers for Disease Control [CDC] 1990). More recently, neuropsychiatric illness, or HIV encephalopathy, known as the AIDS dementia complex, has also met the CDC case surveillance definition for AIDS (CDC 1989e; Rubin 1988). Estimates of the number of Americans likely to meet diagnostic criteria for AIDS over the next 5 years have varied widely. It has been estimated that 270,000 Americans may be diagnosed with AIDS by 1991. In any event, large numbers of patients are likely to present for medical-psychiatric evaluation over the next several years.

Initially, the epidemic appeared to be concentrated among white homosexual men, but in recent years, the rate of new cases has leveled off in this population. Increasingly, HIV infection has become a disorder of poor minority men and women, often burdened with other health problems, and strongly associated with intravenous and other drug abuse. The routes of transmission, however, have remained constant: sexual contact, including vaginal intercourse and anal intercourse; congenital acquisition; and transfusions or blood product exchange either secondary to medical treatment or from intravenous drug abuse. No evidence has been found for casual transmission of the virus outside these routes (CDC 1989e; Rubin 1988). In particular, close social contact including kissing would not be expected to transmit the disease.

Neuropsychiatric Manifestations

A wide variety of neuropsychiatric manifestations of the infection have been reported. Of these, the AIDS dementia complex is probably the most important both in clinical burden and frequency (Gabuzda and Hirsch 1987; Levy et al. 1985b; McArthur 1987; Navia et al. 1986a; Snider et al. 1983). The AIDS dementia complex is characterized by evidence of an insidious dementia, difficulties in motor function, and mood and behavioral disturbances. As described by Navia and colleagues in their review of 46 patients at Memorial Sloan Kettering in New York, patients with AIDS dementia complex present initially with memory impairment and poor concentration. Patients develop increased difficulties with attention and a feeling of slowed mental functioning. Many patients have early motor difficulties, including leg weakness, loss of balance, or impaired coordination. Patients frequently show social withdrawal, and apathy and depression are common features. Patients have been reported as having irritability, lability, or mood disorder with psychotic symptoms early in their course. These symptoms occur as the first manifestation of HIV infection in up to one-third of reported cases (Navia et al. 1986a). Occasionally, no other evidence of immune compromise has been found (Navia and Price 1987).

In most cases, the disorder progresses in an indolent but steady fashion to evidence of greater immune compromise. In a minority of cases, the disorder may have an abrupt onset or accelerate after a previously slow course (Morgan et al. 1988; Navia and Price 1987; Navia et al. 1986a). As the disorder progresses, many patients become profoundly ill with global dementia, marked slowing of mental processes, hypertonia, incontinence, hyperreflexia, and weakness. Terminally, patients may become paraplegic and remain in a bedridden, mute state. However, some patients continue to have prominent psychotic symptoms, including visual hallucinations and delusions. Agitation, myoclonus, and seizures also are encountered (McArthur 1987; Navia et al. 1986a).

Between 40 and 70% of patients with AIDS will develop the AIDS dementia complex during the course of their illness (Levy et al. 1988; McArthur 1987; Navia et al. 1986a; Petito et al. 1986). However, exact percentages of those that will develop AIDS dementia complex are not known, and predictors of who will progress to a severely debilitated state have not been identified. In general, the degree of neuropsychiatric illness covaries with the systemic illness, but this finding is not invariably true.

It has been suggested that AIDS dementia complex may represent a form of subcortical dementia. Subcortical dementias, so named by Martin Albert (Albert et al. 1974), are characterized by memory disturbance and slowed mental function, often with significant affective symptoms bearing some similarity to depressive disorders. Subcortical dementias have been reported in a variety of neuropsychiatric conditions, including Parkinson's disease, Huntington's disease, and Binswanger's disease (Cummings and Benson 1984, 1988; Summergrad and Peterson 1989). We review issues related more specifically to psychiatric symptoms below.

One area of current controversy regards early manifestations of AIDS dementia complex. There have been varied reports regarding the presence or absence of neuropsychiatric symptoms in patients with early AIDS-related infection or HIV seropositivity. In one commonly cited study, Grant and colleagues (1987) found evidence of an increased rate of neuropsychiatric disturbance in patients who had HIV seropositivity, ARC, or AIDS, although there are several methodologic weaknesses in this study. Available studies and abstracts have been reviewed by Marotta and Perry (1989). They suggest that the recent literature supports evidence of neuropsychiatric impairment in patients who are already mildly systemically ill with HIV infection. However, neuropsychological studies of completely asymptomatic seropositive patients have not as yet convincingly demonstrated significant differences from seronegative control subjects. A recent study comparing asymptomatic seropositive patients and seronegative control subjects failed to show evidence of neuropsychological impairment in these clinically well individuals. Of interest, however, is the finding that 67% of the seropositive patients had abnormalities on EEG (generally slowing and anterior theta) and otoneurologic testing, compared with 10% of control subjects ($P < .00005$) (Koralnik et al. 1990). Methodologic difficulties in these studies, as well as failure of groups to use the same batteries of neuropsychological tests or standards for interpretation, have made comparisons across a large number of studies difficult. The clinical issues related to this controversy will be reviewed in greater detail below. A variety of other conditions are associated with the direct effects of HIV infection.

Aseptic Meningitis

Aseptic meningitis is a flulike illness associated with rash, lymphadenopathy, headache, and stiff neck at the time of seroconversion. The illness is generally brief; cerebrospinal fluid (CSF) reveals a pleocytosis, generally mononuclear with mild elevations of protein and normal glucose (Gabuzda and Hirsch 1987; McArthur 1987).

Vacuolar Myelopathy

Patients with vacuolar myelopathy often present with progressive gait ataxia, leg weakness, hyperreflexia, and sensory loss referable to

the posterior columns. This picture is usually associated with dementia, and neuropathological studies show evidence of vacuolization of
the white matter of the posterior and lateral columns of the spinal cord
(Gabuzda and Hirsch 1987; McArthur 1987).

Peripheral Neuropathy

A wide variety of peripheral neuropathies have been related to HIV
infection, including distal polyneuropathy, often causing paresthesias
in the hands and feet. Some patients have also developed demyelinating
polyneuropathies or mononeuritis multiplex. In addition, patients may
develop a Guillain-Barré type of ascending polyneuritis although without the albumino-cytological dissociation classically seen in typical
Guillain-Barré patients (Gabuzda and Hirsch 1987; McArthur 1987).

Pathogenesis

A range of studies suggest that HIV itself is the cause of the AIDS
dementia complex. Studies of affected areas of human brain have shown
the presence of HIV by immunofluorescent in situ hybridization,
Southern blotting, and antigen expression studies. Elevated intrathecal
synthesis of HIV-specific immunoglobulin G (IgG) and isolation and
growth of the virus from the CSF of affected patients have been reported
(Bukasa et al. 1988; Gabuzda et al. 1986; Ho et al. 1985; Koenig et al.
1986; Levy et al. 1985a; Shaw et al. 1985). Some controversy still exists
about the contribution of cytomegalovirus infection to the development of the AIDS dementia complex. Most authorities agree that the
pattern and type of neuropathological involvement, as well as the evidence from antigen and molecular studies, do not support cytomegalovirus as the causative agent (de la Monte et al. 1987).

While a number of types of cells are affected in the CNS, monocyte
and/or macrophage lines appear to be particularly important (de la
Monte et al. 1987; Koenig et al. 1986). It is unclear whether there is
direct viral spread to the CNS (as during the period of aseptic meningitis) or whether the primary route of entry to the CNS is via mon-
ocytes and macrophages. Pathologic studies have revealed a subacute
encephalitis in 30–90% of patients dying of AIDS. (The range of frequencies is most likely a function of sampling differences in studies
as well as variable pathologic criteria.) Most studies report evidence of
white matter pallor, demyelination, microglial nodules, and multi-

nucleated cells, primarily in subcortical gray and white matter. Not all patients with pathologic abnormalities have had clinical evidence of neuropsychiatric disorders during life (Anders et al. 1986; de la Monte et al. 1987; Navia et al. 1986b; Petito et al. 1986).

Neuroradiologic Features

Most patients with the AIDS dementia complex have evidence of cortical and central atrophy on computed tomography (CT) scanning. Magnetic resonance imaging (MRI) also reveals evidence of white matter abnormalities in some cases. EEG studies commonly show generalized slowing.

Psychiatric Disturbances

A wide variety of psychiatric disorders have been reported in association with HIV infection, including mood and schizophreniform disorders with psychotic features, paranoia, mania, and irritable-anxious states. Most of these have been case reports, although some series have been noted (Beckett et al. 1987; Buhrich et al. 1988; Cummings et al. 1987; Faulstich 1987; Holland and Tross 1985; Joffe et al. 1986; Navia et al. 1986a; Perry and Jacobsen 1986; Rundell et al. 1986). In a review of published literature on HIV-related patients with psychotic illness, Harris and co-workers (1989) found that 31% of all reported patients with HIV-related psychosis had psychotic symptoms as the presenting manifestation of their HIV infection.

In addition to these more severe conditions, a number of other disorders have also been noted. A high frequency of depression and dysthymic symptoms have been reported in patients with HIV infection (Dilley et al. 1985; Holland and Tross 1985; Perry and Tross 1984). Other researchers have noted frequent anxiety disorders and obsessional concerns regarding risk of AIDS both in traditional risk groups and in others at significantly lower risk (Brotman and Forstein 1988; Jenike and Pato 1986). Studies attempting to control for premorbid psychiatric disturbance have been performed with groups of homosexual men. Atkinson and colleagues (1988) found high rates of anxiety and depressive disorder in seropositive homosexual men at various stages of illness, with especially high levels of anxiety in men with ARC. High lifetime prevalence rates were also observed for anxiety and depression in homosexual men who were seronegative for HIV. It is unclear whether these findings reflect the general impact of the AIDS epidemic on homosexual men, differential rates of anxiety and depressive disorder among homosexual men compared with the general population, or other methodological factors specific to this study. In a multicenter study, Ostrow and co-workers (1989) reported an association between psychological distress and self-reports of nonspecific but possible HIV-related physical symptoms, such as fatigue, new skin rash, night sweats, or new or unusual dry cough. In this study, HIV serological status did not discriminate between seropositive and seronegative men on either self-report of physical symptoms or measures of psychological distress. These studies suggest caution in the attribution of all psychiatric symptoms to direct CNS effects of HIV infection (Atkinson et al. 1988; Ostrow et al. 1989).

In a commonly cited study in New York, the rate of suicide among men with AIDS was significantly higher than among the age-matched general population or those with other medical disorders, including cancer (Glass 1988; Marzuk et al. 1988).

Other Central Nervous System Processes in HIV-Related Illness

Neuropsychiatric illness in patients with AIDS is not necessarily a function of the AIDS dementia complex or related disorders. In approximately 30% of patients, other opportunistic infections or malignancies will complicate the course of HIV infection. Among these complications are cerebral toxoplasmosis, primary CNS lymphoma, cryptococcal meningitis, herpes simplex encephalitis, cytomegalovirus infection, progressive multifocal leukoencephalopathy, tuberculous meningitis, and infections with atypical mycobacterial species (Dalakas et al. 1989; Gabuzda and Hirsch 1987; Levy et al. 1985b; McArthur 1987; Snider et al. 1983). Other viral, fungal, and parasitic disorders have been reported to afflict patients with AIDS. Additionally, patients with Kaposi's sarcoma metastatic to the brain have been reported.

Patients with AIDS may also suffer from cerebrovascular complications, including intracerebral hemorrhage, thromboembolic disease, hemorrhagic infarction, and infarction secondary to nonbacterial thrombotic endocarditis (Dalakas et al. 1989; Levy et al. 1985b; Snider et al. 1983). While it is not in the scope of this chapter to review these disorders in detail, the psychiatrist needs to be continually alert to the possible development of other AIDS-related CNS diseases. Changes in mental status, particularly increased confusion, should not be presumed to be secondary to direct HIV CNS effects or metabolic phenomena alone. In patients with many of the above disorders, levels of alertness may diminish and patients may develop focal neurologic signs, including hemisyndromes. Such patients who come to psychiatric attention need prompt neurological evaluation, and in most cases evaluation of CSF, unless evidence of increased intracranial pressure or severe thrombocytopenia makes a lumbar puncture unwise. Many of these disorders will appear as lesions on CT scanning, such as single or multiple ring-enhancing lesions in cerebral toxoplasmosis or areas of white matter hypodensity in progressive multifocal leukoencephalopathy. Lesions of CSF lymphoma generally show more uniform enhancement on contrast CT studies. Patients with AIDS-related illness who develop acute mental status changes with abnormalities on CT scanning or neurological examination should have prompt infectious disease and neurologic consultation, especially given the treatable nature of many of the above conditions.

Serologic Studies

More than 90% of patients with AIDS or HIV infection have evidence of antibodies to HIV, usually within 6 months of infection. Tests generally available for the detection of AIDS antibodies include the enzyme-linked immunosorbent assay (ELISA), which is used for initial screening, and the Western blot, which is used to confirm positive ELISAs.

The ELISA has low false-positive and false-negative rates of approximately 1 and 3%, respectively. False-positive ELISAs are most common in patients with a history of multiple prior transfusions, organ transplants, or multiple pregnancies. Western blotting has very low false-negative and false-positive rates and will generally screen out weakly reactive ELISAs. The CDC recommends that no results of serologic testing be reported to patients unless a screening test such as ELISA has been reactive on two or more tests, and those initial results have been confirmed by the Western blot. Occasionally, the Western blot may be reported as indeterminate, reflecting a partial or atypical banding pattern. In some such cases, the patient is in the process of seroconverting. However, if the Western blot remains indeterminate on repeat testing for 6 months, that person is "almost certainly *not* infected with HIV-1" unless other clinical or historical factors support the diagnosis (CDC 1989a, p. 5). As with all diagnostic tests, the predictive value of ELISAs and Western blotting is diminished in a population of low disease prevalence. It is unclear what percentage of patients actually infected with HIV will be seronegative on repeated antibody testing. That possibility needs to be considered in patients at high risk, especially if they have symptoms consistent with HIV infection (CDC 1988a, 1989a; Rubin 1988).

Other molecular, antigen capture, and antibody detection methods are available or under development but are generally not in routine clinical use. Increases in the P24 antigen level appear to be related to disease activity but are not a particularly useful screening measure. Serial T cell measures are recommended for initiation of prophylaxis against Pneumocystis carinii pneumonia, but T cell measures have not yet been linked to neuropsychiatric illness (CDC 1989b). (We review issues related to the diagnosis and treatment of syphilis in HIV-infected individuals in the section on syphilis below.)

Approach to Patients With Possible HIV Infection

When should a psychiatrist initiate an evaluation for possible HIV-neuropsychiatric illness, and what tests should be ordered? Answers to these questions will depend, in part, on the desire of patients to know their HIV status and the clinical urgency of having accurate information.

While the current epidemiology of AIDS and HIV infection may be of some benefit in these considerations, any patient with a history of frequent heterosexual or homosexual contact, drug abuse, or other sexually transmitted disease can be considered to be at increased risk for HIV infection. Patients without a personal or family history of psychiatric illness who present with new-onset psychosis, mania, or major depression accompanied by cognitive impairment or any focal neurologic deficit deserve thorough evaluation. All patients with new psychiatric illness should be specifically asked about symptoms of forgetfulness, mental slowing, difficulty concentrating, and minor neurologic complaints such as clumsiness, diminished fine motor capacity, or gait disturbance. Patients who show evidence of such abnormalities by either history or examination should be considered for further evaluation. A careful history of changes in physical health should also be obtained, with special reference to symptoms of fatigue, fever, night sweats, diarrhea, skin changes, swollen lymph glands, new dry cough, weight loss, shortness of breath, and history of sexually transmitted diseases or genital ulcers. Careful physical, neurologic, and bedside cognitive examinations also are important. Patients, even those with

Table 7-1. Initial evaluation of the psychiatric patient with possible HIV-related illness

1. Careful medical and neurologic history and examination.
2. HIV serology (after informed consent), enzyme-linked immunosorbent assay (ELISA). If reactive two times, ELISA should be confirmed with Western blot.
3. Venereal Disease Research Laboratories (VDRL) test; hepatitis serology; CBC, platelets, BUN, creatinine, electrolytes, liver function tests, thyroid function tests.
4. Magnetic resonance imaging (MRI) of the brain. If evidence of mass lesions are noted on MRI, patients should have contrast-enhanced computed tomography (CT) or MRI.
5. Lumbar puncture with studies including cell counts, protein, glucose, VDRL, IgG, oligoclonal bands, HIV cerebrospinal fluid culture, and other bacteriological, cytological, and fungal studies as indicated.
6. Neuropsychological testing including Wechsler Adult Intelligence Scale—Revised (WAIS-R) and verbal subtests, Trailmaking B, cancellation test, grooved pegboard test.
7. Assessment of capacity for activities of daily living.
8. Follow-up examination including repeated neuropsychological and neuroimaging testing with medical or neuropsychological decline or possibly every 6 months.

a long history of psychiatric illness, should be evaluated for HIV-related illness if they undergo new cognitive or neurologic changes and fall within known high-risk categories.

How should the physician proceed if a patient's symptoms arouse concern? All patients should have HIV serology obtained after consent is obtained (Table 7-1). In addition, complete blood count (CBC) and platelet count are valuable because they may reveal lymphopenia, anemia, or thrombocytopenia. Serology for hepatitis and syphilis should be obtained since these disorders are associated with significant neuropsychiatric abnormalities and with increased risk for HIV infection. In addition, other general laboratory measures, such as liver function tests, thyroid functions, and screening chemistries, should be obtained because of the high rate of occult medical illness among psychiatric patients.

Neuroradiologic testing should begin with MRI whenever possible. MRI is more sensitive than CT to the periventricular white matter abnormality seen in the AIDS dementia complex; it will also screen for mass lesions such as CNS lymphoma, toxoplasmosis, or brain abscess. If mass lesions are observed on MRI, then further evaluation by contrast-enhanced CT may be of benefit. Patients with positive findings should have prompt infectious disease and neurologic consultation.

If patients do not have a mass lesion that might preclude CSF examination, they should have a lumbar puncture. In addition to the usual cell, protein, and glucose studies, patients should have a CSF Venereal Disease Research Laboratory (VDRL) test; IgG level determination; oligoclonal bands; HIV CSF cultures; cryptococcal antigen, fungal, and tuberculosis cultures; and cytology. McArthur and co-workers (1988) found increased rates of pleocytosis, elevated IgG, oligoclonal bands, and positive CSF HIV culture in men with clinical neuropsychiatric abnormalities.

Neuropsychological testing should be performed to provide evidence of current impairment and a baseline for later studies. Because of the variability in the current literature, specific tests have not uniformly provided evidence of cognitive impairment. However, timed tests of subcortical or frontal lobe function, such as Trailmaking B, the cancellation test, and the grooved pegboard test, have been reported as abnormal in patients with HIV infection. The Wechsler Adult Intelligence Scale—Revised (WAIS-R) and its verbal subtest may also be of some value (Marotta and Perry 1989). Serial measures demonstrating deterioration over time may offer more convincing evidence of decline than a single assessment, no matter how elaborate. Moreover, patients with fatigue may be unable to tolerate prolonged testing sessions; therefore, optimal neuropsychological testing will rely on relatively brief batteries of repeatable measures. To some extent, the choice of tests will depend on the expertise of the (neuro)psychological consultant.

In obtaining baseline measures of neuropsychological function, it is important to gather data on daily functioning from patients, relatives, significant others, and close friends. Such data can be particularly important in discharge planning. In a recent San Francisco General Hospital study of psychiatric inpatients with HIV-related illness, none of the 18 patients with dementia could be discharged to outpatient care (Baer 1989). Follow-up studies for patients with documented HIV neuropsychiatric impairment should be obtained if there is deterioration in clinical status expressed as impaired activities of daily living, new cognitive difficulties, new or recurrent psychiatric difficulties, or focal neurologic events. At present, many clinics repeat neuropsychological and neuroimaging measures every 6 months. Whether such anticipatory care will result in differences in clinical outcome is unknown at present.

Pharmacologic Treatment

Treatment for the AIDS dementia complex is limited at present. Zidovudine (AZT) may reduce the progression or cause partial remission of cognitive neurologic disorder. The findings of two U.S. AIDS clinical trials have been reported by the Secretary of Health and Human Services and the lay press. Early indications suggest diminished disease progression in asymptomatic and mildly symptomatic patients with CD4+ T cell counts of less than 500 cells/µl treated prophylactically with AZT. It is not clear from these reports whether this slowed disease progression included diminished neuropsychiatric symptoms. Until these studies have been fully reported in the medical literature and long-term risks and benefits of early AZT treatment have been evaluated, it is not established that AZT therapy will prevent asymptomatic patients or patients with mild neuropsychiatric symptoms from developing the AIDS dementia complex.

AZT has been reported to cause confusion, anxiety, tremulousness, seizures, and a syndrome similar to Wernicke's encephalopathy among patients receiving it and may be limited in its utility because of these and hematologic side effects. Newer drugs may offer more hope of arresting CNS involvement. Preliminary reports have suggested potential CNS efficacy of peptide T (Bridge et al. 1989; Clinical trials of zidovudine in HIV infection 1989; Schmitt et al. 1988; Yarchoan et al. 1987, 1988, 1989).

Symptomatic treatment of neuropsychiatric disorders in HIV-positive patients is at present empiric. Some patients have been reported to show positive response, including improved cognitive function, to psychostimulants (Fernandez et al. 1988, 1989; Holmes et al. 1989). This latter finding may have been related in part to increased speed of performance, which has also been observed in other subcortical dementias treated with antidepressant or stimulant agents. Dextroamphetamine appears to be of less utility than methylphenidate because of the higher frequency of dyskinesias associated with dextroamphetamine use (Fernandez et al. 1988). The benefits of stimulant use must be weighed carefully against the possibility that these drugs may be abused, especially in patients with a preexisting drug-abuse history. Improved mood and speed of cognitive performance appear to be useful endpoints in monitoring continued prescription of stimulant agents.

Anecdotal reports have suggested that AIDS patients may have increased frequency of tricyclic-related side effects including confusion. Fernandez and colleagues (1989) noted a high rate of confusion complicating tricyclic treatment of patients with AIDS, especially in those taking more potent anticholinergic agents such as amitriptyline. Studies using newer agents and agents with less anticholinergic activity are currently under way. Fernandez and colleagues (1989) found that depressed patients with ARC (as opposed to AIDS) had a better treatment response. Schaerf and co-workers (1989) have reported successful

electroconvulsive therapy (ECT) treatment of four HIV-positive depressed inpatients, one of whom had AIDS.

Treatment of anxiety disorders and psychosis in patients with HIV
infection should be guided at present by the cautious use of standard
agents for these syndromes. Anecdotal evidence suggests that patients
may be very sensitive to the side effects of psychotropic agents; therefore, doses should be initially low and titrated upward cautiously, unless an unstable clinical state requires more aggressive pharmacotherapy.
There have been some reports of neuroleptic malignant syndrome and
of increased extrapyramidal side effects of neuroleptics in patients with
HIV infection. The likelihood of these reactions may be greater in
patients with AIDS, especially if they are treated with higher-potency
neuroleptics (Baer 1989; Bernstein and Scherokman 1986).

Special Considerations in HIV-Related Illness

A number of ethical, legal, and clinical dilemmas arise in the treatment of HIV-infected patients. Adler and Beckett (1989) have reviewed
many of these issues in outpatient psychotherapy settings. Binder (1987)
and others have reviewed difficulties that arise on inpatient units.
Issues of staff countertransference antibody testing, confidentiality,
and transfer of patients have been of particular concern in the inpatient
setting. Psychiatrists in hospital settings are likely to be concerned
with the ability of patients to isolate their bodily secretions and the
psychiatric staff's ability to manage AIDS-related medical illness.
Somewhat more problematic are HIV patients, or patients in very high-
risk groups, who attempt to harm themselves or others by exposure
to blood as well as patients with impaired judgment secondary to neuropsychiatric illness who engage in high-risk behavior, such as sexual
contact with HIV-positive patients or patients in high-risk groups.

While these problems can occur on open units, they are more likely
to occur on involuntary units, especially those in state hospitals. Providing sophisticated medical care is often difficult in such settings,
making the medical management of HIV-positive patients problematic.
Because of the demographics of state hospitals, with their high rate
of homeless and drug-abusing patients, and the association of certain
diagnostic groups (borderline or bipolar) with impulsive high-risk
behavior, these settings may harbor a disproportionate number of high-
risk patients. Recent studies suggest that severe mental illness, substance abuse, and medical illness are all highly prevalent among homeless patients and that HIV-positive patients likely may be overrepresented

in state hospitals (Breakey et al. 1989; Susser et al. 1989). Psychiatrists working in such facilities need to be alert to HIV-related issues as well as related infection-control issues, such as the increased rate of tuberculosis among HIV-positive patients (Ruder et al. 1989).

SYPHILIS

Syphilis occupies a unique position in psychiatry. In the late 19th century, neurosyphilis was responsible for a significant minority of admissions to psychiatric hospitals. The early 20th century saw the identification of the causative agent, *Treponema pallidum*, and the introduction of ameliorative treatments. Syphilis was among the first common neuropsychiatric illnesses to have a specific organic etiology demonstrated. In this section, we do not review in detail all aspects of syphilitic manifestations. However, an understanding of the stages of syphilis is critical for clinical diagnosis and for determining the value of serologic and other diagnostic tests. (We review the stages of syphilis below.)

Epidemiology

Syphilis affected 14.7 per 100,000 persons in the United States as of 1987 (Larsen and Beck-Sague 1988). This prevalence rate has increased since the nadir in the late 1950s (CDC 1988b; Relman et al. 1988a). In the early 1970s, the rate of syphilis increased primarily because of an increase in infection among homosexual white males. Since the AIDS epidemic, rates of syphilis infection have decreased among this group. However, rates have been increasing significantly among heterosexuals, especially in inner city areas (CDC 1988b; Relman et al. 1988a).

Syphilis is spread primarily via sexual contact with an infected individual in the primary or secondary stage of infection. Blood transmission occurs rarely.

Pathogenesis

Syphilis is caused by a spirochete, *Treponema pallidum*. The organism enters the skin after direct contact with an active syphilitic lesion, such as a chancre. In approximately 25–40% of cases, syphilis invades the CNS during the primary, secondary, or early latent stages (Holmes and Lukehart 1987; Lukehart et al. 1988; Relman et al. 1988a), which may occur as part of the widespread dissemination of the bacteria during the secondary stage. We outline the clinical manifestations during the stages of syphilis below.

Primary Syphilis

Primary syphilis occurs 3–6 weeks after contact with the organism. The usual symptoms are a chancre at the point of entry and local lymphadenopathy. During this stage, *Treponema pallidum* can be directly demonstrated in lesions by dark field examination, and patients are infectious (Holmes and Lukehart 1987; Larsen and Beck-Sague 1988; Relman et al. 1988a).

Secondary Syphilis

Secondary syphilis occurs 6–8 weeks after the end of the primary stage. Its hallmark is a widely disseminated maculopapular rash over the trunk, extremities, and later the palms and soles. Other mucocutaneous lesions may also be present. Patients are often systemically ill during this period with fever, generalized lymphadenopathy, fatigue, sore throat, headache, and meningismus. Secondary syphilis occasionally may be asymptomatic, especially if its rash is not noted. The frequency of asymptomatic secondary syphilis is unknown. The secondary stage persists for 2–6 weeks and is followed by the stage of latent syphilis (Holmes and Lukehart 1987; Larsen and Beck-Sague 1988; Musher 1978; Relman et al. 1988a).

Latent Syphilis

Latent syphilis is defined by a normal physical examination; absence of cardiac, neurologic, or CSF evidence of syphilis; a prior history of primary or secondary syphilis; and a positive treponemal serology. This period is divided into early latent syphilis, which occurs during the first year after infection, and late latent syphilis thereafter. Patients whose CSF is normal (i.e., without pleocytosis, elevated protein, or positive VDRL) at 2 years after infection are at low risk of progression to neurosyphilis.

Late Syphilis

Late syphilis is caused by ongoing inflammatory disease, most often in the aorta (syphilitic aortitis) or the nervous system (neurosyphilis), although other organs may also be involved. Neurosyphilis, which occurs in approximately 10% of patients, can take one of several forms.

Asymptomatic neurosyphilis. This is characterized by a normal neurologic examination despite evidence of ongoing meningeal inflammation—pleocytosis, elevated protein, and/or reactive VDRL. (We review the use of lumbar puncture in early or possible asymptomatic neurosyphilis in the "Clinical Dilemmas in the Evaluation of Neurosyphilis" section below.) Some patients will have clinical evidence of syphilitic meningitis in the early or latent stage—headache, confusion, and possibly some cranial nerve findings.

Meningovascular syphilis. This generally occurs 6–7 years after infection although in studies from the Boston City Hospital, it occurred as early as within 6 months, and as late as 10–12 years (Adams and Victor 1989). Symptoms include stroke syndromes of subacute onset with a preceding encephalitic picture, including psychiatric disturbances such as lability or personality changes (Lishman 1988; Simon 1985; Swartz 1984). There is significant inflammation of the meninges as well as vasculitis that can lead to vascular occlusion. Meningovascular syphilis should always be considered in a young person with new onset of stroke, especially in the face of positive syphilis serology.

Parenchymal neurosyphilis. This is divided into two major forms: general paresis (also known as the general paralysis of the insane or dementia paralytica), and tabes dorsalis.

General paresis usually begins 20 years after infection. Its initial symptoms are a dementia with memory disturbance, dysarthria, myoclonus, and hyperreflexia. Changes in personality and irritability are frequently noted. The development of more severe mental decline is associated with worsening dementia, motor function, and psychosis. In the pre-penicillin era, it was estimated that two-thirds of patients would become psychotic during this phase. These psychoses were typically either an expansive, grandiose, manic psychosis or a psychotic depression with somatic delusions. The end-stage of the illness left untreated patients in a bedridden, nonfunctional state (Adams and Victor 1989; Hooshmand et al. 1972; Lishman 1988; Simon 1985; Swartz 1984).

In contradistinction to general paresis, tabes dorsalis usually develops 25–30 years after initial infection. The cardinal findings in tabetic neurosyphilis include a loss of position and vibration sense, absent lower-extremity reflexes, ataxia, incontinence, and sharp, rapidly occurring pains in many areas of the body, often called lancinating or lightning pains. Perhaps because of prior treatment with antibiotics, patients may present with combinations of the above presentations. Some authorities believe that atypical presentations are the rule in modern neurosyphilis (Adams and Victor 1989; Hooshmand et al. 1972; Lishman 1988; Simon 1985; Swartz 1984). (We review these presentations further in the section "Clinical Dilemmas in the Evaluation of Neurosyphilis.")

Serology and Diagnosis

Serologic tests for syphilis are divided into two general groups: nonspecific reaginic tests and specific treponemal tests. Both types of tests have important functions to play in the diagnosis of syphilis but provide very different types of information (see Tables 7-2 and 7-3).

Nonspecific reaginic tests. The nonspecific reaginic tests in most frequent use are the rapid plasma reagin test and the VDRL. These tests measure IgG and IgM antibodies against a lipoidal antigen produced by organism-host interaction. Of these tests, the VDRL has been the most widely studied. The VDRL generally becomes positive within several weeks of primary infection and has generally been thought to be positive in virtually all patients with secondary syphilis. It usually continues to remain positive in latent and late syphilis, although it may become negative in serum in up to 20–30% of patients with late disease (Larsen and Beck-Sague 1988; Relman et al. 1988a; Sparling 1971). The VDRL is particularly useful as an index of disease activity and treatment and as an indicator of CNS infection. VDRL results are reported as reactive or nonreactive, and if reactive, the dilution titer is reported as well, for example, 1:8, 1:32, and so on. In general, patients with primary or active syphilis show an increase in titer of fourfold or greater in the 4–8 weeks between initial conversion and the height of the secondary stage. Patients with secondary syphilis usually have a titer of 1:32 or greater. The VDRL titer can also be used as a guide to treatment efficacy. Falling titers of reaginic antibodies provide evidence

Table 7-2. Syphilis—stages and serology

Stage	Time from infection	Duration	VDRL (Serum)	FTA-ABS (Serum)
Primary syphilis	3–6 weeks	1–5 weeks	80–100% positive	90% positive
Secondary syphilis	6–8 weeks	2–6 weeks	Nearly 100% positive Titer >1:32	Nearly 100% positive
Latent syphilis	>1 year	Variable	Decreasing titer 75–90% positive	95–100% positive
Meningovascular syphilis	6 months to 10 years	Variable (months)	70–75% positive	95–100% positive
Parenchymal neurosyphilis	20–30 years	Years, especially if untreated	70–75% positive	95–100% positive

Note. FTA-ABS = fluorescent treponemal antibody–absorbed test. VDRL = Veneral Disease Research Laboratory test.

Table 7-3. False-positive and false-negative syphilis serology

False-positive	
VDRL	FTA-ABS
Titers <1:8	Usually borderline reactive
20–40% false-positive	15% of patients with SLE are positive,
Viral illnesses	often with atypical banding patterns
Mycoplasma	
Hepatitis	
Systemic lupus erythematosus (SLE)	
Other connective tissue disorders	
Aging	
Pregnancy	
Other autoimmune disorders	
Infectious mononucleosis	
Malaria	

False-negative	
VDRL	FTA-ABS
Late syphilis 20–30%	
Latent syphilis 10–25%	Rare
Concurrent HIV infection?	

Note. VDRL = Venereal Disease Research Laboratory test. FTA-ABS = fluorescent treponemal antibody–absorbed test.

of successful treatment, although some patients may remain reactive (Larsen and Beck-Sague 1988). In the CSF, the presence of a positive VDRL is considered diagnostic of neurosyphilis. (We review this finding further below.)

Unfortunately, reaginic tests are liable to false-positive reactions. In general, false-positive reactions are rare in patients whose titers are greater than 1:8 (Holmes and Lukehart 1987; Larsen and Beck-Sague 1988; Relman et al. 1988a). The range of false-positive tests is variable but may be as high as 40%. In particular, patients with connective tissue disorders, especially systemic lupus erythematosus, may be at risk for false-positive results, but these results can also occur with other recent infections and other treponemal disorders. We found no reports of Lyme disease causing false-positive syphilis serology. (We review other issues related to Lyme disease and its diagnosis in patients who have syphilis in the section "Lyme Disease" below.) The concern over the false-positive VDRLs has led, in part, to increased use of specific treponemal tests.

Specific treponemal tests. Many specific treponemal tests are available, including the fluorescent treponemal antibody–absorbed test (FTA-ABS), hemagglutination assays, and treponemal pallidum immobilization. Of these, the FTA-ABS is the most widely used and studied. These tests measure the presence of antibodies specific for *Treponema pallidum*. The FTA-ABS has a far lower level of false positives than the VDRL although it may still show abnormalities in patients with connective tissue disorders, particularly lupus (Holmes and Lukehart 1987; Larsen and Beck-Sague 1988; Relman et al. 1988a). The FTA-ABS is reported as nonreactive, borderline, or reactive, but reactive sera are not reported quantitatively. Thus, the FTA-ABS is not helpful for determining disease activity or response to treatment.

The FTA-ABS generally becomes positive during the primary stage and has a sensitivity of 98% (Larsen and Beck-Sague 1988). It then remains positive for life despite treatment. Classically, the FTA-ABS has been thought to be nearly always reactive in secondary syphilis, although this finding has been questioned in patients with concurrent HIV infection (see below). The number of individuals with false-negative FTA-ABS in late syphilis is very low, certainly lower than the 20–30% false-negative VDRL rate in late syphilis.

Thus, the VDRL or other reaginic tests are best used as initial screening tests because of lower expense and ease of performance and as indicators of disease activity and of response to treatment. The VDRL has a special role in CSF evaluation, which we review further below. The VDRL's major drawbacks are its high rate of false-positive results and its tendency to become negative in late neurosyphilis.

The FTA-ABS is more specific and sensitive than the VDRL but does not provide information about the degree of disease activity or response to treatment. Its role in CSF evaluation is more controversial.

Cerebrospinal Fluid Evaluation

The evaluation of CSF is critical in the treatment of syphilis of prolonged duration (Adams and Victor 1989). Upward of 40% of patients with primary or secondary syphilis have CSF abnormalities, and in approximately 30% the organism can be directly demonstrated (Lukehart et al. 1988). Of untreated patients, asymptomatic neurosyphilis was observed in up to 30% of those with disease duration of 2 or more years (Holmes and Lukehart 1987). Untreated, a significant fraction of these patients progress to symptomatic neurosyphilis. Therefore, patients with asymptomatic neurosyphilis must be evaluated to prevent further disease progression (Adams and Victor 1989).

In general, CSF of patients with active disease shows a pleocytosis of between 10 and 200 cells/mm³ (generally lymphocytes or mononuclear cells), elevated proteins of up to 200 mg/100 ml, and a reactive VDRL. It is rare for glucose to be reported as abnormally low. All patients will not show all findings in CSF at the same time, and the degree of pleocytosis and protein elevation in general closely parallels the degree of disease activity (Adams and Victor 1989; Relman et al. 1988a; Simon 1985).

The VDRL is the gold standard for the diagnosis of CSF neurosyphilis. If the CSF VDRL is reactive in a well-performed, nontraumatic lumbar puncture, the patient has neurosyphilis. In the vast majority of patients with late syphilis who have CNS involvement, the VDRL will be reactive. However, in a significant minority, especially those with very late syphilis, the VDRL may be nonreactive (Davis and Schmitt 1989; Simon 1985). Unfortunately, the FTA-ABS cannot replace the VDRL for evaluation of neurosyphilis. The presence of a positive FTA-ABS may simply reflect passive transfer of antibody from serum to CSF (Jaffe et al. 1978). Treatment generally returns CSF parameters to normal, although a small minority of patients who otherwise appear fully treated still have a weakly reactive VDRL. Whether this group requires further treatment remains controversial (Adams and Victor 1989).

Clinical Dilemmas in the Evaluation of Neurosyphilis

Several clinical problems may confront the psychiatrist dealing with a patient with possible syphilitic infection, including inadequacy of prior treatment, a remote history of syphilis and new psychiatric illness, and CSF VDRL in the "dementia workup."

Prior treatment for primary or secondary syphilis, even with currently recommended standard regimens, does not guarantee that a patient will not develop neurosyphilis even if serum VDRL titers are low. Current recommendations for treatment of primary or secondary syphilis have come under sharp attack (Bayne et al. 1986; Guinan 1987; Lukehart et al. 1988; Markovitz et al. 1986; Moskovitz et al. 1982; Musher 1988). The demonstration of *Treponema pallidum* in the CSF of patients previously treated for primary or secondary syphilis has increased concern that standard treatment regimens may be inadequate, which is further supported by pharmacologic studies suggesting that benzathine penicillin achieves very low penetration of the CSF (Jaffe and Kabins 1982; Lukehart et al. 1988). As such, patients must still be considered at some risk for neurosyphilis if previous low-dose benzathine penicillin or oral antibiotic treatment were used. In addition, patients whose VDRL titer fell after treatment for primary or secondary syphilis by less than fourfold to eightfold are probably at increased risk for treatment failure (Guinan 1987).

In general, patients with syphilis of unknown duration or of greater than 1-year duration who present for psychiatric treatment should undergo a CSF evaluation to detect asymptomatic neurosyphilis. A negative CSF examination, which is acellular with normal protein and serology at that time, makes active CNS disease unlikely and progression to later symptomatic neurosyphilis rare (Adams and Victor 1989; Relman et al. 1988a).

Older patients presenting with some combination of neurologic and psychiatric disturbances (as can occur in all forms of late neurosyphilis) need a CSF examination if they have evidence of prior syphilitic infection documented by reactive serum VDRL, FTA-ABS, or a reliable clinical history. Clinical dilemmas may arise when patients have a nonreactive CSF VDRL. The mere presence of a positive CSF FTA-ABS is not enough to warrant treatment in a patient who has no other CSF abnormalities and a neuropsychiatric examination not suggestive of neurosyphilis. Conversely, patients with a negative CSF VDRL, but with other CSF abnormalities on examination consistent with neurosyphilis, deserve presumptive treatment, especially if they have evidence of prior syphilitic infection by serum FTA-ABS (Adams and Victor 1989; Davis and Schmitt 1989; Simon 1985). Because of the significant false-negative VDRL rate in late syphilis, a serum FTA-ABS should be obtained when clinical suspicion of neurosyphilis is high (Larsen and Beck-Sague 1988; Sparling 1971).

Primary or Secondary Syphilis

The need for CSF examination in primary or secondary syphilis is unclear. Some authorities are now recommending a standard, higher-dose initial therapy to decrease the risk of later progression to neurosyphilis (Musher 1988).

Human Immunodeficiency Virus

Of particular concern to psychiatrists are recent reports of the unusual behavior of syphilitic infections in patients co-infected with HIV.

Johns et al. (1987) reported four cases of neurosyphilis in patients with concomitant HIV infection who had fallen ill despite standard treatment for neurosyphilis. Subsequent studies have amplified these reports and describe a wide variety of other abnormalities in the presentation of syphilis in patients with HIV infection (Berry et al. 1987). Furthermore, HIV-positive patients with secondary syphilis were seronegative for syphilis antibodies but were later found to have the disease (Hicks et al. 1987). It is unknown whether abnormalities in humoral immunity may occur during other stages of syphilis as well. At present, the degree to which these abnormalities represent a true change in the behavior of neurosyphilis in the face of HIV infection is unknown. However, because of the substantial co-morbidity between HIV and syphilis and the evidence that genital ulcers (as in syphilis) promote the acquisition of HIV infection, psychiatrists need to be particularly watchful in these populations (CDC 1988b). Patients with late syphilis should also be evaluated for syphilitic aortitis because it is a frequent cause of morbidity and death (Holmes and Lukehart 1987; Relman et al. 1988a).

Treatments

As noted above, the recommendations for treatment of primary and secondary syphilis have been undergoing modifications (Musher 1988). In general for neurosyphilis, the most effective regimen uses aqueous penicillin G ($12–24 \times 10^6$ units per day) in divided intravenous doses for at least 10–14 days, followed by weekly benzathine penicillin G (2.4×10^6 units/week) intramuscularly for 3 weeks (Adams and Victor 1989; Holmes and Lukehart 1987). Other regimens, especially those using oral agents or nonaqueous penicillin, are likely to be less effective (Lukehart et al. 1988; Musher 1988). The Jarisch-Herxheimer reaction, consisting of fever, chills, headache, and rash, occurs briefly after initial penicillin treatment; it is less likely to occur with late syphilis infections (Relman et al. 1988a). Efficacy of treatment for neurosyphilis is documented by observing the return of CSF parameters to normal within 1 year (Adams and Victor 1989; Relman et al. 1988a). As noted above, the CSF VDRL may remain weakly reactive, and it is unclear whether this is an indication for further pharmacotherapy. The return of pleocytosis, an increase in protein, and/or an increase in VDRL titer is indicative of failed treatment. Pharmacotherapy is empiric for psychiatric disturbances associated with syphilis and should follow principles outlined above for HIV infection, especially in regard to conservative dosage, and close observation for neuropsychiatric side effects.

LYME DISEASE

In 1975, an unusual cluster of arthritis among children and adults in Lyme, Connecticut, led to the characterization of a new form of arthritis called Lyme arthritis (Steere et al. 1977). Since its initial discovery, the clinical presentation of the illness, including neuropsychiatric symptoms, epidemiology, pathogenesis, serology, and treatment, has been well described (Steere 1987, 1989; Steere et al. 1977).

Epidemiology

Lyme disease has been found in 40 states in the United States and has been reported in Europe, Australia, and other countries. Since 1982, 13,825 cases of Lyme disease have been reported in the United States. Most of the U.S. cases have clustered in the Northeast, Northwest, and upper Midwest (CDC 1989d; Relman et al. 1988b; Schmid et al. 1985; Steere 1987, 1989). The vast majority of cases begin in May, June, July, or August and peak in July. Most victims live in or have traveled through heavily wooded areas during these months, increasing the likelihood of encountering the vector, although infected ticks have also been reported on lawns in endemic areas (Falco and Fish 1988).

Pathogenesis

Lyme disease is caused by the spirochete *Borrelia burgdorferi. Borrelia burgdorferi* is carried by mature deer ticks *Ioxides dammini, I. pacificus,* and *I. ricinus.* The deer tick transmits the spirochete via a bite. Clinical symptoms are associated with replication of the spirochete and dissemination to other organ systems. The role that immune complexes may play in the pathogenesis of specific symptoms is unclear (Harden et al. 1979; Steere 1987).

Clinical Description

For 60–80% of patients, the first manifestation of Lyme disease is a distinctive rash, erythema chronicum migrans (ECM). Other patients may not recall a rash or may not have had one. The rash appears within 3–32 days after a tick bite and appears first at the site of the bite (Berardi et al. 1988; Steere 1987, 1989; Steere et al. 1983a). The rash is annular, red, and may be up to 56 cm in diameter. Over time, there is central clearing of the rash, leaving an erythematous ring in a so-called bull's-eye pattern. Many patients will then develop secondary lesions, primarily on the thighs and trunk (Steere et al. 1978). Associated symptoms include fever, fatigue, myalgia, and headache. In patients who develop more severe constitutional symptoms, including stiff neck, CSF will show lymphocytic pleocytosis, elevated protein, and normal glucose (Steere et al. 1983b). Three months after infection, approximately 15% of patients will go on to a second phase of illness, which can include significant neurologic symptoms such as meningitis, encephalitis, radiculitis, central or peripheral neuropathy, and myelitis. In 8% of patients, cardiac symptoms occur (Relman et al. 1988b; Steere 1987). In some cases, there are symptoms and signs of subacute meningoencephalitis, including headaches, stiff neck, irritability, depression, confusion, and emotional lability. Patients may also have an associated facial palsy or another peripheral manifestation of illness. If not treated with high-dose antibiotics, symptoms may persist for up to 1 year (Steere et al. 1983b). CSF findings are similar to those described above.

Cardiac symptoms most commonly include conduction system abnormalities, including first-degree atrioventricular block, second-degree block (both type 1 and type 2), and complete (third degree) atrioventricular block. Patients may also develop left ventricular dysfunction. Valvular disease has not been reported (McAlister et al. 1989; Relman et al. 1988b; Steere 1987; Steere et al. 1980).

A third phase of illness occurs approximately 6 months after the initial infection. This phase consists of an oligoarthritis (which can begin earlier), primarily affecting the knees but also affecting the small joints in a symmetrical pattern. In some cases, patients may experience a migratory arthritis or migratory myalgic symptoms (Steere 1987; Steere et al. 1977, 1979).

The classic stages described above may not occur in a typical fashion because some patients may not have any symptoms until stage 2 or 3. In addition, patients may not have neurologic symptoms until stage 3 but may have arthritic symptoms as early as stage 2. In a modified staging system, stage 1 occurs early and is associated with ECM. Stage 2 occurs in days to weeks after stage 1, and sometimes symptoms do not develop until months later. Stage 3 is defined as late infection, beginning 1 year after infection (Steere 1989).

Neuropsychiatric Manifestations

Recent studies have reported that mild encephalopathic states, characterized by subjective and objective evidence of difficulty in memory orientation, calculation, and construction, are among the most frequent presentations at Lyme disease clinics (Halperin et al. 1989). These states may occur late in the course of illness after other manifestations of Lyme disease have cleared, making diagnosis more difficult. Of 13 patients with encephalopathy who had *Borrelia burgdorferi* specific IgG measured in CSF, 10 patients had evidence of increased specific IgG production in the CNS compared with the periphery (Halperin et al. 1989). Of 17 encephalopathic patients examined by MRI, 7 had white matter abnormalities, 3 of which cleared on repeat MRI after appropriate antibiotic therapy.

Pachner and colleagues also found variable CNS manifestations of Lyme disease often occurring months or years after initial infection. These manifestations have included psychiatric syndromes, including violent behavior, emotional lability with inappropriate laughter, depression, and compulsive behavior. High-dose intravenous antibiotics were associated with clearing of psychiatric symptoms in at least two cases (Pachner et al. 1989). Cases of Lyme CNS illness have also been reported to end in a chronic dementing syndrome (Steere 1989).

Serodiagnosis

Serologic studies may aid in the diagnosis of Lyme disease. However, because most patients with early Lyme disease lack evidence of antibody to *Borrelia burgdorferi*, clinical diagnosis of early disease remains critical.

Serologic studies commonly performed for Lyme disease include ELISA or indirect immunofluorescence assay for IgG. Standard ELISA can detect antibody in approximately 40–50% of early cases (Barbour 1989; Grodzicki and Steere 1988; Relman et al. 1988b; Shrestha et al. 1985; Steere 1987). In patients with later manifestations of Lyme disease, serologic testing is more useful, with a sensitivity of 60%. Major sources of false-positive findings include patients infected with other spirochetal organisms, including other *Borrelia* species, *Treponema pallidum*, and *Leptospira* species (Magnanelli et al. 1987). An antibody-capture enzyme immunoassay test may improve the serologic yield in early Lyme disease to 67% and in convalescence to 93%, but this test is not clinically available at present (Berardi et al. 1988). Variable reference standards and lack of inter- and intralaboratory reliability are another source of potential error in serologic testing. False-negative results, even with IgM-capture assays, are common, especially in early illness. Patients previously treated with oral antibiotics for Lyme disease have been reported to have undetectable antibodies but a demonstrable T cell response to *B. burgdorferi* (Datwyler et al. 1988; Diagnosis of Lyme disease 1989). False-positive results can occur in autoimmune disorders, neurologic disorders, and other spirochetal illnesses including syphilis. A confirmatory test to eliminate false-positive findings is not currently available (Steere 1989).

Issues in Neuropsychiatric Diagnosis

In patients with classic symptoms of Lyme disease such as ECM, diagnosis becomes a somewhat simpler matter. A patient with a history of ECM, meningoencephalitis with facial nerve palsy, and oligoarthritis is likely to have Lyme disease (Barbour 1989). However, because of the nonspecific nature of many early complaints of Lyme disease, patients who lack a history of ECM (up to 40% of patients) are more difficult to diagnose. Clues to the diagnosis include travel in wooded, endemic areas and onset of illness during the summer months.

Patients with irritability, confusion, or lability as a sole or secondary manifestation of Lyme disease are more likely to come to psychiatric attention (Pachner and Steere 1985; Reik et al. 1979, 1986). The presence of symptoms of meningoencephalitis in association with cranial nerve palsy, including bilateral facial nerve palsy or with a radiculoneuritis, is suggestive of Lyme disease. In patients without rash, it is easy to confuse the diagnosis with that of aseptic meningitis; in the latter disease, however, symptoms are usually acute. In Lyme disease, there is an acute phase of illness followed by symptoms of chronic headache, stiff neck, etc. Serologic studies performed during this phase of illness are significantly more likely to be abnormal (Pachner and Steere 1985; Reik et al. 1979, 1986). Particular diagnostic uncertainty may occur in those patients who experience late-onset encephalopathic or psychiatric symptoms (Halperin et al. 1989; Pachner et al. 1989). Because of the limited knowledge about the cognitive changes in Lyme disease, the absence of pathognomonic neuropsychiatric findings, and the small number of confirmed psychiatric cases, psychiatrists must rely on the history and the CSF examination in a patient with less clear-cut or questionable Lyme disease symptoms.

In addition to gathering a detailed history of prior travel, rashes, and other symptoms, evidence of active infection may be inferred from several CSF abnormalities. Patients with stage 2 focal neurologic Lyme disease should have a lumbar puncture. In stage 3 encephalopathic or psychiatric cases where patients are seropositive, or seronegative with a clear history of Lyme disease, especially as documented by ECM, CSF also should be examined. Evidence of pleocytosis and elevated protein represent nonspecific evidence of CNS infection, as may MRI evidence of white matter hyperintensity. CSF that shows evidence of an increase specific IgG CSF index for *B. burgdorferi* is probably the strongest currently available evidence for ongoing CNS infection. Further confirmatory evidence is suggested by clearing white matter lesions on MRI after appropriate antibiotic therapy (Halperin et al. 1989; Pachner et al. 1989; Steere 1989).

Treatment

The treatment of Lyme disease depends on adequate antibiotic therapy of the causative organism. Patients with early disease will generally respond well to tetracycline, 250 mg po qid for 10–20 days. Alternative regimens with erythromycin or penicillin are also useful but associated with a higher rate of late illness. Patients who have evidence of active CNS disease should be treated with 20×10^6 units of aqueous penicillin G per day intravenously in divided doses for 14 days. This regimen is associated with a rapid resolution of meningeal signs and symptoms, although focal neurologic symptoms may persist (Steere 1987; Steere et al. 1983c). Ceftriaxone (2 g iv daily for 14 days or more) is also an effective regimen for Lyme disease–related neurologic illness, although longer courses of treatment may be required (Steere 1989).

Lyme disease is rarely fatal, but when fatalities do occur they are most often due to cardiac complications, including complete heart block, acute myopericarditis, and cardiomegaly. Some patients may require temporary pacing wires until conduction deficits normalize (McAlister et al. 1989; Steere 1989). As such, all patients who present for psychiatric attention with a possible diagnosis of Lyme disease should have evaluation of their cardiac status, including an ECG. Cardiology consultation and follow-up ECGs are indicated if abnormalities are found.

CHRONIC FATIGUE SYNDROME

Reports of focal epidemics of a syndrome characterized by prolonged fatigue, low-grade fever, lymphadenopathy, impaired concentration, and confusion appeared in the medical literature in the 1980s (Jones et al. 1985; Straus et al. 1985; Tobi et al. 1982). Because a number of these cases were associated with elevated antibodies to Epstein-Barr virus or occurred after acute infectious mononucleosis, the syndrome rapidly became known as the chronic Epstein-Barr virus syndrome, or the chronic mononucleosis syndrome (Dubois et al. 1984; Jones et al. 1985). Popularization of this syndrome in the media led to a large number of patients being examined for complaints of chronic fatigue and requesting evaluation of antibodies to Epstein-Barr virus. The high frequency of psychiatric, especially depressive, symptoms among these patients and reports of an association between affective illness and reactivation of Epstein-Barr virus also led to psychiatrists being asked to obtain Epstein-Barr virus serologies on their patients. Recent studies have cast doubt on the association of this syndrome with reactivation of prior Epstein-Barr virus infection and have led a CDC working group to rename this condition chronic fatigue syndrome. CDC has also defined strict criteria for this syndrome as an aid to clinical diagnosis and research (Gold et al. 1990; Holmes et al. 1988) (Table 7-4).

Clinical Diagnosis

Chronic fatigue syndrome bears close similarity to earlier reports of disabling fatigue either after an infectious event, as in the chronic brucellosis reports of the 1950s, or without an inciting cause, as in epidemic neuromyasthenia (Henderson and Shelokov 1959). The hallmark of chronic fatigue syndrome is chronic disabling fatigue often so severe that patients report that they are unable to continue normal household or occupational activities. Patients may report a feeling of feverishness; sore, tender, or enlarged lymph nodes; recurrent sore throat; and feelings of depression. Many patients report the onset of the fatigue after a severe flulike syndrome and say that they feel as if they simply never recovered (CDC 1989c; Holmes et al. 1988; Jones et al. 1985). Because of the nonspecificity of the presenting complaints, attempts to document the severity of the syndrome objectively have proven difficult. In one study on the effect of acyclovir on symptoms of chronic fatigue syndrome, investigators could find no evidence of elevated temperature despite their patients' subjective reports of feverishness (Straus

Table 7-4. Centers for Disease Control (CDC) working case definition for chronic fatigue syndrome

A patient must meet both major criteria and 6 of the 11 symptom criteria plus 2 or more of the 3 physical criteria or 8 or more of the 11 symptom criteria.

Major criteria

1. New persistent fatigue lasting 6 months or more and reducing patient's activity to below 50% of premorbid functioning
2. Full evaluation, including laboratory studies to rule out other causes of fatigue infection such as malignancy, localized or systemic infection, HIV-related illness, chronic psychiatric illness, inflammatory disorders, acute immune disorder, endocrine disease, substance abuse, other chronic medical illness

Minor criteria

Symptom criteria

1. Mild fever: oral temperature 37.5°–38.6°C
2. Sore throat
3. Painful lymph nodes and anterior or posterior cervical or axillary areas
4. Generalized muscle weakness
5. Myalgia
6. Prolonged fatigue (>24 hours) after moderate exercise
7. Generalized headaches
8. Migratory arthralgias
9. Neuropsychologic complaints
10. Sleep disturbance
11. Rapid development of main symptom complex (hours to few days)

Physical criteria (documented by physician on two occasions, 1 month apart or more)

1. Low-grade fever and oral temperature 37.6°–38.6°C
2. Nonexudative pharyngitis
3. Palpable or tender anterior or posterior cervical or axillary nodes (<2 cm in diameter)

et al. 1988). In addition, a study of muscle strength in patients with chronic fatigue syndrome found no evidence of diminished muscle strength or easy fatigability despite patients' reports of weakness (Lloyd et al. 1988). When diagnosed by stricter CDC criteria for chronic fatigue syndrome, patients must fulfill the two major criteria and eight or nine minor criteria for diagnosis (Holmes et al. 1988). In addition, other disorders, including malignancy, infection, autoimmune disease, endocrinopathies, sleep apnea, and other assorted conditions, need to be ruled out. Sleep studies may be of value in patients who are suspected of sleep apnea (Holmes et al. 1988). Of particular importance to the psychiatrist, patients with evidence of a primary psychiatric diagnosis, including major depressive disorder, anxiety disorder, histrionic personality disorder, and schizophrenia, and those who use lithium, antipsychotic, or antidepressant medication qualify for exclusion under the new criteria (Holmes et al. 1988).

In a recent study of 135 patients evaluated at a university clinic for chronic fatigue, only 6 patients could be diagnosed with chronic fatigue syndrome after strict application of the new criteria (Manu et al. 1988). In 7 patients, fatigue was secondary to medical diagnoses including sleep apnea, seizures, polymyalgia rheumatica, and panhypopituitarism. Ninety-one patients were excluded secondary to psychiatric diagnoses, including major depression, panic disorder, somatization disorder, and dysthymia (Manu et al. 1988). Therefore, most excluded patients had treatable psychiatric disorders. In practice, these patients should be treated for their psychiatric disorders and then reevaluated for chronic fatigue symptoms. Residual physical symptoms following adequate psychiatric treatment may require further investigation.

Serologic Studies

Early case series reported unusual profiles of Epstein-Barr virus antibodies in patients with chronic Epstein-Barr virus (Jaffe et al. 1978; Moskovitz et al. 1982). Epstein-Barr virus infects nearly all adults (CDC 1989c). When individuals are infected in adolescence or early adulthood, 30–45% develop infectious mononucleosis, a severe flulike syndrome characterized by intense sore throat, fatigue, lymphadenopathy, and often splenomegaly. During this period of acute infection, patients can be diagnosed by the production of Paul-Bunnell (heterophile) antibodies (CDC 1989c; Schooley 1987).

A number of other antibodies are also characteristically produced during early and late phases of Epstein-Barr virus infections. During the early replicative phase of infection, patients initially show high titers of IgM antibody to Epstein-Barr virus capsid antigen (VCA), which disappears 1–2 months after infection. The development of IgG to VCA also occurs early and then persists at lower titers. Shortly after infection, patients also develop antibodies to early antigens, which may persist at low levels for many years. Several months after infection, patients begin to produce antibodies to Epstein-Barr nuclear antigens (EBNA 1&2), which then persist for life. Therefore, usually an adult with prior exposure to Epstein-Barr virus, but no active infection, will have no IgM to VCA, low IgG to VCA, a low titer of antibody to early antigen, and lifetime antibodies to EBNA 1&2 (Sumaya 1986).

In contrast, patients thought to have chronic Epstein-Barr virus infection had elevated levels of replicative enzyme antibodies (VCA and early antigens) and in some cases absent EBNA 1&2 antibodies (Jones et al. 1985; Straus et al. 1985). Similar to several reported cases of a chronic severe form of infectious mononucleosis with pneumonitis and hematologic abnormalities, this pattern suggested that chronic Epstein-Barr virus might represent an ongoing replication of the virus leading to clinical symptoms (Henle et al. 1987; Miller et al. 1987; Schooley et al. 1986). However, other studies have cast doubt on this hypothesis. While levels of replicative antibodies are higher in chronic fatigue syndrome patients than in controls, this finding only rarely reaches statistical significance, and there is significant overlap in antibody level between patients and asymptomatic controls (Buchwald et al. 1987).

A related study has also found elevated antibody levels to a variety of viruses in patients believed to have chronic Epstein-Barr virus infection, including cytomegalovirus, herpes simplex, and measles, suggesting a general change in immune functioning possibly causing reactivation of these viruses (Holmes et al. 1987). There has been a report of an association with human herpes virus 6, a recently discovered herpes virus. Whether this association will be seen in a larger series of patients with chronic fatigue syndrome is unknown at present. In addition, a variety of other subtle changes in immune functioning have been noted in patients with chronic fatigue, including changes in T helper/suppressor levels (in both directions), mild IgA deficiencies, decreased natural killer cell activity, and other abnormalities. These changes have been inconsistent among studies and are of uncertain significance (CDC 1989c; Straus 1988).

Psychiatric Diagnoses

A number of clinicians have noted a high frequency of psychiatric symptoms, particularly depression, in patients being evaluated for chronic fatigue syndrome (Manu et al. 1988). Kruesi and colleagues (1989) found 75% of patients with chronic fatigue syndrome to have DSM-III (American Psychiatric Association 1980) diagnoses when evaluated by the Diagnostic Interview Schedule. Of these patients, 35% had diagnoses that preceded the onset of their fatigue. Lifetime rates of depression exceeded those for patients with diabetes. Major depression, dysthymia, simple phobia, and somatization disorder were the most frequent diagnoses (Kruesi et al. 1989).

In a treatment study using acyclovir, a correlation was observed between changes in the Profile of Mood States and symptoms of chronic fatigue syndrome (Straus et al. 1988). However, the relationships between affective symptoms and chronic fatigue are complex, and the direction of the causation is unclear (Straus et al. 1988). In a well-designed (for that time) prospective study, Imboden et al. (1961) found increased rates of depression by the Minnesota Multiphasic Personality Inventory (MMPI) in patients who later had delayed recovery from influenza. (We discuss clinical issues related to this observation further below.) There is no evidence that Epstein-Barr virus is a necessary or causative agent for mood disorder (Amsterdam et al. 1986). There have been reports of white matter hyperintensity on MRI in patients with chronic fatigue. Whether this finding will correlate with neuropsychiatric symptoms in a larger series is unknown at present (Straus 1988).

Treatment

Specific treatments for chronic fatigue syndrome are not available. Straus and colleagues (1988) studied acyclovir infusions in a double-blind treatment study of patients with chronic fatigue syndrome. There was no significant difference in objective outcome or subjective well-being between patients in the treatment and the placebo group (Straus et al. 1988). Treatment aimed at reducing symptomatology is warranted whether for psychiatric or other symptoms. Use of antidepressants or other psychopharmacologic agents may be helpful for specific psychiatric syndromes, although studies of this treatment are not available. Patients often are highly reluctant to consider a psychiatric diagnosis but may accept psychopharmacological assistance for specific symptoms if presented in a matter-of-fact, nonthreatening manner.

Clinical Dilemmas in Chronic Fatigue Syndrome

Clinicians need to be wary of foreclosing judgment on patients with chronic fatigue syndrome. Clearly, the complaint of fatigue is common among patients seen in general medical practice, and, in unselected samples of patients with fatigue, psychiatric disorders are common (Buchwald et al. 1987; Holmes et al. 1987). The new criteria for chronic fatigue syndrome are drawn in a purposefully narrow fashion, in part to select patients with a syndrome of homogeneous etiology for research purposes. However, psychiatrists need to be cautious in ascribing all psychiatric symptoms to primary psychiatric illness. The diagnostic criteria for major depression in the setting of medical illness are unclear. Further, the evidence of abnormal immune activation in patients with chronic fatigue syndrome suggests that at least for some patients symptoms may be secondary to the syndrome itself, whatever its ultimate etiology proves to be. Finally, psychiatrists need to be alert to the wide variety of other medical disorders associated with chronic fatigue and to ensure that patients have an adequate evaluation for other etiologies. Whether serologic tests have any clinical role in the evaluation of chronic fatigue syndrome other than for research purposes is unclear (Holmes et al. 1988; Manu et al. 1988).

REFERENCES

Adams R, Victor M: Principles of Neurology, 4th Edition. New York, McGraw-Hill, 1989, pp 573–580

Adler C, Beckett A: Psychotherapy of the patient with an HIV infection: some ethical and therapeutic dilemmas. Psychosomatics 30:203–208, 1989

Albert ML, Feldman RG, Willis AL: "Subcortical dementia" of progressive supranuclear palsy. J Neurol Neurosurg Psychiatry 37:121–130, 1974

American Psychiatric Association: Diagnostic and Statistical Manual of Mental Disorders, 3rd Edition. Washington, DC, American Psychiatric Association, 1980

Amsterdam JD, Henle W, Winoner A: Serum antibodies to Epstein-Barr virus in patients with major depressive disorder. Am J Psychiatry 143:1593–1596, 1986

Anders KH, Guerra WF, Tomiyasu U, et al: The neuropathology of AIDS: UCLA experience and review. Am J Pathol 124:537–558, 1986

Atkinson JH, Grant I, Kennedy CJ, et al: Prevalence of psychiatric disorders among men infected with human immunodeficiency virus: a controlled study. Arch Gen Psychiatry 45:859–864, 1988

Baer JW: Study of 60 patients with AIDS or AIDS related complex requiring psychiatric hospitalization. Am J Psychiatry 146:1285–1288, 1989

Barbour AG: The diagnosis of Lyme disease: rewards and perils. Ann Intern Med 110:501–502, 1989

Bayne LL, Schmidley JW, Goodin DS: Acute syphilitic meningitis: its occurrence after clinical and serologic cure of secondary syphilis with penicillin G. Arch Neurol 43:137–138, 1986

Beckett A, Summergrad P, Manschreck T, et al: Symptomatic HIV infection of the central nervous system in a patient without evidence of immune deficiency. Am J Psychiatry 144:1342–1344, 1987

Berardi VP, Weeks KE, Steere AC: Serodiagnosis of early Lyme disease: analysis of IgM and IgG antibody responses by using an antibody-capture enzyme immunoassay. J Infect Dis 158:754–760, 1988

Bernstein WB, Scherokman B: Neuroleptic malignant syndrome in a patient with acquired immunodeficiency syndrome. Acta Neurol Scand 73:636–637, 1986

Berry CD, Hooton TM, Collier AC, et al: Neurologic relapse after benzathine penicillin therapy for secondary syphilis in a patient with HIV infection. N Engl J Med 316:1587–1589, 1987

Binder RL: AIDS antibody tests on inpatient psychiatric units. Am J Psychiatry 144:176–181, 1987

Breakey WR, Fischer PJ, Kramer M, et al: Health and mental health problems of homeless men and women in Baltimore. JAMA 262:1352–1357, 1989

Bridge TP, Heseltine PNR, Parker ES, et al: Improvement in AIDS patients on peptide T. Lancet 2:226–227, 1989

Brotman AW, Forstein M: AIDS obsessions in depressed heterosexuals. Psychosomatics 29:428–431, 1988

Buchwald D, Sullivan JL, Komaroff AL: Frequency of chronic active Epstein-Barr virus infection in a general medical practice. JAMA 257:2302–2307, 1987

Buhrich N, Cooper DA, Freed E: HIV infection associated with symptoms indistinguishable from functional psychosis. Br J Psychiatry 152:649–653, 1988

Bukasa KS, Sindic CJM, Bodeus M, et al: Anti-HIV antibodies in the CSF of AIDS patients: a serologic and immunoblotting study. J Neurol Neurosurg Psychiatry 51:1063–1068, 1988

Centers for Disease Control Update: Serologic testing for antibody to human immunodeficiency virus. MMWR 36:833–840, 845.4, 1988a

Centers for Disease Control: Continuing increase in infectious syphilis—United States. MMWR 37:35–38, 1988b

Centers for Disease Control: Interpretation and use of the Western blot assay for serodiagnosis of human immunodeficiency virus type 1 infections. MMWR 38 (No S-7):1–7, 1989a

Centers for Disease Control: Guidelines for prophylaxis against Pneumocystis carinii pneumonia for persons infected with human immunodeficiency virus. MMWR 38(S-5):1–9, 1989b

Centers for Disease Control: Chronic Fatigue Syndrome. Atlanta, GA, Centers for Disease Control, 1989c, pp 1–10

Centers for Disease Control: Lyme disease—United States, 1987 and 1988. MMWR 38:668–672, 1989d

Centers for Disease Control: Update: Acquired immunodeficiency syndrome—United States 1981–1988. MMWR 38:229–236, 1989e

Centers for Disease Control: HIV/AIDS Surveillance Report. Atlanta, GA, Centers for Disease Control, October 1990, pp 1–18

Clinical trials of zidovudine in HIV infection (editorial). Lancet 2:483–484, 1989

Cummings JL, Benson DF: Subcortical dementia: review of an emerging concept. Arch Neurol 41:874–879, 1984

Cummings JL, Benson DF: Psychological dysfunction accompanying subcortical dementias. Annu Rev Med 39:53–61, 1988

Cummings MA, Cummings KL, Rapaport MH, et al: Acquired immunodeficiency syndrome presenting as schizophrenia. West J Med 146:615–618, 1987

Dalakas M, Wichman A, Sever J: AIDS and the nervous system. JAMA 261:2396–2399, 1989

Dattwyler RJ, Volkman DJ, Luft BJ, et al: Dissociation of specific T and B lymphocyte responses to *Borrelia burgdorferi.* N Engl J Med 319:1441–1446, 1988

Davis LE, Schmitt JW: Clinical significance of cerebrospinal fluid tests for neurosyphilis. Ann Neurol 25:50–55, 1989

de la Monte SM, Ho DD, Schooley RT, et al: Subacute encephalomyelitis of AIDS and its relation to HTLV-III infection. Neurology 37:562–569, 1987

Diagnosis of Lyme disease (editorial). Lancet 2:198–199, 1989

Dilley JW, Ochitill HN, Perl M, et al: Findings in psychiatric consultations with patients with acquired immune deficiency syndrome. Am J Psychiatry 142:82–86, 1985

Dubois RE, Seeley JK, Brus I, et al: Chronic mononucleosis syndrome. South Med J 77:1376–1382, 1984

Falco RC, Fish D: Prevalence of *Ixodes daminni* near the homes of Lyme disease patients in Westchester County, New York. Am J Epidemiol 127:826–830, 1988

Faulstich ME: Psychiatric aspects of AIDS. Am J Psychiatry 144:551–556, 1987

Fernandez F, Levy JK, Galizzi H: Response of HIV-related depression to psychostimulants: case reports. Hosp Community Psychiatry 39:628–631, 1988

Fernandez F, Levy JK, Mansell PWA: Response to antidepressant therapy in depressed persons with HIV infection. Abstract presented at the 5th International AIDS Conference, Montreal, Canada, June, 1989

Forstein M: The psychosocial impact of the acquired immunodeficiency syndrome. Semin Oncol 11:77–82, 1984

Friedman-Kien A, Laubastein L, Rubinstein P, et al: Disseminated Kaposi's sarcoma in homosexual men. Ann Intern Med 96:693–700, 1981

Gabuzda DH, Hirsch MS: Neurologic manifestations of infections with human immunodeficiency virus: clinical features and pathogenesis. Ann Intern Med 107:383–391, 1987

Gabuzda DH, Ho DD, de la Monte SM, et al: Immunohistochemical identification of HTLV-III antigen in brains of patients with AIDS. Ann Neurol 20:289–295, 1986

Glass RM: AIDS and suicide. JAMA 259:1369–1370, 1988

Gold D, Bowden R, Sixbey J, et al: Chronic fatigue: a prospective clinical and neurologic study. JAMA 264:48–53, 1990

Gottlieb MS, Schroff R, Shanker HM, et al: Pneumocystis carinii pneumonia and mucosal candidiasis in previously healthy homosexual men: evidence of a new acquired cellular immunodeficiency. N Engl J Med 305:1425–1431, 1981

Grant I, Atkinson JH, Hesselink JR, et al: Evidence for early central nervous system involvement in the acquired immunodeficiency syndrome (AIDS) and other human immunodeficiency virus (HIV) infections: studies with neuropsychological testing and magnetic resonance imaging. Ann Intern Med 107:828–836, 1987

Grodzicki Rl, Steere AC: Comparison immunoblotting and indirect enzyme-linked immunosorbent assay using different antigen preparations for diagnosing early Lyme disease. J Infect Dis 157:521–525, 1988

Guinan ME: Treatment of primary and secondary syphilis: defining failure at three and six month follow up. JAMA 257:359–360, 1987

Halperin JJ, Luft BJ, Anand AK: Lyme neuroborreliosis: central nervous system manifestations. Neurology 39:753–759, 1989

Harden JA, Steere AC, Malawista SE: Immune complexes in the evolution of Lyme arthritis dissemination and localization of abnormal C1q binding activity. N Engl J Med 301:1358–1363, 1979

Harris MJ, Gleghorn A, Jeste DV: HIV-related psychosis. Presented at the 142nd meeting of the American Psychiatric Association, San Francisco, CA, May 1989

Henderson DA, Shelokov A: Epidemic neuromyasthenia: a clinical syndrome? N Engl J Med 260:757–764, 1959

Henle W, Henle G, Andersson J, et al: Antibody responses to Epstein-Barr virus determined nuclear antigen (EBNA)-1 and EBNA-2 in acute and chronic Epstein-Barr virus infection. Proc Natl Acad Sci USA 84:570–574, 1987

Hicks CB, Benson AM, Lipton GP: Seronegative secondary syphilis in a patient infected with the human immunodeficiency virus (HIV) with Kaposi sarcoma: a diagnostic dilemma. Ann Intern Med 107:492–495, 1987

Ho DD, Roth TR, Schooley RT, et al: Isolation of HTLV-III from cerebrospinal fluid and neural tissues of patients with neurologic syndromes related to the acquired immunodeficiency syndrome. N Engl J Med 313:1493–1497, 1985

Holland JC, Tross S: The psychosocial and neuropsychiatric sequence of the acquired immunodeficiency syndrome and related disorders. Ann Intern Med 103:760–764, 1985

Holmes GP, Kaplan JE, Stewart JA, et al: A cluster of patients with a chronic mononucleosis-like syndrome. JAMA 57:2297–2302, 1987

Holmes GP, Kaplan JE, Gantz NM, et al: Chronic fatigue syndrome: a working case definition. Ann Intern Med 108:387–389, 1988

Holmes KK, Lukehart SA: Syphilis, in Harrison's Principles of Internal Medicine, 11th Edition. Edited by Braunwald E, Isselbacher KJ, Petersdorf RG, et al. New York, McGraw-Hill, 1987, pp 639–649

Holmes VF, Fernandez F, Levy JK: Psychostimulant response in ARC patients. J Clin Psychiatry 50:5–8, 1989

Hooshmand H, Escobar MR, Kopf SW: Neurosyphilis: a study of 241 patients. JAMA 219:726–729, 1972

Imboden JB, Canter A, Cluff LE: Convalescence from influenza: a study of the psychological and clinical determinants. Arch Intern Med 108:393–399, 1961

Jaffe HW, Kabins SA: Examination of cerebrospinal fluid in patients with syphilis. Review of Infectious Diseases 4:S842–S847, 1982

Jaffe HW, Larsen SA, Peters M, et al: Tests for treponemal antibody in CSF. Arch Intern Med 138:252–255, 1978

Jenike MA, Pato C: Disabling fear of AIDS responsive to imipramine. Psychosomatics 27:143–144, 1986

Joffe RT, Rubinow DR, Squillace K, et al: Neuropsychiatric aspects of AIDS. Psychopharmacol Bull 22:684–688, 1986

Johns DR, Tierney M, Felsenstein D: Alteration in the natural history of neurosyphilis by concurrent infection with the human immunodeficiency virus. N Engl J Med 316:1569–1572, 1987

Jones JF, Ray G, Minnich LL, et al: Evidence for active Epstein-Barr virus infection in patients with persistent, unexplained illnesses: elevated anti-early antigen antibodies. Ann Intern Med 102:1–6, 1985

Koenig S, Gendelman HE, Orenstein JM, et al: Detection of AIDS virus in manophages in brain tissue from AIDS patients with encephalopathy. Science 233:1089–1093, 1986

Koralnik IJ, Beaumanoir A, Hausler R, et al: A controlled study of early neurologic abnormalities in men with asymptomatic human immunodeficiency virus infection. N Engl J Med 323:864–870, 1990

Kruesi MJP, Dale J, Straus SE: Psychiatric diagnosis in patients with chronic fatigue syndrome. J Clin Psychiatry 50:53–56, 1989

Larsen SA, Beck-Sague CM: Syphilis, in Laboratory Diagnosis of Infectious Diseases: Principles and Practice, Vol 1. Edited by Balows A, Hausler WT, Okaski M, et al. New York, Springer-Verlag, 1988, pp 490–503

Levy JA, Hollender H, Shimabukuro J, et al: Isolation of AIDS associated retroviruses from cerebrospinal fluid and brain of patients with neurologic symptoms. Lancet 2:586–588, 1985a

Levy RM, Bredesen DM, Rosenblum ML: Neurologic manifestations of the acquired immunodeficiency syndrome (AIDS): experience at UCSF and review of the literature. J Neurosurg 62:475–495, 1985b

Levy RM, Bredesen DM, Rosenblum ML: Opportunistic central nervous system pathology in patients with AIDS. Ann Neurol 23 (suppl):S7–S12, 1988

Lishman WA: Organic Psychiatry, 2nd Edition. London, Blackwell, 1988

Lloyd AR, Phales J, Gandevia SC: Muscle strength, endurance, and recovery in the post infection fatigue syndrome. J Neurol Neurosurg Psychiatry 51:1316–1322, 1988

Lukehart SA, Hook EW, Baker-Zander SA, et al: Invasion of the central nervous system by Treponema pallidum: implications for diagnosis and treatment. Ann Intern Med 109:855–862, 1988

Magnanelli LA, Anderson JF, Johnson RC: Cross reactivity in serological tests for Lyme disease and other spirochetal infections. J Infect Dis 156:183–188, 1987

Manu P, Lane TJ, Matthews DA: The frequency of chronic fatigue syndrome in patients with symptoms of persistent fatigue. Ann Intern Med 109:554–556, 1988

Markovitz DM, Beutnar KR, Maggio RP, et al: Failure of recommended treatment for secondary syphilis. JAMA 255:1767–1768, 1986

Marotta R, Perry S: Early neuropsychological dysfunction caused by human immunodeficiency virus. Journal of Neuropsychiatry 1:225–235, 1989

Marzuk PM, Tierney H, Tardiff K, et al: Increased risk of suicide in persons with AIDS. JAMA 259:1333–1337, 1988

Masur H, Michelis MA, Greene JB, et al: An outbreak of community acquired Pneumocystis carinii pneumonia: initial manifestation of cellular immune dysfunction. N Engl J Med 305:1431–1438, 1981

McAlister HF, Klementowitz PT, Andrews C, et al: Lyme carditis: an important cause of reversible heart block. Ann Intern Med 110:339–345, 1989

McArthur JC: Neurologic manifestations of AIDS. Medicine 66:407–437, 1987

McArthur JC, Cohen BA, Farzedegan H, et al: Cerebrospinal fluid abnormalities in homosexual men with and without neuropsychiatric findings. Ann Neurol 23 (suppl):S34–S37, 1988

Miller G, Grogan E, Rowe D, et al: Selective lack of antibody to a component of the EB nuclear antigen in patients with chronic active Epstein-Barr virus infection. J Infect Dis 156:26–35, 1987

Morgan MK, Clark ME, Hartman WL: Aids related dementia: a case report of rapid cognitive decline. J Clin Psychol 44:1024–1028, 1988

Moskovitz BL, Klinch JJ, Goldman RL, et al: Meningovascular syphilis after "appropriate" treatment of primary syphilis. Arch Intern Med 142:139–140, 1982

Musher DM: Evaluation and management of an asymptomatic patient with a positive VDRL reaction. Current Clinical Topics in Infectious Diseases 9:147–157, 1978

Musher DM: How much penicillin cures early syphilis? Ann Intern Med 109:849–850, 1988

Navia BA, Price RW: The acquired immunodeficiency syndrome dementia complex as the presenting or sole manifestation of human immunodeficiency virus infection. Arch Neurol 44:65–69, 1987

Navia BA, Jordan BD, Price RW: The AIDS dementia complex, I: clinical features. Ann Neurol 19:517–524, 1986a

Navia BA, Cho ES, Petito CU, et al: The AIDS dementia complex, II: neuropathology. Ann Neurol 525–535, 1986b

Nurnberg HG, Prudic J, Fiori M, et al: Psychopathology complicating acquired immune deficiency syndrome. Am J Psychiatry 141:95–96, 1984

Ostrow DG, Monjan A, Joseph J, et al: HIV-related symptoms and psychological functioning in a cohort of homosexual men. Am J Psychiatry 146:737–742, 1989

Pachner AR, Steere AC: The triad of neurologic manifestations of Lyme disease, meningitis, cranial neuritis, and radiculoneuritis. Neurology 35:47–53, 1985

Pachner AR, Duray P, Steere AC: Central nervous system manifestations of Lyme disease. Arch Neurol 46:790–795, 1989

Perry S, Jacobsen P: Neuropsychiatric manifestations of AIDS-spectrum disorders. Hosp Community Psychiatry 37:135–141, 1986

Perry SW, Tross S: Psychiatric problems of AIDS inpatients at the New York Hospital: a preliminary report. Public Health Rep 99:200–205, 1984

Petito CK, Cho ES, Lemann W, et al: Neuropathology of acquired immunodeficiency syndrome (AIDS): an autopsy review. J Neuropathol Exp Neurol 45:635–646, 1986

Reik L, Steere AC, Bartenhagen NH, et al: Neurologic abnormalities of Lyme disease. Medicine 58:281–294, 1979

Reik L, Burgdorfer W, Donaldson JO: Neurologic abnormalities in Lyme disease without erythema chronicum migrans. Am J Med 81:73–78, 1986

Relman DA, Schoolnik GK, Swartz MN: Syphilis in nonvenereal treponematoses, in Scientific American Medicine, Vol 7. Edited by Rubenstein E, Federman DD. New York, Scientific American, 1988a, pp 1–10

Relman DA, Schoolnik GK, Swartz MN: Lyme disease, in Scientific American Medicine, Vol 7. Edited by Rubenstein E, Federman DD. New York, Scientific American, 1988b, pp 6–11

Rubin RH: Acquired immune deficiency syndrome, in Scientific American Medicine, Vol 7. Edited by Rubenstein E, Federman DD. New York, Scientific American, 1988, pp 1–19

Ruder HL, Cauthen GM, Kelly GD, et al: Tuberculosis in the United States. JAMA 262:385–389, 1989

Rundell JR, Wise MG, Ursano RJ: Three cases of AIDS-related psychiatric disorders. Am J Psychiatry 143:777–778, 1986

Schaerf FW, Miller RR, Lipsey JR, et al: ECT for major depression in four patients infected with human immunodeficiency virus. Am J Psychiatry 146:782–784, 1989

Schmid GP, Horsley R, Steere AC, et al: Surveillance of Lyme disease in the United States, 1982. J Infect Dis 151:1144–1149, 1985

Schmitt FA, Bigley JW, McInnis R, et al: Neuropsychological outcome of zidovudine (AZT) treatment of patients with AIDS and AIDS related complex. N Engl J Med 319:1573–1578, 1988

Schooley RT: Epstein-Barr virus infection, including infectious mononucleosis, in Harrison's Principles of Internal Medicine, 11th Edition. Edited by Braunwald E, Isselbacher RJ, Petersdorf RG. New York, McGraw-Hill, 1987, pp 699–703

Schooley RT, Carey RW, Miller G, et al: Chronic Epstein-Barr virus infection associated with fever and interstitial pneumonitis: clinical and serologic features and response to antiviral chemotherapy. Ann Intern Med 104:636–643, 1986

Shaw GM, Harper ME, Hahn BH, et al: HTLV-III infection in brains of children and adults with AIDS encephalopathy. Science 227:177–182, 1985

Shrestha M, Grodzicki RL, Steere AC: Diagnosing early Lyme disease. Am J Med 78:235–240, 1985

Siegal FP, Lopez C, Hammer GS, et al: Severe acquired immunodeficiency in male homosexuals, manifested by chronic perianal ulcerative herpes simplex lesion. N Engl J Med 305:1439–1444, 1981

Simon RP: Neurosyphilis. Arch Neurol 42:606–613, 1985

Snider WD, Simpson DM, Nielsen S, et al: Neurologic complications of acquired immune deficiency syndrome: analysis of 50 patients. Ann Neurol 14:403–418, 1983

Sparling PF: Diagnosis and treatment of syphilis. N Engl J Med 284:642–653, 1971

Steere AC: Lyme disease, in Harrison's Principles of Internal Medicine, 11th Edition. Edited by Braunwald E, Isselbacher RJ, Petersdorf RG. New York, McGraw-Hill, 1987, pp 657–659

Steere AC: Lyme disease. N Engl J Med 321:586–596, 1989

Steere AC, Malawista SE, Snydman DR, et al: Lyme arthritis: an epidemic of oligoarticular arthritis in children and adults in three Connecticut communities. Arthritis Rheum 20:7–17, 1977

Steere AC, Broderick TF, Malawista SE: Erythema chronicum migrans and Lyme arthritis: epidemiologic evidence for a tick vector. Am J Epidemiol 108:312–321, 1978

Steere AC, Hardin JA, Ruddy S, et al: Lyme arthritis: correlating serum and cryoglobulin IgM with activity and serum IgG with remission. Arthritis Rheum 22:471–483, 1979

Steere AC, Batsford WP, Weinberg M, et al: Lyme carditis: cardiac abnormalities of Lyme disease. Ann Intern Med 93 (part I):8–16, 1980

Steere AC, Bartenhagen NH, Craft JE, et al: The early clinical manifestations of Lyme disease. Ann Intern Med 99:76–82, 1983a

Steere AC, Pachner AR, Malawista SE: Neurologic abnormalities of Lyme disease: successful treatments with high dose intravenous penicillin. Ann Intern Med 99:767–772, 1983b

Steere AC, Hutchinson GJ, Rahn DW, et al: Treatment of the early manifestation of Lyme disease. Ann Intern Med 99:22–26, 1983c

Straus SE: The chronic mononucleosis syndrome. J Infect Dis 157:405–412, 1988

Straus SE, Trosato G, Armstron G, et al: Persisting illness and fatigue in adults with evidence of Epstein-Barr infection. Ann Intern Med 1:7–16, 1985

Straus SE, Dale JK, Tobi M, et al: Acyclovir treatment of the chronic fatigue syndrome: lack of efficacy in a controlled trial. N Engl J Med 319:1697–1698, 1988

Sumaya CV: Epstein-Barr virus serologic testing: diagnostic indications and interpretations. Pediatric Infectious Disease 5:337–341, 1986

Summergrad P, Peterson B: Binswanger's disease (Part I): the clinical recognition of subcortical arteriosclerotic encephalopathy in elderly neuropsychiatric patients. Journal of Geriatric Psychology and Neurology 2:123–133, 1989

Susser E, Struening EL, Conover S: Psychiatric problems in homeless men: lifetime psychosis, substance use, and current distress in new arrivals at New York City shelters. Arch Gen Psychiatry 46:845–850, 1989

Swartz M: Neurosyphilis, in Sexually Transmitted Diseases. Edited by Holmes KK. New York, McGraw-Hill, 1984, pp 313–314

Tobi M, Morag A, Ravid Z, et al: Prolonged atypical illness associated with serologic evidence of persistent Epstein-Barr virus infection. Lancet 1:61–64, 1982

Yarchoan R, Berg G, Prowers P, et al: Response of human immunodeficiency virus associated neurologic disease to 3' azido-2',3' dideoxythimidine. Lancet 1:132–134, 1987

Yarchoan R, Thomas RV, Graftman J, et al: Longterm administration of 3' azido, 2',3' dideoxythymidine to patient with AIDS related neurological disease. Ann Neurol 23 (suppl):S82–S87, 1988

Yarchoan R, Mitsuya H, Myers CE, et al: Clinical pharmacology of 3'-azido-2'-3' dideoxythymidine (zidovudine) and related dideoxynucleosides. N Engl J Med 321:726–738, 1989

Chapter 8

Dermatology

David G. Folks, M.D.
F. Cleveland Kinney, M.D., Ph.D.

A number of dermatologic syndromes are associated with psychiatric illness or are aggravated by psychological factors. Doran and colleagues (1985) reviewed dermatologic disorders that are either directly or indirectly influenced by psychiatric factors (Table 8-1). Furthermore, psychiatric factors are known to precipitate, aggravate, or perpetuate nonspecific dermatoses (Table 8-2).

Psychosocial stressors, interpersonal maladjustment, self-esteem, and social stigma are common factors among dermatologic populations. Thus, the need for psychiatric consultation and the judicious use of psychotherapy, relaxation, cognitive, behavioral, and psychodynamic techniques, together with psychotropics (especially antidepressants and anxiolytics) are often indicated.

In this chapter, we review clinical syndromes encompassing psychiatry and dermatology, including 1) investigations of psychiatric aspects of specific dermatoses, e.g., urticaria, eczema, psoriasis, and acne; 2) evaluation of drug reactions; and 3) analyses of dermatologic involvement in somatoform, factitious, anxiety, mood, and personality disorders. We also discuss mechanisms by which skin diseases that involve psychologic factors or stressors may become chronic.

We greatly appreciate the invaluable help of Julian Thomas, M.D., Assistant Professor, Department of Dermatology, University of Alabama School of Medicine, in his critique of this chapter.

Table 8-1. Dermatologic disorders and psychiatric factors

Disorder	DSM-III-R Axis I diagnosis
Psychogenic disturbance dermatoses (e.g., neurodermatosis)	Psychological factors affecting physical condition
Hypersensitivity reactions (e.g., pruritus, eczema, or urticaria)	Psychological factors affecting physical condition
Stress-induced dermatoses (e.g., shingles, herpes zoster)	Psychological factors affecting physical condition
Metabolic or drug-induced dermatosis (e.g., lithium-induced psoriasis)	None
Neurotic dermatosis (e.g., trichotillomania)	Anxiety disorder
Body image disturbances (e.g., acne, seborrhea, and psoriasis)	Adjustment disorder

Source. Based on Doran et al. 1985.

SPECIFIC DERMATOLOGIC DISORDERS

Urticaria

Of the U.S. population, 15–20% will develop urticaria on at least one occasion. The terms urticaria and "hives" are used synonymously and refer to a typical skin reaction that has been classically described as a "wheal and flare" response. The mechanism for cutaneous anaphylaxis, or hive formation, is similar to systemic anaphylaxis and occurs when histamine or histamine-like substances are released into the skin and produce changes in the permeability of the skin's vascular supply (Sell 1990). Allergens or antigens react with immunoglobulin E (IgE) antibodies fixed to mast cells, which then release pharmacologically active substances. In humans, histamine and arachidonic acid metabolites appear to be the most important of these substances. In cutaneous reactions, the response is localized to the skin because of the fixation of antibodies within the skin. Some urticarial formations probably are not IgE mediated; the mechanism for these formations is currently unknown. However, many potential factors are thought to be responsible for the occurrence of urticaria. Specific etiologic factors implicated in the development of chronic urticaria (symptoms that persist for more than 12 weeks) are difficult to determine, and clear etiologic relationships for the development of urticaria can be established in at most 25% of patients (Monroe 1988).

Table 8-2. Psychodermatologic syndromes

Syndrome	Psychiatric mechanism	Clinical approach
Pruritus	Stress-related (histamine, prostaglandin E, and endopeptidase mediated)	Antihistamines, local preparations, psychotherapy, anxiolytics
Hyperhydrosis	Stress-related Excessive eccrine function	Psychotherapy, psychotropics
Atopic dermatitis (eczema)	Stress-related Familial/developmental	Local preparations, psychotherapy, anxiolytics
Urticaria	Allergic factors (acute) Psychosomatic (chronic)	Topical drugs, psychotropics, psychotherapy, antihistamines, systemic steroids
Rosacea	Environmental factors Stress Foodstuffs	Psychotropics, stress management and environmental manipulation
Alopecia	Unknown Psychosomatic	Stress management, psychotherapy
Psoriasis	Stress Sequelae of infection	Topical drugs, environmental manipulation
	Environmental factors Drug reaction (especially lithium)	Psychotherapy, anxiolytics

A review of 236 cases of urticaria specified psychological factors as the most frequent primary cause of urticaria, with 25% of the cases classified as primarily "psychogenic" and an additional 25% thought to be at least exacerbated by psychiatric factors (Guess et al. 1965; Shertzer and Lookingbill 1987). The existence of a relationship between stress and urticaria is well established, but the pathophysiological mechanisms are not well understood. Fjellner and Arnetz (1985) subjected 10 healthy volunteers to two stressors: a color word conflict test and a forced arithmetic problem. Pulse rate and systolic and diastolic blood pressure were recorded in concert with itching. The authors concluded that there is impressive evidence both clinically and experimentally that pruritus is influenced by mental stress (Fjellner and

Arnetz 1985). Future studies on stress and pruritus, as well as urticaria, are needed to consider more specific objectively measurable psycho-physiologic, psychosocial, and personality factors operative in these types of reactions.

Any drug can induce urticaria at any point during the course of treatment, and urticaria is the second most common dermatologic adverse drug reaction. Clinicians should discontinue a specific pharmaceutical agent if it is unequivocally implicated in the appearance of an acute urticarial reaction, regardless of the severity. If the urticaria persists or worsens, or evidence for more serious medical complications emerges, a formal dermatologic consultation is usually indicated.

Traditional antihistamines often used in the treatment of urticaria have anticholinergic side effects that may cause delirium in geriatric patients. Terfenadine (Seldane) is an H1 antagonist that does not exhibit the prominent anticholinergic side effects seen with diphenhydramine and hydroxyzine. Therefore, terfenadine should be considered as an alternative drug to more traditional medications, particularly in patients at risk for anticholinergic side effects. Systemic steroids, with their attendant side effects, are rarely needed in the treatment of urticaria. The antidepressant doxepin, which is a competitive blocker of both H1 and H2 receptors, is widely used by dermatologists in doses of 25–75 mg per day for the treatment of chronic urticaria.

Psoriasis

Psoriasis is a chronic, often intractable hyperproliferative skin disease characterized most commonly by coalescing dry patches with erythema covered by abundant grayish-white scales. The prevalence in the general population varies geographically from 1 to 2.8% (Ginsburg and Link 1989). Psoriasis is estimated to affect 1–3 million people in the United States. Studies of twins have shown that approximately 30% of monozygotic twin pairs are concordant for psoriasis, indicating that both environmental and genetic factors lead to the expression of the disorder. In 60% of patients, psoriasis starts before age 30 years.

The chronicity and visibility of the disorder and the need for ongoing treatment may make it a crucial factor in the patient's quality of life. Ginsburg and Link (1989) have studied the feelings of stigmatization commonly present in patients with psoriasis. In-depth interviews with 100 adults with psoriasis revealed five dimensions of stigma, including 1) anticipation of rejection, 2) feelings of being flawed, 3) sensitivity to the attitudes of others, 4) guilt and shame, and 5) secretiveness. Some patients described positive attitudes toward their illness. Positive attitudes in psoriasis patients result from denial and/ or detoxifying negative feelings through religious connections or some other means of acceptance. Marked variability was noted in the presence and magnitude of these categories of feelings. The presence of bleeding psoriatic lesions proved to be the strongest correlate of experienced stigma.

Despair and feeling stigmatized may lead to noncompliance with treatment, possibly worsening the prognosis of psoriasis. Ramsay and O'Reagan (1988) studied 104 patients and observed that social and emotional morbidity were present for many patients, despite access to modern treatment. Of these patients, 55% had never experienced a complete remission from their psoriasis; a large percentage avoided common social activities such as swimming and sports; 50% felt that psoriasis had inhibited their sexual relationships; 11% said they would avoid having children in case their offspring should develop the condition; 36% felt that their physician spent most of the consultation time writing prescriptions; and 59% had never been given an explanatory pamphlet or booklet about their psoriasis.

Various "stress" factors have been reported to affect the course of psoriasis. Gupta and colleagues (1989) reported that "high stress reactors" with psoriasis had more disfiguring disease and significantly more recurrences than "low stress reactors." In this study, high stress reactors were simply determined by subjective responses from those patients with psoriasis who stated that stressful events either did or did not exacerbate their psoriasis. Payne and colleagues (1985) also noted the relationship between psychological stress and exacerbations of psoriasis in a series of patients with psoriasis who were matched for age, sex, and marital status with control patients suffering from small cutaneous neoplasms, viral warts, and fungal infections. However, evidence from this controlled study did not support the hypothesis that exacerbations of psoriasis always follow stress, but did show that stress may contribute at least in part to vulnerability to relapse.

Gaston and associates (1987) found a possible relationship between stress and psoriasis, which was evident only by fusing retrospective nonstandardized measures that examined the relationship between psoriasis and stress over a 20-week period. A multivariate statistical method indicated that a positive correlation existed between the severity of psoriasis with psychological distress ($P < .01$) and adverse life events ($P < .05$). Based on these results, stress reduction was suggested as a treatment option for patients suffering from more severe forms of psoriasis.

Seville (1977) examined 132 psoriasis patients who were in complete remission from their disorder. Participants were assessed and then followed over a 3-year period (39%). The prognosis for those patients who were able to recall a specific stress 1 month before the onset of symptoms was significantly better than for those who were unable to relate specific stressors.

Psoriasis has been associated with suicide and an increased prevalence of alcoholism (Gupta et al. 1989). Disturbances in body image and the effect of psoriasis on interpersonal, social, and occupational functioning contribute to the patient's overall psychiatric morbidity, especially if psoriasis begins during a developmentally critical period such as adolescence. When added to overall treatment strategies, outcome may be improved for those patients with psoriasis who have been identified early in the course of their treatment as "stress reactors" by implementation of specific psychosocial interventions directed toward reducing stress or improving coping skills (Gupta et al. 1989). These findings suggest the need for psychiatric consultation and a comprehensive psychiatric approach in the treatment of psoriatic patients with unusually severe, chronic, or stress-related symptoms.

Dermatitis: Eczematous, Atopic, and Pruritic

The association between dermatoses and anxiety and mood disorders (as well as migraine headache, neurodermatitis, and other psychological factors) has been noted frequently in the dermatologic literature, and a possible common role for abnormalities of serotonergic mechanisms has been suggested for these disorders (Garvey and Tollefson 1988). Analyses of atopic dermatitis in children indicated that the measures of stress in the family environment were important predictors of symptom severity even after controlling for demographic and medical status variables, such as age and serum IgE levels (Gil et al. 1987). These results have practical implications for clinicians evaluating children with neurodermatitis syndromes. Faulstich and colleagues (1985) compared 10 atopic dermatitis patients with active symptomatology and 10 control subjects, matched for age, sex, and race, who were given a stress test. Atopic dermatitis subjects had greater electromyograph and heart rate activity as well as higher anxiety scores on the Symptom Checklist-90—Revised. Chronic intractable atopic eczema has been traditionally conceptualized as a physical sign of impaired parent-child relationships and psychological developmental arrest; improvements have been claimed from parent insight and patient education (Koblenzer and Koblenzer 1988). Evidence supporting the role for psychological factors in the pathogenesis of childhood eczema is, however, not consistent. For example, Solomon and Gagnon (1987) considered characteristics of the mother-child dyad in families of very young children with eczema. Neither mothers nor children nor their interaction satisfied the descriptions or hypotheses regarding traditional psychodynamic etiologies discussed in the literature. Thus, it is now difficult to support the notion that childhood eczema is the result of a disturbed mother-child relationship hypothesized to be caused by the lack of physical affection extended to the child from the mother. Further study is needed to confirm generalizations about the psychological contributions to the etiology or maintenance of childhood eczema.

Pruritus

Pruritus is a very common sensation found in conjunction with several of the dermatoses. The current literature suggests that virtually all forms of itching, whatever the cause, may be intensified by emotional stress. Fjellner and Arnetz (1985) studied psychological predictors of pruritus during mental stress. Exposure to mental stressors in healthy volunteers under experimental circumstances activates the psychoneuroendocrine system without any effects on cutaneous responsiveness to intradermal injections of histamine. Interindividual differences were pronounced and partly related to urinary epinephrine levels. Epinephrine appeared to have a suppressive effect on itching and an enhancing effect on flare responses. Pulse rates correlated positively with magnitude of the flare response. During the control period, subjects listened to relaxation tapes; after this, they were exposed to mental stressors with the color word conflict test and forced arithmetic problems for 50 minutes with measured changes in pulse rate and diastolic and systolic blood pressure. This was followed by another 40-minute recovery phase. The results confirmed that pruritus is influenced by subjective mental stress, albeit with major individual variability (Fjellner and Arnetz 1985).

Many of the different psychobiological mechanisms by which skin diseases become chronic appear to be associated strongly with psychological or biobehavioral influences. Pruritus most commonly complicates the course of psoriasis. A prospective study of pertinent psychiatric and dermatologic correlates among 82 inpatients with psoriasis yielded 67% (55 patients) reporting moderate or severe pruritus (Gupta et al. 1988). In this study, the degree of depressive symptoms was identified and differentiated between the mild, moderate, and severe pruritic groups at admission using the Carroll Rating Scale for Depression, the Spielberger State-Trait Personality Inventory, and the Symptom Checklist-90—Revised. Pruritis severity did not correlate significantly with stressful life events, age at onset, present age, sex, marital status, or average reported daily alcohol consumption. Intrapsychic factors, such as severity of depression, rather than external psychosocial or narrowly defined dermatologic factors, were noted as the most significant correlates of pruritus in psoriasis (Gupta et al. 1988).

Psychological factors have also been noted to predict more severe symptoms of recurrent genital herpes infection associated with pruritus. For example, Levenson and co-workers (1987) studied patients with recurrent genital herpes infection; they measured symptoms (pain and itching), psychological factors (depression, anxiety, somatization, interpersonal sensitivity, and life change), and objective indices of disease (number of recurrences in the previous year, total number of recurrences, duration of recurrences, and number of lesions per recurrence). Psychological factors were more strongly associated with pain and itching than were somatic indices, even after considering the patient's gender.

Pruritus, ranging from low-grade pain to a very painful experience, can often be alleviated by pharmacotherapy with the antihistamines, antidepressants, or certain antipsychotics. The use of psychotropic agents must be individualized and employed only after a risk-benefit ratio has been calculated clinically.

Patients experiencing chronic, seasonal, or recurrent episodes of pruritus (especially with rash, respiratory, or systemic signs or symptoms) should have skin testing and allergy consultation. An eosinophil count, sedimentation rate, and other appropriate testing for parasitic infestation (e.g., scabies, lice) should be considered. Recent reports of eosinophilic myalgia with tryptophan illustrate the need to consider drugs and food supplements in the clinical assessment of such patients.

Self-induced Dermatoses

Factitious dermatoses have been recognized at least since 1863 when Gavin first reported a case of factitious scabies in a sailor who rubbed gun powder into needle punctures on his wrist. According to DSM-III-R (American Psychiatric Association 1987), the incidence of dermatitis artefacta, or factitial dermatitis, is thought to be about 0.3%

Table 8-3. Aspects of Munchausen's syndrome and other factitious illnesses amenable to treatment

- Presence of treatable psychiatric syndromes, including
  Affective disorders
  Anxiety disorders
  Psychotic disorders
  Conversion disorders
  Substance-abuse disorders
  Organic mental disorders

- Personality organization closer to compulsive, depressive, or histrionic rather than borderline, narcissistic, or antisocial

- Stability in psychosocial support system as manifested by marriage, stable occupation, and family ties as opposed to the single, unemployed wanderer

- Ability to cope with confrontation or some redefinition of the illness behavior

- Capability of establishing and maintaining rapport with the treating clinicians

Reprinted with permission from Folks DG, Freeman AM: Munchausen's syndrome and other factitious illness. Psychiatr Clin North Am 8:263–278, 1985.

among dermatologic patients. These cases present more frequently in teaching hospitals and tertiary care facilities (Folks and Freeman 1985). Dermatitis artefacta occurs predominantly among females, with a female-to-male ratio of at least 4:1. Age at onset ranges from 9 to 73 years. The lesions have wide-ranging morphologic features and often appear bizarre, with sharp geometric borders surrounded by normal-looking skin. Self-inflicted dermatologic lesions have been associated with mental retardation, psychosis, factitious disorder (including Munchausen's syndrome), and malingering. Folks and Freeman (1985) have reviewed factitious illness and outlined the principles of assessment relevant to dermatologic cases. Psychiatric consultation and psychological testing, along with Amytal interview or hypnosis, are often useful in the evaluation of suspected cases (see Table 8-3).

Gupta and colleagues (1987) reviewed the self-inflicted dermatoses per se, namely dermatitis artefacta, neurotic excoriations, and trichotillomania, and noted specific associations with varying degrees of psychopathology; however, these disorders have received surprisingly little systematic study in the psychiatric literature other than scattered case reports and occasional reviews. This paucity of data probably reflects the fact that the majority of patients may initially deny psychological problems and many patients do not receive psychiatric consultation or intervention; in addition, many patients may present in clinical settings in which a lack of adequate collaboration exists between psychiatry and dermatology. However, self-induced dermatologic disorders may be associated with serious sequelae, such as suicide and inappropriate polysurgery. Effective treatment is often primarily psychiatric, and knowledge of these disorders and access to a psychiatric consultant are critical to the care of such patients.

Gupta and associates (1986) studied neurotic excoriations that are often associated with underlying anxiety, mood, or personality disorders. A 2% incidence of neurotic excoriations was observed among dermatology clinic patients, and a 9% prevalence was observed among dermatologic inpatients with pruritus. A predominance among females has been observed, ranging from 52 to 92% in various studies of patients with neurotic excoriations (Gupta et al. 1986). Most studies report a mean age at onset between 30 and 45 years, although others have reported a peak incidence among middle-aged persons. Perfectionism or obsessive-compulsive personality traits, anxiety, depressive symptoms, conversion reactions, hypochondriasis, and psychoses (including schizophrenia) have all been reported in association with neurotic excoriations.

These excoriations, unlike factitial dermatitis, are usually produced by repetitive self-excoriating behavior, which is initiated by pruritis or other disturbing sensations in the skin or by an uncontrollable urge to excoriate a benign skin irregularity. This sequence initiates and perpetuates the itch-scratch cycle, which in some patients becomes a compulsive ritual. The lesions vary in number ranging from a few to several hundred, and on occasion, the syndrome is associated with suicide or other more severe consequences. Unlike the frequently bizarre-looking lesions of dermatitis artefacta, neurotic excoriations do not stand out as being unusual and do not have the potential to mimic other dermatologic disorders.

Unlike patients with dermatitis artefacta, patients with neurotic excoriations typically acknowledge the self-inflictive nature of their lesions. In a study of controlled psychiatric examinations of 68 patients with neurotic excoriations (the *primary* form) who had contacted a dermatologist within a 5-year period, Fruensgaard (1984) found "low self-esteem or lack of self-confidence, hypersensitivity, meticulous or perfectionist traits, and sexual dysfunction" in a significant number. There was a dominant tendency to depressive moods. Most significantly, in 90% of patients with relapses, distressing psychosocial factors were noted which preceded the recurrence after healing.

Trichotillomania.   Trichotillomania, or traumatic alopecia, is a nonscarring alopecia resulting from a compulsion to pluck out one's own hair. The extracted hair may be chewed or swallowed. Patients typically deny that the alopecia is self-induced, and this disorder is distinguished from hair pulling that may be associated with thumb sucking and nail biting in children. Trichotillomania appears to be a relatively rare disorder with a prevalence of approximately 5 per 10,000 in a child psychiatry setting (Gupta et al. 1987). Among self-inflicted dermatoses, this disorder probably is the best known by psychiatrists because numerous reports of the disorder appear in the literature. Most patients are female, and the mean age at onset is typically between 5 and 12 years. The hair of the scalp, eyebrows, eyelashes, and pubic area are usually affected as is facial hair in moles. The hair plucking is accomplished by twisting the strands around the fingers, followed by pulling the hair. Most patients with trichotillomania manifest anxiety, mood, or adjustment disorders or present with personality disorders. Depressive symptomatology has been reported in a significant number of adolescents with this symptom. Most commonly, stressful life situations have preceded the onset of symptoms (Gupta et al. 1987). A recent report by Swedo and co-workers (1989) describes a double-blind comparison of the efficacy of desipramine and clomipramine for trichotillomania. Clomipramine at doses of 75–225 mg were used, and a possible relationship between trichotillomania and obsessive-compulsive disorder has been suggested. The researchers concluded, "clomipramine appears to be effective in the short-term treatment of trichotillomania," although longer-term follow-up studies are needed to fully evaluate the efficacy of this treatment (Swedo et al. 1989, p. 205).

Acne

A relationship between dermatologic and psychological factors in acne has been observed frequently. Acne patients have often shown the presence of negative self-image as well as greater anxiety and depression than in age-matched controls (Rubinow et al. 1987). Anxiety, depression, insecurity, psychic suffering, and social withdrawal may occur as the more common complications of acne vulgaris. Psychological and behavioral improvement after effective treatment has also been reported (Rubinow et al. 1987). Certain personality factors including "neuroticism, psychosomatic condition, social extraversion, and self-defensive attitude" (Van der Meeren et al. 1985, p. 85), which are more likely complications rather than causes of acne, have been found to be elevated in patients compared with controls.

Garrie and Garrie (1978) hypothesized that subjects with different dermatoses including acne would have different levels of anxiety and compared atopic dermatitis, cystic acne, noncystic acne, tinea versicolor, and pityriasis rosea. Among these dermatologic subgroups, both A-state and A-trait anxiety symptoms were most elevated in subjects with disfiguring acne (cystic) and intolerable pruritic eczema (atopic dermatitis). Wu and associates (1988) examined the possible role of personality and emotional factors in acne patients, noting that studies have been inconsistent and yielded contradictory results. Patients with self-rated severe acne were found to experience significantly higher levels of trait anxiety than did patients with mild and moderate conditions or control subjects. Patients with dermatologist-rated severe acne showed higher states of anxiety and "anger-in and anger-out" characteristics than did other patients. No other significant differences in terms of severity emerged, supporting the view that acne patients are not markedly "neurotic." However, these results support the notion that anxiety and anger are indeed the more common emotional complications experienced by acne patients. Rubinow and colleagues (1987) noted reduced anxiety and depression in acne patients after successful treatment with oral isotretinoin. Substantial evidence of psychological distress was observed before treatment in 72 patients. Significant reductions in anxiety were observed on several measures of anxiety after treatment; mitigation of anxiety and depression were the most robust in those patients with the greatest dermatologic improvement.

Systematic studies that seek to evaluate the psychiatric implications for the treatment of acne with isotretinoin (Accutane) are largely lacking in the literature; local treatments and antibiotics have also not been addressed. Supportive psychotherapy for patients with severe acne who have symptoms of an adjustment disorder should always be considered. For those patients who suffer from disfiguring disease with subsequent disturbances in body image, it would also be appropriate to initiate both supportive psychotherapy and encourage participation in group therapy to maintain or improve self-esteem and socialization skills.

PSYCHOTROPIC MEDICATIONS AND DERMATOLOGY

Lithium

Several psychotropic drugs, especially lithium and antidepressants, are associated with adverse dermatologic reactions. Alvarez and Freinhar (1984) noted the association between lithium and a diverse spectrum of bothersome side effects and identified evidence for a lithium-induced psoriasis or psoriasis-like syndrome.

The lithium-psoriasis association is now well established. Lithium increases both circulating and marginal polymorphonuclear leukocyte pools and enhances their turnover and migration. Concurrently, lithium inhibits the enzyme adenylate cyclase, thereby lowering levels of cyclic AMP, which has the effect of enhancing neutrophil chemotaxis (Heng 1982; Jefferson et al. 1983; Lazarus and Gilgor 1979). These changes, in turn, can result in epidermal cell proliferation, leading to a nonpustular form of psoriasis.

Sarantidis and Waters (1983) compared the incidence of a variety of cutaneous conditions among 19 lithium-treated patients with 44 patients treated with other non-neuroleptic medications. Data were obtained using structured interviews, demographics, medication histories, and personal and family histories. A significantly greater proportion of the lithium-treated patients reported a cutaneous condition that may have been secondary to treatment; that is, the dermatosis developed for the first time after medication or appeared to have been exacerbated by the medication. Among the study group, 28 patients developed psoriasis, 17 acne, 12 folliculitis, and 7 described a maculopapular rash. The remaining patients developed a variety of other dermatoses. The effects were found significantly more often among females. On the other hand, male lithium-treated patients reported the same rate of secondary cutaneous conditions as did both male and female comparison patients, indicating the possibility of a hormonal or gender influence.

Psoriasis is known to be exacerbated by lithium; however, psoriasis does not usually cause hair loss unless the scalp involvement is so severe that clumps of hair are lost with the attached hyperkeratotic scaling. In these circumstances, hair loss will only occur from areas of scalp affected by psoriasis. Based on seven subsequent reports after the initial report of loss of hair associated with lithium by Vacaflor and associates in 1970, Mortimer and Dawber (1984) found that hair loss with lithium therapy may remit, and hair regrows despite continuation of treatment.

Silvestri and colleagues (1988) reported a case of alopecia areata during lithium therapy. A case of total alopecia areata was encountered in a patient who had received lithium for 2 months. In this case, there was a close temporal relationship between the lithium treatment and the appearance of the disease, and an equally close temporal relationship between the suspension of therapy and hair regrowth.

Clark and Jefferson (1987) reported a case in which lithium exacerbated a preexisting biopsy-confirmed Darier's disease, or keratosis follicularis, a rare hereditary disease. This papulosquamous disorder usually begins in late childhood, progresses slowly with age, and is inherited as an autosomal dominant trait that affects both sexes equally. The primary lesion is a scaly papule that may occur in hair follicles, between follicles, or on areas of the body devoid of follicles. The observed exacerbation of this skin disorder with lithium appears to remit with discontinuation of lithium. Recurrence or exacerbation after secondary exposure to lithium carbonate was also reported. The mechanism of action, similar to that proposed with psoriasis, is lithium's ability to inhibit cyclic AMP and in vivo increase in the proliferative rate of epidermal cells. Thus, Darier's disease, as well as psoriasis and other cutaneous disorders, may be exacerbated by lithium.

There have been other rare and isolated reports of the association between lithium and alopecia, exfoliative dermatitis, maculopapular rash, ulcer, stomatitis, ichthyosis, xerosis, eczema, pruritus (Bakker and Pepplinkhuizen 1980; Mortimer and Dawber 1984), and a single case report of dermatitis herpetiformis by Ghadirian and Lalinec-Michaud (1986). These researchers reported a 56-year-old woman who suffered from alopecia and psoriasis, both of which developed for the first time in concert with lithium treatment; however, the psoriasis disappeared, and the alopecia resolved despite continuation of the lithium therapy.

Skerritt (1987) encountered a case of psoriasis occurring de novo during lithium therapy that progressed to psoriatic arthritis. Although exacerbation of preexisting psoriasis during lithium treatment has been commonly observed, this case was the first description of the arthritic component of the syndrome apparently developing secondary to lithium. Lithium-related dermatologic reactions as well as the use of lithium in the medically ill are discussed elsewhere (DasGupta and Jefferson 1990; Stoudemire and Fogel 1987).

Exacerbation of psoriasis from lithium among bipolar disorder patients, as well as other psychiatric and dermatologic patient populations, raises the question of alternative treatments. In such situations, neuroleptics (thioridazine and chlorpromazine) and anticonvulsants known to have mood-stabilizing effects (carbamazepine and valproate) may be considered as alternative agents (see Chapter 2).

Antidepressants

Cutaneous reactions to antidepressants include acneform eruptions, seborrhea dermatitis, contact dermatitis, nonspecific pruritic eruptions, urticaria, and photosensitivity reactions. Most of these conditions are benign and self-limited. Although transient photosensitivity reactions have been documented with tricyclics (as well as with the structurally related phenothiazines), persistent light-sensitive cutaneous reactions appear to be rare. Walter-Ryan and colleagues (1985) reported a case of a healthy 38-year-old patient with depression and anxiety who developed a reversible rash with imipramine treatment. Withdrawal of the drug resulted in resolution of the rash, and subsequent challenge with maprotiline was uneventful. The authors reviewed proposed mechanisms for drug-induced photosensitivity reactions, including 1) the parent drug may produce phototoxicity or photoallergy; (2) drug photosensitivity products produced in the skin by ultraviolet light may be toxic; or (3) fixed-drug eruptions may occur in which the drug or its metabolites form complexes with nucleic acids and are bound in the skin.

Erythema multiforme is usually an acute, self-limited syndrome with distinctive skin lesions with or without mucosal erosions. However, the classical mild form described in the mid-1800s can progress to a more severe and sometimes fatal form first described by Stevens and Johnson in 1922. Ford and Jenike (1985) reported the case of a 63-year-old woman with treatment-resistant depression who was given trazodone and who subsequently developed erythema multiforme, with lesions predominantly located on the distal parts of the limbs, i.e., involvement of the hands, feet, palms, and soles. This particular patient was also taking lithium, which has not been implicated in erythema multiforme.

Barth and Baker (1986) noted severe psoriasis in a patient treated with trazodone. Although severe psoriasis is commonly associated with depression and best treated with doxepin at 75- to 300-mg dosages, the hazards of treating psoriasis patients with lithium are well established, and antidepressants also may destabilize psoriasis. In their case of a 37-year-old man who had suffered from stable plaque psoriasis for 19 years, trazodone provoked a generalized pustular psoriasis. The precipitation of this exacerbation by a serotonin reuptake blocker suggests an alternative mechanism in addition to the generally accepted mechanism of interference with cyclic AMP activity.

Antidepressant medication is effective in certain dermatologic conditions, such as neurodermatitis and chronic urticaria (Neittaanmaki and Fraki 1988). Antidepressants may also be effective in diverse "psychosomatic" or stress-related conditions, such as migraine headache and peptic ulcer disease. These psychophysiologic conditions have a close relationship to the stress responses in the skin (Rosenthal 1984; Yeragani et al. 1987). Eedy and Corbett (1987) described a patient who presented with facial hyperhidrosis in a bilateral malar distribution precipitated by olfactory stimuli and was successfully treated with amitriptyline. Yeragani and colleagues (1988) discussed a 30-year-old man with major depression who had a coexisting skin disease diagnosed as dyshidrosis. The patient had 1- to 2-mm papules on the palmar surfaces of both hands which had been present continuously for about 2.5 years. With desipramine treatment, at a blood level of 150 ng/ml, marked improvement in the skin condition was reported. Since the effect was unlikely to be due to the antihistaminic or anticholinergic effects of desipramine, a common pharmacological action leading to a decrease in autonomic instability resulting from decreased psychological stress was proposed as a possible mechanism.

Oral ingestion of the antidepressant fluoxetine may result in dermatologic side effects (Dista Pharmaceuticals, 1990, personal communication). Infrequently observed side effects include acne, alopecia, contact dermatitis, dry skin, herpes simplex, maculopapular rash, and urticaria. Other dermatologic complications are more rarely observed. In placebo-controlled clinical trials, 2.7% of patients taking fluoxetine developed a rash compared to 1.8% taking placebo; pruritus was documented in 2.4% taking fluoxetine compared to 1.4% taking placebo (Dista Pharmaceuticals, 1990, personal communication). As stated earlier in this chapter, we believe that medications clearly implicated in the occurrence of an urticarial rash should be discontinued, regardless of the severity of the urticaria. A skin biopsy or laboratory investigation of a patient with urticaria may be necessary to rule out a collagen vascular disease.

Neuroleptics

Chlorpromazine-induced discoloration of skin areas exposed to sunlight were first described in 1964 by Greiner and Berry. Incidence rates from 1 to 3% are reported; many cases are believed irreversible. Lovell and co-workers (1986) noted a case of photocontact urticaria from chlorpromazine. Although chlorpromazine is well recognized as a cause of delayed photosensitive eczema, in this patient, the urticarial reaction was not due simply to an alteration in the molecular structure of the drug to render it allergenic. Positive photopatch testing and recurrence of a generalized maculopapular eruption after testing were also identified in the case of a patient treated with thioridazine, 60 mg daily (Rohrborn and Brauninger 1987). These researchers noted that phototoxic and photoallergic reactions to the derivatives of the phenothiazines are well known, but that the precise mechanisms for their other adverse skin reactions remain a viable topic of further study. Some clinicians have reported that the replacement of chlorpromazine or thioridazine with haloperidol results in complete disappearance of the abnormal skin pigmentation; however, a multinational study suggested that other neuroleptics, including haloperidol, may also cause this pigmentation (Ban et al. 1985). In contrast, four chronic psychiatric patients received prolonged high-dosage chlorpromazine, and in each case, cutaneous pigmentation resolved when haloperidol was substituted (Thompson et al. 1988). However, despite the disappearance of the skin pigmentation in these four cases, drug-induced corneal and lenticular opacities persisted. Although any neuroleptic may induce an allergic or idiosyncratic reaction, the high-potency neuroleptics are believed to be the least dermatotoxic, for example, pimozide, haloperidol, thiothixene, fluphenazine, and trifluoperazine. With the more novel agent clozapine, the incidence of dermatologic complications is reportedly 1–3% (Sandoz Pharmaceuticals, 1990, personal communication).

Reports of allergic reactions, including anaphylaxis-delayed hypersensitivity, and more generalized dermatologic conditions following the use of lithium preparations are well represented in the literature (Clark and Jefferson 1987). Some reports suggest the possibility of reactions to inert ingredients that may be used as fillers or excipients. Of the inert ingredients contained in lithium preparations, several are known or suspected allergens. Coal tar derivatives are often cited in the cases of allergic reactions. The best known of these is tartrazine (FD&C yellow no. 5), first reported to evoke allergic reaction by Lockey (1959). Many of the anticonvulsants have been used with increasing frequency to treat psychiatric disorders as an alternative to the neuroleptics and in patients who have not responded to more conventional pharmacotherapies. Carbamazepine especially has proven to be useful in the treatment of bipolar disorder, in the management of certain organic delusional disorders, and in the control of intermittent explosive disorder. The dermatologic complications encountered in the use of carbamazepine include hypersensitivity reactions and dermatitis. As has already been stated, medications should be discontinued if there is a temporal association between a specific drug and the onset of urticaria and/or other dermatologic manifestations.

Psychotropic Allergens

As noted above, tartrazine and other dye sensitivities have been estimated to result in skin reactions in as many as 6 in 1,000 cases.

Adverse reactions to tartrazine occur more frequently in people with aspirin sensitivity, but chronic urticaria without aspirin intolerance has also been reported. Pohl and colleagues (1987) described five cases of apparent allergy to tartrazine in 170 patients exposed to the dye, a much higher frequency than the above-reported frequency of 6 per 1,000. Tartrazine has been removed from two brand-name drugs, Tofranil (imipramine) and Norpramin (desipramine). In addition to this allergic reaction, urticaria, bronchospasm, and nonthrombocytopenic papular rash have also been associated, and other reports suggest that angioedema, rhinitis, and anaphylaxis may be precipitated by tartrazine (Pohl et al. 1987; see Chapter 2).

Neittaanmaki and Fraki (1988) have reported two patients with a rare combination of localized heat urticaria and cold urticaria. Doxepin effectively suppressed the whealing response on the heat-challenged skin. Greene and associates (1985) studied 50 patients with chronic idiopathic urticaria, comparing the responses with treatment with doxepin (10 mg tid) and diphenhydramine (25 mg tid). All patient evaluations failed to disclose a cause for the disease. Therapeutic response was assessed according to suppression of symptoms that were reported by symptom diary scores of daily itching and the frequency, number, size, and duration of hives. Total clearing of the pruritus and urticarial lesions occurred in 43% of patients receiving doxepin and in 5% of patients receiving diphenhydramine ($P < .001$). Partial or total control of the pruritus and hives was noted in 74% of patients receiving doxepin and in 10% of patients receiving diphenhydramine ($P < .001$). In addition, doxepin induced markedly less sedation than diphenhydramine (22 versus 46%; $P < .05$). Neittaanmaki and colleagues (1984) had earlier noted the usefulness of doxepin in the treatment of idiopathic urticaria in a randomized double-blind trial, using doxepin and several conventional antihistamines.

SUMMARY

The study of dermatologic conditions and psychiatric factors in the last decade has strengthened some of the concepts regarding stress, mood (anxiety and depression), psychosocial factors (family constellation, coping, and interpersonal relationships), psychobiologic factors (histamines, prostaglandins, serotonin, noradrenaline, dopamine, and psychoimmunology), and personality factors (hostility, perfectionism, and self-esteem) as they relate to dermatologic illness. In addition, several drug-induced dermatologic syndromes and reactions have been reported and confirmed. Follow-up studies and multivariate analyses of course of illness, psychobiologic mechanisms, and genetic and personality predispositions are logical next steps in the future investigation of the psychiatry of dermatologic disorders.

REFERENCES

Alvarez WA, Freinhar JP: Direct evidence for a lithium-induced psoriasis syndrome. Int J Psychosom 31:21–22, 1984

American Psychiatric Association: Diagnostic and Statistical Manual of Mental Disorders, 3rd Edition, Revised. Washington, DC, American Psychiatric Association, 1987

Bakker JB, Pepplinkhuizen L: Cutaneous side-effects of lithium, in Handbook of Lithium Therapy. Edited by Johnson FN. Baltimore, MD, University Park Press, 1980, pp 372–381

Ban TA, Guy W, Wilson WH: Neuroleptic-induced skin pigmentation in chronic hospitalized schizophrenic patients. Can J Psychiatry 30:406–408, 1985

Barth JH, Baker H: Generalized pustular psoriasis precipitated by trazodone in the treatment of depression. Br J Dermatol 115:629–630, 1986

Clark KJ, Jefferson JW: Lithium allergy (letter). J Clin Psychopharmacol 7:287–289, 1987

DasGupta K, Jefferson JW: The use of lithium in the medically ill. Gen Hosp Psychiatry 12:83–97, 1990

Doran AR, Roy A, Wolkowitz OM: Self-destructive dermatoses. Psychiatr Clin North Am 8:291–298, 1985

Eedy DJ, Corbett JR: Olfactory facial hyperhidrosis responding to amitriptyline. Clin Exp Dermatol 12:298–299, 1987

Faulstich ME, Williamson DA, Duchmann EG, et al: Psychophysiological analysis of atopic dermatitis. J Psychosom Res 29:415–417, 1985

Fjellner B, Arnetz BB: Psychological predictors of pruritus during mental stress. Acta Derm Venereol (Stockh) 65:504–508, 1985

Folks DG, Freeman AM: Munchausen's syndrome and other factitious illness. Psychiatr Clin North Am 8:263–278, 1985

Ford HE, Jenike MA: Erythema multiform associated with trazodone therapy: case report. J Clin Psychiatry 46:294–295, 1985

Fruensgaard K: Neurotic excoriations: a controlled psychiatric examination. Acta Psychiatr Scand [Suppl] 312:1–52, 1984

Garrie SA, Garrie EV: Anxiety and skin diseases. Cutis 22:205–208, 1978

Garvey MJ, Tollefson GD: Association of affective disorder with migraine headaches and neurodermatitis. Gen Hosp Psychiatry 10:148–149, 1988

Gaston L, Lassonde M, Bernier-Buzzanga J, et al: Psoriasis and stress: a prospective study. J Am Acad Dermatol 17:82–86, 1987

Gavin H: Feigned and Fictitious Diseases, Chiefly of Soldiers and Seamen. London, J & A Churchill, 1863

Ghadirian AM, Lalinec-Michaud M: Report of a patient with lithium-related alopecia and psoriasis. J Clin Psychiatry 47:212–213, 1986

Gil KM, Keefe FJ, Sampson HA, et al: The relation of stress and family environment to atopic dermatitis symptoms in children. J Psychosom Res 31:673–684, 1987

Ginsburg IH, Link BG: Feelings of stigmatization in patients with psoriasis. J Am Acad Dermatol 20:53–63, 1989

Greene SL, Reed CE, Schroeter AL: Double-blind crossover study comparing doxepin with diphenhydramine for the treatment of chronic urticaria. J Am Acad Dermatol 12:669–675, 1985

Greiner AC, Berry K: Skin pigmentation and corneal and lens opacities with prolonged chlorpromazine treatment. Can Med Assoc J 90:663–665, 1964

Guess G, Koelsche G, Kurline R: Etiology and pathogenesis of chronic urticaria. Ann Allergy 23:30–36, 1965

Gupta MA, Gupta AK, Haberman HF: Neurotic excoriations: a review and some new perspectives. Compr Psychiatry 27:381–386, 1986

Gupta MA, Gupta AK, Haberman HF: The self-inflicted dermatoses: a critical review. Gen Hosp Psychiatry 9:45–52, 1987

Gupta MA, Gupta AK, Kirkby S, et al: Pruritus in psoriasis: a prospective study of some psychiatric and dermatologic correlates. Arch Dermatol 124:1052–1057, 1988

Gupta MA, Gupta AK, Kirkby S, et al: A psychocutaneous profile of psoriasis patients who are stress reactors. Gen Hosp Psychiatry 11:166–173, 1989

Heng MCY: Cutaneous manifestations of lithium toxicity. Br J Dermatol 106:107–109, 1982

Jefferson JW, Griest JH, Ackerman DL: Lithium Encyclopedia for Clinical Practice. Washington, DC, American Psychiatric Press, 1983

Koblenzer CS, Koblenzer PJ: Chronic intractable atopic eczema. Arch Dermatol 124:1673–1677, 1988

Lazarus GS, Gilgor RS: Psoriasis, polymorphonuclear leukocytes, and lithium carbonate: important clue. Arch Dermatol 115:1183–1184, 1979

Levenson JL, Hamer RM, Myers T, et al: Psychological factors predict symptoms of severe recurrent genital herpes infection. J Psychosom Res 31:153–159, 1987

Lockey SD: Allergic reactions due to FD&C yellow no. 5 tartrazine, an aniline dye used as a coloring and identifying agent in various steroids. Ann Allergy 17:719–721, 1959

Lovell CR, Cronin E, Rhodes EL: Photocontact urticaria from chlorpromazine. Contact Dermatitis 14:290–291, 1986

Monroe EW: Urticaria, in Common Problems in Dermatology. Edited by Green KE. Year Book Medicine, 1988, pp 402–407

Mortimer PS, Dawber RPR: Hair loss and lithium. Int J Dermatol 23:603–604, 1984

Neittaanmaki H, Fraki JE: Combination of localized heat urticaria and cold urticaria: release of histamine in suction blisters and successful treatment of heat urticaria with doxepin. Clin Exp Dermatol 13:87–91, 1988

Neittaanmaki H, Myohanen T, Fraki JE, et al: Comparison of cinnarizine, cyproheptadine, doxepin and hydroxyzine in the treatment of idiopathic cold urticaria: usefulness of doxepin. J Am Acad Dermatol 11:483–489, 1984

Payne RA, Payne CME, Marks R: Stress does not worsen psoriasis?—a controlled study of 32 patients. Clin Exp Dermatol 10:239–245, 1985

Pohl R, Balon R, Berchou R, et al: Allergy to tartrazine in antidepressants. Am J Psychiatry 144:237–238, 1987

Ramsay B, O'Reagan M: A survey of the social and psychological effects of psoriasis. Br J Dermatol 118:195–201, 1988

Rohrborn W, Brauninger W: Short communications. Contact Dermatitis 17:241–261, 1987

Rosenthal SH: Does phenelzine relieve aphthous ulcers of the mouth? N Engl J Med 311:1442, 1984

Rubinow DR, Peck GL, Squillace KM, et al: Reduced anxiety and depression in cystic acne patients after successful treatment with oral isotretinoin. J Am Acad Dermatol 17:25–32, 1987

Sarantidis D, Waters B: A review and controlled study of cutaneous conditions associated with lithium carbonate. Br J Psychiatry 143:42–50, 1983

Sell S: Immunopathology (hypersensitivity diseases), in Anderson's Pathology, 9th Edition. Edited by Kissane JE. St Louis, MO, CV Mosby, 1990, pp 487–545

Seville RH: Psoriasis and stress. Br J Dermatol 97:297–302, 1977

Shertzer CL, Lookingbill DP: Effects of relaxation therapy and hypnotizability in chronic urticaria. Arch Dermatol 123:913–916, 1987

Silvestri A, Santonastaso P, Paggiarin D: Alopecia areata during lithium therapy: a case report. Gen Hosp Psychiatry 10:46–48, 1988

Skerritt PW: Psoriatic arthritis during lithium therapy. Aust N Z J Psychiatry 21:601–604, 1987

Solomon CR, Gagnon C: Mother and child characteristics and involvement in dyads in which very young children have eczema. J Dev Behav Pediatr 8:213–220, 1987

Stevens AM, Johnson FC: A new eruptive fever associated with stomatitis and ophthalmia. Am J Dis Child 24:526–533, 1922

Stoudemire A, Fogel BS: Psychopharmacology in the medically ill, in Principles of Medical Psychiatry. Edited by Stoudemire A, Fogel BS. Orlando, FL, Grune & Stratton, 1987, pp 79–112

Swedo SE, Rapoport JL, Lenane MC, et al: A double-blind comparison of clomipramine and desipramine in the treatment of trichotillomania (hair pulling), in Digest of Neurology and Psychiatry. Edited by Webb WL Jr. Hartford, CT, The Institute of Living, 1989, p 205

Thompson TR, Lai S, Yassa R, et al: Resolution of chlorpromazine-induced pigmentation with haloperidol substitution. Acta Psychiatr Scand 78:763–765, 1988

Vacaflor L, Lehmann HE, Ban TA: Side effects and teratogenicity of lithium carbonate treatment. J Clin Pharmacol 10:387, 1970

Van der Meeren HLM, Van der Schaar WW, Van den Hurk CMAM: The psychological impact of severe acne. Cutis 36:84–86, 1985

Walter-Ryan WG, Kern EE, Shiriff JR, et al: Persistent photoaggravated cutaneous eruption induced by imipramine (letter). JAMA 254:357–358, 1985

Wu SF, Kinder BN, Trunnell TN, et al: Role of anxiety and anger in acne patients: a relationship with the severity of the disorder. J Am Acad Dermatol 18:325–333, 1988

Yeragani VK, Pohl R, Keshavan MD, et al: Are tricyclic antidepressants effective for aphthous ulcer? (letter). J Clin Psychiatry 48:6, 1987

Yeragani VK, Patel H, Keshavan MD: Effectiveness of desipramine in the treatment of dyshidrosis. J Clin Psychopharmacol 8:76–77, 1988

Chapter 9

Heart and Liver Transplantation

Anne Marie Riether, M.D.
J. Wesley Libb, Ph.D.

During the past 30 years, organ transplantation surgery has developed from a daring, radical attempt to save lives into an accepted treatment for end-stage organ failure. Kidney transplantation is now routine, and in the United States, in 1988 alone, 1,272 hearts and 1,098 livers were transplanted (House et al. 1990). Because of sophisticated pharmacological regimens and improved surgical techniques, heart and liver transplant patients not only survive but report an improved quality of life. The 1- and 5-year survival rates now approach 80% and 70%, respectively, for heart transplants, and 74% and 64% for liver transplants.

As transplantation becomes an option for more patients, issues of psychological and psychiatric morbidity of transplantation are beginning to be addressed. In this chapter, we address the psychiatric complications of heart and liver transplantation and the psychiatric screening of transplant recipients.

Much of the material in this chapter is based on Chapter 7 from Smith SL (ed): Tissue and Organ Transplantation: Implications for Professional Nursing Practice. St. Louis, MO, Mosby–Year Book, 1990.

309

GENERAL CONCERNS OF TRANSPLANT RECIPIENTS

Patients who face transplantation report common concerns, regardless of the organ transplanted. These include fear of the unknown, fear of not getting a donor, fear of the pain of surgery, fear of transplant rejection, lack of confidence in rehabilitation, and fear of long-term health problems (Gulledge et al. 1983; Riether and Stoudemire 1987). The psychological difficulties typical of transplant patients include guilt for burdening their families, depression, behavioral problems, loss of self-esteem, changes in body image, sexual dysfunction, marital conflicts, and a sense of isolation. Patients may experience hopelessness or helplessness, dependency and regression, financial stresses, organic mental disorders, psychotic states, cognitive changes, and, occasionally, suicidal ideation (House and Thompson 1988).

SELECTION OF TRANSPLANT CANDIDATES

Careful psychiatric evaluation of transplant candidates may substantially enhance their survival rate and their subsequent quality of life and may decrease complication rates. The overall medical evaluation, of which psychiatric evaluation is a part, is designed to assess the patient's current physical condition, determine whether the current medical problems can be helped by medical treatment, assess the suitability of the patient's condition for transplantation, share with the patient and the family honest information regarding the patient's prognosis, develop a rehabilitation program, and allow the patient to make an informed decision about the surgery (Christopherson 1987).

The limited availability of suitable organs for transplantation intensifies the already highly competitive recipient selection process. In 1988, 929 and 522 patients were waiting for heart and liver transplants, respectively (House et al. 1990). Selection committees must choose among terminally ill patients according to variable and sometimes subjective criteria.

The increasing number of critically ill patients being kept alive for transplant, coupled with the continuing shortage of donor organs, may force committees to practice "lifeboat ethics" (Surman 1989). This critical situation is exacerbated by the federal licensure provisions of transplant centers, which require that each center perform a minimum number of transplantations per year and maintain the survival rate set by national standards. Active transplant centers are subject to review if their survival rates are in the lowest 5% (Surman 1989). Therefore, patients who are considered at risk for noncompliance or psychiatric complications are likely to be eliminated as transplant candidates, especially in the smaller and newer programs, because these patients may decrease the transplant center's survival statistics.

The Initial Assessment

The patient often considers the psychiatric interview as the most subjective part of the evaluation for transplantation. Patients may joke with the psychiatrist about the doctor's vote as a member of the "God squad." They often feel that they must convince the "organ gatekeepers" of their motivation, worthiness, and suitability for transplantation (Christopherson 1987). Because of their need to please, some patients may downplay their fears or uncertainty about the surgery (Allender et al. 1983), which can interfere with an accurate assessment.

Although specifics of the evaluation process differ from one institution to another, several features are common to all centers. All evaluations begin with a complete history, with special emphasis on past psychiatric illness or substance abuse problems and on developmental issues and premorbid emotional problems that may influence the patient's coping. Transplant centers are becoming increasingly quantitative and standardized in their evaluations of potential candidates, supplementing the interview with psychometric tests to assess overall functioning, anxiety, depression, family support, cognitive functioning, and personality traits (see Table 9-1). Because transplant candidates are seriously ill, interviewing and testing sessions should generally be limited to less than 90 minutes. Sometimes patients cannot tolerate even this length of time because of short attention span, poor concentration, or debilitation.

At one transplant center, the psychosocial assessment of candidates has been quantified with the Psychosocial Assessment of Candidates for Transplantation (PACT), a rating scale that has been shown to have high interrater reliability (intraclass correlation = .85) (Olbrisch et al. 1989; Table 9-2). The PACT was designed to organize and structure the clinical judgments of the screeners rather than to directly measure the personal characteristics of the patients. It takes into account the candidate's social support, psychological health, history of compliance, life-style, alcohol or other drug use, and understanding of the transplant. The predictive validity of the PACT currently is being studied.

Table 9-1. Psychometric testing instruments for assessing transplant candidates

- **Overall functioning assessment**

  General Current Quality of Life Scale (Young and Longman 1983)
  Minnesota Multiphasic Personality Inventory—2 (MMPI-2) (Hathaway and McKinley 1989)
  Psychosocial Adjustment to Illness Scale (PAIS) (De-Nour 1982; Derogatis 1983, 1986)
  Psychosocial Assessment of Candidates for Transplantation (PACT) (Olbrisch et al. 1989)
  Quality of Well-Being (QWB) Scale (Bush 1984)
  Sickness Impact Profile (Bergner et al. 1976)
  Simmons Scale (How Are You Feeling?) (McNair et al. 1981)

- **Anxiety assessment**

  State-Trait Anxiety Inventory (STAI) (Spielberger 1983)

- **Depression/mood states assessment**

  Beck Depression Inventory (BDI) (Beck et al. 1961)
  Hamilton Rating Scale for Depression (Hamilton 1960)

- **Cognitive functioning assessment**

  Auditory Verbal Learning Test (AVLT) (Rey 1964; Taylor 1959)
  Conceptual Level Analogy Test (CLAT) (Willner 1976; Willner et al. 1976)
  Mini-Mental State Exam (MMSE) (Folstein et al. 1975)
  Trailmaking Tests A and B (Lezak 1983; Reitan 1958)
  Wechsler Adult Intelligence Scale—Revised (WAIS-R) (Block Design and Vocabulary subtests) (Wechsler 1981)

- **Family support assessment**

  Family Cohesion, Adaptability, Change, and Communication (FACES) (Olson et al. 1983)
  Family Environment Scale (Moos 1986)

- **Alcohol and other drug history assessment**

  Addiction Severity Index (ASI) (McLellan et al. 1983)
  Alcoholism Prognosis Scale for Major Organ Transplant Candidates (Beresford et al., in press)
  CAGE Questionnaire (Ewing 1984)
  Criteria for the Diagnosis of Alcoholism (National Council on Alcoholism 1972)
  Michigan Alcoholism Screening Test (MAST) (Selzer 1971)
  Substance Use Disorder Diagnostic Schedule (SUDDS) (Ramsey Clinic 1985)

- **Personality assessment**

  Millon Clinical Multiaxial Inventory II (MCMI-II) (Millon 1987; Millon et al. 1979)
  The Personality Diagnostic Questionnaire (PDQ) (Hyler et al. 1982)
  The Self-Report Psychopath (SRP) Scale (Hare 1985)
  Impact Message Inventory (Kiesler 1987)
  Personality Disorder Examination (Loranger 1988)
  Structured Clinical Interview for DSM-III-R (SCID) (Spitzer et al. 1990)
  Triphasic Personality Questionnaire (TPQ) (Cloninger 1987)

After history taking, the psychiatrist elicits the patient's attitudes toward, motivations for, and expectations of transplantation and reviews with the patient his or her social support system and other resources. The psychiatrist also evaluates the patient's competency to make decisions and to give informed consent if there is reason to doubt the patient's judgment or cognitive intactness.

When family members are available for direct interview, it is useful to assess the support they plan to provide during and after transplantation. The defense mechanisms and coping strategies that patients use to deal with their chronic illness can be explored with both the patient and the family; they are predictive of a patient's reaction to transplantation (Levenson and Olbrisch 1987; Thompson 1983; Van Thiel et al. 1982). A successful transplant patient needs a stable sense of self and fairly good ego strength, because he or she will be required to integrate the organ from another person into his or her own internal body image.

An assessment of cognitive functioning before transplantation is important because a patient with moderate to severe cognitive deficits may not understand instructions, may not be able to consent, and may lack an overall understanding of the proposed surgery. Baseline cognitive assessments, performed systematically, will also permit evaluation of the transplant's effect on cognitive function. Evaluation for moderate to severe impairment can employ the Mini-Mental State Exam (Folstein et al. 1975) or equivalent, but detection of milder deficits in higher-functioning patients will require more extensive testing, often supplemented with standardized neuropsychological tests.

Cognitive functioning during the immediate preoperative period has been assessed with several different standardized tests (see Table 9-1). These instruments reveal heart transplant patients' preoperative cognitive functioning to be only minimally impaired (Hecker et al. 1989). In contrast, nearly 20% of liver transplant candidates show cognitive signs of delirious or nondelirious hepatic encephalopathy (Trzepacz et al. 1989). Both heart and liver transplant candidates may show difficulty in sustaining concentration and short-term memory impairment (Hecker et al. 1989) or impairment in abstract reasoning.

Illiteracy is not a contraindication for transplantation, but modifications in consent and patient education procedures, such as audio or videotaped instructions or the use of pictures instead of words, must be made for these patients. Our clinical experience is that, with appropriate management, patients with borderline intellectual functioning usually show excellent compliance with treatment recommendations.

A patient whose mental capacity shows a sudden and unexplained

Table 9-2. The Psychosocial Assessment of Candidates for Transplantation (PACT)

Patient Name _____ Date _____

Rater _____

Psychosocial Assessment of Candidates for Transplantation (PACT)
Initial Rating of Candidate Quality (use categories 1–4 only for those patients you think should be accepted for surgery)

0	1	2	3	4
poor, surgery contraindicated	borderline, acceptable under some conditions	acceptable with some reservations	good candidate	excellent candidate

I. SOCIAL SUPPORT

1. Family or Support System Stability

1	2	3	4	5	
no strong interpersonal ties or highly unstable relationships		some stable relationships, some problems evident		stable, committed relationships, strong family commitment, good mental health in supporters	unable to rate

2. Family or Support System Availability

1	2	3	4	5	
support unavailable		support availability limited by emotional or geographical factors		in town with patient thru process, emotionally supportive	unable to rate

II. PSYCHOLOGICAL HEALTH

3. Psychopathology, Stable Personality Factors

1	2	3	4	5	
severe ongoing psychopathology (e.g., schizophrenia, recurrent depression, personality disorder)		moderate personality or adjustment/coping problems (e.g., significant reactive anxiety, situational depression)		well-adjusted	unable to rate

4. Risk For Psychopathology

1	2	3	4	5	
strong family history of major psychopathology, previous significant psychiatric history in patient		periods of poor coping, some psychological sensitivity to medications, some family history of major psychopathology		no history of major psychopathology in family, self, no periods of poor coping	unable to rate

III. LIFESTYLE FACTORS

5. Healthy Lifestyle, Ability to Sustain Change in Lifestyle

1	2	3	4	5	
	sedentary lifestyle; major dietary problems; ongoing smoking; reluctant to change	some lifestyle change; may require further education to reduce controllable risk		major, sustained changes in lifestyle, no major risk factors, willing to change	unable to rate

6. Drug and Alcohol Use

1	2	3	4	5	
	dependence, reluctant to change	moderate, non-daily use, willing to discontinue		abstinence or rare use	unable to rate

7. Compliance With Medications and Medical Advice

1	2	3	4	5	
	unreliable compliance; unconcerned, does not consult physician	knowledgeable re meds; near adequate compliance; not vigilant; usually consults physician		knowledgeable re meds; vigilant, keeps records; consults physician	unable to rate

IV. UNDERSTANDING OF TRANSPLANT AND FOLLOW-UP

8. Relevant Knowledge and Receptiveness to Education

1	2	3	4	5	
	no idea of what is involved: views transplant as cure, no long-range picture	some knowledge gaps or denial, generally good understanding		able to state risks and benefits; realistic	unable to rate

Final Rating of Candidate Quality (Do not average above responses)

(Use categories 1–4 only for those patients you think should be accepted for surgery)

0	1	2	3	4
poor, surgery contraindicated	borderline, acceptable under some conditions	acceptable with some reservations	good candidate	excellent candidate

Which of the above items contributed most heavily to your final rating? (Circle) 1 2 3 4 5 6 7 8

List any factors that went into your final rating other than those included above: _____

_____

Source. Reprinted with permission from Olbrisch ME, Levenson JL, Hamer R: The PACT: a rating scale for the study of clinical decision-making in psychosocial screening of organ transplant candidates. Clinical Transplantation 3:164–169, 1989. Copyright 1988, Mary Ellen Olbrisch.

deterioration needs more extensive neurological and often neuropsychological evaluation. The patient may have new cognitive impairment due to cerebrovascular disease, alcohol or drug effects, or another neurological process. Depending on the etiology and severity of the decline in cognitive function, the patient may be removed from further consideration for transplantation.

Relevance of Psychiatric Factors in Recipient Selection

The importance of psychiatric evaluation is now stressed by many transplant centers. Survival rates and qualitative outcomes can be substantially improved, and complication rates decreased, by judicious selection of recipients and by preventive interventions with recipients at high risk for poor outcome because of psychiatric disorders or maladaptive personality traits (Freeman et al. 1988; Kuhn et al. 1988).

Although some authors (Freeman et al. 1988; Kuhn et al. 1988) have found personality disorder to be a preoperative risk factor that predicts postoperative surgical or psychiatric complications, the postoperative outcome for many patients with preoperative psychiatric disorders is successful. Therefore, the emphasis in preoperative evaluation should be on recommending appropriate psychiatric intervention to prevent complications, rather than on "inappropriate denial of transplantation to those who can benefit medically" (Didlake et al. 1988; Surman 1989).

Compliance Issues

Although preoperative noncompliance with prescribed medical treatment cannot always predict postoperative noncompliance, it is a good indicator. Noncompliance with medication, missed appointments, inattention to failing health, unexplained low blood levels of medications, and failure to report new symptoms to physicians are among the most serious forms of noncompliance.

Patients with a history of noncompliance are excluded as candidates at many centers, although some studies have failed to show valid and reliable indicators for organ failure due to noncompliance. In one series, noncompliance contributed to graft failure or death in 21% of all patients who underwent heart transplantation and contributed to 26% of all deaths. According to this study, the risk for noncompliance increased for patients who had less family support, patients who were single or divorced, and patients who were younger than age 40 years (Cooper et al. 1984).

Perhaps the most severe form of noncompliance is total hopelessness and attempted suicide. In the Emory experience, one patient committed suicide by cutting his wrists 3 months after a successful liver transplant. Schizotypal personality disorder was documented during his preoperative psychiatric evaluation, but he had not been hospitalized previously for psychiatric indications, did not abuse alcohol or other drugs, and seemingly showed good motivation and compliance. A decision was made to offer the patient a transplant for his end-stage liver disease resulting from chronic active hepatitis. While waiting for the transplant, he suffered an acute psychotic decompensation that responded to a brief psychiatric hospitalization and low-dose neuroleptics. The patient's postoperative medical course was not remarkable. He had been seen in outpatient psychiatric follow-up approximately 3 weeks before his suicide, at which time he asked extensive questions about his psychotic break and expressed shame about "being out of control." Approximately 1 week before his suicide, he was seen in the posttransplant medical clinic and gave no indication of his distress.

Another patient, assessed preoperatively to be a high risk, had been given a diagnosis of dysthymia and borderline personality; she had limited psychosocial supports and had been hospitalized at least once because of an overdose. Despite a chaotic social situation, she appeared motivated and was compliant with preoperative medical treatment and individual psychotherapy. After successful transplantation, however, she refused to participate in the liver transplant support groups or individual psychiatric treatment, and she overdosed nearly 1 year after her surgery. She survived, but she again refused follow-up psychiatric care, although she remained compliant with her immunosuppressant regimen. She died nearly 2 years after her transplant from medical complications related to her transplant.

Realizing that psychiatric and psychosocial variables play an important role in mediating quality of life, and that compliance is regarded as essential to successful transplantation, those factors that can optimize good outcomes must be identified. Examining psychiatric risk factors preoperatively may help to identify those patients at risk for increased psychiatric morbidity and, to the greatest extent possible, permit intervention before an adverse outcome ensues.

The importance of these considerations was highlighted by a tragic experience at Emory, in which a 20-year-old man died from multisystem organ failure after his third liver transplant. After a 7-month stay in the hospital, he died 23 days after discharge with undetectable levels of cyclosporine in his blood.

As organ transplantation becomes more available and more patients who are at risk for psychiatric morbidity receive transplants, it is likely that suicide in this population will increase. According to one study of 292 renal transplant patients, 92 developed depression and 7 attempted suicide (Penn et al. 1971). Further, relationships between preoperative psychiatric problems and postoperative complications may become more evident as systematic outcome data accrue.

These cases illustrate an important point about compliance. The pretransplant patient is often desperate to accept all treatment recommendations in exchange for transplant, so it is often difficult to assess compliance without evaluating the patient's history. A history of poor follow-up, dietary noncompliance, and poor coping skills indicates potential problems.

Although few studies have systematically examined compliance in transplant patients, commonly cited predictors for good compliance are the abilities to tolerate adverse conditions and to establish emotional support and good personal relationships. Conversely, noncompliers are said to have a low tolerance for frustration and an inability to delay gratification (Stewart 1983). Some clinicians have identified "educated patients in professional positions" and those "with manual skills" as better able to comply with the demands of the posttransplant regimen than others (Cooper et al. 1984).

Evaluation of Addicted Patients

Patients with substance abuse and dependence are being referred with increasing frequency for organ transplant evaluation. Traditionally, these patients were deemed unsuitable for transplant, and if they were considered at all, the guidelines about who should be transplanted and how long a patient needed to be sober before transplant were often quite arbitrary.

Unfortunately, these guidelines were not often based on empirical studies. The 1983 Consensus Development Panel of the National Institutes of Health stated that alcoholic liver disease was an indication for transplant only in a "small portion of cases." They further stated that only those patients who had "established clinical indicators of fatal outcome" and who were judged "likely to abstain from alcohol" should be considered (Beresford et al. 1990).

Preoperative evaluation of these patients begins with a careful clinical history and a diagnosis of abuse or dependence based on DSM-III-R criteria (American Psychiatric Association 1987). Screening questionnaires such as the CAGE (Ewing 1984), the Michigan Alcoholism Screening Test (Selzer 1971), the PACT (Olbrisch et al. 1989), and the Alcoholism Prognosis Scale (Beresford et al. 1990) are sometimes used.

Beresford and associates (1990) have developed a prognostic scale to evaluate transplant candidates who meet the criteria for alcohol dependence. This simple scoring system offers a method of quantifying clinical impressions. The six areas of functioning assessed were based in part on the criteria of Valliant and associates (Valliant 1983; Valliant et al. 1983), which they consider important for a patient to become "securely abstinent" (more than 3 years of sobriety). The Alcoholism Prognosis Scale (Beresford et al. 1990) (Table 9-3) assesses the patient's and the family's acceptance of alcoholism, the presence or absence of substitute activities, the patient's understanding of the behavioral consequence of his or her drinking, the presence or absence of hope and self-esteem, the presence or absence of social relationships, and the patient's social stability. Each area is weighted to permit statistical comparison. Each area of the scale has been shown to be critical in maintaining abstinence. A good prognosis by the Alcoholism Prognosis Scale can be used in place of an arbitrary period of sobriety before considering a patient for transplantation.

Patients with iatrogenic drug addiction but without a prior history of drug abuse or dependence usually do not continue to abuse drugs once they are detoxified. On the other hand, patients with a strong family history of drug dependence and patients who continue to abuse mood-altering substances despite adverse consequences usually need formal chemical dependency treatment and involvement in a support network such as Alcoholics Anonymous.

Some centers have transplant recipients with few or no periods of documented sobriety and have reported surprisingly good outcomes (Starzl et al. 1988). Unfortunately, documentation of the patient's sobriety in these studies is based on patient reports not corroborated by the patient's family, so caution must be used in interpreting the results.

Regarding the purely physical prognosis, alcoholic cirrhosis does not imply a poor outcome from liver transplantation. The 2-year survival rate for transplanted alcoholic cirrhotic patients in one recent large study was 73%, not statistically different from the rate for non-alcohol-related liver failure patients (Beresford et al. 1990; Van Thiel et al. 1989).

Despite these encouraging findings, addicted patients are at in-

Table 9-3. Alcoholism Prognosis Scale for major organ transplant candidates

Subscale	Yes/No	Points	Description
1. Acceptance of alcoholism	Yes	4	Patient and family
		3	Patient alone
		2	Family alone
	No	1	Neither patient nor family

The patient and a family member or another person with a strong personal commitment to the patient's welfare clearly acknowledge the patient's alcoholism (the inability to control drinking alcohol) as a disease beyond the patient's control.

2. Substitute activities	Yes	3	
	No	1	

The patient engages in time-consuming, constructive activities during the time he or she would otherwise have been drinking. Examples include extensive involvement with Alcoholics Anonymous, community volunteer activities, gainful employment or educational pursuits. They must make up a major portion of the patient's average day. For severely debilitated patients, use appropriate historical data when he or she last felt well.

3. Behavioral consequences	Yes	3	
	No	1	

The patient understands that by resuming drinking he or she will incur specific and unpleasant consequences that will significantly alter the ability to function. Examples include being asked to leave the home by his or her family, immediate and severe medical consequences such as severe pain or imminent death or immediate incarceration (relatively subtle or nonimmediate consequences such as kidney or liver failure do not count nor do the results of failing to care for the transplanted organ).

4. Hope/self-esteem	Yes	3	
	No	1	

The patient spontaneously describes a new or renewed interest in an activity from which he or she derives a personal sense of hope for his or her own future or an improved sense of personal worth irrespective of the future. Examples include active participation in a religion or religious organization or in the spiritual program of the Twelve Steps of Alcoholics Anonymous.

5. Social relationship	Yes	3	
	No	1	

The patient reports, and the object of his or her affection confirms, the existence of a new or renewed relationship involving the patient's affection that has existed with the knowledge and understanding of the patient's alcoholism on the part of both parties and in the specific absence of active addictive drinking by either party. Examples include a spouse, a mentor, a close friend, or a psychotherapist.

continued

Table 9-3. Continued

Subscale	Yes/No	Points	Description
6. Social stability		0–4	
The patient had a steady job for the past 3 years, one to which he or she may return following surgery. For women this may include household or child-rearing duties and tasks.		1	
The patient has had a stable residence for the 2 years preceding evaluation for surgery.		1	
The patient does not live alone.		1	
The patient is currently married or lives with a spouse.		1	
Total of items 1–6		20 points	

Note. This scale is intended for research purposes only. Its use presupposes that the clinician has made a diagnosis of alcohol dependence as described in DSM-III-R for any patient under study. The scoring system offers a method of quantifying clinical impressions for the purposes of statistical comparison. Neither the scale nor any part thereof should be used in isolation as a means of offering or declining to offer medical or surgical assistance.
Source. Reprinted with permission from Beresford TP, University of Michigan Alcohol Research Center, 400 East Eisenhower Parkway, Suite A, Ann Arbor, MI 48104.

creased risk for graft rejection if they abuse alcohol or drugs after the transplant because substance abuse is associated with poor medical compliance. The transplant team at Massachusetts General Hospital (Gastfriend et al. 1989) retrospectively reviewed 407 transplantations between 1983 and 1988. Most (340) were kidney transplants, 53 were liver transplants, and 14 were heart transplants. Of the 40 patients who had histories of substance abuse or dependence, 65% (26) continued to abuse chemicals, including alcohol, after transplantation; of the 26, 15 were noncompliant with postoperative care. Serious rejection occurred in 4 of the 40 patients with substance abuse, and graft loss occurred in 5 (12.5%). In contrast, only 2 of the non-substance-abusing patients had graft loss from noncompliance, for a total of 7 grafts lost out of 407 (1.7%) (Gastfriend et al. 1989).

PSYCHOLOGICAL ADJUSTMENT IN THE PREOPERATIVE PERIOD

For most patients and families, organ failure is the end point of months or years of living with a chronic illness; acute stress is superimposed on chronic stress. While patients and their families wait for a suitable donor predictable psychological stages or psychological rites of passage occur: denial, anger, accentuation of personality character-istics, magical expectations, idealization, and acceptance. Psychiatric intervention may be helpful when a patient has difficulty negotiating a particular stage.

The first stage, denial, generally takes the form of the patient's disbelief that he or she is "that sick" or that a transplant is needed. Unless this stage is worked through and the rationalizations and min-imizations confronted, the patient may reject the possibility for trans-plant or may be noncompliant with the recommendations of the treatment team.

A combination of anger, depression, and grief may follow. The patient is often angry at his or her illness (or at God) and may displace this anger. A patient rarely displaces this anger and aggression onto the transplant team, however, since this group will decide whether the patient is a suitable candidate for transplantation. Instead, members of the nursing staff or family caretakers may be the target of displaced anger, hostility, and sarcasm. Some researchers have noted that older patients tend to express less anger and more depression than do younger patients (Stewart 1983).

Transplant patients of all ages experience progressive, physically restrictive symptoms that serve as a reminder of mortality and make treatment an urgent issue. Formerly independent, these patients must now rely on family members for help with routine daily tasks, and their symptoms frequently isolate them from previous social contacts (Riether and Rubenow 1989a). Helping a patient work through grief over the loss of an organ often involves dealing with the patient's anger over changes imposed by the transplant, with its attendant medical regimen.

The next stage that may be observed is a period of accentuation of premorbid personality characteristics. Nearing transplantation, each potential recipient reacts according to his or her own personality style. Patients with pronounced maladaptive personality traits or subclinical personality disorders may develop clinically significant behavioral dis-turbances. The next phase of the patient's psychological adjustment may involve "magical expectations." When these occur, the patient has accepted the illness and the need for a transplant, but has unreal-istic expectations about the future course. The patient minimizes the time it will take to find a compatible donor, the cost of the surgery, and the possibility of rejection. The patient may see the transplant as a panacea for life's problems. Patients experiencing this stage need help in assessing their situations realistically. The psychiatrist can offer disillusionment in tolerable doses in the context of a supportive relationship.

A period of idealization may at times also be observed. Patients idealize the surgeon and the hospital, frequently dreaming about their physician, boasting to family and friends about their doctor's accomplishments, training, and surgical "cures." They may worry about their surgeon's health and tend to see him or her as a man or a woman with an "M deity" rather than an M.D.

During the final psychological stage of the waiting period, the acceptance stage, patients realistically acknowledge their illness and await their transplant. They are aware of the risks and potential benefits but have made an informed decision to proceed with the surgery.

Special Stresses of the Waiting Period

As the availability of transplants and the number of eligible candidates have increased, waiting times have increased (Busuttil 1986; Casscells 1986; Tisza et al. 1976). The pretransplant period may be accompanied by increased anxiety, depression, fear, anger, and competition among those waiting for an organ (Levenson and Olbrisch 1987). Patients may become frustrated at the delay and wonder whether they are "really" on the list. One patient poignantly described the waiting period this way: "It's like being on a long-distance phone call and being placed on hold; the longer you wait, the more it costs you." Patients who are able to remain at home and carry on their daily lives may adapt better to a lengthy wait. All patients experience some distress at "never knowing when the beeper will go off." Most find it difficult to leave town or make long-term commitments.

A morbid type of humor may be openly verbalized during the preoperative period (Levenson and Olbrisch 1987). Patients may joke about inclement weather because fatal accidents are more likely (Frierson and Lippmann 1987). One patient expressed embarrassment and guilt after blurting out that he was glad the legal speed limit had been raised to 65, because "more people will die in accidents." After waiting 7 months for a suitable liver, another patient was heard asking a new medical student her blood type as casually as if he were asking her about the weather.

Family members may also show increased distress during the waiting period. Mindful that their relative may be emotionally vulnerable, they may feel the need to appear strong. Hopeful for the future yet afraid of the present, they may need the opportunity to ventilate their expectations, hopes, and fears. At times family members also need the reassurance that everything possible is being done to find a donor and to keep their loved one alive while waiting.

Psychiatric Disorders

For many patients with organ failure, frequent hospitalizations and a worsening quality of life lead to depression, anxiety, or other mental symptoms. Some degree of anxiety is expected and may actually help the patient mobilize resources and prepare for the transplant. However, excessive anxiety is uncomfortable and interferes with decision making and problem solving. For patients with more severe adjustment reactions, supportive psychotherapy usually is effective.

Depression. Most patients awaiting transplants have some depressive symptoms. These may represent major depression, dysthymia, organic mood disorder, or adjustment disorder. It is therefore important to quantify the extent and duration of symptoms. Patients who are clinically depressed appear to be at increased risk for surgical morbidity (Surman 1978), and it has been suggested that depression negatively affects posthospital adjustment and survival (Beidel 1987). Although specific experience with heart and liver transplants is limited, Lowry and Atcherson's (1979) and Reichsman and Levy's (1972) experience with patients in renal failure demonstrated that nearly 50% of these patients with depression remain untreated for their depression and usually continue to be depressed (Hong et al. 1987). Some of these patients may actually become more depressed after the transplant, independent of any signs of organ rejection (Abram and Buchanan 1976–77). Patients with alcoholic cardiomyopathy and cirrhosis are also reported to have increased prevalence of depressive symptoms (Levenson and Olbrisch 1987).

Anxiety. Patients awaiting transplantation also have increased rates of anxiety (Levenson and Olbrisch 1987). These patients may meet the criteria for an adjustment disorder with anxiety, as noted above, or may be suffering exacerbations of generalized anxiety or panic disorder. Somatic symptoms of anxiety, such as shortness of breath, hyperventilation, diaphoresis, palpitations, chest pain, nausea, and vomiting, may be due to the patient's somatic illness, so that differential diagnosis is subtle. Sometimes a therapeutic trial of pharma-cotherapy for anxiety is diagnostically useful.

Delirium. Clinicians working with patients awaiting transplantation recognize a high prevalence of organic mental disorders in this population. Unfortunately, delirium goes unrecognized in as many as 65% of patients in general hospitals (Levine et al. 1978). Although differentiating organic from functional causes is difficult and not always relevant in transplant patients, psychiatrists are nonetheless often asked to assess the etiology of a patient's change in mental status. Delirium may appear as a combination of incoherence, altered psychomotor activity, disorientation, perceptual disturbances, attention deficits, memory impairment, and sleep-wake alterations (American Psychiatric Association 1987). Its manifestation may be as obvious as a hepatic coma or as subtle as a difficulty in concentrating or an inability to complete customary tasks.

Patients with liver failure are especially susceptible to delirium. Liver transplant candidates show signs of encephalopathy secondary to hepatic failure, metabolic abnormalities, and medications. A prospective study evaluating 247 consecutive liver transplant candidates showed an 18% prevalence rate of delirium (Trzepacz et al. 1989). Not surprisingly, these patients' altered mental states had a negative impact on their overall adaptive functioning and quality of life. Delirious candidates had poorer adaptive functioning, more occupational impairment, and lower social-scale ratings as measured on the Brief Evaluation Form (Mezzich et al. 1986; Trzepacz et al. 1989).

Heart transplant candidates also are at risk for delirium secondary to low cardiac output, drug side effects, metabolic abnormalities, and infection. Although a great deal of the transplant literature examines postcardiotomy delirium, no large prospective studies have examined the incidence of delirium in heart transplant candidates.

Serial mental status testing, physical examinations, and careful history taking are important in making the diagnosis, since mild delirium may go unrecognized. Because no specific diagnostic test for delirium exists, the diagnosis is made on clinical features.

Regarding laboratory assessment, low serum albumin levels correlated better with diffuse cognitive dysfunction in liver-diseased patients than did the results of routine serum liver function tests (Trzepacz et al. 1988). EEG usually shows a characteristic slowing of the dominant posterior rhythm below alpha (8–13 Hz) frequency or an increase in the amount of diffuse theta (4–7 Hz) activity. Sometimes, in more severe cases of delirium, there are generalized bursts of slower activity, primarily in the theta and occasionally in the delta (<4 Hz) frequencies (Trzepacz et al. 1988) (see also Chapter 5). Occasionally, computed tomography or magnetic resonance imaging may be necessary to rule out gross neurological causes for an acute change in mental status.

THE POSTOPERATIVE PERIOD

Psychiatric Disorders

Psychiatric disorders in postoperative transplant patients are common and include organic mental disorders such as delirium, organic mood disorders with depression or mania, anxiety disorders, and psychotic disorders.

Depression.   Immediately after surgery, many patients are mildly euphoric, grateful for having survived the surgery, and looking forward to a full life. Rapid increases in steroid medication during this time may lead to reversible psychotic episodes that may include hallucinations, paranoid delusions, hypomania, depersonalization, and dissociation (Kraft 1971). On the other hand, reduction of steroid dose may produce a mild dysphoric state. Mild depression is not uncommon, beginning on postoperative day 4 or 5. This dysphoric reaction usually resolves without specific treatment.

Survivor guilt may contribute to depression. Patients may feel guilty for having wished that a potential donor would die while they were waiting for their transplant. They may also feel guilty for benefiting from another's misfortune or have difficulty assimilating an organ from someone of the opposite sex or a different ethnic background. This survivor guilt is increased, in our experience, when the recipient has knowledge of the donor and the circumstances of the donor's death.

Recent observation of postsurgical cardiac transplant patients reveals that feelings of depression may occur when the patient encounters the unpleasant side effects of the immunosuppressant drugs (Freeman et al. 1984; McAleer et al. 1985; O'Brien 1985; Watts 1984). After transplantation, patients may talk about a "fear of life" rather than a fear of death (Kemph 1966). Among the factors that negatively influence transplant adjustment are depressive symptoms, including hopelessness and helplessness, and psychosomatic complaints (Lefebvre et al. 1973).

Some patients who have looked forward to returning to work after transplantation become depressed when they cannot do so. Other patients on long-term disability before the surgery cannot afford to lose this financial support since a new salary usually will not pay their monthly medical bills. Still others become discouraged at trading one set of body changes for another: although no longer jaundiced or edematous, many patients complain about weight gain, hirsutism, acne, and moon facies, which are characteristic side effects of steroids and cyclosporine.

Anxiety. The first biopsy after transplantation often evokes significant anxiety and fear. The patient wonders "how the organ is doing" and whether the body is rejecting this lifesaving organ. Although a patient may minimize the biopsy procedure (having just gone through a transplantation and survived), the procedure bears tremendous emotional and symbolic significance. Threatened rejection obviously is cause for grave concern, and anxiety and depression often accompany an unfavorable biopsy report. Patients also often report an increase in anxiety when transferred to the general surgical floor from the intensive care unit, and again when they are discharged home, unconsciously hopeful that they will continue to receive intensive care and treatment.

Most often, anxiety symptoms decrease as the patient's physical health improves. In our experience, however, family members may show increased anxiety as the patient nears discharge. Family roles have been altered by the sickness, and members may look upon the transplant recipient with fear and awe. Having lived through many years of the patient's disability, they may become overprotective, anxious that the patient will die once he or she comes home. Patients often report increased family stress as they attempt to regain former positions in their families. (See Chapter 14 for comments on families' adaptation to a member's chronic illness.)

Delirium. Posttransplant delirium has been reported by some to be the most frequent psychiatric complication in transplant patients (Freeman et al. 1988). Numerous studies have reported high prevalence rates of delirium in the week after transplantation (Freeman et al. 1984, 1988; Mai et al. 1986). Generally, the patient's delirium can be traced to electrolyte abnormalities or medications, and it is usually self-limiting. Sometimes no cause for the patient's confusion can be found, and short-term empiric treatment with low-dose neuroleptics is begun if the patient's mental state is interfering with postoperative care.

Psychosis. The literature contains numerous reports about psychotic symptoms in transplant patients (Freeman et al. 1984, 1988).

Medications frequently are the primary cause of psychotic symptoms. According to a recent review of 70 cardiac transplant patients (Freeman et al. 1988), 10 manifested psychotic symptoms thought to be secondary to steroids. Steroid psychosis is observed in about 7% of transplant recipients but generally clears as the steroid dosage is reduced (Helfrich et al. 1980).

Psychotic reactions after surgery also may be related to sensory deprivation, metabolic disturbances, other medications, or emotional events (Castelnuovo-Tedesco 1971). They may be secondary to an organic, manic, or depressive state, or they may be the result of disintegration of the patient's defenses due to overwhelming anxiety. Others have suggested that a patient's difficulty in assimilating a stable internal body image after transplantation may be responsible for a psychotic reaction after surgery (Castelnuovo-Tedesco 1973).

Patients with more severe personality disorders are, in our experience, at higher risk for psychiatric decompensation after surgery because of poor coping mechanisms, inability to ask for or accept psychiatric help, limited support networks, or difficulty modulating their intense affects. These patients are at risk for self-destructive acts, and unfortunately, they may stir up negative reactions in the transplant team, which may lead to diminished attention or even avoidance by some team members.

Neurologic disorders.   Neurologic complications of transplantation may produce organic mental disorders. In a retrospective study of 83 patients after cardiac transplantation, 54% had at least one neurologic complication, 16% had more than one, and 20% died of neurologic complications (Hotson and Pedley 1976). Because of the high doses of steroids that they are given, transplant patients are at risk for opportunistic infections. Patients may contract fungal infections such as aspergillosis with the potential for metastatic abscesses or meningeal involvement. Many patients with early infections have only mild signs of cognitive impairment and may have normal EEGs. In this situation, mental disturbances are sometimes believed to be of psychological origin, and the infection is found only on postmortem inspection.

Neuropsychiatric Side Effects of Immunosuppression

Immunosuppressants obviously are lifesaving for transplant patients, but the side effects often affect a patient's postoperative adjustment and lead to psychiatric complications. Euphoria, depression, and psychotic reactions are the common manifestations of corticosteroid-induced mental disturbances (Ling et al. 1981). Psychiatric symptoms are most common in patients receiving over 40 mg/day of corticosteroids, and the incidence of symptoms is dose related (Boston Collaborative Drug Surveillance Program 1972). However, neither the dosage nor the duration of corticosteroid treatment has any effect on the time of onset, duration, type, or severity of the disturbances (Ling et al. 1981). As mentioned, organic mood and organic delusional disorders are frequently observed in patients receiving corticosteroids. Patients may show symptoms of hypomania or depression (Borman and Schmallenberg 1951; Clark et al. 1952); others may experience acute psychotic reactions (Baloch 1974; Glaser 1953). Although no correlation can be found between age groups and the incidence of mental disturbances (Ling et al. 1981), it seems that women may be at higher risk for developing adverse side effects than men (Nielsen et al. 1963).

During periods of threatened rejection, transplant patients are frequently given high bolus doses of corticosteroids. They may exhibit psychiatric symptoms of depression, agitation, anxiety, and psychotic reactions at those times or during any sudden increase or decrease in steroid dosage.

Since the advent of cyclosporine (Sandimmune), transplant patients have the possibility for longer-term survival. However, cyclosporine is associated with numerous neuropsychiatric side effects. Mental status changes have been seen in approximately 25% of liver transplant patients who have received cyclosporine (deGroen et al. 1987; House et al. 1990), and mania has been associated with cyclosporine use after transplantation (Wamboldt 1984). Patients frequently complain about cyclosporine-induced tremor, hirsutism, acne, and gum hyperplasia; physicians worry about cyclosporine-induced renal dysfunction and neurotoxicity.

Cyclosporine-induced neurotoxicity is characterized by motor impairment, confusion, impaired memory, tremors, grand mal seizures, dysarthria, and vestibular and cochlear toxicity (Atkinson et al. 1984; Labar et al. 1986). Cyclosporine also caused toxicity to the central nervous system in 3 of 15 patients receiving prophylaxis with the drug after allogenic bone marrow transplantation (Labar et al. 1986).

Neurological findings are most often reversed when cyclosporine levels are reduced, which suggests that levels should be monitored carefully (see Table 9-4). There is particular risk for cyclosporine toxicity in the presence of electrolyte disturbances, recent high-dose steroid treatment (Durrant et al. 1982; Kahan 1985; Thompson et al. 1984),

Table 9-4. Commonly used immunosuppressive agents for transplantation

Name	Indication	Dosage	Drug interactions	Adverse reactions	Comments
Azathioprine (Imuran)	Adjust therapy in management of allograft rejection	3–5 mg/kg daily beginning day 1	Allopurinol: inhibition of azathioprine metabolism	Hematologic: bone marrow depression, pancytopenia GI: nausea, vomiting, anorexia, diarrhea Hepatic: hepatotoxicity, drug-induced hepatitis	
Cyclosporine (Sandimmune)	Prevention of allograft rejection	Initial: 15 mg/kg 4–12 hours before transplantation Maintenance: titrated to maintain radioimmunoassay cyclosporine blood levels (250–800 mg/ml)	Nephrotoxic agents: additive nephrotoxicity Ketoconazole: decreased cyclosporine clearance Erythromycin: decreased cyclosporine clearance	CNS: delirium, tremor, seizure Renal: nephrotoxic CV: hypertension Hepatic: hepatotoxic	Not a bone marrow suppressant

Drug	Indications	Dosage	Drug Interactions	Adverse Effects	Mechanism
Muromonab-CD3 (Orthoclone OKT3)	Rescue from acute rejection	5 mg iv daily for 10–14 days	Potassium-sparing diuretics: enhanced hyperkalemia; Other immunosuppressant agents: additive effects	Dermatologic: hirsutism, gingival hyperplasia, photosensitivity; Allergic: anaphylaxis; Fever; Myalgia; Pulmonary edema	Monoclonal murine antibody CD3 cell marker on T cells
Prednisone	Adjunct therapy in management of allograft rejection	Pharmacologic: 5–15 mg daily tapered to the lowest dose possible to achieve effect		CNS: psychosis, pseudotumor cerebri, euphoria, depression, insomnia; Metabolic: water and salt retention, glucose intolerance, iatrogenic Cushing syndrome, acne, striae, hirsutism	

Note. GI = gastrointestinal. CNS = central nervous system. CV = cardiovascular.

or low magnesium levels (Thompson et al. 1984). Children may be especially susceptible to cyclosporine-related seizures (Durrant et al. 1982; Joss et al. 1982), and seizures occur more often with parenteral use (Adams et al. 1987).

The most serious side effects from azathioprine (Imuran) are hematologic and gastrointestinal, although the risks of secondary infections and mental status changes are also present. Orthoclone OKT3, a monoclonal antibody to the T3 antigen of human T cells, is also capable of producing psychiatric symptoms. This treatment is used at our institution for acute allograft rejection, a time when patients frequently report increased symptoms of depression and anxiety. Patients most often report feeling as if they have the flu, feeling tired, with fever and chills. Concomitant steroid therapy is lowered during Orthoclone treatment, which may also account for reported symptoms of depression. Intravenous hydrocortisone sodium succinate, 100 mg 30 minutes after Orthoclone, decreases the incidence of reactions to the first dose. Acetaminophen and antihistamines also reduce the incidence of fever and chills.

A new experimental drug, FK-506, believed to be 100 times more potent than cyclosporine, is currently undergoing drug trials. This drug is reported to be virtually free of neuropsychiatric and life-threatening side effects and has the potential to increase survival rates as well as eliminate the adverse reactions of the other immunomodulators (Starzl et al. 1989).

TREATMENT OF PSYCHIATRIC DISORDERS IN TRANSPLANT RECIPIENTS

Organic Mental Disorders

The management of an organic mental disorder has to be individualized to target specific symptoms. An attempt should be made to treat the underlying cause of the delirium, and conservative measures should be tried first. As most psychiatrists are familiar with basic environmental strategies to orient delirious patients, these will not be discussed here in detail (Goldstein 1987).

Individual assessments must be made on the use of psychotropic medications in the management of delirium. Haloperidol is useful for the agitation that often accompanies delirium, and it offers the advantage of minimal side effects. This medication is especially useful in cardiac transplant candidates because it has almost no effect on pulmonary or cardiovascular dynamics (Goldstein 1987; Slaby and Cullen 1987). Hypotensive and anticholinergic side effects are less common with this high-potency drug than with the lower-potency neuroleptics such as chlorpromazine. Haloperidol is useful in the intensive care unit setting because it can be given intravenously, intramuscularly, or by mouth (Dudley et al. 1979).

Parenteral haloperidol is preferred for extreme agitation in the intensive care unit because this route leads to a faster response and more reliable blood levels than do other routes (Goldstein 1987). Because their muscle perfusion is poor, critically ill patients may have poor absorption from intramuscular injections. Intravenous haloperidol may cause fewer acute extrapyramidal side effects than do comparable intramuscular injections; the explanation for this phenomenon is not known (Goldstein 1987; Tesar et al. 1985).

Mild agitation usually responds to a parenteral (including intravenous) dose of 0.5–2.0 mg of haloperidol and moderate agitation to 2.0–10.0 mg; for severe agitation, 10.0 mg or more may be used (Goldstein 1987). It is safer to begin with the lower dosage; if agitation persists unchanged 20–30 minutes after the parenteral dose, another dose, double the amount of the first, can be given. For patients with severe liver disease, one-half the usual dose is given since metabolism may be slowed.

It is frequently helpful to prescribe a routine dose of haloperidol that is one-half the initial total dose given over the first 24 hours. This dose should be divided into a three-times-a-day schedule. A routine bedtime dose helps regulate sleep while the clinician uncovers and then treats the etiology of the psychosis.

Treatment of delirious or psychotic reactions sometimes must be instituted while the etiology of the psychosis is still unknown. The first step is to protect the patient from harm to self or others. This patient may be at risk for suicidal behavior because of his or her distorted reality and impaired judgment. One-to-one nursing care, and physical restraints in acute situations, may be necessary to protect the patient and the staff. Pharmacologic restraint is indicated if the patient becomes disruptive or out of control. Undermedication with inadequate supervision is more hazardous than the commonly feared overdosing (Groves and Manschreck 1987). Typical neuroleptic therapy for psychotic or agitated behavior would be similar to that described above (see Table 9-5).

For patients with a history of steroid-induced psychosis, short-term lithium prophylaxis is often useful (Falk et al. 1979). Close follow-up of renal functioning is imperative because cyclosporine can be neph-

Table 9-5. Treatment guidelines for the starting-dose use of intravenous haloperidol in the intensive care setting

Degree of agitation	Dose (mg)
Mild	0.5–2.0
Moderate to severe	2.0–10.0

Titration and maintenance

1. Allow 20–30 minutes before the next dose.
2. If agitation is unchanged, administer double dose every 20–30 minutes until patient begins to calm.
3. If patient is calming down, repeat the last dose at next dosing interval.
4. Adjust dose and interval to patient's clinical course. Gradually increase the interval between doses until the interval is 8 hours, then begin to decrease dose.
5. Once stable for 24 hours, give doses on a regular schedule and supplement with PRN doses.
6. Once stable for 36–48 hours, begin attempts to taper dose.
7. When agitation is very severe, very high dose boluses (up to 40 mg) may be required. Decreased doses may be needed in patients with decreased liver metabolism.

Source. Reprinted with permission from Goldstein: Intensive care unit syndromes, in Principles of Medical Psychiatry. Edited by Stoudemire A, Fogel BS. Orlando, FL, Grune & Stratton, 1987, p 412.

rotoxic and can impair creatinine clearance. Lithium levels initially should be determined biweekly, and a serum level of 0.8–1.2 meq/L should be maintained if tolerated.

If the patients continue to need higher doses of primary or adjunctive neuroleptic medication, extrapyramidal side effects may develop. Diphenhydramine, 25 mg im, rapidly treats these effects. Although relatively safe, it does cause sedation and, because of its anticholinergic action, should be used with caution in patients awaiting heart transplant. Continued oral administration of an anticholinergic agent may be required if the patient needs continuing antipsychotic medications.

Amantadine may be used in combination with neuroleptic therapy. The clearance of amantadine is reduced and plasma levels are increased in patients with renal failure and in patients over age 65; dosages should thus be adjusted according to the individual's renal function and general medical condition (see Table 9-6). Heart transplant candidates with congestive heart failure should be monitored closely since amantadine has been reported to aggravate symptoms of cardiac failure.

Depression

If depression interferes with treatment management or is pronounced, pharmacologic intervention should be considered. For all

Table 9-6.   Amantadine doses for impaired renal function

Creatine clearance levels (ml/min per 1.73 m^2)	Dose of amantadine
30–50	200 mg first day and 100 mg each day thereafter
15–29	200 mg first day followed by 100 mg on alternate days
<15	200 mg every 7 days

Source. Data from Physicians' Desk Reference 1989.

transplant candidates, starting doses should be low (e.g., 10 mg of desipramine or nortriptyline) and may be increased every 2–5 days to reach therapeutic levels only if the patient tolerates the current dose (Levenson 1987; Stoudemire and Fogel 1987).

After a successful transplant, with a healthy liver to metabolize the medication or a strong denervated heart, patients generally tolerate the usual therapeutic doses of antidepressants unless orthostatic hypotension is a problem. However, monitoring of serum levels is still recommended because of individual differences in metabolism. In theory, heart transplant recipients are a safer population for antidepressants than the general population since vagal blockade and atrioventricular conduction effects are of no concern in their denervated and sometimes externally paced hearts (Kay 1988).

Tricyclic antidepressants, such as nortriptyline and trazodone, offer sedation at relatively low doses of 25–50 mg to help with sleep disturbances. Desipramine, fluoxetine, and trazodone are less anticholinergic (Schoonover 1987). Impaired left ventricular function may potentiate tricyclic-induced orthostatic hypotension (Levenson 1987; Stoudemire and Fogel 1987).

Fluoxetine shows great promise for use with heart transplant candidates because, at least in preliminary studies, no intraventricular conduction delays were noted (Fisch 1985) and the drug has minimal if any effects on blood pressure. Because the half-life is prolonged in liver failure patients, an every-other-day dosing (20 mg qod or 20 mg Monday, Wednesday, Friday) may be preferable. In cases in which antidepressant therapy has proven unsuccessful or is contraindicated, electroconvulsive therapy has been safely used in transplant recipients (House et al. 1990). Bupropion also has a very favorable cardiac profile; however, there are no published reports as yet of its use in cardiac or liver transplant patients.

Psychostimulant medications can be prescribed when traditional antidepressants have not been helpful or are contraindicated. Psychostimulants act rapidly and improve motivation, energy, psychomotor activity, and mood. Side effects include tachycardia, hypertension, and nausea, which is usually transient (Riether and Rubenow 1989b). Although the mood-elevating effects may diminish with continued use, stimulatory activity persists with chronic low-dose administration. Abrupt withdrawal frequently precipitates a recurrent depression accompanied by hypersomnia and lethargy (Riether and Rubenow 1989b).

Anxiety

For anxiety accompanied by marked motor restlessness, tension, autonomic hyperactivity, and apprehension that does not respond to supportive treatment, anxiolytic therapy is useful (Watts et al. 1984). Many transplant candidates complain of a sense of losing control or of impending doom. For some patients who have mild to moderate anxiety, relaxation techniques combined with imaging techniques, hypnotherapy, or biofeedback are helpful.

For severe anxiety or for patients unresponsive to nonpharmacologic intervention, benzodiazepines or low-dose neuroleptics may be helpful. The benzodiazepines are largely protein bound; that is, they depend on liver metabolism for degradation and are then excreted by the kidneys. Metabolites can accumulate in transplant candidates with renal or hepatic insufficiency; therefore anxiolytics with short or intermediate half-lives (3–18 hours) or those with no active metabolites are preferred. Midazolam, lorazepam, temazepam, and oxazepam are most frequently used for transplant candidates because they accumulate less with multiple doses and are more rapidly cleared after the medication is stopped (Cutler and Narang 1984).

For patients unable to take oral medications, lorazepam and midazolam can be given parenterally. Lorazepam may be helpful when given before painful procedures, although it has anterograde amnestic properties (Stoudemire and Fogel 1987).

For transplant candidates who complain of difficulty sleeping, temazepam and triazolam may be particularly helpful. Triazolam, because of its ultrashort half-life, is often used for patients who have difficulty falling asleep; but it has been associated with dissociative, confusional states, with rebound insomnia (Stoudemire and Fogel 1987), and, as noted earlier, with anterograde amnesia. If it is used, the 0.125-mg dose is generally preferable, although it may not provide coverage for the duration of an entire night's sleep.

POSTOPERATIVE ADJUSTMENT AND QUALITY OF LIFE

Although most patients seem to adjust fairly well after transplant, all patients need to incorporate and integrate the new organ into their body image (Lefebvre and Crombez 1977). This integration, which has been called the "psychological transplant" (Mulsin 1971), is said to depend on the real as well as the fantasized qualities of the donor and on the relationship, if any, between the donor and the recipient (Gulledge et al. 1983). Patients also need to grieve for their lost organ. Although it may have been no longer functional, it was keeping them alive; if asked, patients may relate elaborate restorative fantasies about what happened to their organ. One patient in our practice was sure that his heart was being used to teach hundreds of medical students and scientists about heart disease.

As these patients adjust to their lives after transplant, there is an initial stage during which they may react to their transplanted organ as a foreign body, reporting that it "feels funny." They may worry that the organ will "fall out" or "get loose." Next, a stage of partial incorporation may be observed, during which the patient is less preoccupied with the foreignness of the organ. Finally, during the complete incorporation stage, the organ is completely psychologically assimilated (Mulsin 1971).

Early research on postoperative adjustment after orthotopic transplant dealt almost exclusively with questions of patient survival. Issues of infection, immunosuppression, and rejection were paramount (Jamieson et al. 1982). As procedures have been refined and the rate of survival has improved, however, research interest has shifted to include aspects of life after transplantation, referred to as quality of life. Other health-related medical problems and emotional, sexual, social, marital, and vocational adjustment have become more central.

By definition, health-related quality of life refers to the impact of health conditions on the person's functional status, including subjective state. As an all-pervasive, all-encompassing, yet highly subjective concept, the definition of quality of life or health quality, as well as its measurement, has been somewhat elusive. Numerous quality-of-life measures have been proposed in the past 20 years (see Table 9-1).

Separate measures for the many dimensions that are assumed to be components of overall quality of life may be measured, or an attempt may be made to weigh the various dimensions of health status to provide a single measure of health status (Bush 1984; Kaplan 1988). In the former approach, anxiety, depression, cognitive dysfunction, or memory loss might be measured. Such focused approaches leave the clinician to make assumptions about the overall life quality experienced by the patient.

In more comprehensive approaches, a weighted model for assessing the range of functions considered to constitute quality of life is used. The Quality of Well-Being Scale (Bush 1984), developed out of the RAND Corporation framework, is an example of such a model. The overall aggregate score yielded by this approach has obvious merit in comparing outcomes of treatment. On the other hand, the multidimensional psychometric approach permits the comparison of individuals to normative populations on psychometric procedures that have been correlated with successful coping. A combination of these two approaches seems ideal.

Most research on the quality of life after transplant has emphasized psychometric approaches. The findings of several investigators (Allender et al. 1983; Lough et al. 1985; Najman and Levine 1981) suggest that a complicated medical course after surgery, including drug side effects, rejection episodes, infection, and the necessity for recurrent hospitalizations, can adversely affect the quality of life.

Retrospective review of subjective quality-of-life measures has shown that patients who refuse to talk openly about death, who view the surgery as a mutilating assault on their bodies, and who have little family support have more difficulty and less significant quality-of-life changes than those patients who are realistic yet hopeful about their situations and who want to prolong life to do specific things (Christopherson and Lunde 1971).

Most cardiac transplant patients achieve improved status postsurgery and tend to rate their quality of life as good to excellent (Freeman et al. 1988; Jones et al. 1988; Lough et al. 1985). However, some patients report difficulty adjusting (Freeman et al. 1988). Lough and associates (1985) have observed that more than 25% of a sample of heart transplant patients felt that life had become less rewarding after surgery. Negative changes were noted most frequently in physical appearance, sexual functioning, and finances. Immunosuppressant-induced symptoms and the distress associated with them were also tied to poorer quality of life.

Sometimes we do not meet the rehabilitative needs of transplant candidates or recipients because we are unaware of the services these patients require. Recently, transplant recipients were asked to list those services they felt would have improved the quality of their lives during transplant and postsurgical recovery (Wolcott, personal communication, 1989). Their lists included services for nutritional counseling and weight loss, financial counseling, advice on returning to work, and vocational rehabilitation. Patients also felt that ongoing psychiatric therapy and, at times, medication for depression and insomnia would have improved their recovery. Transplant recipients also listed specific counseling for sexual concerns and ongoing group therapy as helpful (Wolcott, personal communication, 1989).

Long-term follow-up of transplant patients is necessary for an accurate evaluation of selection criteria, psychiatric outcomes, and adjustment after transplant. Subjective quality-of-life measures and appropriate ratings of psychiatric, intellectual, and social functioning will help psychiatrists better understand and provide intervention and support for patients undergoing transplantation.

REFERENCES

Abram HS, Buchanan DC: The gift of life: a review of the psychological aspects of kidney transplantation. Int J Psychiatry Med 7:153–164, 1976–1977

Adams DH, Gunson B, Honigsberger L, et al: Neurological complications following liver transplantation. Lancet 1:949–951, 1987

Allender J, Shisslak C, Kaszniak A, et al: Stages of psychological adjustment associated with heart transplantation. Heart Transplantation 2:228–231, 1983

American Psychiatric Association: Diagnostic and Statistical Manual of Mental Disorders, 3rd Edition, Revised. Washington, DC, American Psychiatric Association, 1987

Atkinson K, Biggs J, Darveniza J, et al: Cyclosporine-associated central nervous system toxicity after allogenic bone marrow transplantation. Transplantation 38:34–37, 1984

Baloch N: Steroid psychosis–a case report. Br J Psychiatry 124:545–546, 1974

Beck AT, Ward CH, Mendelson M, et al: An inventory for measuring depression. Arch Gen Psychiatry 4:561–571, 1961

Beidel DC: Psychological factors in organ transplantation. Clinical Psychology Review 7:677–694, 1987

Beresford TP, Turcotte JG, Merion R, et al: A rational approach to liver transplantation for the alcoholic patient. Psychosomatics 31:241–254, 1990

Bergner M, Bobbitt RA, Pollard WE, et al: The Sickness Impact Profile: validation of a health status measure. Med Care 14:57–67, 1976

Borman MC, Schmallenberg HC: Suicide following cortisone treatment. JAMA 146:337–338, 1951

Boston Collaborative Drug Surveillance Program: Acute adverse reactions to prednisone in relation to dosage. Clin Pharmacol Ther 13:694–698, 1972

Bush JW: General Health Policy Model/Quality of Well-Being (QWB) Scale, in Assessment of Quality of Life in Clinical Trials of Cardiovascular Therapies. Edited by Wenger WK, Mattson ME, Furberg CD, et al. La Jolla, CA, LeJacq, 1984, pp 170–199

Busuttil RW (moderator): Liver transplantation today. Discussants: Goldstein LI, Danovitch GM, Ament ME, et al. Ann Intern Med 104:377–389, 1986

Casscells W: Heart transplantation: recent policy developments. N Engl J Med 315:1365–1368, 1986

Castelnuovo-Tedesco P: Cardiac surgeons look at transplantation—interviews with Drs. Cleveland, Cooley, DeBakey, Hallman, and Rochelle. Seminars in Psychiatry 3:5–16, 1971

Castelnuovo-Tedesco P: Organ transplant, body image, psychosis. Psychoanal Q 42:349–363, 1973

Christopherson LK: Cardiac transplantation: a psychological perspective. Circulation 75:57–62, 1987

Christopherson LK, Lunde DT: Selection of cardiac transplant recipients and their subsequent psychological adjustment. Seminars in Psychiatry 3:36–45, 1971

Clark LD, Bauer W, Cobb S: Preliminary observations on mental disturbances occurring in patients under therapy with cortisone and ACTH. N Engl J Med 246:205–216, 1952

Cloninger CR: A systematic method for clinical description and classification of personality variants: a proposal. Arch Gen Psychiatry 44:573–588, 1987

Cooper DKC, Lanza RP, Barnard CN: Noncompliance in heart transplant recipients: the Cape Town experience. Heart Transplantation 3:248–253, 1984

Cutler NR, Narang PK: Implications of dosing tricyclic antidepressants and benzodiazepines in geriatrics. Psychiatr Clin North Am 7:845–861, 1984

deGroen PC, Aksamit AJ, Rakela J, et al: Central nervous system toxicity after liver transplantation: the role of cyclosporine and cholesterol. N Engl J Med 317:861–866, 1987

De-Nour AK: Psychosocial Adjustment to Illness Scale (PAIS): a study of chronic hemodialysis patients. J Psychosom Res 26:11–22, 1982

Derogatis LR: The Psychosocial Adjustment to Illness Scale (PAIS and PAIS-SR) Scoring Procedures and Administration Manual I. Baltimore, MD, Clinical Psychometric Research, 1983

Derogatis LR: The Psychosocial Adjustment to Illness Scale (PAIS). J Psychosom Res 30:77–91, 1986

Didlake RH, Dreyfus K, Kerman RH, et al: Patient noncompliance: a major cause of late graft failure in cyclosporine-treated renal transplants. Transplant Proc 20 (suppl 3):63–69, 1988

Dudley DL, Rowlett DE, Loebel PJ: Emergency use of intravenous haloperidol. Gen Hosp Psychiatry 1:240–246, 1979

Durrant S, Chipping PM, Palmer S, et al: Cyclosporine A, methylprednisolone, and convulsions (letter). Lancet 2:829–830, 1982

Ewing J: Detecting alcoholism: the CAGE questionnaire. JAMA 252:1905–1907, 1984

Falk WE, Mahnke MW, Peskanzer DC: Lithium prophylaxis of corticotropin-induced psychosis. JAMA 241:1011–1012, 1979

Fisch C: Effect of fluoxetine on the electrocardiogram. J Clin Psychiatry 46:42–44, 1985

Folstein MF, Folstein SE, McHugh P: "Mini-Mental State": a practical method for grading the cognitive state of patients for the clinician. J Psychiatr Res 12:189–198, 1975

Freeman AM, Watts D, Karp R: Evaluation of cardiac transplant candidates: preliminary observations. Psychosomatics 25:197–207, 1984

Freeman AM, Folks DG, Sokol RS, et al: Cardiac transplantation: clinical correlates of psychiatric outcome [issue title]. Psychosomatics 29:47–54, 1988

Frierson RL, Lippmann SB: Heart transplant candidates rejected on psychiatric indications. Psychosomatics 28:347–355, 1987

Gastfriend DR, Surman OS, Gaffey GK, et al: Substance abuse and compliance in organ transplantation. Substance Abuse 10:149–153, 1989

Glaser GH: Psychotic reactions induced by corticotropin (ACTH) and cortisone. Psychosom Med 15:280–291, 1953

Goldstein MG: Intensive care unit syndromes, in Principles of Medical Psychiatry. Edited by Stoudemire A, Fogel BS. Orlando, FL, Grune & Stratton, 1987, pp 403–421

Groves JE, Manschreck TC: Psychotic patients, in Massachusetts General Hospital Handbook of Psychiatry, 2nd Edition. Edited by Hackett TP, Cassem NH. Littleton, MA, PSG, 1987, pp 208–226

Gulledge AD, Buszta C, Montague DK: Psychosocial aspects of renal transplantation. Urol Clin North Am 10:327–335, 1983

Hamilton M: A rating scale for depression. J Neurol Neurosurg Psychiatry 23:56–62, 1960

Hare R: Comparison of procedures for the assessment of psychopathology. J Consult Clin Psychol 53:7–16, 1985

Hathaway SR, McKinley JC: Minnesota Multiphasic Personality Inventory—2. Minneapolis, MN, University of Minnesota, 1989

Hecker JE, Norvell N, Hills H: Psychological assessment of candidates for heart transplantation: toward a normative data base. Heart Transplantation 8:171–176, 1989

Helfrich GB, Chu-Aquino B, Pechan W, et al: Are there too many complications from renal transplantation? in Controversies in Nephrology. Edited by Schreiner GE. Washington, DC, Georgetown University Hospital, 1980

Hong BA, Smith MD, Robson AM, et al: Depressive symptomatology and treatment in patients with end-stage renal disease. Psychol Med 17:185–190, 1987

Hotson JR, Pedley TA: The neurological complications of cardiac transplantation. Brain 99:673–694, 1976

House RM, Thompson TL: Psychiatric aspects of organ transplantation. JAMA 260:535–539, 1988

House RM, Trzepacz PT, Thompson TL II: Psychiatric consultation to organ transplant services, in American Psychiatric Press Review of Psychiatry, Vol 9. Edited by Tasman A, Goldfinger SM, Kaufman CA. Washington, DC, American Psychiatric Press, 1990, pp 515–536

Hyler S, Rieder R, Spitzer R, et al: The Personality Diagnostic Questionnaire (PDQ). New York, New York State Psychiatric Institute, 1982

Jamieson SW, Oyer PE, Bieber CP, et al: Transplantation for cardiomyopathy: a review of the results. Heart Transplantation 2:28, 1982

Jones BM, Chang VP, Esmore D, et al: Psychological adjustment after cardiac transplantation. Med J Aust 149:116–122, 1988

Joss DV, Barrett AJ, Kendra JR, et al: Hypertension and convulsions in children receiving cyclosporine. Lancet 1:906, 1982

Kahan BD: Individualization of cyclosporine therapy using pharmacokinetic and pharmacodynamic parameters. Transplantation 40:457–476, 1985

Kaplan RM: Health-related quality of life in cardiovascular disease. J Consult Clin Psychol 56:382–392, 1988

Kay J: Psychiatric qualifiers for heart transplant candidates (letter to the editor). Psychosomatics 29:143–144, 1988

Kemph JP: Renal failure, artificial kidney and kidney transplant. Am J Psychiatry 122:1270–1274, 1966

Kiesler DJ: Manual for the Impact Message Inventory. Palo Alto, CA, Consulting Psychologists Press, 1987

Kraft IA: Psychiatric complications of cardiac transplantation. Seminars in Psychiatry 3:58–69, 1971

Kuhn WF, Myers B, Brennan AF, et al: Psychopathology in heart transplant candidates. Heart Transplantation 7:223–226, 1988

Labar B, Bogdanic V, Plavsic F, et al: Cyclosporine neurotoxicity in patients treated with allogenic bone marrow transplantation. Biomed Pharmacother 40:148–150, 1986

Lefebvre P, Crombez J: The one-day-at-a-time syndrome in posttransplant evolution. Presented at the World Congress of Psychiatry, Honolulu, Hawaii, Aug 1977

Lefebvre P, Crombez JC, Lebeuf J: Psychological dimension and psychopathological potential of acquiring a kidney. Can J Psychiatry 18:495–500, 1973

Levenson JL: Cardiovascular disease, in Principles of Medical Psychiatry. Edited by Stoudemire A, Fogel BS. Orlando, FL, Grune & Stratton, 1987, pp 477–493

Levenson JL, Olbrisch ME: Shortage of donor organs and long waits. Psychosomatics 28:399–403, 1987

Levine PM, Silberfarb PM, Lipowski ZJ: Mental disorders in cancer patients: a study of 100 psychiatric referrals. Cancer 42:1385–1391, 1978

Lezak MD: Neuropsychological Assessment, 2nd Edition. New York, Oxford University Press, 1983

Ling MHM, Perry PJ, Tsuang MT: Side effects of corticosteroid therapy. Arch Gen Psychiatry 38:471–477, 1981

Loranger AW: Personality Disorder Examination Manual. Yonkers, NY, DV Communications, 1988

Lough ME, Lindscy AM, Shinn JA, et al: Life satisfaction following heart transplantation. Heart Transplantation 4:446–449, 1985

Lowry MR, Atcherson E: Characteristics of patients with depressive disorder on entry into home hemodialysis. J Nerv Ment Dis 167:748–751, 1979

Mai FM, McKenzie FN, Kostuk WJ: Psychiatric aspects of heart transplantation: preoperative evaluation and postoperative sequelae. Br Med J 292:311–313, 1986

McAleer MJ, Copeland J, Fuller J, et al: Psychological aspects of heart transplantation. Heart Transplantation 4:232–233, 1985

McLellan AT, Luborsky L, Woody GE, et al: Predicting response to alcohol and drug abuse treatments. Arch Gen Psychiatry 40:620–625, 1983

McNair DM, Lorr M, Droppleman LF: Manual for the Profile of Mood States. San Diego, CA, Educational and Industrial Testing Service, 1981

Mezzich JE, Munetz M, Ganguli, et al: Computerized initial and discharge evaluations, in Clinical Care and Information Systems in Psychiatry. Edited by Mezzich JE. Washington, DC, American Psychiatric Press, 1986

Millon T: Millon Clinical Multiaxial Inventory—II: Manual for the MCMI-II. Minneapolis, MN, National Computer Systems, 1987

Millon T, Green C, Meagher R: The MBHI: a new inventory for the psychodiagnostician in medical settings. Professional Psychology 10:529–539, 1979

Moos RH: Family Environment Scale, 2nd Edition. Palo Alto, CA, Consulting Psychological Press, 1986

Mulsin HL: On acquiring a kidney. Am J Psychiatry 127:105–108, 1971

Najman JM, Levine S: Evaluating the impact of medical care and technologies on the quality of life: a review and critique. Soc Sci Med 15:107–115, 1981

National Council on Alcoholism, Criteria Committee: Criteria for the diagnosis of alcoholism. Am J Psychiatry 129:41–48, 1972

National Institutes of Health, Consensus Development Panel: Liver transplantation: consensus conference. JAMA 250:2961–2964, 1983

Nielsen JB, Drivsholm AA, Fischer F, et al: Long-term treatment with corticosteroids in rheumatoid arthritis. Acta Med Scand 173:177–183, 1963

O'Brien VC: Psychological and social aspects of heart transplantation. Heart Transplantation 4:229–231, 1985

Olbrisch ME, Levenson JL, Hamer R: The PACT: a rating scale for the study of clinical decision-making in psychosocial screening of organ transplant candidates. Clinical Transplantation 3:164–169, 1989

Olson DH, Russell CS, Sprenkle DH: Circumplex model of marital and family systems, VI: theoretical update. Fam Process 22:69–83, 1983

Penn I, Bunch D, Olenik D, et al: Psychiatric experience with patients receiving renal and hepatic transplants. Seminars in Psychiatry 3:133–144, 1971

Physicians' Desk Reference, 43rd Edition. Oradell, NJ, Medical Economics, 1989

Ramsey Clinic: Standardized Structured Interview for DSM-III-R: Chemical Dependency Diagnosis, the Substance Use Disorder Diagnosis Schedule (SUDDS). Ramsey Clinic, Department of Psychiatry, 640 Jackson Street, St. Paul, MN 55101, 1985

Reichsman F, Levy NB: Problems in adaptation to maintenance hemodialysis. Arch Intern Med 130:859–865, 1972

Reitan RM: Validity of the Trailmaking Test as an indicator of organic brain damage. Percept Mot Skills 8:271–276, 1958

Rey A: L'Examen Clinique en Psychologie. Paris, Presses de France, 1964

Riether AM: Psychiatric aspects of organ transplantation, in Tissue and Organ Transplantation: Implications for Professional Nursing Practice. Edited by Smith S. St. Louis, MO, CV Mosby, 1990

Riether AM, Rubenow JC: Psychiatric symptomatology in transplant patients. Clinical Advances in Psychiatric Disorders 3:8–10, 1989a

Riether AM, Rubenow JC: Psychiatric treatment of transplant patients. Clinical Advances in Psychiatric Disorders 4:4–10, 1989b

Riether AM, Stoudemire A: Surgery and trauma, in Principles of Medical Psychiatry. Edited by Stoudemire A, Fogel BS. Orlando, FL, Grune & Stratton, 1987, pp 423–449

Schoonover SC: Depression, in The Practitioner's Guide to Psychoactive Drugs. Edited by Bassuk EL, Schoonover SC, Gelenberg AJ. New York, Plenum, 1987, pp 19–77

Selzer ML: The Michigan Alcoholism Screening Test: the quest for a new diagnostic instrument. Am J Psychiatry 127:1653–1658, 1971

Slaby AE, Cullen LO: Dementia and delirium, in Principles of Medical Psychiatry. Edited by Stoudemire A, Fogel BS. Orlando, FL, Grune & Stratton, 1987, pp 135–175

Spielberger CD: Manual for the State-Trait Anxiety Inventory. Palo Alto, CA, Consulting Psychologists Press, 1983

Spitzer RL, Williams JBW, Gibbon M, et al: Structured Clinical Interview for DSM-III-R Personality Disorders (SCID-II). Washington, DC, American Psychiatric Press, 1990

Starzl TE, Van Thiel D, Tzakis AG, et al: Orthotopic liver transplantation for alcoholic cirrhosis. JAMA 260:2542–2544, 1988

Starzl TE, Fung J, Venkataramman R, et al: FK506 for liver, kidney and pancreas transplantation. Lancet 2:1000–1004, 1989

Stewart RS: Psychiatric issues in renal dialysis and transplantation. Hosp Community Psychiatry 34(7), 623–628, 1983

Stoudemire A, Fogel BS: Psychopharmacology, in Principles of Medical Psychiatry. Edited by Stoudemire A, Fogel BS. Orlando, FL, Grune & Stratton, 1987, pp 79–111

Surman O: The surgical patient, in Massachusetts General Hospital Handbook of General Hospital Psychiatry, 1st Edition. Edited by Hackett TP, Casscm NH. St. Louis, MO, CV Mosby, 1978, pp 64–92

Surman OS: Psychiatric aspects of organ transplantation. Am J Psychiatry 146:972–982, 1989

Taylor EM: The appraisal of children with cerebral deficits. Cambridge, MA, Harvard University Press, 1959

Tesar GE, Murray GB, Cassen NH: Use of high-dose intravenous haloperidol in the treatment of agitated cardiac patients. J Clin Psychopharmacol 5:344–347, 1985

Thompson CB, Sullivan KM, June CH, et al: Association between cyclosporine neurotoxicity and hypomagnesaemia. Lancet 2:1116–1120, 1984

Thompson ME: Selection of candidates for cardiac transplantation. Heart Transplantation 3:65–69, 1983

Tisza VB, Dorsett P, Morse J: Psychological implications of renal transplantation. J Am Acad Child Psychiatry 15:709–720, 1976

Trzepacz PT, Brenner RP, Coffman G, et al: Delirium in liver transplantation candidates: discriminant analysis of multiple test variables. Biol Psychiatry 24:3–14, 1988

Trzepacz PT, Brenner R, Van Thiel DH: A psychiatric study of 247 liver transplantation candidates. Psychosomatics 30:147–153, 1989

Valliant GE: The Natural History of Alcoholism. Cambridge, MA, Harvard University Press, 1983

Valliant GE, Clark W, Cyrus C, et al: Prospective study of alcoholism treatment: eight-year follow-up. Am J Med 75:455–463, 1983

Van Thiel DH, Schade RR, Starzl TE, et al: Liver transplantation in adults. Hepatology 2:637–640, 1982

Van Thiel D, Gavaler JS, Tarter RE, et al: Liver transplantation for alcoholic liver disease: a consideration of reasons for and against. Alcoholism 13:181–184, 1989

Wamboldt FW: Cyclosporine mania. Biol Psychiatry 19:1161–1162, 1984

Watts D, Freeman AM, McGriffin DG, et al: Psychiatric aspects of cardiac transplantation. Heart Transplantation 3:243–247, 1984

Wechsler D: Manual for Wechsler Adult Intelligence Scale—Revised. New York, Psychological Corporation, 1981

Willner AE: Conceptual Level Analogy Test. New York, Cognitive Testing Service, 1976

Willner AE, Rabiner CJ, Wisoff BG, et al: Analogical reasoning and postoperative outcome: predictions for patients scheduled for open heart surgery. Arch Gen Psychiatry 33:255–259, 1976

Young KJ, Longman AJ: Quality of life and persons with melanoma: a pilot study. Cancer Nurs 6:219–225, 1983

Section III

Clinical Neuropsychiatry

Chapter 10

Diagnosis and Management of Patients With Frontal Lobe Syndromes

Barry S. Fogel, M.D.
Paul J. Eslinger, Ph.D.

The frontal lobes are thought to play wide-ranging roles in a number of complex human behaviors, from social learning and personality development to the regulation of emotional states (Stuss and Benson 1986). Scientific inquiry into frontal lobe function spans molecular biology, gross and microscopic neuroanatomy, physiology, and the macroscopic clinical analysis of cognition, emotion, and behavior in patients with frontal lobe lesions. Treatment of patients with frontal lobe syndromes is among the most perplexing issues faced by mental health professionals. While not always recognized as such, frontal lobe dysfunction may underlie or contribute to various neuropsychiatric and neurobehavioral disorders throughout the life span. It is frequently encountered as a consequence of closed head injury and is often a major feature of dementing disorders, cerebrovascular disease, and multifocal encephalopathies. Frontal lobe dysfunction may cause an organic personality disorder (Carlson 1977; Grafman et al. 1986; Gross and Herridge 1988; Lahmeyer 1982) or may modify the expression of a concurrent mood disorder or psychosis (McAllister and Price 1987).

Supported in part by Grant 1-P50-NS-26985-01 to P.J.E.

Table 10-1.   Functions impaired by frontal lobe damage and relation to
behavioral signs

Function	Behavioral sign
Linkage of knowledge with action	Impulsiveness; poor judgment
Handling sequential behaviors	Perseveration; disorganization
Establishing or changing a response set	Poor acquisition of new skills; perseveration
Maintaining a mental set	Impersistence; distractibility
Self-monitoring	Unkempt appearance: inappropriate behavior
Motivation	Apathy

Source. Functions are adapted from Stuss and Benson 1984.

While clinical scientists have been recording cases of frontal lobe damage for over a century, the emerging challenge in our era is to assemble the data into workable models of how the brain operates, how its function becomes disturbed, and how to ameliorate untoward consequences. Stuss and Benson (1984) have enumerated six cardinal features of frontal (strictly speaking, *prefrontal*) lobe damage: 1) separation of action from knowledge, 2) impairment of the ability to handle sequential behaviors, 3) impairment of the ability to establish or change response set, 4) impairment of the ability to maintain a response set, 5) impairment of the ability to monitor personal behavior, and 6) production of attitudes of apathy. Frontal lobe functions and behavioral signs of frontal lobe dysfunction are summarized and linked in Table 10-1.

In this chapter, we offer a neuropsychologic perspective on frontal lobe dysfunction. We also show how recent work on the treatment of behavioral syndromes due to anatomic frontal lobe damage can not only be helpful in neuropsychiatric patients, but also can inform a more general approach to general psychiatric patients with deficits in self-regulation, planning, and related executive functions.

ETIOLOGY OF FRONTAL LOBE DYSFUNCTION

Frontal lobe dysfunction occurs in its most isolated form in patients with localized anatomic damage to frontal lobe structures, as in the cases of tumor and stroke. However, frontal lobe dysfunction may be prominent in a variety of other conditions, listed in Table 10-2.

Degenerative diseases, including Pick's disease, Parkinson's dis-

Table 10-2. Etiologies of frontal lobe dysfunction

- **Degenerative diseases**
  Alzheimer's disease
  Huntington's disease
  Parkinson's disease
  Pick's disease
  Wilson's disease
  Pure frontal lobe degeneration

- **Multifocal encephalopathies**
  Binswanger's disease
  Multi-infarct dementia
  Multiple sclerosis
  Head injury
  HIV-related involvement
  Toxic-metabolic encephalopathy

- **Congenital and developmental disorders**
  Attention-deficit hyperactivity disorder
  Hydrocephalus

- **Primary psychiatric illnesses**
  Chronic schizophrenia
  Bipolar disorder
  Major depression

- **Disruption of frontal inputs**
  Thalamic disease
  Basal ganglia disease

ease, Huntington's disease, and hepatolenticular degeneration (Wilson's disease), show cortical involvement disproportionately affecting the frontal lobes (Caltagirone et al. 1985; Knopman et al. 1989; Roos 1986). Also, there has recently been described a dementing syndrome of relatively pure frontal lobe degeneration, with nonspecific pathological features that do not include senile plaques, neurofibrillary tangles, or Pick cells (Brun 1987; Neary et al. 1988). Frontal lobe dysfunction may also be prominent in Alzheimer's disease (Palmer et al. 1987), in which symptoms can range from the inability to make decisions, plan, anticipate, and complete tasks to marked personality change with irritability and withdrawal. Patients with Parkinson's disease, particularly when it is accompanied by depression, may show frontal lobe dysfunction, perhaps due to the loss of crucial dopaminergic and noradrenergic inputs to the frontal lobe from the locus coeruleus and ventral tegmental area (Starkstein et al. 1989; Sudarsky et al. 1989). Patients with Parkinson's disease and unilateral symptoms show lateralized cognitive disturbances

(Starkstein et al. 1987). Patients with progressive supranuclear palsy show intellectual impairment even more often than Parkinson's disease patients, and they have particular difficulty with tests sensitive to frontal lobe dysfunction (Maher et al. 1985).

Multifocal encephalopathies such as multiple sclerosis, progressive multifocal leukoencephalopathy, multi-infarct dementia, and Binswanger's disease may have prominent effects on the frontal lobes because of damage to afferent and efferent white matter tracts connecting the frontal lobes with other brain regions (Caplan 1985; Ishii et al. 1986; Knoefel and Albert 1985). Closed head injury may disproportionately affect frontal regions, both because the frontal lobes are vulnerable to contusion and because of the effect of shearing stresses on long fibers connecting frontal lobes with other regions (Hinebaugh 1986; Levin et al. 1982; Stuss 1987). Cognitive signs of frontal lobe dysfunction also have been observed in patients with acquired immunodeficiency syndrome (AIDS) encephalopathy. A predominance of frontal signs is particularly likely early in the course of human immunodeficiency virus (HIV) central nervous system (CNS) disease (Marotta and Perry 1989; Ochitill and Dilley 1988), perhaps because executive functions, which depend on polysynaptic information processing, are particularly vulnerable to disruption by mild diffuse brain damage.

Congenital and developmental disorders, such as cerebral palsy and some cases of attention-deficit hyperactivity disorder (ADHD), may display prominent signs of frontal dysfunction. In some cases, anatomic evidence of frontal abnormality can be demonstrated; in others, dysfunction is inferred from the pattern of behavior and performance on neuropsychological tests. A recent single-photon emission computer tomography (SPECT) study of ADHD has also indicated hypoperfusion in the neostriatum, which is closely interconnected with the frontal lobes. Furthermore, treatment with methylphenidate tended to increase blood flow to the neostriatum (Lou et al. 1989).

Toxic and metabolic factors may differentially affect functions associated with the frontal lobes. This is true both for chronic conditions, such as alcoholism (Tarter and Edwards 1985), and for acute intoxication, particularly with CNS depressant drugs. In the latter case, although the depression of brain function may be diffuse, the greater complexity of adaptive functions subserved by the frontal lobes and the more complex neuroanatomic pathways that support them may make those functions more vulnerable to disruption by the toxic insult. Neuropsychological tests sensitive to frontal lobe dysfunction sometimes show disproportionate abnormalities in cases of occupational neurotoxic exposure (Hartman 1988).

Hydrocephalus, whether congenital or acquired, affects frontal lobe function by impairing frontal connections that pass near the ventricles. The gait disturbance, incontinence, and cognitive changes associated with normal pressure hydrocephalus can all be regarded as frontal signs. Compared with Alzheimer's disease patients, patients with normal pressure hydrocephalus have more prominent frontal lobe signs relative to their overall degree of cognitive impairment (Alexander and Geschwind 1984).

Primary psychiatric illnesses, particularly chronic schizophrenia (Goldberg 1985; Goldberg et al. 1987; Levin 1984; Morice 1986; Weinberger 1988; Weinberger et al. 1986; Williamson 1987) and the more severe mood disorders (Wilson and Staton 1984), can be associated with impaired frontal lobe function. In these disorders, evidence for frontal lobe dysfunction affecting at least some severely ill patients is supported not only by cognitive findings but also by direct measurements of blood flow or metabolism by positron-emission tomography (PET) or SPECT (Buchsbaum 1987; Buchsbaum et al. 1984; Geraud et al. 1987; O'Connell et al. 1989; Weinberger et al. 1986). Abnormalities in EEG spectral content or evoked potentials over the frontal regions also have been observed in these conditions (Morstyn et al. 1983; Schatzberg et al. 1986; Weinberger 1988).

Finally, frontal lobe dysfunction also can result from *changes in key connections of the frontal lobes*. Diseases of the thalamus and the basal ganglia can produce "frontal" signs even when anatomic pathology of the frontal lobes is minimal (Eslinger and Grattan 1989; Metter et al. 1981; Strub 1989). The former association may be mediated by disruption of corticopetal or corticofugal connections with the thalamus (Jones 1985; Kievit and Kuypers 1977), whereas the latter association is probably due to disruption of the powerful corticostriate projection system (Kemp and Powell 1970; Yeterian and Van Hoesen 1978). A stroke in the parietal lobe may in the acute phase produce signs of frontal dysfunction due to massive disruption of frontal lobe inputs from parietal association areas—a phenomenon called *diaschisis*.

NEUROBIOLOGY OF THE FRONTAL LOBES

The frontal lobes are demarcated clearly in gross anatomy, extending laterally to the Sylvian fissure and caudally to the motor strip and Rolandic fissure (central sulcus). The lateral surfaces of the frontal lobes are extremely prominent, but the orbital and mesial surfaces also are extensive. These areas or regions appear to be distinguishable on anatomical and functional grounds, and damage to each is associated with characteristic clinical syndromes.

The Mesial Frontal Pattern

The mesial frontal lobes have superior, middle, and inferior portions, and each may well be associated with different neurobehavioral sequelae. The most clearly described are those associated with damage to the superior mesial region (Damasio and Van Hoesen 1982; LaPlane and Eslinger 1977). This region includes the supplementary motor area and the anterior cingulate gyrus, which are intimately interconnected with major motor structures and with the limbic system. The most prominent behavioral changes after damage to this region usually involve impaired initiation of behavior, apathy, and loss of emotional expression. Bilateral damage can cause a profound akinesia and mutism, with lesser injury disrupting spontaneity, motivation, and timely responsiveness.

The Dorsolateral Frontal Pattern

Diverse behavioral impairments have been reported with dorsolateral frontal lobe damage. Disturbances of cognition figure most prominently since patients can exhibit aphasia, apraxia, hemispatial neglect, decreased intellect, disorganization, and poor judgment and planning. The often profound "real life" behavioral disorders of these patients, including changes in personality, motivation, grasp of situations, and the ability to plan and complete any daily activities, are thought to be related to the disturbed regulation of the more elementary cognitive processes mediated by posterior (nonfrontal) cortical areas. The elementary cognitive processes, such as visual perception, word finding, etc., usually remain intact.

The Orbital Frontal Pattern

The orbital frontal region of the frontal lobes is richly interconnected with the limbic system, and, in fact, its posterior ventromedial extent is considered a paralimbic area (Mesulam 1985). It also interconnects with the lateral frontal lobes and may be a crucial site of mediation between the high-level cognitive processing of sensory experiences carried out by the dorsolateral regions and the internal states, drives, and motivations determined by the limbic cortex. Not surprisingly, the orbital region plays an important role in regulation of the autonomic nervous system. Recent studies of patients with damage to this region of the frontal lobes have confirmed disturbed autonomic responsiveness, especially in response to social stimuli (Tranel and Damasio 1989). It has been suggested that regulation of autonomic tone is an essential element in judging social stimuli and eliciting appropriate social behavior. Disturbance of autonomic responses may be a matter of concern not only in adults with acquired orbital damage, but also in the social development of children with early frontal damage. The posterior ventromedial extension of the orbital frontal region, characterized histologically as paralimbic cortex, is strongly interconnected with limbic structures concerned with memory. Damage to this region is associated with impaired memory. Emotional lability is also frequent and may be due either to disruption of limbic connections or to involvement of the nucleus accumbens, which lies within this region.

ASSESSMENT OF FRONTAL LOBE DYSFUNCTION

Relation of Cognition and Behavior

Frontal lobe dysfunction is associated with characteristic cognitive problems and behavioral disturbances. Identification of the cognitive problems is helpful diagnostically because their presence helps establish that the behavioral problems have a basis in brain dysfunction. However, cognitive problems of patients with brain dysfunction limited to the frontal lobes often escape attention on casual assessment because they are not detected by common screens for delirium and dementia, such as the Mini-Mental State Exam (Folstein et al. 1975; Nelson et al. 1986), or by many clinicians' usual bedside screening examinations. In fact, patients with profound defects in frontal function may perform within normal limits on even more sensitive cognitive tests, such as the Wechsler Adult Intelligence Scale—Revised (WAIS-R). While cognitive problems can be found in most, but not all, patients with frontal lobe dysfunction, specialized tests usually are needed.

A central cognitive role of the nonmotor parts of the frontal lobes (the prefrontal region) is self-regulation and planning—the executive functions of cognition (Milner and Petrides 1984). The principal role of the prefrontal region in memory function is that of encoding and decoding, rather than of storage. Thus, if cognitive tests focus only on the simpler components of cognition, such as simple calculation, naming, or multiple choice memory, they are unlikely to detect frontal dysfunction. Tests that challenge the patient to "put it together" through problem solving, abstract reasoning, processing conflicting stimuli, or recalling details in the face of distraction are more likely to detect deficits. Specific tests will be detailed below. Regardless of the tests chosen, however, patients with frontal lobe dysfunction will tend to perform better on highly structured tests than on tests that require patients to supply their own structure. They also will do better in formal testing situations than in the real world. For this reason, incidental observations of patients' behavior in the examination area before and after testing and in the face of any unplanned distractions are highly relevant to the diagnosis.

Demonstration of specific and restricted frontal lobe dysfunction often requires proving that the component parts of a cognitive performance are intact although the entire performance is impaired. Thus, an inference of frontal lobe function from a failure of abstract reasoning requires demonstration of sufficient comprehension, verbal fluency, and general intelligence and education to grasp the task. Only under these circumstances can a concrete or impulsive reply be given localizing significance. Likewise, frontal lobe problems can be suspected when free recall is poor under distracting conditions, yet multiple-choice memory and rote memory without distraction are intact.

Performance on frontal lobe tasks and good judgment in the real world depend not only on patients' neurologic equipment but also on their upbringing, education, and emotional makeup—notions captured in such terms as "character" and "ego strength." Because of these other influences on test performance, isolated failures should not be over-interpreted. The greatest weight can be given to findings of abnormal performance on tests that should be well within the patient's capacity, given his or her general intelligence, education, and upbringing, and that use emotionally neutral stimuli in nonthreatening test circumstances. In adjusting for education, it should be considered that educational attainment well below expectations for the patient's social class and parental educational status may be the result of early frontal lobe dysfunction.

Role of Neurodiagnostic Procedures in Assessing Frontal Lobe Dysfunction

Neurologic examination, brain imaging, physiologic tests of brain function (SPECT, PET, and evoked potential mapping), and neuropsychologic examination have complementary roles in establishing the relevance of frontal lobe deficits to a behavioral syndrome (see Chapters 1 and 5). When all tests are abnormal and point to the same region, the diagnosis of organic psychopathology due to frontal lobe dysfunction is established. Often, however, tests may show a cognitive or functional deficit without a detectable anatomic correlate or may show anatomic abnormality with unimpressive cognitive and functional tests. In these cases, it is necessary to assess and weigh various factors in the patient's case.

In assessing frontal lobe dysfunction, the emphasis has been on detecting and characterizing the neuropsychological impairments from disease of the prefrontal region. Located rostral to the motor strip and premotor cortex, this region of granular cortex is considered the most enigmatic and complex of human associative cortices. Damage to the prefrontal region does not produce primary motor, sensory, or cranial nerve findings, with the exception of olfactory disturbance from disruption of the olfactory tracts, which lie along the mesial-orbital surface. However, since these tracts project to the temporal lobe and thalamus (Eslinger et al. 1982), not all olfactory disturbances are referable to disease of the orbital-frontal region. Temporal or orbital frontal lesions can affect olfaction, but parietal, occipital, or dorsolateral frontal lesions cannot (Jones-Gotman and Zatorre 1988). There are, however, numerous signs on neurological examination that may suggest or support a diagnosis of frontal lobe dysfunction; they are detailed below.

Assessment of "executive control" functions has been the longstanding concern of behavioral neuroscientists; preservation of the functions has been taken to imply the integrity of the prefrontal lobes. Diagnostic behavioral markers of prefrontal lobe damage, however, have been more elusive than tests for the function of more posterior cerebral regions. This is because the prefrontal lobe plays a regulatory role with respect to emotions and a wide variety of cognitive functions, including language, perception, memory, praxis, and intellect. Frontal lobe symptomatology, therefore, may involve cognition, emotions, behavioral patterns, and personality.

Extensive damage to the prefrontal region may at times not affect the laboratory-based measurement of many of these neuropsychological functions or, alternatively, may affect all of them (Damasio 1979; Eslinger and Damasio 1985; Stuss and Benson 1986). The reasons for such diversity historically have not been clear and have been much debated (Nauta 1971; Teuber 1964). One such reason is that the prefrontal region is not a homogeneous unit in either a neuroanatomical or a cognitive sense. There is increasing evidence from both human and nonhuman primate research that there are functional subdivisions within the frontal lobe, specifically including the orbital, mesial, and dorsolateral sectors. Symptoms of prefrontal lobe disease will therefore depend to a large extent on which of these more specialized sectors are affected. Another reason is that the type of disease process interacts with the location of damage (Finger 1978). Such characteristics as lesion momentum, edema, mass effect, and irritative phenomena produce differing symptomatology from similarly located lesions. These and other realities of human frontal lobe disease have yet to be reconciled scientifically since the bulk of extant literature combines patients with different disease processes and different locations of damage within the frontal lobe.

Often, psychometric assessment does not ensure the unequivocal diagnosis of prefrontal lobe damage. For instance, one of the most frequently used standardized functions is the Wisconsin Card Sorting Test (WCST). It assesses cognitive flexibility by asking patients to sort a set of cards according to principles that must be inferred from the examiner's feedback that the patient's sorting is correct or incorrect; the hidden rule for sorting is periodically changed during the test administration. (See Heaton 1985 and Milner 1963 for detailed descriptions of procedures and stimuli.) The test requires patients to sort cards according to an abstract principle they must infer and also to switch their responses to a different sorting principle based on the change in the examiner's feedback. Thus, performance depends on abstraction ability, use of examiner feedback to identify correct response categories, sustained attention to maintain a response set over multiple sorts, and the cognitive flexibility to terminate a response set and switch to a different category. Based on available studies, cutoff scores that optimize identification of patients with focal frontal lobe damage are at best about 71% accurate (Heaton 1985). Patients with diffuse cerebral damage and with damage to other cerebral regions can also perform very poorly on the WCST, presumably because of impairments related to various specific requirements of the task, such as sustained attention and visual perceptual discrimination. The discriminating power of the WCST for frontal lobe damage is thus greatest when other brain areas are provably intact.

A battery of several tests is necessary to examine the full range of prefrontal lobe functions (Bornstein 1986; Goodglass and Kaplan 1979; Lezak 1985). In addition to the WCST, they include

1. *Verbal associative fluency measures.* For example, patients are asked to generate words beginning with a certain letter of the alphabet within a specific time limit (Benton 1968). These measures lend themselves very easily to bedside and office evaluation. They may be differentially sensitive to dominant hemisphere frontal dysfunction. Both dorsal and mesial lesions may be associated with impaired fluency. Patients with secondary frontal lobe dysfunction due to basal ganglia disease may also have impaired fluency.

   More elaborate tests of complex linguistic abilities have also been employed to show that patients with frontal lobe damage have impaired verbal abilities (e.g., in composing coherent arguments or in analyzing complex grammatical structures). This is despite conservation of basic language skills, such as naming, to confrontation or comprehension of simple sentences (Novoa and Ardila 1987).

2. *Tests of alternating sequences.* These are also frequently used bedside evaluation techniques and, as described by Strub and Black (1985), they can include visual pattern completion, hand movement patterns, and reciprocal coordination. In addition, neuropsychological evaluation may include the Trailmaking Test (Reitan 1958) and delayed alternation.

3. *Tests of self-regulation.* These may include "go–no go" tasks and conflicting stimuli, such as the Stroop Test, which requires the patient to call out the color in which words are printed, with each word being the name of a different color. Patients with diffuse frontal damage or dorsal involvement may not "get" the task; those with relatively isolated orbital frontal dysfunction may "get" the task but be unable to inhibit inappropriate responses.

4. *Tests of memory.* Memory tests that evaluate free recall after a delay can detect memory problems due to frontal lobe dysfunction (Jetter et al. 1986). Impairment in free recall

after delay or distraction disproportionate to impairment on cued memory or immediate recall suggests frontal dysfunction. Memory disturbance can occur with either posterior ventromedial or dorsal frontal damage (Eslinger and Grattan 1989). Patients with inferior frontal damage make relatively more errors of commission on recall tasks. When required to first organize the information for later recall, patients with frontal damage may show very poor performance (della Rochetta 1986; Freedman and Cermak 1986).

Additional evidence for frontal lobe dysfunction can be provided when memory tests show excessive disruption from interfering stimuli, either external or internally produced by anxiety (Malmo and Amsel 1948; Stuss et al. 1982). Also, specialized memory testing will demonstrate in some frontal lobe patients an inability to judge the temporal ordering of information (Milner 1982). Clinically, the latter phenomenon can be observed in medical histories elicited from patients with frontal lobe damage, which on occasion show striking jumps back and forth in time.

5. *Tests of abstract reasoning.* The ability to observe similarities and differences or to group items in categories is dependent on intact frontal lobe function. This ability is tested formally by such measures as the Category Test (Crockett et al. 1986) and the test of Verbal Concept Attainment (Bornstein and Leason 1985). Informally, it is tested at the bedside by having the patient say how two things are alike (e.g., chair and table, president and king). Failure on these reasoning tasks not explained by poor education or language difficulties suggests dorsolateral frontal dysfunction.

No one test is adequate to diagnose frontal lobe dysfunction; frontal dysfunction is inferred from a typical pattern of performance that suggests impaired "executive functions." However, certain tests are commonly included in neuropsychologic test batteries to augment sensitivity to frontal defects. These are listed in Table 10-3.

Tests of prefrontal lobe function may be failed for various reasons, not all of which are related to prefrontal lobe damage. It is therefore crucial to evaluate a number of neuropsychological processes, including basic language abilities (i.e., naming, repetition, comprehension, writing, speech), immediate and sustained attention, encoding and retention of new information, visuoconstructional ability, visual perception, and intellectual functions such as verbal abstractions, arithmetic

Table 10-3. Commonly used neuropsychological tests for frontal lobe dysfunction

Test (source)	Description	Time to administer (minutes)	Test strengths and weaknesses
Wisconsin Card Sort (Heaton 1981)	Subject must abstract, maintain, and shift card-sorting principles	15–30	Sensitive to frontal lobe dysfunction Yields multivariate measures Normative values available Failure not specific to frontal lobes
Verbal Associative Fluency (Benton 1968)	Subject must generate words beginning with certain letter within limited response time	5	Sensitive to frontal lobe dysfunction Easy to administer and score Normative values available Failure not specific to frontal lobes
Verbal Concept Attainment (Bornstein and Leason 1985)	Subject chooses one word on each line that has conceptual similarity to words on preceding and following lines	30-minute limit	Sensitive to left frontal lesions Normative values available No special equipment needed Failure not specific to frontal lobes
Stroop Test (Perret 1974)	Conflicting stimuli task in which subjects must suppress the reading of color words to name the color in which the words are printed	5	Sensitive top left frontal lesions Easy to administer and score Normative values available
Category Test (Crockett et al. 1986)	Requires subject to abstract similarities and differences (principles) among stimuli and to formulate hypotheses	45	Sensitive to damage in many areas of the brain Not especially sensitive to frontal lobe dysfunction except when impaired in isolation Requires special equipment

Table 10-4.   Frontal lobe signs on neurological examination

Sign	Comment
Snout reflex	Often present in normal elderly people
Grasp reflex	Difficult to distinguish from spasticity
Suck and root reflexes	Low sensitivity
Abnormal gait	"Magnetic gait" most characteristic
Paratonia	May mimic deliberate oppositional behavior
Olfactory loss	Seen in orbital frontal or medial anterior temporal damage
Voluntary lateral gaze defect	May be seen when frontal eye fields are involved: insensitive and nonspecific
Impaired coordination	Nonspecific

reasoning, vocabulary, and general knowledge. In addition to the highly quantified, psychometric evaluation of behavior in the laboratory, increasing attention is being given to the qualitative aspects of human behavior (Goldberg and Costa 1986). Goldberg and Costa (1986) give excellent examples of how to incorporate into the neuropsychologic assessment a systematic observation of patients' problem-solving style. Thus, they combine actuarial analysis and the potentially rich clinical observation of behavior.

Particularly in the domain of frontal lobe dysfunction, neuropsychological evaluation that is based on test scores alone and does not include qualitative analysis of the patient's behavior during the test is not diagnostically adequate (Hagberg 1987; McKay et al. 1985).

Frontal Lobe Signs on Neurologic Examination

Although the fact that the motor strip is in the frontal lobe means that upper motor neuron weakness could be technically regarded as a "frontal" sign, the term is generally reserved for signs of dysfunction of premotor areas—those anterior to the motor strip (see Table 10-4). Furthermore, Broca's aphasia, while due to involvement of the motor speech area in the frontal lobe, is again not regarded as a frontal sign. Instead, many neurologists narrowly use the term *frontal sign* to refer to the grasp reflex, snout reflex, suck reflex, and rooting reflex—all primitive behaviors seen in normal infants and thought to be "released" from inhibition when there is substantial dysfunction of the premotor areas.

Frontal release signs, however, are neither sensitive nor specific.

Normal elderly people show a high prevalence of snout reflexes (Jacobs and Glassman 1980). Grasp reflexes, when bilateral, may be a manifestation of bilateral spasticity of any cause, and while an elaborate grasping behavioral pattern can theoretically be distinguished from simple grasping due to hyperactive finger flexor reflexes, the distinction is not always easy in practice. Transient grasp reflexes have been reported in schizophrenic patients without neuropsychologic evidence of frontal dysfunction (Lohr 1985). The suck and root reflexes, while definitely pathologic, are rarely seen in the absence of profound brain dysfunction that would be evident otherwise (Jenkyn et al. 1977).

There are, however, other neurological signs that suggest frontal lobe dysfunction. Abnormal gait can be produced by bilateral premotor dysfunction or damage; this is seen most typically in hydrocephalus, where enlarged ventricles compromise frontal lobe efferents. The typical gait has been variously described as a gait apraxia, with difficulty placing the feet, or as a "magnetic" gait, with feet grasping the floor and not letting go. Characteristically, the patient can perform leg movements while lying supine that he or she cannot do standing with feet "glued" to the floor (Damasio 1979). Of course, lateralized frontal dysfunction, if it affects the motor strip, will present with a hemiparetic gait. Less specific gait disorders will require a complete neurological evaluation to distinguish sensory, vestibular, cerebellar, extrapyramidal, and frontal lobe contributions to the gait impairment.

Muscle tone may also be abnormal in patients with prefrontal damage, particularly when the damage is in the dorsal lateral frontal lobes, relatively close to the motor strip. The characteristic sign is paratonia. This refers to apparently deliberate opposition to the examiner's efforts to move a limb passively. The patient may or may not be aware of the paratonia but in either case will be unable to suppress the oppositional tendency (Damasio 1979).

On cranial nerve examination, impairment of olfactory function may be due to damage to the orbital frontal region; this is often seen in cases of closed head trauma in which the olfactory bulbs or tracts are damaged by the same trauma that contuses the orbital frontal region. Degenerative diseases such as Alzheimer's disease that involve the frontal lobe or white matter diseases such as multiple sclerosis also can affect either olfactory acuity or the ability to recognize scents accurately. A formal smell identification test is the most reliable way to demonstrate these defects. Pocket "scratch-and-sniff" cards can be used for screening (Doty 1983). Defects in voluntary lateral gaze in the absence of otherwise compromised eye movements can suggest dysfunction of one or both of the frontal eye fields, which are located in the premotor area contralateral to the direction of gaze that is weak (Cogan 1956).

Testing of coordination may reveal defects in fine finger movements or motor sequences in the hand contralateral to the damage. These problems can be brought out by having the patient tap fingers repeatedly in order from index to little finger, or by having the patient alternately tap the fist, the palm, and the edge of the hand on the table (Luria 1980). Impaired coordination in the absence of sensory loss, weakness, cerebellar signs, or extrapyramidal signs—tremor, rigidity, or involuntary movements—is particularly suggestive of frontal dysfunction.

The sensory examination is normal in pure frontal lobe disease. However, there may be some neglect of simultaneous stimulation on the side contralateral to a frontal lobe lesion, particularly when the lesion is on the nondominant side.

FRONTAL LOBE DYSFUNCTION AND PSYCHIATRIC DISORDERS

Relation of Frontal Lobe Dysfunction to Major Psychopathology

Recent literature relates frontal lobe dysfunction to major psychopathology in five general ways.

First, frontal lobe damage may mimic primary psychiatric disorders. For example, a patient with frontal polar or orbital frontal damage may show a personality disorder with antisocial features (pseudopsychopathy). Or patients with apathy due to prefrontal lesions may be mistakenly diagnosed as depressed because their apathy and lack of emotional expression belies the absence of true mood disturbance (Lishman 1987).

Second, frontal lobe dysfunction may be a correlate, either permanent or state dependent, of the major mood disorders and schizophrenia. Laboratory findings on PET, SPECT, and brain electrical activity mapping (BEAM) support the presence of frontal lobe dysfunction in at least some cases of these disorders, in association with neuropsychologic evidence of impaired performance on tests sensitive to frontal lobe dysfunction. Further, ventricular enlargement or cerebral atrophy, sometimes frontally predominant, can be encountered in these disorders (Nasrallah et al. 1989; Shelton et al. 1988).

Third, frontal dysfunction may be a modifying or subtyping feature of psychopathology. For example, among patients with mood disorders, those with ventricular enlargement have a worse prognosis and are more likely to display psychotic features (Nasrallah et al. 1989). Among patients with schizophrenia, cerebral atrophy and ventricular enlargement have been associated with greater cognitive impairment, more negative symptoms, a poor social prognosis, and a less satisfactory response to neuroleptics (Shelton et al. 1988; Smith et al. 1983).

Fourth, frontal lobe damage may be related to the subsequent development of a psychiatric syndrome. For example, strokes in the left frontal lobe are highly likely to produce a syndrome of major depression, and the association is strongest for lesions close to the left frontal pole (Starkstein et al. 1988). Right frontal lesions, on the other hand, have been shown occasionally to produce secondary mania (Robinson et al. 1984, 1988).

Finally, psychopathology not directly related to frontal lobe dysfunction may influence the behavioral manifestation of a comorbid frontal lobe disorder. Greater psychological arousal due to anxiety, hypomania, drug withdrawal, or akathisia may aggravate impulsive behavior in an individual with preexisting frontal lobe damage. Such effects can be of great clinical importance in patients with fixed frontal damage due to prior head injury. Further, psychodynamic issues may influence the type of behavior—for example, sexual versus aggressive—that emerges when a frontal lesion diminishes impulse control.

Frontal Lobe Dysfunction and Attention-Deficit Hyperactivity Disorder

Patients with ADHD may display some behavioral features, such as distractibility, impersistence, and impulsiveness, that also are encountered in patients with structural frontal lobe damage (Chelune et al. 1986). However, not all ADHD patients have a primary frontal lobe dysfunction, let alone damage. The pathophysiology of ADHD is not known, but extrafrontal problems such as primary noradrenergic dysfunction have been proposed (Zametkin and Rapoport 1987).

Nonetheless, clinical experience suggests that a proportion of patients with a clinical syndrome of ADHD have frontal lobe dysfunction, suggested by motor "soft signs" and by neuropsychologic findings showing impairment on frontal tests not requiring sustained attention.

An example of the latter would be a similarities task, in which each individual response could be completed within a few seconds. Difficulty with abstract reasoning on such a task would be hard to attribute to attentional problems in themselves. When such frontal signs are encountered, they suggest that primary dysfunction of the frontal lobes may contribute to the syndrome of ADHD. Stimulants, which ameliorate the symptoms of ADHD, may act via enhancement of frontal lobe function (Evans et al. 1986).

Further, patients with ADHD have an increased risk of injury, including head injury. The head-injured patient with premorbid ADHD would be particularly vulnerable to overt behavioral expression of any frontal lobe damage acquired from the head injury. Treatment of the ADHD might mitigate the behavioral effects of the acquired frontal injury.

Frontal Lobe Dysfunction and Alcoholism

Alcoholic intoxication impairs all cognitive functions, frontal lobe functions included. In patients with relative deficiencies of executive functions, such as individuals with prior structural frontal lobe damage, alcohol may further impair the frontal lobe functions of self-regulation and planning.

Chronic alcoholism is associated with a more long-lasting frontal lobe dysfunction that persists during periods of sobriety (Gorenstein 1987; Tarter and Edwards 1985). The specific mechanism of alcohol-associated cognitive impairment may not be the same in every patient because many alcoholic patients have either confounding influences of head trauma or congenital cognitive problems that predate alcohol use. Nonetheless, the literature on alcoholic cognitive impairment does suggest a direct toxic effect of alcohol on brain functions, with particular effect on memory. The alcoholic memory deficit, best brought out under conditions of delay and distraction and often greatly remedied by cues and context, is typical of the memory dysfunction encountered in patients with frontal lobe damage.

Patients with frontal lobe dysfunction certainly should be counseled to avoid alcohol, and patients' persistence in drinking regularly despite this advice can be regarded as presumptive evidence of a drinking problem. Frontal lobe dysfunction related to alcohol exposure, when it is reversible with sobriety, tends to recover rapidly but not necessarily completely during the first few weeks of abstinence (Tarter and

Table 10-5. Treatment of patients with frontal lobe dysfunction and abnormal behavior

---

- **Neurologic treatment of etiologic and aggravating factors**

- **Specific pharmacological therapy**
  Dopamine agonists for apathy, mutism, and akinesia
  Stimulants for hyperactivity and distractibility
  Carbamazepine for impulsiveness, irritability, and affective lability

- **Environmental modification**
  Family intervention for patients living in families
  Liaison interventions for patients in institutions

- **Cognitive strategies**
  Cuing for apathy or poorly organized behavior
  Self-monitoring practice for impulsive or socially inappropriate behavior
  Psychotherapy for empathic deficits, especially for right frontal deficits

- **Psychiatric treatment of comorbid psychopathology**

Edwards 1985). Deficits not ameliorated after a year of abstinence are likely to persist.

TREATMENT CONSIDERATIONS

General Approach to Treatment

Despite the neural and cognitive complexity of frontal lobe syndromes, there are specific aspects that can be targeted for treatment. Options include drug therapy for the patient and psychological and behavioral interventions for patients and their families. While a few studies have examined one or another of these options in a select few frontally damaged patients (Albert et al. 1987; Ross and Stewart 1987; Sohlberg et al. 1988), rarely have combined approaches been systematically studied in patients with carefully localized frontal lobe lesions and thoroughly described neuropsychological findings.

The treatment of the patient with frontal lobe dysfunction and abnormal behavior has five major components (Table 10-5): 1) treatment of biologic factors causing or aggravating the frontal lobe dysfunction itself; 2) amelioration of frontal dysfunction by biochemical manipulation of neuromodulatory inputs to the frontal lobes; 3) environmental modification, including vocational rehabilitation and family intervention; 4) employment of cognitive and behavioral strategies to enable the patient to exploit preserved brain functions; and 5) treatment of comorbid psychopathology that aggravates either the frontal dysfunction or its behavioral expression. The first of these is the subject matter of neurology; the next three are addressed elsewhere in this chapter. The fifth component, treatment of comorbid psychopathology, is often overlooked, so it is illustrated with the example of left frontal stroke.

Patients with left frontal strokes are particularly likely to develop major depression afterward (Starkstein et al. 1988). This major depression, assuming it is physiologically like a primary major depression, may further compromise frontal lobe blood flow and metabolism (O'Connell et al. 1989) and aggravate the frontal lobe deficits. Even if this does not occur, focal cognitive impairment can be aggravated by depression and alleviated by its treatment (Fogel and Sparadeo 1985). Treatment of the comorbid depression may improve the frontal dysfunction to the point where it is not causing impairment in everyday living, even though it may still be detectable on neuropsychologic examination. Stroke patients might be receiving antihypertensive drugs or anticonvulsants that cause organic mood disorders with depressive features (Pascualy and Veith 1989); changing these drugs might improve cognitive function as well as mood.

Because treatment of comorbid psychopathology, particularly depression and anxiety, can have a powerful effect on both behavior and neuropsychological test performance, assessment of disturbed mood deserves priority in all cases of frontal lobe disorder. This effect, however, complicates the reading of the literature on drug treatment of organic mental syndromes. If a particular agent, such as imipramine or buspirone, appears to benefit a patient with frontal lobe damage, it may be difficult to distinguish between effects mediated by an improvement in mood and those due to a direct biochemical effect of the agent. In discussing specific pharmacologic therapies for frontal lobe dysfunction, we focus on treatments directed at frontal lobe dysfunction itself rather than at associated mood disorder. In practice, however, assessment and treatment of disturbed mood may be the most positive contribution a psychiatrist can make to the treatment of patients with frontal lobe damage.

Neurotransmitters and Frontal Lobe Function

In approaching pharmacologic strategies for enhancing frontal lobe function, it is relevant to note that most neurotransmitters in the cerebral cortex are equally distributed about the brain. Some neurotransmitters, particularly dopamine and Met-enkephalin, have their cortical localization primarily in the frontal lobes and limbic areas (Parnavelas and McDonald 1983). Manipulation of these transmitters might be expected to have differential effects on frontal lobe function. Reported benefits of dopamine agonists and adverse effects of dopamine antagonists on frontal functions are discussed below. However, several considerations should be borne in mind when drawing inferences from neurotransmitter localization to drug choice:

1. Acute and delayed effects of drugs can be substantially different.
2. Drugs not having primary effects on the frontal lobes may have important secondary, transsynaptic effects.
3. The frontal lobes may be differentially sensitive to a particular agent even though it acts throughout the cortex.
4. Different frontal regions may be differentially sensitive to a drug's effects.
5. The benefit of a drug in the case of a gross anatomic lesion depends on the residual capacity of the undamaged brain. This capacity may vary according to premorbid endowment, the nature of incomplete damage near the boundary of the lesion, and the individual's degree of cortical specialization, which, with handedness, varies among individuals.

Combining Treatment Components

In combining the components of therapy, two central themes are setting priorities and monitoring for negative interactions. When setting priorities, simple and inexpensive interventions generally are preferred, as are those whose effectiveness is supported by controlled clinical trials. A paradigmatic high-priority intervention is the substitution of carbamazepine for phenobarbital in patients with epilepsy, frontal lobe dysfunction, and problems with impulsive behavior. Brief therapeutic trials often are helpful in deciding whether to include a particular treatment modality. A patient with frontal lobe disease and disturbed memory who showed substantial improvement with cuing in a laboratory setting would be more likely to benefit from formal memory training than a patient who showed no benefit from cues. Thus, neuropsychologic consultation can be focused on identifying and testing potential rehabilitative strategies.

Monitoring for negative interactions is particularly important for pharmacologic interventions. Potential interactions involving neuroleptics, stimulants, dopamine agonists, and benzodiazepines will be considered.

Neuroleptics may reduce impulsive behavior due to orbital frontal dysfunction by reducing arousal, by reducing anxiety, by diminishing paranoid thinking and psychotic symptoms, or perhaps by a direct effect on dopaminergic modulation of orbital frontal function. However, neuroleptics may impair spontaneity and planning, functions of the frontal convexity, especially if these agents produce akinesia (Rifkin et al. 1975). Further, if neuroleptics cause akathisia, the resulting restlessness may aggravate impulsivity (Herrera et al. 1988). Impairment on neuropsychological tests of frontal function has also been associated with neuroleptic treatment of schizophrenia (Medalia et al. 1988).

Stimulants can enhance some brain functions, such as memory and higher cognitive tasks, both in normal (Rapoport et al. 1978, 1980) and in brain-damaged individuals, perhaps by directly affecting dopaminergic and noradrenergic tone, by bringing about an optimum level of arousal, or in some cases by relieving a depressed mood that interferes with cognition. However, an excessive dose could lead to hyperarousal that would aggravate impulsivity or more quietly disrupt information processing. In this regard, it has been observed that the optimal dose of stimulants in the treatment of hyperactive boys might be different depending on whether cognitive performance or behavioral conformity is the end point (Sprague and Sleator 1977). Further, if paranoid ideation were induced by stimulants, it could lead to inappropriate behavior.

Dopamine agonists, like stimulants, may enhance cognition directly but may also induce or aggravate symptoms of mood disorder or thought disorder (Addonizio 1989), as in the well-known example of levodopa-induced psychosis in parkinsonian patients. In excessive doses or in vulnerable patients, dopamine agonists may produce delirium. Thus, the dose-response curve with cognition as an end point is curvilinear; the shape and location of the curve are not known in general.

Benzodiazepines may reduce impulsive behavior due to hyperarousal and may improve cognition if it is disrupted by severe anxiety. However, benzodiazepines may directly produce disinhibition (Klein et al. 1980) and can impair memory (Curran 1986). The ideal dose of benzodiazepine for a particular patient will depend on the relative importance of anxiety versus other factors in the behavioral expression of brain dysfunction. Because nonbenzodiazepine anxiolytics such as buspirone are now available, particular caution in the use of benzodiazepine in brain-damaged patients is indicated.

Strategy for Monitoring

A high potential for negative interactions in pharmacological treatment is best dealt with by continual and simultaneous monitoring of psychopathology, cognition, and everyday function (instrumental activities of daily living). Such monitoring helps detect when improvement in one area of function has been obtained at the cost of deterioration in another. Specific tests for monitoring frontal lobe cognitive function are detailed elsewhere in this chapter. Appropriate measures for everyday function are those most directly relevant to the patient's actual life and level of independence. These might include qualitative or semiquantitative ratings of the patient's ability to handle money, to shop independently, to be well-groomed, and to use public transportation, among others. For patients at the higher reaches of function, work performance may be the appropriate measure.

Specific Pharmacological Approaches

While there are abundant studies of various agents for syndromes such as agitation, dementia, self-injurious behavior, and severe mental retardation, few studies specifically focus on the consequences of well-defined frontal lesions. An important recent exception is research on dopamine agonists for akinetic mutism associated with organic frontal dysfunction. In one study, Echiverri et al. (1988) reported four children who exhibited akinetic mutism after the course of various neurological diseases. The children were treated with bromocriptine, and the akinetic mute states were reversed in all cases. Catsman-Berrevoets and von Harskamp (1988) reported a 38-year-old woman with bilateral thalamic infarctions with severe apathy whose apathy improved with bromocriptine. (In this case, thalamic inputs to the frontal lobe were disrupted.) Albert et al. (1987) reported improvement in transcortical motor aphasia with bromocriptine; this particular form of aphasia is due to damage to the dominant supplementary motor area or its connections (located in the superior mesial frontal cortex or deep to it). Finally, Crimson et al. (1988) reported three cases of akinetic muteness after severe closed head injury that improved with bromocriptine therapy. In two cases there was bilateral cerebral damage visualized in computed tomography (CT) scans; in the third the injury was believed to be confined largely to the brain stem. Taken together, these studies suggest that at least some states of apathy, mutism, or decreased behavior due to frontal dysfunction might respond to dopamine agonists.

These observations are complemented by studies of neuropsychologic tests of frontal function in patients with Parkinson's disease. In one such study, Gotham et al. (1988) tested frontal functions in patients on and off levodopa. Off levodopa, the Parkinson's disease patients had impaired verbal fluency compared with controls; the difference disappeared when levodopa was given. By contrast, performance on another "frontal" test, the WCST, was impaired in patients both on and off levodopa. The findings suggest that dopamine agonist treatment strategies may work selectively with some forms of frontal dysfunction, perhaps those more related to mesial structures.

Selegiline (deprenyl), a selective monoamine oxidase inhibitor (MAOI) that enhances dopaminergic transmission, might also be expected to improve some frontal lobe cognitive functions. In a trial of 10 mg of selegiline daily in 17 patients with dementia of the Alzheimer type, Tariot et al. (1987) found improvement on a memory and learning task requiring complex information processing and sustained effort. Knowledge memory and other cognitive functions were not altered by selegiline. The improved capacity for sustained effort and information processing might be linked to an enhancement of frontal lobe function by selegiline.

While dopamine agonist treatment has focused on improving attention and reducing apathy, carbamazepine treatment has been directed against symptoms of impulsiveness and affective lability often associated with orbital frontal damage. Two small case series have reported beneficial effects on behavior of patients with known frontal lesions (McAllister 1985; McQuistion et al. 1987). In the first series, McAllister specifically pointed out the existence of concurrent primary psychiatric disorders in his patients.

Propranolol and other beta-blockers have been used extensively to treat violence, aggression, and agitated behavior in brain-injured patients, many of whom have frontal lobe damage (Elliott 1977; Williams et al. 1982; Yudofsky et al. 1981; Yudofsky et al. 1987). They also have been used to treat aggressive behavior in patients with chronic schizophrenia (Sorgi et al. 1986); many of the cases reported are likely to have involved frontal lobe dysfunction. However, we have not found in the literature an analysis of response to beta-blockers based on a careful characterization of regional brain dysfunction, and it is not clear whether beta-blockers alleviate aggression by a general reduction of arousal, by specific effects on the frontal lobe, or by other mechanisms. For example, the high affinity of propranolol for frontal cortical serotonin receptors (Peroutka 1988) could prove relevant to its effects on aggressive behavior, in view of recent associations of altered serotonergic function with suicide, a form of self-directed aggression.

Pharmacology of Stimulants for Attention-Deficit Hyperactivity Disorder

Because there is some overlap between the symptoms of idiopathic ADHD and the attentional disturbances encountered in individuals with demonstrable frontal lobe damage or function, frontal lobe patients with marked attentional disturbances, hyperactivity, and/or distractibility might warrant therapeutic trials of stimulant drugs. The stimulants commonly used to treat ADHD include dextroamphetamine, methylphenidate, pemoline, and the MAOI tranylcypromine. While these drugs share a common action on dopaminergic systems, there are significant differences among them, and patients may respond better to one than to the others. A brief summary is offered here; the reader can consult recent reviews for details (Donnelly 1989; Klein 1987; Wender et al. 1981). In general, adults with ADHD are less likely to respond well to stimulants than are children (Mattes et al. 1984).

Dextroamphetamine (Dexedrine) was the first drug shown to be effective for ADHD. Usual doses in adults range from 5 mg twice a day to 20 mg three times a day. Once-a-day dosing is not feasible because of the relatively short half-life of the drug. With higher doses, and particularly with doses above 60 mg/day, there is an increasing risk of paranoid symptomatology and, at worst, the development of a schizophreniform psychosis. Even in patients who respond well initially, tachyphylaxis may occur, requiring tapering off and discontinuation of the drug, and reinstitution at a lower dose after a washout period of 2 weeks or more. The drug is a Schedule II agent, requiring triplicate prescriptions without refills.

Methylphenidate (Ritalin) is similar to dextroamphetamine in its actions; however, it has somewhat less effect on noradrenergic symptoms and may be less likely to cause paranoid or psychotic phenomena. Like dextroamphetamine, it needs to be given at least two or more times per day, and its dosage range is similar; it is less potent than dextroamphetamine, however, and patients who respond to both drugs may require a somewhat higher dose of methylphenidate. It also can cause tachyphylaxis, which must be handled similarly. It is also a Schedule II drug. Compared with dextroamphetamine, it has a shorter half-life (6–12 hours versus 2–3 hours, with much variability).

Pemoline (Cylert) is less potent than either dextroamphetamine or methylphenidate, but it has a long half-life and may be given once a day. It is listed on Schedule V, so triplicate prescriptions are not required and refills can be given. The dosage in adults ranges from 37.5

mg/day to 150 mg/day. While its pharmacologic features make it a more convenient drug to prescribe, it may be less effective than dextroamphetamine, and a trial of pemoline cannot be regarded as a definitive stimulant trial.

Tranylcypromine (Parnate), an MAOI antidepressant, is also an effective agent for ADHD (Zametkin et al. 1985). Like other nonselective MAOIs, it has effects on other neurotransmitter systems, including norepinephrine and serotonin. It also requires a tyramine-restricted diet and interacts with numerous other drugs. Tranylcypromine usually must be given two or more times per day because postdose orthostatic hypotension occurs if a full day's dose is given at once. Adult doses range from 30 to 60 mg/day, with some patients needing as much as 90 mg/day, although this higher dose is outside the manufacturer's published recommendations. In adult neuropsychiatric practice, we have found tranylcypromine to be particularly useful in patients who have depressive or obsessional symptoms in addition to their disturbance of attention.

Stimulant trials can be discontinued if there is no benefit after 2 weeks for dextroamphetamine or methylphenidate, or after 5 weeks for pemoline (Donnelly 1989).

Cognitive Retraining

A number of rehabilitation specialists offer various kinds of "cognitive retraining" for patients with recent acute frontal lobe injury, particularly younger people with frontal lobe injury from head trauma. Advocates of cognitive retraining believe that frequent practice, often computer assisted, can stimulate functional recovery of undamaged brain tissue. While this is an attractive hypothesis and one in keeping with animal findings that stimulation may improve functional recovery after early brain damage, evidence is lacking for a decisive impact of cognitive retraining on eventual functional outcome. In this respect, cognitive retraining and other specialized occupational therapy programs have the same status as speech therapy for aphasia—they are attractive therapeutic offerings that look hopeful and are often appreciated by patients and families demoralized by brain damage. Cognitive rehabilitation specialists, like speech therapists, can usually point to individuals who appear to do very well with the intervention. However, the specificity of effect remains to be seen. In our opinion, limited resources should be focused first on neurological stabilization and the optimum management of definite psychiatric complications and comorbidities. If resources are abundant, the added stimulation of cognitive retraining programs may be helpful and is unlikely to do harm. If cognitive retraining is undertaken, a time-limited trial with objective outcome measures may help the clinician and family evaluate its usefulness for a specific patient.

Psychological Approaches

Behavior therapy with an external cuing system. Since a portion of the executive control deficit of frontal lobe patients is thought to be the patients' inability to cue themselves and thus modify their behavior, an external cuing system might successfully serve as a mental prosthesis. Sohlberg et al. (1988) recently described such an approach. The subject was a 38-year-old man who had suffered a severe closed head injury 13 months before the experiment. CT revealed evidence of multifocal cerebral injury affecting predominantly the frontal lobes but also the right thalamus and right anterior horn areas. Clinically, the patient was apathetic, aspontaneous, and unmotivated, with a very restricted range of affect and interpersonal behavior. In an attempt to increase the patient's verbal initiation in group therapy sessions, the patient was trained to ask himself, "Am I initiating conversation?" whenever he was handed a card with a geometric figure on it. The card was introduced on a variable interval schedule, within a range of 3–10 minutes. This procedure produced a fivefold increase in his initiation of conversations that apparently fit in with the group conversation. Improvement also was observed when a similar procedure was applied to other behaviors, including making eye contact with the speaker, smiling in a manner appropriate to what another person was saying, and orienting physically toward the speaker.

The report by Sohlberg et al. (1988) raises a number of important issues, such as response maintenance, application to other subjects with frontal lobe damage, and generalizability of behavior to situations outside the training sessions; these remain to be investigated. A particularly interesting question is the potential benefit of combining pharmacotherapy with external cuing, targeting aspontaneity, apathy, and impulsivity. For example, dopamine agonists may improve responsiveness and initiation after mesial frontal damage, but it is not known whether they do so in an overlapping or complementary fashion to behavioral modification procedures. There is, however, a single case report that lithium added nothing to the therapeutic benefits of behavior therapy for inappropriate touching and verbalizations in a patient with frontal lobe damage (Whaley et al. 1986). A summary of treatments for frontal lobe syndromes and links to regions of involvement is presented in Table 10-6.

Psychotherapeutic possibilities. A second major form of psychological intervention after brain injury is individual psychotherapy. Carberry and Burd (1986) addressed this in an interesting way by focusing on neuropsychological impairments that may affect the outcome of psychotherapy. These impairments include several that are highly relevant to frontal lobe syndromes, such as verbal disinhibition, cognitive rigidity, disturbed learning and retention, and decreased empathy and concreteness in thinking. Their suggestions, yet to be subjected to scientific scrutiny, are to deal with these impairments in a straightforward manner, such as interrupting the patient's rambling responses and attempting to refocus the patient; listing alternative views and choices; specifically questioning what the feelings of others are or would be; and communicating literally and precisely rather than abstractly.

There are a number of concepts emerging from neuropsychological research that are potentially important as well. For instance, in recent laboratory research, one of the authors and his colleagues have discovered that changes in empathy after frontal lobe damage can occur as relatively isolated findings, particularly after damage to the orbital frontal region. Empathic changes associated with poor cognitive flexibility may occur after damage to the dorsolateral frontal lobe (Grattan and Eslinger 1989). A loss of empathy following dorsolateral frontal damage may be secondary to cognitive inability to perceive, imagine, or anticipate another person's feelings or state of mind. This inability has implications both in the treatment setting as well as in the better-known "real world" interpersonal situations. As cognitive abilities improve, then, so may empathic behavior. Loss of empathy due to orbital frontal damage does not have a known cognitive correlate and may have an entirely different basis, such as disturbed autonomic function or disconnection of cognitive and autonomic processes.

Changes in empathy after frontal lobe damage may differ depending on lesion laterality (Grattan and Eslinger 1989). Patients with left frontal lobe damage are acutely aware of their empathic change, so flooding them with reminders may be counterproductive. Patients with right frontal lobe damage will often deny changes and may profit from repeated cues and feedback. Finally, time since injury also will influence psychological intervention (Statham et al. 1989). We have observed that many frontally damaged patients (except, of course, those with akinesia and mutism) in the first month after injury are often eager to

Table 10-6. Syndromes and management options for damage to different frontal lobe regions

Region of damage	Associated behavioral and cognitive impairments	Treatment considerations
Superior mesial	Apathy, "pseudodepression," disturbance of initiation, bradykinesia, aspontaneity, decreased speech, performance deficits, superficial cognitive processing, go–no go deficit, decreased attention	Dopamine agonists Therapy to increase stimulation and reactivity: physical, speech, occupational Cuing to action
Dorsal lateral	Significant cognitive impairments that may include decreased intellect, poor memory, apraxia, aphasia, disturbed attention, hemispatial neglect, extinction, poor judgment, impulsivity, lack of planning, decreased empathy, cognitive and emotional rigidity, affective disturbances, irritability	Mood stabilizers Environmental structuring Concrete behavioral therapies Simplified consistent routines
Orbital	"Pseudopsychopathic": impulsiveness, poor planning Disturbed motivation; poor follow-through Emotional lability, lack of empathy, possibly with decreased autonomic responses Primary social deficits: may be entirely normal in IQ, memory, perception, praxis	Mood stabilizers Environmental structuring Behavior therapies
Posterior ventromedial	Prominent memory disturbance Confabulation; emotional lability	Cuing to improve memory Reality orientation Mood stabilizers

discuss their behavior. Once they are at home, confronting the manifold consequences of their interpersonal and cognitive deficits, their willingness to discuss and address emotional changes may be lost. Ironically, this is more likely to be the time when the family initiates contact with a mental health professional.

Involvement of the Family in Treatment

A striking feature of isolated frontal lobe dysfunction is that patients may appear to be cognitively intact to casual observers, yet have impulsiveness, markedly poor judgment, and a lack of both foresight and insight. This can be puzzling or exasperating for families, who cannot understand why their apparently bright relative cannot behave better, take advice, or even learn from experience. At worst, families respond with anger or with misdirected advice that is of no help to the patient.

The demonstration of frontal lobe dysfunction and its explanation to the family by the psychiatrist and/or neuropsychologist can be remarkably helpful in reframing the situation for all concerned. Once the neurological basis for the patient's behavior is demonstrated, there tends to be less blaming and a fresh approach to problem solving can be taken. Furthermore, more realistic expectations can be set, and behavioral strategies can sometimes be adopted that could be perceived as condescending were the nature of the neurological problem not appreciated by both the patient and the family. Groups for family caregivers may be relevant for some categories of patients with frontal lobe disorders, such as those with dementia (Schmidt and Keyes 1985) or closed head injury.

When family therapy is to be undertaken by a therapist not involved in the neuropsychiatric or neuropsychological workup, it is essential that the therapist understand the neurological dimensions of the case. Without this understanding, erroneous attributions of causality can easily be made, with attendant guilt or blame.

Liaison Issues in Patients With Frontal Lobe Dysfunction

Problems encountered by family members who erroneously attribute the behavior of patients with frontal lobe damage can also be encountered by professional caretakers. When such patients are seen in hospital or nursing home settings, their impulsive, thoughtless, or self-defeating behavior may evoke angry or punitive reactions from staff. If the patient with frontal lobe dysfunction tends to perseverate, repeating the same questions or complaints over and over, staff may become irritated and either avoid the patient or respond harshly.

Primary-care physicians without neurologic or psychiatric experience may at times fail to recognize frontal lobe syndromes and may attribute the pathological behavior of patients with frontal lobe damage to a disturbance of personality or even to deliberate intentions to provoke. Positive outcomes are facilitated by liaison interventions that educate institutional staff, and primary-care physicians if necessary, regarding the manifestations of frontal lobe syndromes and the extent to which the patient's behavior is due to organic causes not under the patient's control. The demonstration of specific neurological signs or cognitive deficits is particularly helpful in establishing the organic dimension of the case. Curiously, patients seen as having behavioral disturbance on an organic basis are often treated with greater sympathy and patience than those exhibiting the same behavior without demonstrable organic cause. While this attitude is perhaps regrettable, it certainly should be exploited by liaison psychiatrists working with brain-damaged patients.

AGITATION, VIOLENCE, AND FRONTAL LOBE DISORDERS

Many of the neurological and psychiatric disorders that may give rise to violent or agitated behavior share frontal lobe dysfunction as a common feature. However, large classes of patients with frontal lobe dysfunction—for example, those with frontal lobotomies—are not particularly prone to agitation or violence (Stuss and Benson 1986), and certainly there are numerous violent patients who are intact on all known measures of frontal lobe function. When patients with frontal lobe dysfunction do become violent, there are particular features that suggest an organic basis for the violent behavior. The first is a tendency for the violence to be impulsive rather than planned. Violence carried out in fulfillment of a manipulative threat should not be blamed on frontal lobe pathology. A second feature that may be seen in violent patients with frontal lobe damage is a failure to grasp the circumstances in which the violent action takes place and to realize that the action is inappropriate. For example, a patient with severe frontal lobe damage might physically assault a caretaker in an institution, unaware that the likely consequence would be the application of restraints or some other negative reinforcement. Finally, patients with frontal lobe dysfunction may be unable to resist an impulse, even when they do appreciate intellectually that there may be bad consequences. The failure to appreciate context usually implies involvement of the frontal convexities (dorsolateral region), whereas the inability to inhibit the impulses despite intellectual appreciation of the context usually implies orbital frontal disorder, with relative sparing of the dorsolateral frontal lobes. Patients with major mesial frontal damage tend to be apathetic and therefore not violent.

In addition to the frontal lobe problems associated with anatomic damage, irritative lesions of the frontal lobes that produce frontal lobe seizures may produce agitated and violent behavior as an ictal or post-ictal manifestation (Boone et al. 1988; Rasmussen 1975; Takeda 1988; Williamson et al. 1985). Although not common, frontal lobe seizures may pose particularly difficult problems in differential diagnosis, both because the behavioral patterns of frontal lobe seizures are often complex and not obviously epileptic and because routine EEG recordings may not necessarily show abnormality (Quesney 1987; Spencer et al. 1985; Williamson et al. 1985).

Often, frontal lobe damage or dysfunction serves as a modifier of agitated and violent behavior rather than as its sole cause. For example, an individual with previously paranoid and irascible personality traits might suffer a head injury, leading to the expression of his or her irritable trait as impulsive violence. A head injury might simultaneously damage frontal and temporal regions, with subsequent partial epilepsy leading to angry or fearful emotion, which is then expressed violently because of a lack of inhibition due to orbital frontal damage.

Interestingly, there is some animal evidence for an interaction between personality and orbital frontal damage in the production of violent behavior. In a 1983 study, deBruin et al. performed bilateral orbital frontal lesions in rats and observed them for changes in intermale aggression. Effects of lesions were seen in the more aggressive WEZOB strain, but not in the less aggressive Wistar strain (deBruin et al. 1983). Further evidence for an interaction between frontal cerebral lesions and other causes of violence is reported by Heinrichs (1989), who developed a multivariate predictive model for the frequency of violent incidents in a group of 45 neuropsychiatric patients. A formula combining the presence of focal frontal lesions, the number of inpatient days, and a history of seizure disorder predicted about one-third of the variance. Thus, frontal damage was a relevant contributing factor but not a sole cause of violence.

Violence in patients with schizophrenia may be viewed similarly. The biological basis of schizophrenia probably comprises both frontal and temporal lobe abnormalities (Weinberger 1988), and it is tempting to speculate that the degree of overt behavioral expression of thought disorder due to temporal lobe damage may be partially a function of the degree of frontal lobe involvement.

Pharmacologic and behavioral therapies directed at agitation and violence usually are not specifically targeted on the frontal lobe, and when they are effective, multiple mechanisms are possible. Thus, when carbamazepine is known to be effective for controlling impulsive violence in a patient with frontal lobe damage, it is not certain whether carbamazepine has worked primarily through a direct effect on the frontal lobe or through changes in the level of emotional arousal by its action on limbic structures. As discussed above, the antiaggressive action of propranolol has not been anatomically localized either. The efficacy of behavioral therapies, as well, cannot easily be linked to action on specific brain regions.

Nonetheless, the choice of therapy for a particular patient with known frontal lobe damage or dysfunction might be guided to some extent by the location and severity of the frontal lobe disorder. A patient with known orbital frontal damage who is unable to inhibit behavior even in situations with clear negative consequences ("the policeman at his elbow") is unlikely to respond to a psychotherapeutic or cognitive strategy alone, and will probably do better with medication aimed at reducing arousal, stabilizing mood, or perhaps enhancing the inhibitory function of undamaged frontal lobe neurons. A patient who shows impaired ability to appreciate context, but who has intact ability to inhibit behavior once context is clear, might benefit from cuing or reminding strategies.

Published reports of drug treatments for agitation and violence in brain-damaged individuals cannot be evaluated in this framework unless the areas of regional brain damage and dysfunction are carefully documented. More specific drug therapies for organically based violence may be possible after a generation of studies on patients who are characterized in detail both anatomically and neuropsychologically.

CONCLUSION

The widespread occurrence of frontal lobe dysfunction in a variety of neuropsychiatric disorders makes the assessment and management of frontal dysfunction a central feature of neuropsychiatric practice. Further, assessment of frontal lobe dysfunction is relevant not only for patients with known brain damage but for virtually all patients with severe psychopathology. Evaluation of frontal lobe function adds a valuable dimension to treatment planning even for patients with primary psychiatric diagnoses. In particular, frontal dysfunction may be important in subtyping patients, selecting therapeutic strategies, and evaluating adverse cognitive side effects of psychotropic drugs.

Patients with dorsolateral lesions and patients with orbital frontal lesions who are not extremely impulsive often benefit from environmental changes and cognitive strategies that impose structure and organization on their daily routine and cognitive tasks. Patients with apathy and difficulty initiating speech and action due to mesial lesions or disruption of dopaminergic inputs may be helped by dopamine agonists. Patients with impulsiveness due to orbital frontal lesions may be helped by contingency management and frequent reminders of the consequences if the dysfunction is not too severe. In more severe cases, a totally controlled environment may be needed. Drugs to decrease arousal or increase inhibition also may be helpful. Patients with hyperactivity and distractibility due to known or putative frontal lobe dysfunction might benefit from stimulants.

REFERENCES

Addonizio G: The patient with Parkinson's disease, in Treatments of Psychiatric Disorders, Vol 2. Edited by the American Psychiatric Association Task Force on Treatments of Psychiatric Disorders. Washington, DC, American Psychiatric Association, 1989, pp 860–866

Albert ML, Bachman D, Morgan A, et al: Pharmacotherapy for aphasia. Neurology 37:175, 1987

Alexander MP, Geschwind N: Dementia in the elderly, in Clinical Neurology of Aging. Edited by Albert ML. New York, Oxford University Press, 1984, pp 254–276

Benton AL: Differential behavioral effects in frontal lobe disease. Neuropsychologia 6:53–60, 1968

Boone KB, Miller BL, Rosenberg L, et al: Neuropsychological and behavioral abnormalities in an adolescent with frontal lobe seizures. Neurology 38:583–586, 1988

Bornstein RA: Contribution of various neuropsychological measures to detection of frontal lobe impairment. The International Journal of Clinical Neuropsychology 8:18–22, 1986

Bornstein RA, Leason M: Effects of localized lesions on the verbal concept attainment test. J Clin Exp Neuropsychol 7:421–429, 1985

Brun A: Frontal lobe degeneration of the non-Alzheimer type, I: neuropathology. Arch Gerontol Geriatr 6:193–208, 1987

Buchsbaum MS: Positron emission tomography in schizophrenia, in Psychopharmacology: The Third General of Progress. Edited by Meltzer HI. New York, Raven, 1987

Buchsbaum MS, DeLisi LE, Holcomb HH, et al: Anteroposterior gradients in cerebral glucose use in schizophrenia and affective disorders. Arch Gen Psychiatry 41:1159–1166, 1984

Caltagirone C, Masullo C, Benedetti N, et al: Dementia in Parkinson's disease: possible specific involvement of the frontal lobes. Int J Neurosci 26:15–26, 1985

Caplan LR: Binswanger's disease, in Handbook of Clinical Neurology, Vol 2: Neurobehavioral Disorders. Edited by Frederiks JAM. Amsterdam, Elsevier, 1985, pp 317–322

Carberry H, Burd B: Individual psychotherapy with the brain injured adult. Cognitive Rehabilitation 4:22–24, 1986

Carlson RJ: Frontal lobe lesions masquerading as psychiatric disturbances. Can Psychiatr Assoc J 22:315–318, 1977

Catsman-Berrevoets CE, von Harskamp F: Compulsive pre-sleep behavior and apathy due to bilateral thalamic stroke: response to bromocriptine. Neurology 38:647–649, 1988

Chelune GJ, Ferguson W, Koon R, et al: Frontal lobe disinhibition in attention deficit disorder. Child Psychiatry Hum Dev 16:221–234, 1986

Cogan DG: Neurology of the Ocular Muscles, 2nd Edition. Springfield, IL, Charles C Thomas, 1956, pp 84–117

Crimson ML, Childs A, Wilcox RE, et al: The effect of bromocriptine on speech dysfunction in patients with diffuse brain injury (brain stem). Clin Neuropharmacol 11:462–466, 1988

Crockett D, Bilsker D, Hurwitz T, et al: Clinical utility of three measures of frontal lobe dysfunction in neuropsychiatric samples. Int J Neurosci 30:241–248, 1986

Curran HV: Tranquillising memories: a review of the effects of benzodiazepines on human memory. Biol Psychiatry 23:179–213, 1986

Damasio A: The frontal lobes, in Clinical Neuropsychology. Edited by Heilman KM, Valenstein E. New York, Oxford University Press, 1979, pp 360–412

Damasio AR, Van Hoesen GW: Emotional disturbances associated with focal lesions of the limbic frontal lobe, in The Neuropsychology of Human Emotion. Edited by Heilman KM, Satz P. New York, Oxford University Press, 1982

deBruin JP, Van Oyen HG, Van de Poll NE: Behavioural changes following changes of the orbital prefrontal cortex in male rats. Behav Brain Res 10:209–232, 1983

della Rochetta AI: Classification and recall of pictures after unilateral frontal or temporal lobectomy. Cortex 22:189–211, 1986

Donnelly M: Attention-deficit hyperactivity disorder and conduct disorder, in Treatments of Psychiatric Disorders, Vol 1. Edited by the American Psychiatric Association Task Force on Treatments of Psychiatric Disorders. Washington, DC, American Psychiatric Association, 1989, pp 365–398

Doty RL: The Smell Identification Test Administration Manual. Philadelphia, PA, Sensonics, 1983

Echiverri HC, Tatum WO, Merens TA, et al: Akinetic mutism: pharmacologic probe of the dopaminergic mesencephalofrontal activating system. Pediatric Neurology 4:228–230, 1988

Elliott FA: Propranolol for the control of belligerent behavior following acute brain damage. Ann Neurol 5:489–491, 1977

Eslinger PJ, Damasio AR: Severe disturbance of higher cognition after bilateral frontal lobe oblation. Neurology 35:1731–1741, 1985

Eslinger PJ, Grattan LM: A cortical and subcortical network of structures involved in cognitive flexibility. J Clin Exp Neuropsychol 11:50–51, 1989

Eslinger PJ, Damasio AR, Von Hoesen GW: Olfactory dysfunction in man: anatomical and behavioral aspects. Brain and Cogn 1:259–285, 1982

Evans RW, Gualtieri CT, Hicks RE: Neuropathic substrate for stimulant drug effects in hyperactive children. Clin Neuropharmacol 9:264–281, 1986

Finger S: Lesion momentum and behavior, in Recovery From Brain Damage. Edited by Finger S. New York, Plenum, 1978, pp 135–160

Fogel BS, Sparadeo FR: Single case study: focal cognitive deficits accentuated by depression. J Nerv Ment Dis 173:120–124, 1985

Folstein MF, Folstein SE, McHugh PR: Mini-Mental State. J Psychiatr Res 12:189–198, 1975

Freedman M, Cermak LS: Semantic encoding deficits in frontal lobe disease and amnesia. Brain Cogn 5:108–114, 1986

Geraud G, Arne-Bes A, Guell A, et al: Reversibility of hemodynamics hypofrontality in schizophrenia. J Cereb Blood Flow Metab 7:9–12, 1987

Goldberg E: Akinesia, tardive dysmentia and frontal lobe disorder in schizophrenia. Schizophr Bull 11:255–263, 1985

Goldberg E, Costa LD: Qualitative indices in neuropsychological assessment: an extension of Luria's approach to executive deficits following prefrontal lesions, in Neuropsychological Assessment of Neuropsychiatric Disorders. Edited by Grant I, Adams KM. New York, Oxford University Press, 1986, pp 48–64

Goldberg TE, Weinberger DR, Berman KF, et al: Further evidence for dementia of the prefrontal type in schizophrenia? Arch Gen Psychiatry 44:1008–1014, 1987

Goodglass H, Kaplan E: Assessment of cognitive deficit in the brain-injured patient, in Handbook of Behavioral Neurobiology, Vol 2: Neuropsychology. Edited by Gazzaniga M. New York, Plenum, 1979, pp 3–22

Gorenstein EE: Cognitive-perceptual deficit in an alcoholism spectrum disorder. J Stud Alcohol 48:310–318, 1987

Gotham AM, Brown RG, Marsden CD: 'Frontal' cognitive function in patients with Parkinson's disease 'on' and 'off' levodopa. Brain 111:299–321, 1988

Grafman J, Vance SC, Weingartner H, et al: The effects of lateralized frontal lesions on mood regulation. Brain 109:1127–1148, 1986

Grattan LM, Eslinger PJ: The relationship between cognitive flexibility and empathy after brain damage. J Clin Exp Neuropsychol 11:47, 1989

Gross RA, Herridge P: A manic-like illness associated with right frontal arteriovenous malformation. J Clin Psychiatry 49:119–120, 1988

Hagberg B: Behaviour correlates to frontal lobe dysfunction. Arch Gerontol Geriatr 6:311–321, 1987

Hartman DE: Neuropsychological Toxicology: Identification and Assessment of Human Neurotoxic Syndromes. New York, Pergamon, 1988

Heaton RK: Wisconsin Card Sorting Test Manual. Odessa, FL, Psychological Assessment Resources, 1985

Heinrichs RW: Frontal cerebral lesions and violent incidents in chronic neuropsychiatric patients. Biol Psychiatry 25:174–178, 1989

Herrera JN, Sramek AJ, Costa JF, et al: High potency neuroleptics and violence in schizophrenics. J Nerv Ment Dis 176:558–561, 1988

Hinebaugh FL: Frontal lobe contributions to the psychopathology of closed cranial insults of vehicular origin. Cognitive Rehabilitation, Nov/Dec 1986, pp 24–27

Ishii N, Nishihara Y, Imamura T: Why do frontal lobe symptoms predominate in vascular dementia with lacunes? Neurology 36:3404–3405, 1986

Jacobs L, Glassman MD: Three primitive reflexes in normal adults. Neurology 30:184–188, 1980

Jenkyn LR, Walsh DB, Culver CM, et al: Clinical signs of diffuse cerebral dysfunction. J Neurol Neurosurg Psychiatry 40:956–966, 1977

Jetter W, Poser U, Freeman RB, et al: A verbal long-term memory deficit in frontal lobe damaged patients. Cortex 22:229–242, 1986

Jones EG: The Thalamus. New York, Plenum, 1985

Jones-Gotman M, Zatorre RJ: Olfactory identification deficits in patients with focal cerebral excision. Neuropsychologia 26:387–400, 1988

Kemp JM, Powell TP: The cortico-striate projection in the monkey. Brain 93:525–546, 1970

Kievit J, Kuypers HGJM: Organization of the thalamo-cortical connections to the frontal lobe in the rhesus monkey. Exp Brain Res 29:299–322, 1977

Klein E, Gittelman R, Quitkin F, et al: Diagnosis and Drug Treatment of

Psychiatric Disorders: Adults and Children, 2nd Edition. Baltimore, MD, Williams & Wilkins, 1980, p 573

Klein RG: Pharmacotherapy of childhood hyperactivity: an update, in Psychopharmacology: The Third Generation of Progress. Edited by Meltzer HY. New York, Raven, 1987, pp 1215–1224

Knoefel JE, Albert ML: Secondary dementias, in Handbook of Clinical Neurology, Vol 2: Neurobehavioral Disorders. Edited by Frederiks JAM. Amsterdam, Elsevier, 1985, pp 385–411

Knopman DS, Christensen KJ, Schut LJ, et al: The spectrum of imaging and neuropsychological findings in Pick's disease. Neurology 39:362–368, 1989

Lahmeyer HW: Frontal lobe meningioma and depression. J Clin Psychiatry 43:254–255, 1982

LaPlane D, Eslinger PE: Clinical consequences of corticectomies involving the supplementary motor area in man. J Neurol Sci 34:310–314, 1977

Levin HS, Benton AL, Grossman R: The Neurobehavioral Consequences of Closed Head Injury. New York, Oxford University Press, 1982

Levin S: Frontal lobe dysfunction in schizophrenia, II: impairments of psychological and brain functions. J Psychiatr Res 18:57–72, 1984

Lezak M: Neuropsychological Assessment. New York, Oxford University Press, 1985

Lishman WA: Organic Psychiatry, 2nd Edition. Oxford, Blackwell Scientific, 1987, pp 68–71

Lohr JB: Transient grasp reflexes in schizophrenia. Biol Psychiatry 20:172–175, 1985

Lou HC, Henriksen L, Bruhn P, et al: Striatal dysfunction in attention deficit and hyperkinetic disorder. Arch Neurol 46:48–52, 1989

Luria AR: Higher Cortical Functions in Man, 2nd Edition. New York, Basic Books, 1980

Maher ER, Smith EM, Lees AJ: Cognitive deficits in the Steele-Richardson-Olszewski syndrome (progressive supranuclear palsy). J Neurol Neurosurg Psychiatry 48:1234–1239, 1985

Malmo RB, Amsel A: Anxiety-produced interferences in serial rote learning with observations on rote learning after partial frontal lobectomy. J Exp Psychol [Learn Mem Cogn] 38:440–454, 1948

Marotta R, Perry S: Early neuropsychological dysfunction caused by immunodeficiency virus. Journal of Neuropsychiatry and Clinical Neurosciences 1:225–235, 1989

Mattes JA, Boswell L, Oliver H, et al: Methylphenidate effects on symptoms of attention deficit disorder in adults. Arch Gen Psychiatry 41:1059–1063, 1984

McAllister TW: Carbamazepine in mixed frontal lobe and psychiatric disorders. J Clin Psychiatry 46:393–394, 1985

McAllister TW, Price TR: Aspects of the behavior of psychiatric inpatients with frontal lobe damage: some implications for diagnosis and treatment. Compr Psychiatry 28:14–21, 1987

McKay SE, et al: Assessment of frontal lobe dysfunction using the Luria-Nebraska Neuropsychological Battery—Children's Revision: a case study. International Journal of Clinical Neuropsychology 7:107–111, 1985

McQuistion HL, Adler LA, Leong S: Carbamazepine and frontal lobe syndrome: two more cases (letter). J Clin Psychiatry 48:456, 1987

Medalia A, Gold J, Merriam A: The effects of neuroleptics on neuropsychological test results of schizophrenics. Archives of Clinical Neuropsychology 3:249–271, 1988

Mesulam M-M: Patterns in behavioral neuroanatomy: association areas, the limbic system, and hemispheric specialization, in Principles of Behavioral Neurology. Edited by Mesulam M-M. Philadelphia, PA, FA Davis, 1985, pp 1–70

Metter EJ, Wasterlain CG, Kuhl DE, et al: ^{18}FDG positron emission computed tomography in a study of aphasia. Ann Neurol 10:173–183, 1981

Milner B: Effects of different brain lesions on card sorting. Arch Neurol 9:90–100, 1963

Milner BL: Some cognitive effects of frontal lobe lesions in man. Philos Trans R Soc Lond [Biol] 298:211–226, 1982

Milner B, Petrides M: Behavioral effects of frontal-lobe lesions in man. Trends in Neuroscience, Nov 1984, pp 403–407

Morice R: Beyond language—speculations on the prefrontal cortex in schizophrenia. Aust N Z J Psychiatry 20:7–10, 1986

Morstyn R, Duffy H, McCarley RW: Altered topography of EEG spectral content in schizophrenia. Electroencephalogr Clin Neurophysiol 56:263–271, 1983

Nasrallah HA, Coffman JA, Olson SC: Structural brain-imaging findings in affective disorders: an overview. Journal of Neuropsychiatry and Clinical Neurosciences 1:21–27, 1989

Nauta WJH: The problem of the frontal lobe: a reinterpretation. J Psychiatr Research 8:167–187, 1971

Neary D, Snowden JS, Northen B, et al: Dementia of frontal lobe type. J Neurol Neurosurg Psychiatry 51:353–361, 1988

Nelson A, Fogel BS, Faust D: Bedside cognitive screening instruments: a critical assessment. J Nerv Ment Dis 174:73–83, 1986

Novoa OP, Ardila A: Linguistic abilities in patients with prefrontal damage. Brain Lang 30:206–225, 1987

Ochitill HN, Dilley JW: Neuropsychiatric aspects of acquired immunodeficiency syndrome, in AIDS and The Nervous System. Edited by Rosenblum ML, Levy RM, Bredesen DE. New York, Raven, 1988, pp 315–325

O'Connell, VanHeertum RL, Billick SB, et al: Single photon emission computed tomography (SPECT) with ^{123}I[IMP] in the differential diagnosis of psychiatric disorders. Journal of Neuropsychiatry and Clinical Neurosciences 1:145–153, 1989

Palmer AM, Wilcock GK, Esiri MM, et al: Monoaminergic innervation of the frontal and temporal lobes in Alzheimer's disease. Brain Res 401:231–238, 1987

Parnavelas JG, McDonald JK: The cerebral cortex, in Chemical Neuroanatomy. Edited by Emson PC. New York, Raven, 1983, pp 505–549

Pascualy M, Veith C: Depression as an adverse drug reaction, in Aging and Clinical Practice: Depression and Coexisting Disease. Edited by Robinson RG, Rabins PV. New York, Igaku and Shoin, 1989, pp 132–151

Peroutka SJ: Antimigraine drug interactions with serotonin receptor subtypes in human brain. Ann Neurol 23:500–504, 1988

Perret E: The left frontal lobe of man and the suppression of habitual responses in verbal categorical behavior. Neuropsychologica 12:323–330, 1974

Quesney LF: Extracranial EEG evaluation, in Surgical Treatment of the Epilepsies. Edited by Engel J. New York, Raven, 1987, pp 129–166

Rapoport JL, Buchsbaum M, Zahn T, et al: Dextroamphetamines: cognitive and behavioral effects in normal prepubertal boys. Science 199:560–563, 1978

Rapoport JL, Buchsbaum M, Weingartner H, et al: Dextroamphetamines: cognitive and behavioral effects in normal and hyperactive boys and normal adult males. Arch Gen Psychiatry 37:933–946, 1980

Rasmussen T: Surgery of frontal lobe epilepsy, in Advances in Neurology, Vol 8. Edited by Purpura DP, Penry JK, Walter RD. New York, Raven, 1975, pp 197–204

Reitan RM: Validity of the Trailmaking Test as an indicator of organic brain damage. Conceptual and Motor Skills 8:271–276, 1958

Rifkin A, Quitkin F, Klein D: Akinesia: a poorly-recognized drug-induced extrapyramidal behavioral disorder. Arch Gen Psychiatry 32:672–674, 1975

Robinson RG, Kubos KL, Starr LB, et al: Mood disorders in stroke patients: importance of location of lesion. Brain 107:81–93, 1984

Robinson RG, Boston JD, Starkstein SE, et al: Comparison of mania and depression after brain injury: causal factors. Am J Psychiatry 145:172–178, 1988

Ross ED, Stewart RS: Pathological display of affect in patients with depression and right frontal brain damage: an alternative mechanism. J Nerv Ment Dis 175:165–172, 1987

Roos RAC: Neuropathology of Huntington's disease, in Handbook of Clinical Neurology, Vol 5: Extrapyramidal Disorders. Edited by Vinken PJ, Bruyn GW, Klawans HL. Amsterdam, Elsevier, 1986, pp 315–326

Schatzberg F, Elliott GR, Lerbinger JE, et al: Topographic mapping in depressed patients, in Topographic Mapping of Brain Electrical Activity. Edited by Duffy FH. Boston, MA, Butterworths, 1986, pp 389–392

Schmidt GL, Keyes B: Group psychotherapy with family caregivers of demented patients. Gerontologist 25:347–350, 1985

Shelton RC, Karson CN, Doran AR, et al: Cerebral structural pathology in schizophrenia: evidence for a selective prefrontal cortical deficit. Am J Psychiatry 145:154–163, 1988

Smith RC, Largen J, Calderon M, et al: CT scans and neuropsychological tests as predictors of clinical response in schizophrenics. Schizophr Bull 19:505–509, 1983

Sohlberg MM, Sprunk H, Metzelaar K: Efficacy of an external cuing system in an individual with severe frontal lobe damage. Cognitive Rehabilitation 6:36–41, 1988

Sorgi PJ, Ratey JJ, Polakoff S: β-Adrenergic blockers for the control of aggressive behavior in patients with chronic schizophrenia. Am J Psychiatry 143:775–776, 1986

Spencer SS, Williamson PD, Bridgers SL, et al: Reliability and accuracy of localization by scalp ictal EEG. Neurology 35:1567–1575, 1985

Sprague RL, Sleator EA: Methylphenidate in hyperkinetic children: differences in dose effects on learning and social behavior. Science 198:1274–1276, 1977

Starkstein SE, Leiguarda R, Gershanik O, et al: Neuropsychological disturbances in hemiparkinson's disease. Neurology 37:1762–1770, 1987

Starkstein SE, Robinson RG, Price TR: Comparison of patients with and without post-stroke major depression matched for size and location of lesion. Arch Gen Psychiatry 45:247–252, 1988

Starkstein SE, Bolduc PL, Preziosi TJ, et al: Cognitive impairments in different stages of Parkinson's disease. Journal of Neuropsychiatry and Clinical Neurosciences 1:243–248, 1989

Statham PF, Johnston RA, Mapherson P: Delayed deterioration in patients with traumatic frontal lobe contusions. J Neurol Neurosurg Psychiatry 52:351–354, 1989

Strub RL: Frontal lobe syndrome in a patient with bilateral globus pallidus lesions. Arch Neurol 46:1024–1027, 1989

Strub RL, Black FW: The Mental Status Examination in Neurology, 2nd Edition. Philadelphia, PA, FA Davis, 1985

Stuss DT: Contribution of frontal lobe injury to cognitive impairment after closed head injury: methods of assessment and recent findings, in Neurobehavioral Recovery from Head Injury. Edited by Levin HS, Grafman J, Eisenberg HM. New York, Oxford University Press, 1987, pp 166–177

Stuss DT, Benson DF: Neuropsychological studies of the frontal lobe. Psychol Bull 95:3–28, 1984

Stuss DT, Benson DF: The Frontal Lobes. New York, Raven, 1986

Stuss DT, Kaplan EF, Benson DF, et al: Evidence for the involvement of orbitofrontal cortex in memory functions: an interference effect. Journal of Comparative and Physiological Psychology 96:913–925, 1982

Sudarsky L, Morris J, Morero J, et al: Dementia in Parkinson's disease: the problem of clinicopathological correlation. Journal of Neuropsychiatry and Clinical Neurosciences 1:159–166, 1989

Takeda A: Complex partial status epilepticus of frontal lobe origin. Jpn J Psychiatry Neurol 42:525–530, 1988

Tariot PN, Sunderland T, Weingartner H, et al: Cognitive effects of l-deprenyl on Alzheimer's disease. Psychopharmacology 91:489–495, 1987

Tarter RE, Edwards KL: Neuropsychology of alcoholism, in Alcohol and the Brain: Chronic Effects. Edited by Tarter RE, Van Thiel DH. New York, Plenum, 1985, pp 217–242

Teuber HL: The riddle of frontal lobe function in man, in The Frontal Granular Cortex and Behavior. Edited by Warren JM, Akert K. New York, McGraw-Hill, 1964

Tranel D, Damasio H: Intact electrodermal skin conductance responses after bilateral amygdala damage. Neuropsychologia 27:381–390, 1989

Wechsler D: Wechsler Adult Intelligence Scale—Revised. San Antonio, TX, Psychological Corporation, 1981

Weinberger DR: Schizophrenia and the frontal lobe. Trends in Neuroscience 11:367–370, 1988

Weinberger DR, Berman KF, Zec RF: Physiologic dysfunction of dorsolateral prefrontal cortex in schizophrenia. Arch Gen Psychiatry 43:114–124, 1986

Wender PH, Reimherr FW, Wood DR: Attention deficit disorder. Arch Gen Psychiatry 38:449–456, 1981

Whaley AL, Stanford CB, Pollack IW: The effects of behavior modification vs. lithium therapy on frontal lobe syndrome. J Behav Ther Exp Psychiatry 17:111–115, 1986

Williams DT, Mehl R, Yudofsky S, et al: The effect of propranolol on uncontrolled rage outbursts in children and adolescents with organic brain dysfunction. J Am Acad Child Psychiatry 21:129–135, 1982

Williamson P: Hypofrontality in schizophrenia: a review of the evidence. Can J Psychiatry 32:399–404, 1987

Williamson PD, Spencer DD, Spencer SS, et al: Complex partial seizures of frontal lobe origin. Ann Neurol 18:497–504, 1985

Wilson H, Staton RD: Neuropsychological changes in children associated with tricyclic antidepressant therapy. Int J Neurosci 24:307–312, 1984

Yeterian EH, Van Hoesen GW: Cortico-striate projections in the rhesus monkey: the organization of certain cortico-caudate connections. Brain Res 139:43–63, 1978

Yudofsky SC, Williams D, Gorman J: Propranolol in the treatment of rage and violent behavior in patients with chronic brain syndromes. Am J Psychiatry 183:218–220, 1981

Yudofsky SC, Silver JM, Schneider SE: Psychopharmacologic treatment of aggression. Psychiatric Annals 17:397–407, 1987

Zametkin AJ, Rapoport JL: Noradrenergic hypothesis of attention deficit disorder with hyperactivity: a critical review, in Psychopharmacology: The Third Generation of Progress. Edited by Meltzer HY. New York, Raven, 1987

Zametkin A, Rapoport JL, Murphy DL, et al: Treatment of hyperactive children with monoamine oxidase inhibitors, II: plasma and urinary monoamine findings after treatment. Arch Gen Psychiatry 42:969–973, 1985

Chapter 11

Headache Syndromes

James R. Merikangas, M.D., F.A.C.P.

Headache is the prototypical neuropsychiatric problem. The symptoms are subjective, the signs are few, and the disability produced is extremely variable. Headache is the most common physical complaint in the general population and is the leading chief complaint resulting in neurological consultation. Head pain produces more anxiety than some other types of pain because of the implication that there may be a threat to the brain and therefore to the very essence of the patient's persona. Headache is the subject of a remarkable number of scholarly books and articles, which recently have explored the neurochemical aspects of pain in general and of headache in particular (Dalessio 1980; Olesen and Edvinsson 1988; Pearce 1984; Raskin 1988; Rose 1988; Welch 1987). In this chapter I introduce essential concepts regarding the psychiatric importance of headache and the clinical approaches to the diagnosis and treatment of each of the major categories of head pain. Key points will be illustrated by case examples.

It has been known for generations that headache may be accompanied by psychiatric symptoms, especially in the case of migraine (Moersch 1924). Moreover, headaches are strongly associated with some of the more common psychiatric conditions, particularly depression and anxiety. Referral to psychiatrists is common when the treating physician reaches an impasse in the treatment and diagnosis of headache. There are many reasons why headache patients are referred to psychiatrists, including the suspicion that the headache may be hysterical or "psychosomatic." The frequent occurrence of drug abuse or dependence in people with chronic headache also leads to psychiatric referral.

Most patients with headache are "medically cleared" before they are referred for psychiatric care. However, many are referred to nonmedical psychotherapists, who may not be trained to evaluate and treat headache properly or who may not be alert to the emergence of neurological signs in cases that may represent progressive conditions. Headache is such a common complaint that psychiatrists may discover the symptoms incidentally in the course of taking a psychiatric history. When a headache history is elicited, the question naturally occurs as to when to refer the patient to a neurologist or when the psychiatrist should do the workup for headache. While some psychiatrists are theoretically capable of conducting a sufficiently accurate neurological examination, referring headache patients for medical clearance or routine physicals may be a disappointing and nonproductive experience. Such examinations, if performed by physicians or physicians' assistants who do not have the entire history and who may not follow the patient, are often superficial and not directed to core diagnostic questions in a way that is truly useful. It is therefore essential for every psychiatrist to know what constitutes an appropriate and complete evaluation of a headache sufferer and how to make a differential diagnosis (Merikangas 1977).

CLINICAL HISTORY OF HEADACHE

The differential diagnosis of headache begins with a description of the type and location of pain, timing, precipitants, prodromal events, and associated symptoms. The following information should be elicited in the clinical interview: onset; frequency; location; duration; quality; severity; precipitants; precursors; triggers; phenomena that worsen or relieve the pain; warning signs; prodromal events; specific symptoms including visual changes, gastrointestinal symptoms, or neurologic symptoms; sensitivity to light, noise, sounds, or touch; mood changes; and cognitive changes. Detailed family history, description of course, and previous evaluation and treatment should also be obtained.

An image of the brain is mandatory at some point in the evaluation of every patient with severe or persistent headache. Computed tomography (CT) should be done for the "first" or "worst" headache or when a subdural hematoma is suspected. Magnetic resonance imaging (MRI) should be done when hydrocephalus, brain tumor, sinusitis, vasculitis, or posterior fossa lesions are suspected, or when exposure to electromagnetic radiation is contraindicated (Johnson and Zimmerman 1989).

Case Example 1

A 37-year-old divorced mother of two small children had seen a neurologist for persistent throbbing headaches that were accompanied by nausea and dizziness. She was treated with propranolol but had little relief. Because of increasing depression, she sought psychiatric treatment with the encouragement of her treating neurologist, who suggested the headaches were psychosomatic, caused by her recent divorce and subsequent coping problems. On interview she did indeed appear depressed, but she stated that she actually felt better after the divorce and was convinced that her depression was the result rather than the cause of the headaches.

She had no previous history of migraine and during previous depressive episodes had had no headaches. On neurological examination there were no abnormalities and her laboratory profile was unremarkable. A CT scan of the brain demonstrated a parasagittal meningioma the size of a walnut. This was removed with no complications and no subsequent neurological deficits. Both the headache and the depression resolved with no pharmacologic treatment.

In this case example, there had been no initial CT scan because utilization criteria rather than sound clinical judgment weighed more heavily in the decision to discontinue the workup after neurological "clearance." Had the recommendations contained in this chapter been followed, a brain image would have been obtained.

In addition to history taking, physical examination, and imaging procedures, laboratory examination is also necessary. Table 11-1 lists the laboratory tests that should be performed on the initial visit of a headache sufferer. This may appear to be a large number of tests, but there is no substitute for the information obtained. Even if the results are all negative and do not uncover a metabolic, endocrine, or autoimmune etiology, this information may serve as a baseline for subsequent drug therapy. The listed blood tests should be done in every case because there is simply no other way to gain the differential diagnostic information. Although a general physical examination may disclose anemia or myxedema, it is more likely that the more subtle etiologies would not even be suspected until the return of the laboratory test

Table 11-1. Laboratory tests used in the evaluation of headache

CBC with differential	Urinalysis
Platelet count	Creatinine
Sedimentation rate	Uric acid
VDRL	Serum calcium
TSH	Phosphorus
T3 serum by RIA	Total serum protein
Serum folate	Serum albumin
Vitamin B_{12}	A/G ratio
ANA	Globulin
CPK	Total serum bilirubin
BUN	SGOT
LDH	SGPT
Alkaline phosphatase	SGT
Triglycerides	Cholesterol
Electrolytes	Serum iron

Note. CBC = complete blood count. VDRL = Venereal Disease Research Laboratories test. TSH = thyroid-stimulating hormone. RIA = radioimmunoassay. ANA = antinuclear antibody titer. CPK = creatine phosphokinase. BUN = blood urea nitrogen. LDH = lactic dehydrogenase. A/G ratio = albumin-to-globulin ratio. SGOT = serum glutamic-oxaloacetic transaminase. SGPT = serum glutamic-pyruvic transaminase. SGT = serum glutamine transferase.

values. A physician often can negotiate with a clinical laboratory for a customized profile, including tests for headache (or for other specific indications such as dementia, movement disorder, psychosis, or anxiety), that may cost a great deal less than a smaller number of individually selected tests ordered separately for each patient.

EEGs are required in the evaluation of headache when there is a particularly paroxysmal presentation or if concomitant syncope or seizures occur. EEG may also aid in the detection of drug abuse. Both barbiturates and benzodiazepines produce a pattern of excessive beta activity (see Chapter 5). EEG is also indicated if the headache is associated with altered mental states. Headaches associated with epilepsy suggest intoxication, an underlying infection, hemorrhage, or structural disease. Neuroimaging may identify unexpected lesions and is mandatory in such headache patients.

CLASSIFICATION OF HEADACHE

The International Headache Society recently introduced a new headache classification system for international use. Because the com-

Table 11-2. Headache classification system of the International Headache Society

1. Migraine
2. Tension-type headache
3. Cluster headache and chronic paroxysmal hemicrania
4. Miscellaneous headaches unassociated with structural lesions
5. Headache associated with head trauma
6. Headache associated with vascular disorder
7. Headache associated with nonvascular intracranial disorder
8. Headache associated with substances or their withdrawal
9. Headache associated with noncephalic infection
10. Headache associated with metabolic disorder
11. Headache or facial pain associated with disorder of cranium, neck, eyes, ears, nose, sinuses, teeth, mouth, or other facial or cranial structures
12. Headache associated with cranial neuralgias, nerve trunk pain, and deafferentation pain
13. Headache not classifiable

Source. Olesen J: Classification and diagnostic criteria for headache disorders, cranial neuralgias and facial pain. Cephalalgia 8 (suppl 7):1–96, 1988.

mittee that developed the criteria comprises an international group of headache specialists, these criteria are expected to have widespread utility. The new system not only provides a classification scheme and diagnostic criteria but also serves as a guide to differential diagnosis (Table 11-2). The criteria are intended to be applied to classify headache subtypes based on information obtained from a history, a physical and neurological examination, and appropriate laboratory investigations. There is general agreement that a thorough evaluation is required for all patients presenting with headache complaints (Saper 1987).

In the classification scheme of the International Headache Society, there is no category for "psychosomatic" or "psychogenic" headache because there has never been a valid demonstration that mental illness or life stress causes headaches. Headaches may in very rare cases be a symptom of severe depression or psychosis. However, when headache is attributed to mental illness, periodic reevaluation for organic causes is needed as long as the headache persists. Even though the organic factors present may not be ameliorated, assuring the patient that the pain is "real" and has a specific etiology that is understood by medical science can itself help relieve the pain and suffering. Headaches are very rarely purely psychogenic, and conditions that cause headaches can also cause anxiety, depression, psychosis, dementia, and episodic violent behavior. The clinician should be particularly cautious when a patient is referred for psychotherapy because of a "stress-induced" headache or a "depressive equivalent" headache. Some physicians have a particular blind spot for causes in their own specialty. For example, it is not unusual for a neurosurgeon to refer a psychogenic headache patient who has pseudotumor cerebri or a chronic subdural hematoma, or for an internist to refer a patient who has a vasculitis. It is the obligation of the psychiatrist to be familiar with the evaluation done to date and to complete it, if necessary. If systemic conditions such as lupus or hypoglycemia are not considered and deliberately evaluated, they are frequently overlooked.

Headache in the elderly is of particular concern because the prevalence of primary and metastatic brain tumors increases with age. Whereas most tumors will be primary in persons under age 50, the incidence of metastatic tumors increases sharply thereafter. The incidence of chronic subdural hematoma also increases with age and is much more common in patients taking anticoagulants or aspirin. Subdural hematoma may be remarkably silent except for a dull headache and may be of significant size before any hard neurologic signs are evident.

According to Zilkha (1988, p. 24), "when a patient presents with a headache, the doctor has a chance of practicing the full art and science of medicine." The proper treatment of headache depends on discovering the specific diagnosis. Because headache is such a nonspecific complaint with an enormous number of etiologies ranging from the trivial to the acutely life threatening, a very skillful workup is essential in every case. Such a workup begins with an interview and a complete personal and family history, which often in themselves suggest the correct diagnosis.

Migraine Headache

Migraine is more than a headache. Migraine generally presents with symptoms emanating from one or more systems, including the vascular, neurologic, gastrointestinal, endocrine, and visual. These symptoms are accompanied by a variety of changes in behavior and cognition, including mood alterations and confusion. Migraine is composed of episodic attacks of headache lasting from a few hours to 3 days and is characterized by unilateral location, pulsating quality, aggravation by routine physical activity, gastrointestinal symptoms, and photophobia and phonophobia. Migraine was formerly divided into two major subtypes, common and classic, with the latter being distinguished by the presence of neurologic symptoms that precede the onset of the headache. The new classification of migraine by the International Headache

Table 11-3. International Headache Society diagnostic criteria for migraine

I. Migraine without aura
   A. At least five attacks fulfilling B–D
   B. Headache attacks lasting 4–72 hours (untreated or unsuccessfully treated)
   C. At least two of the following characteristics:

   1. Unilateral location
   2. Pulsating quality
   3. Moderate or severe intensity
   4. Aggravation by walking stairs or similar routine physical activity

   D. During a headache, at least one of the following:

   1. Nausea and/or vomiting
   2. Photophobia and phonophobia

II. Migraine with aura
   A. At least two attacks fulfilling B
   B. At least three of the following four characteristics:

   1. One or more fully reversible aura symptoms indicating focal cerebral cortical and/or brain stem dysfunction
   2. At least one aura symptom developing gradually over more than 4 minutes, or two or more symptoms occurring in succession
   3. No aura symptom lasting more than 60 minutes; if more than one aura symptom is present, accepted duration is proportionally increased
   4. Headache following aura with a free interval of less than 60 minutes (or beginning before or simultaneously with the aura)

Source. Olesen J: Classification and diagnostic criteria for headache disorders, cranial neuralgias and facial pain. Cephalalgia 8 (suppl 7):1–96, 1988.

Society no longer includes the common-classic distinction; instead, migraine is separated by the presence or absence of aura symptoms (reversible neurologic dysfunction). The diagnostic criteria for migraine are shown in Table 11-3.

Migraine is a familial syndrome affecting 4–19% of males and 8–29% of females. The incidence of migraine increases with age, with a peak before age 40 in both males and females. The disorder comprises a great variety of mental symptoms in addition to pain. Although migraine has been postulated to have an autosomal dominant mode of transmission, recent reviews of the genetic studies of migraine indicate that its mode of transmission has not been established. Indeed, a substantial proportion of migraine patients have no family history of this condition (Merikangas 1990).

Migraine may occur with a prolonged aura, and on occasion headache is absent. Migraine can have rather complicated and dramatic symptoms, as in the following case example.

Case Example 2

A 37-year-old man was admitted to the cardiac intensive care unit with epigastric pain and nausea, a left hemiparesis, and severe headache. The ECG showed nonspecific S-T changes, and the CT scan of the brain was normal. He was treated with morphine, which produced some relief of the pain. Neurologic examination was positive for a left hemiparesis with an extensor plantar response and sensory deficit. On interview the patient was asked, "Have you ever had this before?" His reply was, "Several times, it always goes away if I can get to sleep." The diagnosis was hemiplegic migraine.

The hemiparesis that accompanies the aura of hemiplegic migraine may often be prolonged. Because hemiplegic migraine is usually familial, a thorough family history may help to determine the diagnosis. The International Headache Society classification includes familial hemiplegic migraine as a specific subtype of migraine with aura.

Basilar artery migraine is another subtype of migraine with aura. This type of migraine can produce a variety of confusing symptoms that can mimic epilepsy, labyrinthitis, Arnold-Chiari malformation, hypoglycemia, transient ischemic attacks of other etiologies, or hysteria. Patients can present with blindness or vivid visual hallucinations, and with mixtures of brain stem signs of vertigo, difficulty walking, including paraparesis; and difficulty speaking or hearing. They sometimes proceed to unconsciousness or to dissociative episodes. The diagnosis becomes more difficult when attacks are accompanied by seizures. The headache of basilar artery migraine may be accompanied by disorientation or memory loss, so that basilar artery migraine may present as transient global amnesia with headache. (Transient global amnesia without headache has been suspected to be vascular due to vascular spasm.) Like transient global amnesia, basilar migraine is of relatively short duration and rarely leads to stroke. The difference between basilar migraine and transient global amnesia may simply be that the latter lacks other neurological symptoms and signs (Fisher and Adams 1964).

Case Example 3

A 30-year-old keypunch operator, mother of three small children, reported episodes of intense true vertigo accompanied by confusion, loss of muscular tone, and difficulty thinking. The attacks could awaken her from sleep, were not accompanied by convulsive movements, and did not seem to be associated with eating or fasting, position or movement, or time of day. The patient had been evaluated with audiometry, EEG, and routine blood tests, which were all normal. On physical examination she had a I/VI systolic heart murmur, a normal neurological examination, and a great deal of anxiety. Further questioning disclosed that her mother had migraine and that there was no family history of epilepsy. MRI of the brain was normal, as was a 5-hour glucose tolerance test. Treatment with 50 mg/day of atenolol prevented further episodes. The diagnosis was basilar artery migraine.

Other subtypes of migraine include ophthalmoplegic migraine, retinal migraine, and childhood periodic syndromes that may be precursors to migraine.

Although the etiology of migraine is unknown, current evidence favors a neurogenic basis for the disorder (Pearce 1984). That is, migraine has been hypothesized to result from a complex series of events that follow inappropriate fluctuation in the activity of efferent monoaminergic neurons in the brain stem, particularly those containing serotonin and norepinephrine. These changes may result from the response of brain stem nuclei to environmental stimuli. An inflammatory response in vascular walls and the dura mater is induced by complex vasomotor changes in both the intra- and extracranial vasculature (Moskowitz et al. 1988). Pain results from activation of nociceptors tributary to the trigeminal nerve, and it is processed and perceived by neurons in the brain stem, thalamus, and cerebral cortex. The vascular changes and pain of migraine may also result from local release of mediators of inflammation, particularly in and around vascular walls (Blau 1988; Welch 1987).

Treatment of migraine. Treatment of migraine can be prophylactic, with medication taken daily; abortive, with medication taken at the onset of an attack; or palliative, with medication taken after the pain has begun. Prophylactic treatments for migraine are of varying effectiveness. Table 11-4 summarizes the evidence from controlled clinical trials on the efficacy of various classes of drugs in the treatment of migraine (Merikangas and Merikangas 1988a). This table presents the average proportion of subjects across all controlled studies in which there is at least a 50% reduction in frequency and/or severity of headaches. Clinical trials of migraine treatment are complicated by the high placebo response rate among subjects with migraine, the heterogeneity of diagnostic subtypes of headache, the intermittent nature

Table 11-4.   Efficacy of prophylactic treatments of migraine

Drug class	Average effect (%)[a]
Beta-blockers	60
Calcium channel blockers	50
Tricyclic antidepressants	70
Monoamine oxidase inhibitors	80
Prostaglandin inhibitors	40
Serotonin inhibitors	50

[a]Average proportion of patients with greater than 50% diminution of severity and/or frequency of headaches after drug treatment across studies.

of the condition, and the frequent use of additional analgesics to treat headache pain.

The treatment of migraine chosen for an individual depends not only on the diagnosis of migraine headache but also on related factors specific to the patient. Excellent reviews of both the acute and prophylactic treatment of migraine have been presented by Blau (1988), Raskin (1988), and Rose (1988).

The beta-blockers are currently the first-choice treatment in migraine prophylaxis (Daroff and Whitney 1986; Tfelt-Hansen 1986). However, their effect is moderate at best; no study has reported complete elimination of migraine. The average duration and severity of headaches are reduced by about 50% in most subjects (Anthony 1988).

Only those beta-blocking agents that are devoid of sympathomimetic activity and possess membrane-stabilizing properties are efficacious in migraine. Their mechanism of action is unknown. Beta blockade per se is unlikely to be the major factor because dextropropranolol, which does not block beta-adrenergic receptors, also is efficacious. Hypotheses for therapeutic action of beta-blockers include drug-induced decrease in the excessive sympathetic activity often found in migraine patients; blockade of the beta receptors of the cranial vasculature, preventing the vasodilation associated with pain; and serotonergic antagonism. To date, no specific migraine subtypes that are particularly responsive to beta-blockers have been identified (Anthony 1988; Peatfield et al. 1986).

After beta-blockers, the next most frequently used agents to treat migraine are methysergide, naproxen sodium, and calcium channel blockers. Recent clinical trials, however, have not demonstrated calcium channel blockers to be superior to placebo in the treatment of migraine.

It is interesting that the antidepressant drugs, particularly those of the tricyclic class, have demonstrated greater efficacy than the above-cited first-line agents. Tricyclic antidepressants are effective in the prophylaxis of migraine and also in the treatment of depression that often accompanies headache. Because pain is perceived as more onerous or debilitating when a person is depressed, an antidepressant may help both directly and through an action on mood. There does seem to be a direct analgesic effect of amitriptyline and other tricyclics (Spiegel et al. 1983). Relief of migraine by amitriptyline is not contingent on the presence of depression, however. Couch et al. (1976) showed improvement in headache to be independent of patients' change in depression ratings.

Treatment with amitriptyline (or preferably with its metabolite, nortriptyline, which has fewer side effects) should begin with very small doses, such as 10 mg qhs, and dosage should be raised gradually to minimize side effects. Frequently, the drug is given in too large an initial dose, and the patient, discouraged by side effects, does not follow through with it. Both amitriptyline alone and amitriptyline with betablockers have been found in comparative trials to yield a greater than 50% response in more than 70% of subjects (Couch and Hassanein 1979; Couch et al. 1976). This is the highest treatment response of any of the prophylactic agents for migraine.

Although less widely studied, the monoamine oxidase inhibitors (MAOIs) also have been reported to be efficacious in the prophylaxis of migraine headache, particularly in patients who have been nonresponsive to first-line prophylactic treatment, including the beta-adrenergic blocking agents, ergot compounds, and prostaglandin inhibitors (Daroff and Whitney 1986; Raskin 1988). The last-cited study, which employed phenelzine 45 mg/day for periods of up to 2 years, reported at least a 50% reduction in the frequency of migraine in 80% of the subjects. The authors reported no correlation between clinical response and changes in plasma serotonin. In a recent review of prophylactic treatment of migraine, Daroff and Whitney (1986) declared that phenelzine may be the most efficacious antimigraine agent.

The theoretical basis for the use of MAOIs to treat migraine has derived from the suggestion that migraine may result from a depletion of central monoamines, particularly serotonin, leading to the vasodilation associated with pain. The MAOIs are known to increase the accumulation of monoamines, particularly serotonin, dopamine, tryptamine, tyramine, and epinephrine, perhaps thereby preventing uncontrolled vasodilation of cerebral vasculature.

Fear of hypertensive reactions formerly limited the use of MAOIs because noncompliance with the diet or an inadvertent ingestion of a sympathomimetic drug has a potential for causing a hypertensive crisis, but calcium channel blockers have reduced this hazard. Verapamil 80 mg, which is available in tablet form, may be given to the patient on MAOI therapy to carry with the advice that if a severe generalized headache with flushing or hypertension occurs, the verapamil should immediately be taken orally (Merikangas and Merikangas 1988a, 1988b). It need not be dissolved under the tongue or crushed, as it is rapidly effective when swallowed. The patient should also be advised to seek medical attention if a reaction occurs and, if the reaction does not go away in 15 or 20 minutes, to take another dose of verapamil. Oral verapamil is more practical than intravenous phentolamine and is preferable to chlorpromazine, which may incapacitate the patient by sedation or a dystonic reaction.

Combinations of the above classes of drugs have also been used for patients who fail to respond to first-line treatments. Tricyclics plus beta-blockers and tricyclics plus MAOIs are the two most commonly combined preventive treatments of migraine. However, a generally effective drug for migraine prophylaxis has yet to be found. In a recent review of the treatment of migraine, Blau (1988) concluded that although many agents had been found to be effective in migraine prophylaxis, few have stood the test of time.

Migraine and psychopathology.   The existence of a "migraine personality" has been postulated since the earliest descriptions (Wolff 1937) but has not been confirmed (Friedman 1978). Nevertheless, every neurologist has seen obsessional and conscientious migraine patients whose rigidity not only seems characteristic but also makes them ideal treatment subjects because they scrupulously follow diets, medication regimens, and advice to quit smoking.

There is a strong association between migraine and depression in clinical studies of patients in treatment for migraine (Selby and Lance 1960) and patients in treatment for depression (Cassidy et al. 1957; Diamond 1964; Merikangas et al. 1988). An association between migraine and depression has also been found in epidemiologic samples, thereby demonstrating that this association cannot be attributed to increased representation of persons with both conditions in treated samples (Merikangas et al. 1990). Moreover, the prodrome of migraine is generally characterized by symptoms that typically occur in psychiatric syndromes, including acute changes in energy, appetite, mood, and level of anxiety (Blau 1988). Therefore, migraine patients deserve a full psychiatric evaluation with particular attention to the possibility of a comorbid mood disorder.

Given the overlap of symptoms of the actual migraine episode and those on the anxiety-depression spectrum, along with the increased prevalence of anxious and depressive symptoms between migraine attacks in migraine sufferers, it is not surprising that similar pharmacologic agents have been employed in the treatment of both migraine and the symptoms of anxiety and depression.

If the patient has a strong component of anxiety, initial treatment with a beta-blocker is indicated. A good choice might be atenolol, 25 mg to start, adjusting as necessary up to 100 mg in a single dose each day. However, since beta-blockers may be associated with depression and lethargy, patients should be advised to report any increase in depressive symptoms after therapy has begun (Griffin and Friedman 1986). If there is a strong component of depression or an associated panic disorder, initial treatment with an antidepressant is indicated. Phenelzine is more effective than atenolol in the prophylaxis of migraine and will simultaneously treat the anxiety and depression that so frequently co-occur with migraine (Merikangas and Merikangas 1988a).

The diet required for MAOI treatment eliminates foods prepared by fermentation, such as aged cheese or red wine. Since it therefore also eliminates the foods and drinks that commonly are associated with the production of migraine, some of the therapeutic effect also may be attributable to the dietary changes (Monro et al. 1980).

Acute treatment of migraine.   When a patient with an acute severe headache presents to the emergency room with a "first and worst" headache, a CT scan of the brain is mandatory. If the scan is negative, an examination of the spinal fluid to rule out subarachnoid hemorrhage is required. Patients with intracranial bleeds may appear to be intoxicated, severely agitated, or obnoxious. In these cases, countertransference should not obscure the fact that such behavior may be symptomatic of a life-threatening illness. Meningitis often presents with headache; every headache accompanied by fever or stiff neck should alert the clinician to this possibility.

The nausea and vomiting that frequently accompany migraine are partly the result of central stimulation of the medullary vomiting centers. They often are accompanied by gastroparesis. Metoclopramide is, therefore, a logical and effective treatment for migrainous nausea. Chlorpromazine also produces sedation and, in the acute treatment of migraine, may assist the patient in going to sleep. Sleep is nature's remedy for migraine.

Clinicians should be alert to the dangers of abuse of agents used to treat migraine, such as ergotamine and narcotics. Percocet and Percodan are two of the most popular drugs among opiate addicts, who prefer oral narcotics because their narcotic ingredient, oxycodone, is short acting, effective orally, and a euphoriant with a high street value. In acute use, however, narcotics do not produce addiction (Melzack 1990). Narcotics for severe acute migraine may be necessary, and, in those rare cases, morphine usually is a better choice than the synthetic narcotics such as meperidine (Demerol) and hydromorphone (Dilaudid) (Kaiko et al. 1983). Sumatriptin, a serotonergic agonist that is now available in Great Britain and soon will be available in the United States, may be a better choice for parenteral treatment of acute migraine (Humphrey et al. 1990; Palus et al. 1990).

Nonpharmacological treatment of headache. The prophylactic effect of exercise on migraine and the therapeutic effect of exercise on muscle tension headache should be emphasized. Changes in life-style and consideration of the total person and his or her environment are a necessary part of treating the headache patient. Dietary restrictions are important in the prophylaxis of migraine. Smoking, cheese, chocolate, and fermented beverages have all been shown to provoke attacks of migraine (Monro et al. 1980). Patients should be advised to maintain a diary, carefully recording symptoms, timing, duration, and severity of attacks, along with concomitant daily activities, events, diet, and drug use, in order to identify possible environmental triggers of the attacks.

Headache in particularly photosensitive migraine sufferers may be reduced if sufferers wear photosensitive glasses that adjust to brightness by darkening and avoid exposure to fluorescent lights. Lights in the workplace should be incandescent. Cathode-ray tubes or video display terminals may require color filters on a trial-and-error basis to determine which is least likely to precipitate headaches.

Tension Headache

Tension headache is characterized by episodes of bilateral pain lasting several days at a time. The International Headache Society has introduced a set of specific criteria for the diagnosis of tension headache, both chronic and acute types (Table 11-5). It is distinguished from migraine headache by its generally longer duration, the lack of pulsating quality of the pain, the lack of worsening with physical activity, and the absence of gastrointestinal concomitants. However, migraine and tension-type headache may often coexist, either simultaneously or alternating over time.

Table 11-5. International Headache Society diagnostic criteria for tension
headache

I. Episodic tension-type headache
   A. At least 10 previous headache episodes fulfilling criteria B–D listed below;
      number of days with such headache: 180/year
   B. Headache lasting from 30 minutes to 7 days
   C. At least two of the following pain characteristics:

      1. Pressing/tightening (nonpulsating) quality
      2. Mild or moderate intensity
      3. Bilateral location
      4. No aggravation by walking stairs or similar routine physical activity

   D. Both of the following:

      1. No nausea or vomiting (anorexia may occur)
      2. Absence of photophobia and phonophobia, or presence of one but not the
         other

II. Chronic tension-type headache
   A. Average headache frequency >15 days/month for >6 months (180
      days/year) fulfilling criteria B–D listed below
   B. At least two of the following pain characteristics:

      1. Pressing/tightening quality
      2. Mild or moderate severity
      3. Bilateral location
      4. No aggravation by walking stairs or similar routine physical activity

   C. Both of the following:

      1. No vomiting
      2. No more than one of the following: nausea, photophobia, or phonophobia

---

Source. Olesen J: Classification and diagnostic criteria for headache disorders, cranial neuralgias and
facial pain. Cephalalgia 8 (suppl 7):1–96, 1988.

The diagnosis of tension headache requires the exclusion of other
conditions, including brain tumors, pseudotumor cerebri, vasculitis,
hypertension, and extracerebral disease, any of which may be concurrent rather than causal. Tension headache is a syndrome that is too
readily diagnosed in patients who present with mild depressive symptoms.

Imaging procedures include X rays of the jaw for malocclusion,
films of the cervical spine for degenerative changes, and a CT scan or
MRI of the brain and are indicated before attributing headaches to
tension or stress. Indeed, headache may cause stress as frequently as
it may result from it.

Electromyography (EMG) has little to offer in the diagnosis of tension headache or muscle contraction headache because muscle tension

is readily diagnosed with the fingertips palpating the affected muscles, and unless one suspects myotonic dystrophy or amyotrophic lateral sclerosis, EMG has no specific diagnostic value. Even in the case of peripheral nerve injuries or lumbar disc disease, EMG is only positive during specific time periods and after specific types of injury, so a negative test does not rule out neurogenic pain.

Symptoms of tension headache may arise iatrogenically from drugs such as ergotamine used to treat migraine, often as a result of overuse of the drug, as described below. Isler (1988) estimates that more than 40% of chronic headache cases are associated with overuse of drugs intended to alleviate headache. Clinical or subclinical ergotism has been proposed as the sole cause of the transformation of intermittent responsive migraine into chronic intractable headache, perpetuated by rebound headache on withdrawal (Isler 1988). Fiorinal, which is a mixture of butalbital (a short-acting barbiturate), aspirin, and caffeine, is frequently used by non-neurologists for the treatment of headache. However, tolerance and/or drug dependence may occur. Rebound from either caffeine or the barbiturate can be a cause of headache, resulting in a vicious circle of headache relief and rebound headache with ultimate consequences of overuse, abuse, and intoxication. Fiorinal with codeine is particularly pernicious because, in addition to developing dependence on barbiturates, patients may become dependent on narcotics. When tolerance develops, larger doses are required to produce the same relief, so such drugs should never be used to treat a chronic condition.

There is no general agreement as to the pathophysiology of the tension headache syndrome, which is also referred to as "muscle contraction headache" or stress headache. Even in apparently obvious cases, it is a grave mistake to attribute causation to concurrent psychopathology. Saper (1987) noted that although emotional factors are at times very important, emotional phenomena may have been overemphasized in the etiology of headache. Assumption of emotional etiology before a thorough diagnostic evaluation is counterproductive. Moreover, emotional etiology should not be assumed for those residual cases with no known basis.

Treatment of tension headache depends on a specific diagnosis. A headache diary is also useful in assessing the criteria for tension headache. Treatment of tension headache must be individualized, and although biofeedback, massage, relaxation, muscle relaxants, cervical traction, chiropractic manipulation, hot packs, and cold packs have all been reported to be effective, there are no convincing guidelines to suggest one modality rather than another. In a large study of chiropractic in Australia, there was found to be no agreement in diagnosis, treatment, or outcome using manipulation and physical methods (Parker et al. 1980). The use of minor tranquilizers or analgesics containing barbiturates or narcotics should be avoided.

Cluster Headache

Cluster headache is a distinct syndrome characterized by frequent attacks (often several per day) over a 1- to 2-month period, separated by headache-free intervals for as long as 1 or 2 years. Although it is commonly grouped with migraine, current evidence including epidemiological data, treatment response, and clinical features suggests that cluster headache may comprise a distinct syndrome (Dalessio 1980). Cluster headache was first described in the neurological literature by Romberg in 1840, and it has been given over 13 different names, some of them misnomers (Kudrow 1983). Histaminic cephalalgia and sphenopalatine neuralgia are among the better-known alternatives (Dalessio 1980). Migraine headache, cluster headache, and tension headache are frequently confused, and readers are encouraged to learn the new international classification criteria for these conditions.

Cluster refers to a "clustering in time," with the headache bouts coming from every day to several times a day over a period of days to weeks, followed by a headache-free interval. The condition of constantly recurring or chronic migraine described as "status migrainosis" is not cluster but may resemble it until a specific inquiry is made about symptoms. Cluster headache is generally retro-orbital in location and is accompanied by autonomic changes such as lacrimation, rhinorrhea, erythema of the eye, and agitation. Patients with cluster headache do not retire to dark rooms and lie down to avoid the stimulation but may in fact do quite the opposite, appearing almost manic in their agitation. The pain can be so intense that the sufferer may appear to be psychotic because of the screaming and thrashing that may be associated with the pain. "Cluster migraine" is a confusion in terms because cluster and migraine are different conditions with different pathophysiology (based on response to medication) and different characteristics.

Chronic paroxysmal hemicrania is a type of cluster headache, specifically responsive to treatment with indomethacin and characterized by many daily focal attacks of pain lasting for short periods, generally about 15 or 20 minutes per attack (Raskin 1988). The International

Table 11-6.   International Headache Society diagnostic criteria for cluster headache and chronic paroxysmal hemicrania

A. At least five attacks fulfilling B–D
B. Severe unilateral orbital, supraorbital, and/or temporal pain lasting 15–180 minutes untreated
C. Association with at least one of the following signs, which must be present on the pain side:

  1. Conjunctival injection
  2. Lacrimation
  3. Nasal congestion
  4. Rhinorrhea
  5. Forehead and facial sweating
  6. Miosis
  7. Ptosis
  8. Eyelid edema

D. Frequency of attacks from one every other day to eight per day

Source. Olesen J: Classification and diagnostic criteria for headache disorders, cranial neuralgias and facial pain. Cephalalgia 8 (suppl 7):1–96, 1988.

Headache Society diagnostic criteria for cluster headache are given in Table 11-6.

Cluster headache has a very low population prevalence (less than 1% of the general population) and occurs nearly exclusively in males. Acute attacks can be treated with inhalation of oxygen by mask. Ergotamine aerosol is effective about 80% of the time (Raskin 1988). The most efficacious prophylactic agents are lithium (600–900 mg/day) (Raskin 1988; Rose 1988), methysergide (4–10 mg/day), and prednisone (50–80 mg/day) (Ekbom 1981; Kudrow 1978; Watson and Evans 1987). Attacks of cluster headache can be precipitated by alcohol consumption during acute periods but not during remissions; patients with active cluster headache are thus advised to avoid all alcoholic beverages, including wine and beer.

Imipramine and daily ergotamine also have been used for the prophylaxis of cluster headache, which remains very difficult to treat. The use of calcium channel blockers remains controversial for this headache syndrome.

Miscellaneous Headaches Unassociated With Structural Lesions

Another reason for psychiatric referral of headache is the occurrence of unusual symptoms or complaints that may not be familiar to the referring doctor and that therefore suggest a psychiatric etiology. These include some of the types of headache described below, which do not clearly fall within the domain of migraine or tension headache and which are not associated with a specific lesion.

Ice pick pain is an acute, stabbing pain in the head, frequently described as being "like someone jabbed an ice pick into me" or "like someone stuck a knife through my eye." This may sound histrionic or bizarre, and if one did not know that this is quite typical for migraine, it might generate a psychiatric referral. Frequently, "neurotic" or "psychotic" headaches are described in terms like "My head is in a vise" or "There is a steel band around my head and it is shrinking." These descriptions are in fact quite common among migraine sufferers and patients with muscle contraction headaches and are more representative of a capacity for lucid description than of the presence of a mental illness.

Patients who complain of headache during or after sexual intercourse or masturbation may be suspected of having a sexual dysfunction, shame, or guilt; but, in fact, orgasmic cephalalgia is a variant of migraine that responds readily to prophylactic treatment with beta-blocking drugs. These agents are effective if prescribed on a prn basis before intercourse.

"Ice cream headache" is a very severe and sudden pain that occurs within a minute after exposure to cold food. Deep within the head, it is nonthrobbing and generally resolves spontaneously and rather quickly. It has been reported in about one-third of the normal population and in 90% of migraine sufferers (Raskin 1988).

Patches of pain and tenderness on the scalp may be the residual of migraine, but they may also be a sign of temporal arteritis, giant cell arteritis, and neuralgias due to local trauma to peripheral nerves, including the occipital and the supraorbital.

Headache Associated With Head Trauma

Posttraumatic headaches occur quite commonly after seemingly trivial injuries as well as after severe head trauma. These may be of the tension or migrainous variety. In some cases, posttraumatic hemorrhage, demyelination, or hydrocephalus may be invisible on CT scans, and therefore the MRI scan is of greater utility in the evaluation of posttraumatic syndromes of long duration because it may show tiny areas of demyelination secondary to trauma. Even in cases without demonstrable intracranial lesions, headaches may become chronic, although the majority tend to disappear with time. Chronic posttraumatic headache is a syndrome that is difficult to treat (Friedman 1969). Trials of amitriptyline, carbamazepine, beta-blockers, and nonsteroidal anti-inflammatory drugs should be attempted. However, caution in the use of nonsteroidal anti-inflammatory drugs is necessary because of their gastrointestinal side effects and because they may actually cause headache in some patients (Isler 1988). There is frequently a depressive component with postconcussive syndromes, including sleep loss, that is helped by antidepressant treatment.

A common error is to ascribe a posttraumatic headache to compensation neurosis or malingering simply because no signs are present on neurologic examination and because imaging procedures are negative. In these cases, single photon emission computed tomography (SPECT) may be positive when the CT scan and MRI scan are negative (Merikangas J.R. and Caride V., June 1986, unpublished data). (See Chapter 1 for caution regarding overinterpretation of SPECT.)

Headache Associated With Vascular Disorders

A cerebral vascular accident may have headache as a premonitory or "sentinel" sign, and headache may precede or accompany an intracerebral bleed. Ischemia without stroke may be accompanied by a dull headache. Vascular headaches of psychiatric interest also include those caused by systemic lupus erythematosus (SLE) and temporal arteritis. Up to 50% of lupus sufferers have a major psychiatric disorder of an "organic basis," which may mimic schizophrenia, mania, depression, or dementia (Lishman 1987). Autoimmune diseases including temporal arteritis, lupus, and vasculitis must be suspected when the patient has a generalized illness, especially one including arthritis or cutaneous rashes. Tests for erythrocyte sedimentation rate (ESR) and antinuclear antibody (ANA) are recommended for every headache patient; unfortunately, the ESR may be normal in cases of giant cell arteritis and ANA tests may vary from week to week and from laboratory to laboratory, so that low titers do not rule out autoimmune disease, nor do high titers rule it in. False-positive ANAs at low titer are especially common in older people. The anti-double standard DNA test is more specific for SLE.

A high index of suspicion of temporal arteritis does mandate immediate steroid therapy and referral of the patient to a neurologist or rheumatologist. Temporal artery biopsy, a simple procedure that is performed by a variety of surgical specialists including ophthalmologists, may be diagnostic, but in acute cases steroid therapy is necessary to preserve eyesight in the interval before the biopsy results return. Reading the biopsy requires scanning longitudinal slices of the artery with great care. The acute onset of headaches with seizures or psychosis should suggest autoimmune disease.

Case Example 4

A 64-year-old woman with a history of a small stroke that left her with a mild expressive aphasia presented with headache, paranoid psychosis, and an agitated confused state. Neurological examination showed no acute changes, but erythematous skin lesions and a malar rash raised the suspicion of an autoimmune disease. Her ESR was only slightly elevated and was interpreted as normal for her age. Her ANA titer also was considered normal for her age at 1:40, and a skin biopsy of one of the erythematous lesions on her legs was read as nonspecific. Cerebrospinal fluid examination (CSF) was normal. Her mental state cleared dramatically with prednisone treatment. Subsequently, X rays of her hand were read as joint subluxation consistent with lupus arthritis, and a diagnosis of SLE was confirmed.

Case Example 5

A 67-year-old woman was referred by her internist for treatment of depression manifested by insomnia, weight loss, malaise, difficulty concentrating, and feelings of hopelessness and sadness. Depression was attributed to the deteriorating condition of her husband, who was suffering from Parkinson's disease. On interview she met symptom criteria for major depression and had tears in her eyes. She had already been given a trial of amitriptyline, but this drug caused her to become confused and agitated. Neurological examination was normal apart from bilateral palmomental reflexes. Blood was drawn for a neurological profile (see Table 11-1 for tests used in a neurologic profile), with the finding of an ESR of 44, a slightly elevated alkaline phosphatase, and an ANA titer of 1:80. CT of the brain was unremarkable. A diagnosis of arteritis was entertained, but the internist disagreed. Despite symptomatic improvement on 80 mg/day of prednisone, steroids were discontinued because there was no specific diagnosis. The patient deteriorated and died. On autopsy, a diffuse arteritis was demonstrated.

Headache Associated With Nonvascular Intracranial Disorder

One of the major fears of persons who experience their first episode of severe headache is that the etiology is a brain tumor. Although the probability of a brain tumor is low, this condition should always be considered in the differential diagnosis of headache. Early diagnosis is obviously of great value in tumor cases.

Case Example 6

> A 40-year-old, single, sixth-grade female schoolteacher consulted her internist because of headaches and dizziness as well as stiffness in the left neck. On examination she was found to have a disturbance of her eye movements; there was no reflex asymmetry. The examining doctor did not record a sensory examination, corneal reflexes, or the appearance of the optic discs. He suggested that she was suffering from stress, tension, and anxiety and referred her for psychotherapy. The nurse clinician providing the psychotherapy felt the woman was psychologically healthy and recommended a neurological consultation. The woman went back to the internist, who did not order a neurological consultation but again referred her to a psychiatrist for "stress management." The psychiatrist also expressed the opinion that this was not a functional disorder, and it was only after the patient's left leg began to drag and she developed urinary incontinence that a CT scan was done revealing a walnut-sized acoustic neuroma affecting the left ear and causing marked hydrocephalus.

Auditory evoked potentials and audiology are useful in the diagnosis of acoustic neuroma but are not nearly as diagnostic as an MRI scan. They can, however, find cases of eighth nerve dysfunction, which would not be apparent on imaging procedures. Careful assessment of hearing, one ear at a time, should be part of the neurological examination of headache patients because acoustic neuroma often presents with unilateral hearing loss.

A headache in the occiput with pain and stiffness in the neck sometimes exacerbated by turning the head can suggest an acoustic neuroma or other posterior fossa tumor. Acoustic neuroma can produce motor and sensory changes in the face and loss of corneal reflex. Tinnitus, vertigo, and hearing loss could also indicate that diagnosis. Acoustic neuromas are associated with a high CSF protein; this, plus obstruction of the aqueduct by tumor growth, can produce severe hydrocephalus. The development of ataxia, apraxia, incontinence, and Babinski signs, along with restriction of upward gaze or Parinaud's syndrome (which includes retraction nystagmus in the upward gaze position), indicates the need for prompt CT, MRI, and perhaps ventricular shunt placement.

Chronic hydrocephalus in the elderly, the so-called normal pressure or low pressure type, is not usually associated with headache but presents with personality changes, dementia, and gait disturbance with apraxia and incontinence.

Pseudotumor cerebri is a syndrome of brain swelling with generalized headaches seen in obese young women, particularly after hormone treatment or treatment with certain other drugs including tetracycline. The diagnosis is made by the observation of papilledema, sometimes with restricted upward gaze or even skew deviation. CT or MRI shows small ventricles, and CSF pressure is elevated on lumbar puncture. The CSF usually shows a low protein concentration.

Pseudotumor cerebri produces a diffuse headache sometimes accompanied by ophthalmological signs (Merikangas 1978) and should be suspected when CT or MRI reveals very small ventricles. Lumbar puncture must be performed to document high pressure of CSF and low protein. Pseudotumor is precipitated by a number of drugs including tetracyclines, by excess vitamin A, and by recent hormonal changes such as those brought on by pregnancy, birth control pills, or other estrogen treatment. Pseudotumor cerebri is treated with acetazolamide to reduce the production of CSF. Oral glycerol for osmotic shift, as well as steroids, may be needed to reduce intracranial pressure rapidly (Corbett and Thompson 1989). Ventricular shunting is necessary if all else fails. Patients with this condition frequently are quite anxious because they have gone from doctor to doctor and are falsely reassured that nothing is the matter because their CT scans are read as normal, even in the presence of very small ventricles, which are, after all, a normal finding in young people. Few, if any, focal neurologic signs are present.

An unusual headache related to position is produced by colloid cysts of the third ventricle. Bending over or leaning back produces a ball-valve effect that causes a sudden increase in intracerebral pressure accompanied by vomiting and sometimes loss of consciousness. These tumors are slow growing and benign but very difficult to reach surgically. However, surgical removal or shunting is required because they are life threatening. CT or MRI is the only way to diagnose them.

Headache Associated With Substances or Their Withdrawal

Drug abuse is an important consideration in the differential diagnosis of tension headache. The drug of abuse may not be illicit but, ironically, may be a medication prescribed to treat headaches, such as narcotics, acetaminophen, or ergotamine (Saper 1983). The most common drugs that may induce headaches on withdrawal are caffeine and nicotine. Caffeine is a potent cerebral vasoconstrictor which, if used to excess, will produce a withdrawal state accompanied by nervousness, irritability, and severe headache when the drug concentration falls below the usual level. This is likely to happen in the morning before the first cup of the day and in the afternoon before supper time. Many over-the-counter analgesics and many prescription headache compounds contain caffeine, which may contribute to the chronic headache associated with their abuse. Drugs that can cause headaches include nitrates, such as Isordil and nitroglycerin, MAOIs (even in the absence of hypertensive crisis), and tricyclic antidepressants (occasionally by exacerbation of narrow-angle glaucoma).

The headache of chronic analgesic abuse is treated by withdrawal from analgesics and narcotics. The headache of caffeine withdrawal is similarly treated by reduction in caffeine intake, which may be accomplished most satisfactorily by gradual replacement with decaffeinated coffee. There may be other chemicals in coffee besides caffeine that lead to headache, so decaffeinated coffee should also be limited in total amount.

Cigarette smoking is another major factor in chronic headache, partly because of allergic responses to the smoke and partly because of the increased incidence of nasopharyngeal and sinus infections in smokers. It has been suggested that about one-third of "migraine" sufferers will have a marked reduction in frequency and severity if they abstain from tobacco. Carbon monoxide contributes to the headache of cigarette smokers, perhaps by compensatory vasodilation of cerebral vessels.

Cocaine has also been added to the list of substances that may precipitate migraine (Satel and Gawin 1989), a fact that should be obvious to the user. Cocaine may also precipitate strokes and lacunar infarcts and thereby contribute to the personality changes seen in drug abusers. Headache is also a regular feature of narcotic abuse.

Everyone is familiar with the headache that results from overindulgence in alcohol, but this is quite distinct from the precipitation of an attack of migraine by even a small amount of red wine or malty beer in susceptible individuals (Littlewood et al. 1988). The chronic dull headache of hypervitaminosis A occurs among aficionados of vitamins and health food and goes away when excessive doses of vitamin A are withdrawn from the diet. The mechanism is not known.

A number of chemicals, including nitroglycerin, monosodium glutamate, alcohol, tyramine, many organic solvents, and carbon monoxide, may precipitate headaches. Exposure to these substances often will not be discovered on routine laboratory tests or brain images. Each of these headaches requires for diagnosis a careful history and an understanding of the patient's occupation and environment.

Headache Associated With Noncephalic Infection

Because fevers in general—particularly those caused by urinary tract infections or viremias—can cause headaches, measurement of temperature is an important step in the evaluation of headache. Surprisingly, it is often omitted in outpatient evaluations. Patients can be asked to take their temperature during a typical headache to evaluate this possibility. The ESR is an important measure that, if elevated, should lead to a search for the cause.

Headache Associated With Metabolic Disorder

Headaches that occur when the patient awakens in the morning or goes without eating during the day may be precipitated by hypoglycemia. A 5-hour glucose tolerance test may aid in the diagnosis. A high-protein, frequent-feeding diet may prevent the headaches. Hypoglycemia may also be stimulated by some artificial sweeteners or by diet soft drinks.

Pheochromocytoma-induced headache is usually very severe (like the headache of MAOI "cheese reaction") and accompanied by flushing. This headache may be precipitated by beta blockade in patients wrongly diagnosed as suffering from migraine.

Headache or Facial Pain Associated With Disorders of Cranium, Neck, Eyes, Ears, Nose, Sinuses, Teeth, Mouth, or Other Facial or Cranial Structures

Headache after "whiplash" injury can become chronic secondary to muscle strain or sprain. In cases of "fibromyositis"—a syndrome of muscle pain and stiffness frequently seen in women, often after an apparently mild injury and associated with depression—thermography can help to validate the diagnosis by demonstrating areas of abnormal heat corresponding to the "trigger zones" described by physical therapists. The areas of muscle spasm and tenderness are readily palpated in affected individuals. Thermography is also helpful over the temporomandibular joints and lends some credibility to patients who otherwise might be considered "psychosomatic" (Abernathy and Uematsu 1986). Amitriptyline or nortriptyline and exercise can be helpful to this group of patients, as can be reassurance that their headache is not "all in their head."

The so-called TMJ or temporomandibular joint syndrome is probably overdiagnosed, but it does exist. It may be diagnosed by palpating the pterygoid muscles through the patient's open mouth and by palpating the joints themselves while the patient makes chewing motions. Extreme tenderness on palpation is the typical finding. Trauma to the jaw may also cause the TMJ syndrome.

More common is the severe headache caused by acute malocclusion by dental repairs or fillings that shift the bite and cause muscle strain. Malocclusions may be treated by dental restorations, the grinding down of high fillings, or the wearing of a prosthetic bite plate. Serious temporomandibular joint derangements may need to be treated specifically with surgery. When headache appears temporally linked to recent dental work, a focused dental reassessment is indicated.

Sinus headaches may require drainage of sinuses by surgery, antihistamines or decongestants, or antibiotics, as well as by elimination of an offending allergen. However, many self-described sinus headaches actually meet criteria for migraine.

The headache of high cervical disc disease, which gives no other localizing signs, can be mistaken for neurosis or depression, especially if the patient has been accused of malingering for financial gain in a whiplash lawsuit. The MRI scan is useful in the diagnosis of cervical stenosis or bulging discs. Central discs may have few localizing signs except for pain, leg weakness, or urinary incontinence. Of course, cervical muscle strains and sprains are also genuine causes of occipital-parietal pain because of traction on the galea aponeurotica covering the skull. In diffuse head pain, the neck should be carefully examined.

Cervical spine strains, sprains, or chronic fatigue may be treated with exercise, massage, or amitriptyline or nortriptyline given in a single bedtime dose adequate to produce a good night's sleep without daytime sedation. Use of muscle relaxants such as diazepam should be avoided, if possible, because of the sedation produced and because dependence occurs fairly rapidly. If cervical disc derangement is present, wearing a soft cervical collar in the evening and while asleep during the night and home cervical traction is recommended. Neurosurgical referral is indicated if signs of spinal cord compression, weakness, or radicular pain are present.

Headache Associated With Cranial Neuralgias, Nerve Trunk Pain, and Deafferentation Pain

Trigeminal neuralgia is a specific syndrome that should not be mistaken for headache because it is paroxysmal, lancinating, and localized in a particular division of the trigeminal nerve. The syndrome of glossopharyngeal neuralgia should be recognized because it has exactly the same characteristics but a different distribution that occasionally leads to psychiatric referral because the complaint is so bizarre (i.e., severe unilateral pain in the region of the tonsil or the ear, provoked by yawning or eating). Carbamazepine is the drug of choice, although phenytoin, valproic acid, and baclofen also have been used with success. Surgical treatment (i.e., section of the nerve) has been successful in cases refractory to medication. In cases of trigeminal or glossopharyngeal neuralgia, a search should be made for a specific etiology, such as multiple sclerosis, aneurysms, or nerve entrapments.

Atypical facial pain, a pain in trigeminal distribution without the paroxysmal features of trigeminal neuralgia, may respond to antipsychotic or antidepressant medication. If a trial of antidepressants is ineffective, an antidepressant-neuroleptic combination may be useful (Taub and Collins 1974). Amitriptyline or nortriptyline is sometimes effective for other neuralgic head pains, including occipital neuralgia, the neuralgias of diabetic neuropathy, and postherpetic neuralgia.

HEADACHES IN CHILDREN

For discussion of headaches in childhood, the work of Barlow (1984) and Hockaday (1988) is recommended. Hallucinations are not uncommon in childhood migraine with both auditory and, more frequently, visual phenomena ranging from simple patterns and colors to complex scenes or voices. These may be mistaken for hysteria or psychosis. Hemiplegic migraine often begins with the syndrome of alternating hemiplegia occurring in childhood without headache. Motion sickness is a frequent childhood precursor of migraine and should be the subject of inquiry when taking the history. The benign paroxysmal vertigo of childhood may develop into classic migraine in adult life. Because of the high frequency of posterior fossa tumors in childhood, every serious chronic headache in a child requires a CT or MRI scan (Ford 1973). Visual evoked responses in children may prove to be a useful test in the diagnosis of migraine, revealing higher fast-wave amplitude and higher voltage; specificity of 96% has been reported (Mortimer et al. 1990).

Visual phenomena in migraine can be mistaken for hysteria if one is not aware of retinal migraine as a cause of apparently "nonphysiological" visual loss and the occurrence of scintillating scotomas and fortification spectra. Childhood migraine may be accompanied by marked changes in sensorium, as the following case example illustrates.

Case Example 7

A 16-year-old boy was referred by the neurosurgical service for psychiatric treatment for schizophrenia after having received an evaluation including lumbar puncture, EEG, and arteriography of the cerebral vasculature. He was a previously healthy high school football player who one morning awakened aphasic with a right hemiparesis. The symptoms had resolved shortly after he was transferred by helicopter from an outlying emergency room to the university hospital. When again able to speak, he told examining physicians that the voice of God had spoken to him that night and warned him that he was going to die. When he awakened he was certain that the prophecy was coming to pass.

On psychiatric interview he was an apparently normal young man without any sign of psychopathology that might lead one to consider either schizophrenia or a conversion reaction. A review of the family history, however, revealed that his mother suffered from classic migraine for many years, but that this had resolved after menopause. His mother also reported that the patient never had headaches but as a small child suffered from carsickness.

The patient was given no specific treatment at that time but was advised to call if there were any further problems. In a matter of weeks he called to report severe headaches consistent with migraine. During some of these, one or the other of his arms would occasionally feel weak. Prophylactic treatment with propranolol prevented any further symptoms.

SUMMARY

In summary, headache has numerous possible etiologies, many of which require specific treatment and some of which are life threatening or potentially disabling conditions. The success of therapy depends on identification of the cause. Thorough clinical and family histories, laboratory examinations, and imaging procedures should be completed in persons seeking treatment for headache. Application of the diagnostic criteria recently introduced by the International Headache Society will aid in the differential diagnosis and facilitate communication among professional caregivers. A high "up-front" cost of evaluation is warranted if a truly definitive diagnosis can be made.

Most headaches may be relieved or prevented unless the complicating factor of drug abuse is present. The famous sinus headache is frequently common migraine, and the true sinus headache may respond to amitriptyline because that medication is a very good antihistamine. Even if a patient is quite bizarre, attributing a headache to a primary psychiatric disorder is risky, and repeating neurologic evaluation at regular intervals if headaches persist is recommended to avoid diagnostic mistakes.

Psychiatric disorders are strongly associated with some subtypes of headache (especially migraine and atypical facial pain) and are rarely considered by specialists outside the field of psychiatry. These conditions should be considered in the selection of treatment for headaches, both to minimize psychiatric side effects of headache treatments and to achieve concomitant amelioration of psychiatric and headache symptoms whenever possible.

REFERENCES

Abernathy M, Uematsu S (eds:): Medical Thermology. Washington, DC, American Academy of Thermology, Georgetown University Medical Center, 1986

Anthony M: Review of beta-adrenoceptor blocking agents in migraine, in Migraine and Beta-Blockade. Edited by Carroll JD, Pfaffenrath V, Sjaastad O. Mölndal, Sweden, AB Hässle, 1988, pp 193–199

Barlow C: Headaches and Migraine in Childhood. Philadelphia, PA, JB Lippincott, 1984

Blau JN: Premonitory symptoms of migraine, in Basic Mechanisms of Headache. Edited by Olesen J, Edvinsson L. New York, Elsevier, 1988, pp 345–352

Cassidy WL, Flanagan NB, Spellman ME: Clinical observations in manic-depressive disease. JAMA 164:1535–1546, 1957

Corbett JJ, Thompson TH: The rational management of idiopathic intracranial hypertension. Arch Neurol 16:1049–1051, 1989

Couch JR, Hassanein RS: Amitriptyline in migraine prophylaxis. Arch Neurol 36:695–699, 1979

Couch JR, Ziegler DK, Hassanein R: Amitriptyline in the prophylaxis of migraine: effectiveness and relationship of antimigraine and antidepressant effects. Neurology 26:121–127, 1976

Dalessio DJ: Cluster headache, in Wolff's Headache and Other Head Pain. Edited by Dalessio DJ. New York, Oxford University Press, 1980, pp 163–170

Daroff RB, Whitney CM: Treatment of vascular headaches. Headache 26:470–472, 1986

Diamond S: Depressive headaches. Headache 4:255–258, 1964

Ekbom K: Lithium for cluster headache: review of the literature and preliminary results of long-term treatment. Headache 21:132–139, 1981

Fisher CM, Adams RD: Transient global amnesia. Acta Neurol Scand [Suppl] 9:183, 1964

Ford FR: Diseases of the Nervous System in Infancy, Childhood and Adolescence, 6th Edition. Springfield, IL, Charles C Thomas, 1973

Friedman AP: The so-called posttraumatic headache, in The Late Effects of Head Injury. Edited by Walker AE, Caveness WF, Critchley M. Springfield, IL, Charles C Thomas, 1969, pp 55–71

Friedman AP: Migraine. Med Clin North Am 62(3):481–494, 1978

Griffin SJ, Friedman MJ: Depressive symptoms in propranolol users. J Clin Psychiatry 47:453–457, 1986

Hockaday J: Headaches in children, in The Management of Headache. Edited by Rose FC. New York, Raven, 1988, pp 149–166

Humphrey PPA, Feniuk W, Perren MJ: Amitriptyline drugs in development: advances in serotonin receptor pharmacology. Headache 30 (suppl 1):12–16, 1990

Isler H: Migraine treatment as a cause of chronic migraine, in Advances in Migraine Research and Therapy. Edited by Rose FC. New York, Raven, 1982, pp 159–164

Isler H: Headache drugs provoking chronic headache: historical aspects and common misunderstandings, in Drug-Induced Headache. Edited by Diener H, Wilkinson M. Heidelberg, Springer-Verlag, 1988, pp 87–94

Johnson CE, Zimmerman RD: Imaging decisions in the evaluation of headache. MRI Decisions, May/June, 1989, pp 2–16

Kaiko RF, Foley KM, Grabinski PY, et al: Central nervous system excitatory effects of meperidine in cancer patients. Ann Neurol 13:180–185, 1983

Kudrow L: Comparative results of prednisone, methysergide, and lithium therapy in cluster headache, in Current Concepts in Migraine Research. Edited by Greene R. New York, Raven, 1978, pp 159–163

Kudrow L: Cluster headache: new concepts. Neurol Clin 1:369, 1983

Lishman WA: Organic Psychiatry, 2nd Edition. Oxford, Blackwell Scientific, 1987, pp 363–366

Littlewood J, Glover V, Davies PTG, et al: Red wine as a cause of migraine. Lancet 1:558–559, 1988

Melzack R: The tragedy of needless pain. Sci Am 262:27–33, 1990

Merikangas JR: Common neurologic syndromes in medical practice. Med Clin North Am 61:723–736, 1977

Merikangas JR: Skew deviation in pseudotumor cerebri. Ann Neurol 4:583, 1978

Merikangas K: Genetic epidemiology of migraine, in Migraine: A Spectrum of Ideas. Edited by Sandler M, Collins G. London, Oxford University Press, 1990, pp 40–50

Merikangas JR, Merikangas KR: Advances in pharmacologic treatment of migraine. Psychopharmacology 96 (suppl):14a, 1988a

Merikangas JR, Merikangas KR: Calcium channel blockers in MAO-I induced hypertensive crisis. Psychopharmacology 96 (suppl):229, 1988b

Merikangas KR, Risch N, Merikangas JR, et al: Migraine and depression: association and familial transmission. J Psychiatr Res 22:119–129, 1988

Merikangas K, Angst J, Isler H: Psychopathology and migraine: results of the Zurich Cohort Study of Young Adults. Arch Gen Psychiatry 47:849–853, 1990

Moersch FP: Psychic manifestations in migraine. Am J Psychiatry 80:698–716, 1924

Monro J, Bronstoff J, Carini C, et al: Food allergy in migraine. Lancet 2:1–4, 1980

Mortimer MJ, Good PA, Marsters JB, et al: Visual evoked responses in children with migraine: a diagnostic test. Lancet 1:75–77, 1990

Moskowitz MA, Henrickson BM, Markowitz S, et al: Intra- and extracranio vascular nociceptive mechanisms and the pathogenesis of head pain, in Basic Mechanisms of Headache. Edited by Olesen J, Edvinsson L. Amsterdam, Elsevier, 1988, pp 429–438

Olesen J, Edvinsson L: Basic Mechanisms of Headache. Amsterdam, Elsevier, 1988

Olesen J: Classification and diagnostic criteria for headache disorders, cranial neuralgias and facial pain. Cephalalgia 8 (suppl 7):1–96, 1988

Palus W, Botzel K, Plendl H, et al: Specificity of sumatriptin for abortion of migraine attacks. Lancet 1:51, 1990

Parker GB, Pryor DS, Tupling H: Why does migraine improve during clinical trial? Further results from a trial of cervical manipulation for migraine. Aust N Z J Med 10:192–198, 1980

Pearce JMS: Migraine: a cerebral disorder. Lancet 2:86–89, 1984

Peatfield RC, Fozard JR, Rose FC: Drug treatment of migraine, in Handbook of Clinical Neurology, Vol 48. Edited by Rose FC. Amsterdam, Elsevier, 1986, pp 173–216

Raskin NH: Headache. New York, Churchill Livingston, 1988, pp 183–187

Rose CF (ed): The Management of Headache. New York, Raven, 1988

Saper JR: Drug overdose among patients with headache. Neurol Clin 1:465–477, 1983

Saper JR: Drug treatment of headache: changing concepts and treatment strategies. Seminars in Neurology 7:178–192, 1987

Satel SL, Gawin FH: Migrainelike headache and cocaine use. JAMA 26:2995–2996, 1989

Selby G, Lance JW: Observations on 500 cases of migraine and allied vascular headache. J Neurol Neurosurg Psychiatry 23:23–32, 1960

Spiegel K, Kalb R, Pasternak GW: Analgesic activity of tricyclic antidepressants. Ann Neurol 13:462–465, 1983

Taub A, Collins WF: Observations on the treatment of denervation dysesthesia with psychotropic drugs, in Advances in Neurology, Vol 4. Edited by Bonica JJ. New York, Raven, 1974, pp 309–315

Tfelt-Hansen P: Efficacy of β-blockers in migraine: a critical review. Cephalalgia 6 (suppl 5):15–24, 1986

Watson CPN, Evans RJ: Chronic cluster headache: a review of 60 patients. Headache 27:158–165, 1987

Welch KMA: Migraine: a biobehavioral disorder. Arch Neurol 44:323–327, 1987

Wolff HG: Personality features and reactions of subjects with migraine. Archives of Neurology and Psychiatry 37:895–921, 1937

Zilkha K: Differential diagnosis of headache, in Management of Headache. Edited by Rose FC. New York, Raven, 1988, pp 21–24

Chapter 12

Neuroleptic Malignant Syndrome: Clinical Presentation, Pathophysiology, and Treatment

Daniel D. Sewell, M.D.
Dilip V. Jeste, M.D.

Occasionally, the practice of psychiatry involves making vital treatment decisions rapidly. Usually these decisions concern the management of a physical illness in a psychiatric patient. One such situation, the diagnosis and treatment of neuroleptic malignant syndrome (NMS), involves the psychiatrist in decisions with a substantial risk of mortality if errors are made. In this chapter, we provide current information regarding NMS.

HISTORICAL OVERVIEW

Documentation of clinical syndromes that sound very similar to NMS dates back to 1832 when Calmeil described psychotic patients

This work was supported, in part, by the Department of Veterans Affairs and by NIMH Grants 5R37-MH-43693, 1R01-MH-45131, 1P50-MH-45294, and 5R01-MH-45298.

who suddenly changed from agitated states to profound stupor and then died a short time later with hyperthermia (Ladame 1919). In retrospect, it seems likely that Calmeil was describing lethal catatonia.

Although Delay and co-workers (1960) are usually credited with the first descriptions of NMS, a case reported by Ayd (1956) appears very similar to those Calmeil described except that the patient Ayd described had been treated with a neuroleptic, chlorpromazine. This patient, a 41-year-old man with chronic schizophrenia, received treatment with increasing doses of chlorpromazine (up to 2,500 mg daily). After 3 weeks of treatment, he suddenly collapsed, developed a temperature of 108°F, experienced seizures, and died 9 hours later. The environmental temperature was high, and based on the information provided in the published report, it is difficult to know if this patient had only hyperpyrexia or NMS. Nonetheless, Ayd's case report seems to have special historical significance because it is the first published example of a patient developing a malignant febrile illness while receiving neuroleptic treatment (Sewell and Jeste 1989). The temporal association between the use of chlorpromazine and the development of the illness certainly does not prove causation, but it does require that chlorpromazine be considered as a possible cause.

NOMENCLATURE

The term *neuroleptic malignant syndrome* is unsatisfactory for several reasons: 1) NMS can occur in patients being withdrawn from dopamine-agonist drugs (Simpson and Davis 1984; Toru et al. 1981) as well as during the course of administration of dopamine-blocking drugs; 2) NMS has also occurred with the use of dopamine-depleting drugs (Burke et al. 1981) and with the use of metoclopramide (Friedman et al. 1987; Robinson et al. 1985); 3) it appears that the course of NMS in all cases is not always "malignant." However, the term NMS is so deeply rooted that it will not be discarded easily.

Some researchers, for example, Levinson and Simpson (1986), believe that NMS is frequently erroneously diagnosed. They propose that the term *extrapyramidal syndrome with fever* be used to describe a heterogeneous syndrome in which a primary cause of fever other than NMS can be found in a majority of patients. This issue of nomenclature is likely to remain unresolved for some time. For scientific reasons, we recommend the use of standardized diagnostic criteria (Keck et al. 1989b; Levenson 1985). However, although diagnostic precision is quite important for valid scientific research, clinically it is not always possible or relevant to treatment decisions. For example, if a patient with preexisting fever or delirium or both develops rigidity and an elevated creatine phosphokinase (CPK), an unequivocal diagnosis of NMS may not be possible. Nonetheless, we would recommend instituting the treatment protocol for NMS (see Table 12-4) as a part of the interventions provided to the patient. We discuss differential diagnosis and treatment issues in more detail in subsequent sections.

FREQUENCY OF NEUROLEPTIC MALIGNANT SYNDROME

The actual frequency of NMS remains unclear. We found eight retrospective studies of the frequency of NMS (Addonizio et al. 1986; Delay et al. 1960; Keck et al. 1989b; Mohan et al. 1985; Neppe 1984; Pope et al. 1986b; Shalev and Munitz 1986; Shalev et al. 1988). The frequencies reported in these studies ranged from 0.02–1.9%.

There have also been three prospective assessments of the frequency of NMS. Keck and associates (1987) completed an 18-month prospective study and found 6 cases of NMS out of approximately 679 patients receiving neuroleptics—a frequency of 0.9%. Using the criteria developed by Pope et al. (1986b), Gelenberg et al. (1988) identified only 1 case of NMS out of 1,470 patients treated with neuroleptics in a private psychiatric hospital over a 1-year period. They calculated the frequency of NMS to be 0.07%, much lower than most other published estimates. Deng et al. (1990) recently published the results of a prospective study conducted between January 1980 and December 1986 of the prevalence of NMS in patients hospitalized at a 700-bed psychiatric hospital in China. The authors identified 12 cases of NMS out of an estimated 9,792 inpatients treated with neuroleptic medication. Based on these results, Deng et al. estimated the prevalence of NMS to be 0.123%.

Regional differences in neuroleptic use, including average total daily dose, and differences in study methodology, including diagnostic criteria, account for these large differences in the reported frequency of NMS. In addition, institutions vary in their therapeutic response to milder extrapyramidal syndromes that may be prodromal to NMS.

Table 12-1.   Putative risk factors for neuroleptic malignant syndrome (NMS)

Affective illness
Concurrent lithium treatment
Dehydration
Depot fluphenazine
Discontinuation of dopaminergic drugs
Exhaustion
Intramuscular injections
Male gender
Preexisting medical or neurologic illness
Previous history of NMS
Psychomotor agitation
Rapid neuroleptization
Rapid reintroduction of neuroleptic following an episode of NMS
Use of high-potency neuroleptic

RISK FACTORS

There are no published prospective studies of possible risk factors for NMS. However, a number of retrospective studies including a case-control study (Keck et al. 1989a) have identified clinical factors that appear to be associated with the development of NMS. The absence of prospective studies requires that these factors be considered potential or presumptive risk factors rather than proven risk factors. Table 12-1 lists putative risk factors in alphabetical order.

One putative risk factor is preexisting medical and neurologic illness. In a case report review of 53 cases published between 1979 and 1984, Levenson (1985) found 18 patients whose primary or secondary diagnosis was a medical or neurologic illness. Lazarus and colleagues (1989) analyzed 195 case reports of NMS and found 25 patients with organic brain syndrome (13%) and 12 (6%) with mental retardation. Of 203 case reports reviewed by Shalev and associates (1989), 41 patients had a concurrent diagnosis of organic central nervous system (CNS) disease. The most common diagnoses were alcoholism ($n = 7$), brain damage and/or trauma ($n = 5$), and mental retardation ($n = 4$). HIV-positive psychotic patients may be unusually sensitive to neuroleptics and have a greater risk of various side effects including NMS (Baer 1989; Harris and Jeste 1989). In addition, a number of medical problems, such as dehydration and exhaustion, have been discussed as potential risk factors for NMS. These findings suggest that NMS is not uncommon in medical settings.

A number of authors including Caroff (1980) and Levenson (1985) found that published cases of NMS in men outnumber cases in women by a ratio of 2:1. Individuals with mood disorders may be at greater risk for NMS just as they may have increased susceptibility to tardive dyskinesia. In a review of 330 cases, Pearlman (1986) found that at least 40% of the reported diagnoses involved affective conditions. In case reports reviewed by Addonizio and colleagues (1987) that included a psychiatric diagnosis, 44% of patients suffered from some form of affective illness.

A past history of NMS, especially a recent episode, has also been suggested as a risk factor. In a recently published study of neuroleptic rechallenge after NMS, Rosebush and co-workers (1989) found that successful rechallenge was significantly related to the length of time since resolution of an episode of NMS. Specifically, they reported that "neuroleptics were successfully reintroduced in virtually all cases in which there was an interval of at least 2 weeks following resolution of the previous NMS episode, whereas neuroleptics were poorly tolerated when less than 2 weeks had elapsed" (Rosebush et al. 1989, p. 296). In their recently published case-control study, Keck et al. (1989a) reported that patients with psychomotor agitation were overrepresented in the NMS group.

Shalev and Munitz (1986) studied the effect of neuroleptic loading rate on the development of NMS and found that antipsychotic dose increases regularly preceded the development of NMS. Keck and colleagues (1989a) found that patients with NMS received significantly higher doses of neuroleptics, and that dose increases were more rapid in the NMS group. They also found an association between the number of intramuscular injections and the occurrence of NMS. The use of high-potency neuroleptics and concurrent lithium treatment have been suggested as risk factors; however, findings of a recent study (Sewell and Jeste 1990) did not confirm this suggestion. Deng et al. (1990) found that depot fluphenazine decanoate, especially when used without an antiparkinsonian agent, was a risk factor. The abrupt discontinuation of dopaminergic drugs is one last putative treatment-related risk factor (Simpson and Davis 1984; Toru et al. 1981).

CLINICAL PRESENTATION

NMS can present in a number of different medical and psychiatric settings. The setting in which NMS is most likely to present is not known, but because patients with preexisting medical or neurologic illness may be at greater risk, a fair number of cases can be expected among patients hospitalized on medical or neurologic inpatient units. In addition, patients from outpatient psychiatry clinics or state psychiatric hospitals with suspected NMS often are immediately transferred to general hospital emergency rooms. NMS is also likely to be seen in settings in which relatively large doses of antipsychotics are used, such as acute inpatient psychiatry wards.

In a retrospective study of 120 case reports, NMS occurred as soon as 45 minutes or as late as 65 days after the administration of a new neuroleptic (Shalev and Munitz 1986). In most cases, NMS appeared within 10 days of administration of a new drug.

The rate of evolution of symptoms in NMS is controversial. Resolution of this controversy is difficult because increased recognition of NMS has led to earlier intervention and this intervention has altered the natural history of the syndrome. The study conducted by Shalev and Munitz (1986, p. 339) revealed that "in more than 90% of the cases the full syndrome was present within 48 hours of the first symptoms." However, Addonizio and associates (1987) reported that NMS may not necessarily be a fulminant reaction. Although 67 of the 85 cases for whom they had sufficient data developed fulminant NMS within 3 days, in the remaining 18 cases (21%), the full-blown syndrome took 4–30 days to appear.

Addonizio and colleagues (1987) analyzed all the case reports in the English-language literature up to 1987 ($n = 115$). Tachycardia was present in 97% of the reported patients. A temperature over 38°C (100.4°F) was reported in 92% of the cases. Rigidity was present in 91% of the cases, and diaphoresis was present in 57%. Systolic blood pressure greater than 140 mmHg occurred in 55%; diastolic pressure greater than 90 mmHg occurred in 49%.

Addonizio and colleagues (1987) analyzed laboratory data and noted that CPK was elevated in 97% of the case reports that included CPK values. Leukocytosis was present in 78% of the cases. Most of the cases that included lumbar punctures had normal cerebrospinal fluids. Similarly, most computed tomography scans were normal, and most of the EEGs were normal or showed nonspecific slowing.

DIAGNOSIS AND DIFFERENTIAL DIAGNOSIS

Although the diagnostic criteria for NMS used by different researchers are not currently identical, most criteria include the following four features: hyperthermia, extrapyramidal symptoms, autonomic instability, and mental status changes. Levenson (1985) and Pope and co-workers (1986b) have proposed operational criteria for establishing the diagnosis of NMS.

Levenson (1985) borrows the format used in the revised Jones criteria (American Heart Association 1965) for diagnosing rheumatic fever to organize criteria for NMS. Levenson classifies fever, rigidity, and elevated CPK as major manifestations, and lists the following minor manifestations: tachycardia, abnormal blood pressure, tachypnea, altered consciousness, diaphoresis, and leukocytosis. According to Levenson (1985), if all three major or two major and four minor manifestations are present and if the clinical history is appropriate, the diagnosis of NMS should be made.

The criteria developed by Pope and co-workers (1986b) and recently revised by Keck and associates (1989b) require the following three items for a definite diagnosis: 1) oral temperature of at least 38.0°C in the absence of another known etiology; 2) at least two extrapyramidal side effects from the following list: lead-pipe muscle rigidity, pronounced cogwheeling, sialorrhea, oculogyric crisis, retrocollis, opisthotonos, trismus, dysphagia, choreiform movements, dyskinetic movements, festinating gait, and flexor-extensor posturing; and 3) autonomic dysfunction characterized by two or more of the following: hypertension, tachycardia, tachypnea, prominent diaphoresis, and incontinence. According to these criteria, if the diagnosis is being made retrospectively and if one of the above items is missing, the diagnosis of NMS should still be made if clouded consciousness, leukocytosis (>15,000 white blood cells/mm³), or elevated serum CPK (>1,000 units/ml) is present.

NMS-like symptoms generate an extensive differential diagnosis. A thorough, but not exhaustive, list of differential diagnoses for NMS would include lethal catatonia (also called "Stauder's lethal catatonia"), malignant hyperthermia, serotonin syndrome, lithium toxicity, monoamine oxidase inhibitor (MAOI)–associated toxicity, central anticholinergic syndrome, extrapyramidal symptoms with fever from an identifiable medical cause, strychnine poisoning, tetany, heatstroke, and rhabdomyolysis. We limit our discussion of the differential diagnosis to the following four conditions: lethal catatonia, heatstroke, malignant hyperthermia, and other drug-induced conditions including serotonin syndrome. Table 12-2 lists important diagnostic differences among some of these disorders.

Table 12-2. Differential diagnosis of neuroleptic malignant syndrome (NMS)

	Lethal catatonia	Heatstroke	Malignant hyperthermia	Serotonin syndrome	NMS
Clinical setting					
Ambient temperature	May be elevated	Always elevated	Rarely elevated	Rarely elevated	May be elevated
Previously recognized psychiatric illness	Almost always	Not necessarily	Not necessarily	Almost always	Almost always
Onset of symptoms	May have had weeks or months of manic or schizophrenic symptoms	No prodrome; symptoms develop over several hours	Symptoms develop rapidly within hours of administration of anesthesia	No prodrome; usually within days to months of serotonergic drug use	No consistent prodrome; usually within hours to months of neuroleptic use
Antecedent pharmacologic treatment					
Anesthesia	Never	Never	Always	Never	Never

Muscle cell depolarizing agents	Never	Never	Always	Never	Never
Neuroleptics	Sometimes	Sometimes	Sometimes	Sometimes	Usually
Serotonergic agents	Sometimes	Sometimes	Sometimes	Always	Sometimes
Clinical features					
Autonomic dysfunction	Sometimes	Rarely	Rarely	Rarely	Always
Alternating episodes of stupor/posturing with catatonic excitement/agitation	Often	Never	Never	Never	Rarely
Diaphoresis	Sometimes	Absent	Sometimes	Sometimes	Commonly
Rigidity	Intermittently	Absent	Present	Present	Present
Flaccid paralysis with curare	Always	Always	Never	Always	Always

Lethal Catatonia

Catatonia literally means a lowering of tension (Hinsie and Campbell 1974). Clinically, the term refers to a syndrome characterized by either stupor or overactivity, resulting from a number of different conditions. *Lethal catatonia* is also a nonspecific term that is used to describe a syndrome caused occasionally by identifiable brain disease but more often appearing as an end-stage heat exhaustion syndrome in cases of uncontrolled manic or catatonic excitement (Caroff 1980).

Differentiation between NMS and lethal catatonia is not easy. However, Guzé and Baxter (1985) suggest that autonomic dysfunctions or involuntary movements are more common in NMS. In their review, Castillo and colleagues (1989) challenged the notion that lethal catatonia is clinically indistinguishable from NMS. They describe differences in mode of onset, signs and symptoms, and outcome; for example, no consistent prodromal phase has been described for NMS. However, some researchers believe that severe dystonia that does not respond to conventional treatment may represent a prodrome for NMS (B. Fogel, December 1989, personal communication). With this possibility in mind, we would amend the observation by Castillo and co-workers (1989) in the following way: A characteristic and invariably present prodrome has not been consistently described for NMS. In addition, Castillo and colleagues point out that periods of catatonic excitement alternating with periods of stupor are not characteristic of NMS.

Addonizio and Susman (1987) suggest that electroconvulsive therapy (ECT) may deserve a trial when it is difficult to distinguish between NMS and an evolving catatonic state.

Neuroleptic-induced catatonia.   Neuroleptic-induced catatonia is a relatively rare condition that develops particularly after the use of high-potency neuroleptic medication (Lohr et al., in press). The clinician may fail to recognize neuroleptic-induced catatonia because it may look exactly like the catatonia associated with the underlying psychiatric illness. The temporal relationship between the onset of catatonic symptoms and the initiation of neuroleptic treatment may help to identify the etiology of the catatonia. For example, if the patient did not have catatonic symptoms before neuroleptic treatment, then the catatonic symptoms may have been caused by the neuroleptic. The syndrome may also occur with metoclopramide. Successful treatment with amantadine and anticholinergics has been reported, although Lohr and colleagues (in press) reported successful treatment with lorazepam. In general, this syndrome should be considered a profound extrapyramidal reaction to neuroleptics and treated as such. Treatment should usually begin with amantadine, 100 mg bid. It may take 2–3 weeks for the syndrome to resolve (Stoudemire and Luther 1984).

Heatstroke

Heatstroke and NMS share some clinical features. In addition, neuroleptics increase the risk of heatstroke by reducing peripheral heat loss. Clinical features that distinguish heatstroke from NMS include the absence of diaphoresis, the absence of rigidity, low or normal rather than elevated blood pressures, and the absence of a markedly increased CPK (Haggerty and Gillette 1987). Finally, heatstroke is likely to occur in hot, humid weather or following heavy exercise or agitation and is more likely in patients on anticholinergic drugs. These clinical features are not common precipitants of NMS.

Malignant Hyperthermia

Malignant hyperthermia is a genetic disorder characterized by a hypermetabolic state of skeletal muscles and typically follows the administration of halogenated anesthetic agents and succinylcholine. Presenting features include tachycardia, hypertonicity, hyperpyrexia, and elevated CPK. Curare and pancuronium, which are peripherally acting, nondepolarizing, neuromuscular blocking agents, produce a flaccid paralysis in NMS but not in malignant hyperthermia. These agents usually produce an intensification of rigidity when administered to patients with malignant hyperthermia (Britt 1983).

Other Drug-Induced Conditions, Including Serotonin Syndrome

Drug interactions between drugs that increase effective CNS concentrations of serotonin (such as certain antidepressants including clomipramine, fluoxetine, various MAOIs, and tryptophan) may cause a syndrome that resembles NMS. Features of this syndrome commonly include fever, resting tremor, rigidity, myoclonus, and generalized seizures. This syndrome has been called the serotonin syndrome (Gerson and Baldessarini 1980). A careful history, physical examination, and urine and blood toxicology usually help to distinguish between NMS and serotonin syndrome. However, in cases in which both serotonergic drugs and neuroleptics have been administered, it is difficult to distinguish between these two syndromes, as the recent case report by Kline and colleagues (1989) demonstrates. Appropriate treatment of serotonin syndrome includes discontinuation of all serotonergic medications. In more severe cases, the use of a serotonin antagonist, such as cyproheptadine, may be considered (Warner 1987).

Patients with anticholinergic toxicity have dry, flushed skin, but patients with NMS have episodes of prominent diaphoresis. Other characteristics of patients with anticholinergic toxicity distinguishing them from patients with NMS include dry mucous membranes, decreased bowel sounds, and urinary retention. Although patients with anticholinergic toxicity have dilated pupils, pupillary size is not a reliable way to distinguish between these two conditions because patients with NMS may also have dilated pupils. A brief symptomatic improvement with physostigmine is usually seen in anticholinergic toxicity; however, this treatment should not be used to differentiate between NMS and anticholinergic toxicity because physostigmine may cause complications in a patient who is already quite ill.

CLINICAL COURSE

Respiratory failure and renal failure are the two most common medical complications of NMS. Respiratory failure may occur secondary to tachypneic hypoventilation, aspiration, infection, pulmonary embolism, shock (Lavie et al. 1986), or adult respiratory distress syndrome. Rhabdomyolysis with extremely high serum CPK levels, hyperkalemia, myoglobinuria, and acute renal insufficiency has been reported in 26% of cases (Levenson 1985).

The mortality rate reported for NMS varies between 4% and 25%. Wider recognition and more rapid and effective interventions may be decreasing the mortality rate (Pearlman 1986; Shalev et al. 1989). Shalev and associates (1989) studied the mortality of NMS by reviewing 202 published case reports and observed a decrease in mortality—25% before 1984 and 11.6% after 1984. This decrease in mortality occurred independently of treatment with dopamine agonists and dantrolene. In addition, the rate of mortality was lower from NMS induced by haloperidol compared with other agents (7%, $P < .001$) and the rate of mortality was relatively higher among patients with organic mental syndrome (38.5%). However, diagnoses and reports of milder forms of NMS may also contribute to the reported decreases in mortality rate.

Reported causes of death in NMS include cardiorespiratory arrest, pneumonia, pulmonary embolism, sepsis, and hepatorenal failure. Shalev and associates (1989) reported that myoglobinemia and renal failure are strong predictors of mortality; the presence of either condition was associated with a mortality risk of approximately 50%.

PATHOPHYSIOLOGY

The pathophysiology of NMS remains unclear. Two categories of theories have appeared in the literature: those that provide an explanation for the fever associated with NMS and those that provide a pathophysiologic basis for all features of the syndrome.

Explanation of the Fever

There are several possible explanations for the fever seen in patients with NMS: 1) disordered central thermal regulation, 2) heat generation by muscle contraction, 3) nonshivering thermogenesis, 4) impairment of heat dissipating mechanisms, and 5) medical factors such as concurrent infection or dehydration. The first explanation, disordered central thermal regulation, suggests that dopamine plays an important role in the thermoregulatory centers of the hypothalamus. For more information about these hypotheses, see our recently published review (Sewell and Jeste 1989).

Pathophysiologic Hypotheses

Table 12-3 lists several hypotheses suggested by the literature as possible pathophysiologic explanations of NMS and relevant literature citations. We limit the discussion of these proposed theories to the two hypotheses that have generated the most interest: 1) decreased function of dopamine neurons and 2) pathophysiologic processes similar to those seen in malignant hyperthermia. For additional information about the other three theories, see the literature cited in Table 12-3 and Sewell and Jeste (1989).

Decreased function of dopamine neurons.   NMS may result from

Table 12-3.   Pathophysiologic hypotheses for neuroleptic malignant
syndrome

Theory	Relevant citations in the literature
Decreased dopamine function	Addonizio et al. 1987 Burke et al. 1981 Caroff 1980 Cox and Lee 1977 Harris et al. 1987 Hashimoto et al. 1984 Kashihara and Ishida 1988 Kurlan et al. 1985 Lazarus 1985 Levenson 1985 Levinson and Simpson 1986 Norman et al. 1987 Pearlman 1986 Smego and Durack 1982 Ungvari 1987
Pathophysiologic processes similar to malignant hyperthermia	Addonizio et al. 1987 Burke et al. 1981 Caroff 1980 Caroff et al. 1983, 1987 Downey et al. 1984 Hermesh et al. 1988, 1989 Lazarus 1985 Levenson 1985 Levinson and Simpson 1986 Scarlett et al. 1983 Tollefson 1982 Tollefson and Garvey 1984 Yamawaki et al. 1986
Serotonergic hyperfunction in the hypothalamus	Yamawaki et al. 1986
Excessive catecholamine secretion	Addonizio et al. 1987 Feibel and Schiffer 1981 Hashimoto et al. 1984 Levenson 1985 Schibuk and Schachter 1986
Relative gamma-aminobutyric acid (GABA) deficiency	Addonizio et al. 1987 Lew and Tollefson 1983 Pearlman 1986

diminished dopaminergic function in specific brain areas such as the hypothalamus, nigrostriatal system, and corticolimbic tracts. This theory explains all of the major manifestations associated with NMS: decreased dopamine in the hypothalamic tracts to explain fever and autonomic instability, lowered functional dopamine levels in the nigrostriatal system to explain rigidity, and diminished dopamine in the corticolimbic tracts to explain mental status changes. The evidence in support of this theory is mostly indirect. For example, antipsychotics are known to be dopamine-blocking agents. In addition, dopamine agonists, such as bromocriptine, carbidopa, and levodopa (Harris et al. 1987), may help to resolve NMS.

Although dopamine receptors are located in the periphery (Clark 1985), it is unlikely that they play a role in the development of NMS. Peripheral dopamine receptors have been detected on smooth muscle cells in blood vessels and certain exocrine glands and on cell bodies and terminal varicosities of sympathetic nerves (Clark 1985); however, dopamine receptors have not been found on skeletal muscle cells.

Pathologic processes similar to those seen in malignant hyperthermia. The shared clinical features of malignant hyperthermia and NMS, such as fever, muscular rigidity, and elevated CPK, have led a number of investigators to compare NMS and malignant hyperthermia. Thus, muscle biopsy specimens from NMS patients, like those from patients susceptible to malignant hyperthermia, exhibited increased muscle tension when exposed to halothane or caffeine (Caroff et al. 1983, 1987; Downey et al. 1984). However, other researchers could not confirm these findings (Krivosic-Horber et al. 1987; Scarlett et al. 1983; Tollefson 1982).

Hermesh and co-workers (1989) studied the relationship between these two disorders by conducting a retrospective study and tried to elucidate the risk of malignant hyperthermia in psychiatric patients who suffered from NMS. Of 20 patients who had NMS and their 108 first-degree relatives, none of the patients or their first-degree relatives had ever experienced malignant hyperthermia. The researchers concluded that patients with a history of NMS are not at a considerably greater risk for developing malignant hyperthermia (Hermesh et al. 1989). However, this study has been criticized by Caroff and colleagues (1989). In retrospective studies, up to 70% of patients susceptible to malignant hyperthermia had not developed hyperthermia during general anesthesia administered on previous occasions (Caroff et al. 1989).

Yamawaki and co-workers (1986) have attempted to demonstrate a pathophysiologic link between NMS and malignant hyperthermia by using a third approach, which was inspired because dantrolene has been successfully used in the treatment of both conditions (Yamawaki 1986). The approach also incorporates the theory that both dopaminergic and serotonergic mechanisms are involved in thermoregulation (Yamawaki et al. 1983).

The pathophysiologic mechanism in malignant hyperthermia is believed to be an abnormality of calcium metabolism in skeletal muscle. Calcium ions play an important role in regulating neurotransmitter release, and Yamawaki and colleagues (1986) believe that an abnormality of calcium metabolism in hypothalamic cells leads to serotonergic hyperfunction, which, in turn, leads to the development of NMS. Yamawaki and co-workers hypothesized that dantrolene corrects an abnormality in intraneuronal handling of calcium, which leads to a decrease in serotonin release and a subsequent resolution of NMS.

To gather support for their theories, Yamawaki and colleagues (1988) developed an animal model of NMS and then examined the effects of dantrolene on serotonin release in the hypothalamus. Their model involves the microinjection of veratrine, an intracellular calcium releaser, into the preoptic anterior hypothalamus. These injections induced hyperthermia and other abnormal behaviors in rats pretreated with haloperidol but not in saline-treated rats. The hyperthermia induced by veratrine plus haloperidol was blocked by dantrolene in a dose-dependent manner. In addition, cyproheptadine, a serotonin antagonist, partially blocked the hyperthermia induced by veratrine plus haloperidol.

TREATMENT

There have been no controlled studies of the treatments of NMS, and as a result, the efficacy of various treatments or combinations of treatments remains unclear.

In lieu of a prospective study, retrospective studies of the efficacy of various treatments have been conducted. However, these studies have also been limited by methodological problems. For example, in the published case reports, there is marked variability in the time between onset of NMS and the initiation of treatment, the dosages of medication given, the use of concomitant medications, and the duration of treatment.

General Measures

Early recognition of NMS and immediate discontinuation of dopamine-blocking agents are of crucial importance. It has been our and others' experience (B.S. Fogel and A. Stoudemire, October 1990, personal communication) that appropriate treatment for NMS is sometimes delayed because of uncertainty over the accuracy of the diagnosis. Because of the seriousness and potential lethality of NMS, the NMS treatment algorithm (Table 12-4) should be instituted quickly in probable cases, even if the diagnosis is not certain.

Important supportive measures include antipyretic medications, intravenous fluids, and serial monitoring of pertinent laboratory values, including serum electrolytes, serum creatinine, blood urea nitrogen (BUN), CPK, and urine myoglobin. Depending on the severity of the episode, patients may require transfer to an intensive care unit.

Relevant laboratory tests should be obtained daily as long as the patient is experiencing the signs and symptoms of NMS. Daily CPK determinations provide a means of monitoring the impact of treatment efforts. Measuring electrolyte values on a daily basis is necessary because of the likely occurrence of hyperkalemia if rhabdomyolysis is present (Flamenbaum et al. 1983), the administration of intravenous fluids, and the possibility of diminished renal function. Regular measurements of serum CPK, BUN, and urine myoglobin permit an estimation of renal damage and residual renal function.

Research by Eneas and associates (1979) showed that hydration, bicarbonate therapy, and diuresis with mannitol and/or loop diuretics may help prevent acute renal failure in patients with severe rhabdomyolysis and myoglobinuria; these complications are common in NMS (Lavie et al. 1986). Fluid intake and output should be closely monitored. Urine output that is consistently less than 400 ml/day (oliguria) suggests the presence of significant renal injury (Rudnik et al. 1983).

If agitation is a clinically significant problem, initial interventions should include minimizing environmental stimulation, providing frequent reassurance, observing closely, and setting firm limits on inappropriate behaviors. If these efforts are unsuccessful in managing the agitation, pharmacologic treatment with a medium- to long-acting benzodiazepines may be necessary.

Drug Treatments

Dopamine agonists—bromocriptine. The possibility that decreased function of dopamine neurons in various specific brain regions

Table 12-4.   Flow chart for the treatment of neuroleptic malignant
syndrome (NMS)

Step 1: Review patient medication regimen

  A. Discontinue dopamine antagonists
  B. Resume treatment with any recently discontinued dopamine agonists

Step 2: Initiate and maintain supportive measures

  A. Monitor vital signs
  B. Intravenous fluids
  C. Cooling blankets
  D. Antipyretic medications
  E. Mannitol or loop diuretics for oliguria or myoglobinuria

Step 3: If patient is severely ill or does not improve within 12–24 hours after the
interventions above and if patient can take medication orally, begin treatment
with bromocriptine

  A. Initial dose: 5 mg po tid
  B. Increase dose daily in 5-mg increments tid until positive response is
      noted; then fix dose
  C. Continue "fixed dose" for 10 days; then gradually withdraw over a 1-week
      period
  D. During withdrawal, monitor closely for relapse of NMS, especially if
      patient had been receiving depot neuroleptics
  E. If symptoms recur, return to lowest dose at which the patient was
      symptom free, continue this dose for 1 week, then resume tapering

Step 4: If patient cannot take medication orally or if bromocriptine causes intolerable
nausea or other severe side effects, begin treatment with intravenous
dantrolene

  A. Initial dose 1–2 mg/kg body weight
  B. If the patient responds, give the same dose qid
  C. If no response is observed after several hours, give another dose 25%
      larger than the initial dose
  D. Continue to give gradually increasing doses every several hours until a
      response is observed. The dose at which a response occurs should then be
      given qid
  E. Doses higher than 10 mg/day are usually not necessary and are relatively
      contraindicated because of hepatotoxicity

Step 5: As soon as patient can take medication orally, add bromocriptine

  A. Follow procedure outlined in Step 3
  B. Once patient demonstrates global improvement in the symptoms of NMS,
      discontinue dantrolene

Step 6: If patient's condition has not improved at all after 3–4 days despite the
interventions outlined above, consider electroconvulsive therapy

---

underlies the development of NMS provides the theoretical basis for the use of dopamine agonists in the treatment of NMS. Our discussion is limited to the dopamine agonist most commonly used in the treatment of NMS, bromocriptine. The reported proportion of NMS patients who have been helped by bromocriptine ranges from 87 to 100% (Addonizio et al. 1987; Lavie et al. 1986; Levinson and Simpson 1986). However, it is not clear if bromocriptine actually resolves the underlying pathology in NMS or if it provides only symptomatic treatment.

For NMS patients who are able to swallow, bromocriptine is the best initial drug treatment because it appears to be more consistently effective than other drug treatments such as dantrolene. (See discussion on dantrolene below.) Although bromocriptine could be administered via nasogastric tube for patients who are unable to swallow, this treatment is not recommended because of the risk of aspiration. The recommended starting dose is 15 mg daily in three doses (Mueller 1985). The dosage should be increased daily in 5-mg increments given three times daily (a total daily increase of 15 mg) until a positive response is noted or until side effects preclude further dose increases. Because of physiologic changes associated with aging, in older patients we recommend a starting dose of 7.5 mg daily in three doses, with total daily dose increases of no more than 7.5 mg if necessary. Once an optimal dose has been established, it should be continued for 10 days and then gradually withdrawn over a 1-week period while the patient is closely monitored for a recurrence of NMS symptoms. If signs or symptoms of NMS reappear, the dose should be returned to the lowest dose at which no signs or symptoms were present. This dose should be continued for several days before resuming the taper.

Dantrolene.   Dantrolene is a directly acting muscle relaxant and was helpful in 75–89% of the cases in which it was administered (Addonizio et al. 1987; Lavie et al. 1986; Levinson and Simpson 1986). The exact mechanism of action of dantrolene in NMS, whether central or peripheral, is not known.

If a patient is unable to swallow, if bromocriptine causes poorly tolerated side effects, or if bromocriptine is ineffective and the patient is severely ill, then intravenous infusion of dantrolene is indicated. Published recommendations regarding the appropriate dose of dantrolene for the treatment of NMS have varied from 0.25–3 mg/kg four times daily (Mueller 1985) to 4–10 mg/kg daily (Bismuth et al. 1984). We recommend administering a an initial dose of 1–2 mg/kg. If the patient responds, this dose should then be administered four times daily. If no response is noted after several hours, a 25%-larger dose than the original dose should be given. Gradually increasing doses of dantrolene should be continued every several hours until a response is observed. The dose at which a response occurs should then be administered four times daily. According to Mueller (1985), individual doses of greater than 3 mg/kg usually are not needed. Doses higher than 10 mg/kg/day usually are not necessary and are contraindicated because of hepatotoxicity.

Mueller (1985) recommends that as soon as the patient's musculature relaxes sufficiently to permit the use of oral medication, treatment with bromocriptine should be initiated. Controversy exists regarding whether dantrolene is as effective as bromocriptine at relieving the CNS symptoms of NMS. Mueller (1985) and others believe that dantrolene is not as effective as bromocriptine for CNS symptoms and that bromocriptine should be started as soon as possible and dantrolene be discontinued once bromocriptine has begun to relieve the CNS symptoms. One case report (Granato et al. 1983) described prolonged, continued use of both bromocriptine and dantrolene. Concurrent administration of dantrolene and bromocriptine may be an effective and rational strategy for treating NMS (Granato et al. 1983), but we hesitate to recommend this combined treatment until more scientific information demonstrates that continued combined treatment is more effective and no less safe than treatment with a single agent.

The most serious adverse reaction associated with dantrolene is dose-related liver toxicity, which has an incidence of 0.1%. Patients who appear to be at greatest risk for hepatotoxicity are those who are over age 30 years and who have received more than 300 mg daily for more than 60 days. Hepatotoxicity is not likely when total daily doses of 200 mg or less have been administered. Baseline liver function tests (serum glutamic-oxaloacetic transaminase [SGOT] or serum glutamic-pyruvic transaminase [SGPT] and alkaline phosphatase) should be obtained before beginning therapy with dantrolene and then repeated monthly. Dantrolene is contraindicated in patients with active hepatic disease (AMA Division of Drugs 1983).

Anticholinergics. The hypothesis that NMS may represent an extreme form of an extrapyramidal reaction provides the rationale for using anticholinergic drugs to treat NMS. However, evidence shows they are only minimally helpful in the treatment of NMS (Lavie et al. 1986). Because anticholinergics may worsen hyperthermia by inhibition of sweating (Pearlman 1986), anticholinergics may actually be contraindicated in febrile patients.

Electroconvulsive Therapy

ECT is believed to be effective in the treatment of NMS because it increases dopamine turnover in the brain (Pearlman 1986). Published clinical reports and opinions regarding the appropriateness of treating NMS with ECT are mixed. ECT may be indicated for the persistently psychotic and agitated patient in whom it is difficult to distinguish between NMS and lethal catatonia and when there appears to be significant risk of recurrence of NMS on restarting neuroleptics (Addonizio and Susman 1987; Addonizio et al. 1987). However, careful monitoring of cardiac function is very important because of a possibly increased risk of cardiac arrest in patients with autonomic instability (Pearlman 1986).

MANAGEMENT OF PSYCHOSIS IN PATIENTS WITH A HISTORY OF NEUROLEPTIC MALIGNANT SYNDROME

It is not yet known how often and when NMS is likely to recur. Only limited scientific evidence is available regarding when neuroleptics can be safely readministered to a patient who has experienced an episode of NMS. Challenge with the same drug resulted in recurrence in six of the eight patients in whom it was attempted (Shalev and Munitz 1985). Recurrence was rare in cases rechallenged with a low-potency antipsychotic.

Susman and Addonizio (1988) observed that 16 of 20 patients with recurrence had been given neuroleptics within the first 2 weeks after the development of NMS. Unlike Shalev and Munitz (1985), Susman and Addonizio (1988) found no clear relationship between the potency of the neuroleptic administered and recurrence of NMS; specifically, both high-potency and low-potency neuroleptics triggered recurrence.

Rosebush and associates (1989) studied reintroduction of neuroleptics in 15 patients with a history of NMS. Of them, 13 patients were eventually able to resume neuroleptic treatment safely. Some of these findings mirror previous work by Susman and Addonizio (1988). Rosebush et al. (1989) found that successful rechallenge was significantly related to the time that had elapsed following resolution of the NMS episode. In 7 instances, treatment with neuroleptic medication was resumed within 2 weeks of resolution of the NMS episode, and 6 of these instances resulted in immediate relapse. On 13 occasions, the neuroleptic was restarted after 2 or more weeks had elapsed since the resolution of NMS, and relapse occurred only once. Because of the relatively small sample size of this study, caution is indicated when using these findings to establish treatment guidelines. For example, the risk of relapse if neuroleptic treatment is reinstituted exactly 2 weeks after an episode of NMS could still be relatively large.

Rosebush and colleagues (1989) reported that using a lower-potency neuroleptic than that which precipitated the original episode did not significantly affect outcome. They also reported that using a lower dose of neuroleptic (measured in milligrams of chlorpromazine equivalents) than that which precipitated the original episode did not significantly decrease the probability of recurrence. The recurrence of NMS may be significantly delayed for long periods, even a year or longer (Levenson and Fisher 1988).

A number of pharmacologic strategies for preventing recurrence have been proposed, but in most cases, little scientific evidence exists to support these strategies. For example, it is not known whether prophylactic administration of amantadine, low-dose bromocriptine, or oral dantrolene would decrease the likelihood of recurrence. In addition, the question of whether clozapine is safe regarding NMS remains unanswered. Evidence suggests that clozapine may be relatively free of extrapyramidal side effects (Kane et al. 1988) so that it may be much less likely to cause NMS. We are aware of two case reports of NMS associated with the use of clozapine, but in neither was clozapine used alone. In one report (Müller et al. 1988), clozapine was used in conjunction with carbamazepine; in the other report (Pope et al. 1986a), clozapine was used with lithium. Based on these two case reports of NMS associated with clozapine, it appears that clozapine treatment is not free from the risk of NMS although the incidence of clozapine-associated NMS has not yet been determined and could be lower than the risk with conventional neuroleptics. However, one case has been reported of successful use of clozapine without recurrence of NMS in a patient with a history of NMS induced by haloperidol, mesoridazine, and lithium as single agents (Stoudemire and Clayton 1989).

SUMMARY

The information presented above yields the following recommendations regarding the treatment of psychosis in patients with a history of NMS. Treatment alternatives other than neuroleptics (e.g., ECT, lithium, carbamazepine, benzodiazepines, propranolol, and nonpharmacologic treatments) should be considered especially within 2 weeks of resolution of an episode of NMS. Risk factors, such as dehydration, should be identified and averted. Reintroduction of a neuroleptic should be avoided for as long as possible. If a neuroleptic is essential, a low-potency drug is preferred and should be used in low doses. If they develop early, drug-induced parkinsonism or dystonia should be treated promptly, and amantadine is preferred over anticholinergics if amantadine is effective and tolerated. Signs suggesting recurrence of NMS should be closely monitored, and serum CPK levels should be obtained several times during the first week of reinstitution of neuroleptic treatment.

REFERENCES

Addonizio G, Susman VL: ECT as a treatment alternative for patients with symptoms of neuroleptic malignant syndrome. J Clin Psychiatry 48:102–105, 1987

Addonizio G, Susman VL, Roth SD: Symptoms of neuroleptic malignant syndrome in 82 consecutive inpatients. Am J Psychiatry 143:1587–1590, 1986

Addonizio G, Susman VL, Roth SD: Neuroleptic malignant syndrome: review and analysis of 115 cases. Biol Psychiatry 22:1004–1020, 1987

AMA Division of Drugs: AMA Drug Evaluations, 5th Edition. Chicago, IL, American Medical Association, 1983, pp 358–359

American Heart Association: Jones criteria (revised) for guidance in the diagnosis of rheumatic fever. Circulation 32:664–668, 1965

Ayd FJ: Fatal hyperpyrexia during chlorpromazine therapy. Journal of Clinical Experimental Psychopathology and Quarterly Review of Psychiatry and Neurology 17:2:189–192, 1956

Baer JW: Study of 60 patients with AIDS or AIDS-related complex requiring psychiatric hospitalization. Am J Psychiatry 146:1285–1288, 1989

Bismuth C, de Rohan-Chabot P, Goulon M, et al: Dantrolene: a new therapeutic approach to the neuroleptic malignant syndrome. Acta Neurol Scand [Suppl] 100:193–198, 1984

Britt BA: Malignant hyperthermia, in Complications in Anesthesiology. Edited by Orkin FK, Cooperman LH. Philadelphia, PA, JB Lippincott, 1983, pp 291–313

Burke RE, Fahn S, Mayeux R, et al: Neuroleptic malignant syndrome caused by dopamine-depleting drugs in a patient with Huntington disease. Neurology 31:1022–1026, 1981

Caroff SN: The neuroleptic malignant syndrome. J Clin Psychiatry 41:79–83, 1980

Caroff S, Rosenberg H, Gerber JC: Neuroleptic malignant syndrome and malignant hyperthermia. J Clin Psychopharmacol 3:120–121, 1983

Caroff SN, Rosenberg H, Fletcher JE, et al: Malignant hyperthermia susceptibility in neuroleptic malignant syndrome. Anesthesiology 67:20–25, 1987

Caroff SN, Mann SC, Rosenberg H, et al: The relationship between malignant hyperthermia and neuroleptic malignant syndrome. Anesthesiology 70:172–173, 1989

Castillo E, Rubin RT, Holsboer-Trachsler E: Clinical differentiation between lethal catatonia and neuroleptic malignant syndrome. Am J Psychiatry 146:324–328, 1989

Clark BJ: The role of dopamine in the periphery, in The Dopaminergic System. Edited by Flückiger E, Müller EE, Thorner MO. Berlin, Springer-Verlag, 1985, pp 27–39

Cox B, Lee TF: Do central dopamine receptors have a physiologic role in thermoregulation? Br J Pharmacol 61:83–86, 1977

Delay J, Pichot P, Lemperiere T: Un neuroleptique majeur non phenothiazine et non reserpinique, l'haloperidol, dans le traitement des psychoses. Ann Med Psychol 118:145–152, 1960

Deng MZ, Chen GQ, Phillips MR: Neuroleptic malignant syndrome in 12 of 9,792 Chinese inpatients exposed to neuroleptics: a prospective study. Am J Psychiatry 147:1149–1155, 1990

Downey GP, Rosenberg M, Caroff S, et al: Neuroleptic malignant syndrome: patient with unique clinical and physiologic features. Am J Med 77:338–340, 1984

Eneas JF, Schoenfeld PY, Humphreys MH: The effect of infusion of mannitol-sodium bicarbonate on the clinical course of myoglobinemia. Arch Intern Med 139:801–805, 1979

Feibel JH, Schiffer RB: Sympathoadrenomedullary hyperactivity in the neuroleptic malignant syndrome: a case report. Am J Psychiatry 138:1115–1116, 1981

Flamenbaum W, Gehr M, Gross M, et al: Acute renal failure associated with myoglobinuria and hemoglobinuria, in Acute Renal Failure. Edited by Brenner BM, Lazarus JM. Philadelphia, PA, WB Saunders, 1983, pp 269–282

Friedman LS, Weinrauch LA, D'Elia TA: Metoclopramide-induced neuroleptic malignant syndrome. Arch Intern Med 147:1495–1497, 1987

Gelenberg AJ, Bellinghausen B, Wojcik JD, et al: A prospective survey of neuroleptic malignant syndrome in a short-term psychiatric hospital. Am J Psychiatry 145:517–518, 1988

Gerson SC, Baldessarini RJ: Motor effects of serotonin in the central nervous system. Life Sci 27:1435–1451, 1980

Granato JE, Stern BJ, Ringel A, et al: Neuroleptic malignant syndrome: successful treatment with dantrolene and bromocriptine. Ann Neurol 14:89–90, 1983

Guzé BH, Baxter LR: Current concepts of neuroleptic malignant syndrome. N Engl J Med 313:163–166, 1985

Haggerty JJ, Gillette GM: Neuroleptic malignant syndrome superimposed on tardive dyskinesia. Br J Psychiatry 150:104–105, 1987

Harris MJ, Jeste DV: Evaluation and management of HIV/AIDS and psychosis. Clinical Advances in the Treatment of Psychiatric Disorders 3(2):8–9, 1989

Harris M, Nora L, Tanner CM: Neuroleptic malignant syndrome responsive to carbidopa/levodopa: support for a dopaminergic pathogenesis. Clin Neuropharmacol 10:186–189, 1987

Hashimoto F, Sherman CB, Jeffery WH: Neuroleptic malignant syndrome and dopaminergic blockade. Arch Intern Med 144:629–630, 1984

Hermesh H, Aizenberg D, Lapidot M, et al: Risk of malignant hyperthermia among patients with neuroleptic malignant syndrome and their families. Am J Psychiatry 145:1431–1434, 1988

Hermesh H, Aizenberg D, Lapidot M, et al: The relationship between malignant hyperthermia and neuroleptic malignant syndrome. Anesthesiology 70:171–173, 1989

Hinsie LE, Campbell RJ: Psychiatric Dictionary, 4th Edition. London, Oxford University Press, 1974, p 113

Kane J, Honigfeld G, Singer J, et al: Clozapine for the treatment-resistant schizophrenic. Arch Gen Psychiatry 45:789–796, 1988

Kashihara K, Ishida K: Neuroleptic malignant syndrome due to sulpiride. J Neurol Neurosurg Psychiatry 51:1109–1110, 1988

Keck PE, Pope HG, McElroy SL: Frequency and presentation of neuroleptic malignant syndrome: a prospective study. Am J Psychiatry 144:1344–1346, 1987

Keck PE, Pope HG, Cohen BM, et al: Risk factors for neuroleptic malignant syndrome: a case-control study. Arch Gen Psychiatry 46:914–918, 1989a

Keck PE, Sebastianelli J, Pope HG, et al: Frequency and presentation of neuroleptic malignant syndrome in a state psychiatric hospital. J Clin Psychiatry 50:352–355, 1989b

Kline SS, Mauro LS, Scala-Barnett DM, et al: Serotonin syndrome versus neuroleptic malignant syndrome as a cause of death. Clin Pharmacol 8:510–514, 1989

Krivosic-Horber R, Adnet P, Guevart E, et al: Neuroleptic malignant syndrome and malignant hyperthermia. Br J Anaesth 59:1554–1556, 1987

Kurlan R, Hamill R, Soulson I: Neuroleptic malignant syndrome. Clin Neuropharmacol 7:109–120, 1985

Ladame C: Psychose aiguë idiopathique ou foudroyante. Schweiz Arch Neurol Psychiatr 5:3, 1919

Lavie CJ, Olmstead TR, Ventura HO, et al: Neuroleptic malignant syndrome: an underdiagnosed reaction to neuroleptic agents? Postgrad Med 80:171–178, 1986

Lazarus A: Neuroleptic malignant syndrome: detection and management. Psychiatric Annals 15:706–712, 1985

Lazarus A, Mann SC, Caroff SN: The neuroleptic malignant syndrome and related conditions. Washington, DC, American Psychiatric Press, 1989, p 14

Levenson JL: Neuroleptic malignant syndrome. Am J Psychiatry 142:1137–1145, 1985

Levenson JL, Fisher JG: Long-term outcome after neuroleptic malignant syndrome. J Clin Psychiatry 49:154–156, 1988

Levinson DF, Simpson GM: Neuroleptic-induced extrapyramidal symptoms with fever. Arch Gen Psychiatry 43:839–848, 1986

Lew T, Tollefson G: Chlorpromazine-induced neuroleptic malignant syndrome and its response to diazepam. Biol Psychiatry 18:1441–1446, 1983

Lohr JB, Jeste DV, Harris MJ, et al: Treatment of agitation and psychosis, in Clinical Geriatric Psychopharmacology, 2nd Edition. Edited by Salzman C. Baltimore, MD, Williams & Wilkins (in press)

Mohan KS, Gangadhar BN, Pradhan N, et al: The description of the malignant neuroleptic syndrome. NIMHANS Journal 3:109–113, 1985

Mueller PS: Neuroleptic malignant syndrome. Psychosomatics 26:654–662, 1985

Müller T, Becker T, Fritze J: Neuroleptic malignant syndrome after clozapine plus carbamazepine. Lancet 2:1500, 1988

Neppe VM: The neuroleptic malignant syndrome: a priority system. S Afr Med J 65:523–525, 1984

Norman AB, Wylie GL, Prince AK: Supersensitivity of d-amphetamine-induced hyperthermia in rats following continuous treatment with neuroleptics. Eur J Pharmacol 140:349–351, 1987

Pearlman CA: Neuroleptic malignant syndrome: a review of the literature. J Clin Psychopharmacol 6:257–273, 1986

Pope HG, Cole JO, Choras PT, et al: Apparent neuroleptic malignant syndrome with clozapine and lithium. J Nerv Ment Dis 174:493–495, 1986a

Pope HG, Keck PE, McElroy SL: Frequency and presentation of neuroleptic malignant syndrome in a large psychiatric hospital. Am J Psychiatry 143:1227–1233, 1986b

Robinson MB, Kennett RP, Harding AE, et al: Neuroleptic malignant syndrome associated with metoclopramide. J Neurol Neurosurg Psychiatry 40:1304, 1985

Rosebush PI, Stewart TD, Gelenberg AJ: Twenty neuroleptic rechallenges after neuroleptic malignant syndrome in 15 patients. J Clin Psychiatry 50:295–298, 1989

Rudnik MR, Bastl CP, Elfinbein IB, et al: The differential diagnosis of acute renal failure, in Acute Renal Failure. Edited by Brenner BM, Lazarus JM. Philadelphia, PA, WB Saunders, 1983, pp 176–222

Scarlett JD, Zimmerman R, Berkovic SF: Neuroleptic malignant syndrome. Aust N Z J Med 13:70–73, 1983

Schibuk M, Schachter D: A role of catecholamines in the pathogenesis of neuroleptic malignant syndrome. Can J Psychiatry 31:66–68, 1986

Sewell DD, Jeste DV: Neuroleptic malignant syndrome: a review. Jpn J Psychopharmacol 9:319–333, 1989

Sewell DD, Jeste DV: Neuroleptic malignant syndrome: a study of 30 cases. Presented at the 143rd annual meeting of the American Psychiatric Association, New York, May 17, 1990

Shalev A, Munitz H: The neuroleptic malignant syndrome: agent and host interaction. Acta Psychiatr Scand 73:337–347, 1986

Shalev A, Hermesh H, Munitz H: The role of external heat load in triggering the neuroleptic malignant syndrome. Am J Psychiatry 145:110–111, 1988

Shalev A, Hermesh H, Munitz H: Mortality from neuroleptic malignant syndrome. J Clin Psychiatry 50:18–25, 1989

Simpson DM, Davis GC: Case report of neuroleptic malignant syndrome associated with withdrawal from amantadine. Am J Psychiatry 141:796–797, 1984

Smego RA, Durack DT: The neuroleptic malignant syndrome. Arch Intern Med 142:1183–1185, 1982

Stoudemire A, Clayton L: Successful use of clozapine in a patient with a history of neuroleptic malignant syndrome. Journal of Neuropsychiatry and Clinical Neurosciences 1:303–305, 1989

Stoudemire A, Luther JS: Neuroleptic malignant syndrome and neuroleptic-induced catatonia: differential diagnosis and treatment. Int J Psychiatry Med 14:57–63, 1984

Susman VL, Addonizio G: Recurrence of neuroleptic malignant syndrome. J Nerv Ment Dis 176:234–241, 1988

Tollefson G: A case of neuroleptic malignant syndrome: in vitro muscle comparison with malignant hyperthermia. J Clin Psychopharmacol 2:266–270, 1982

Tollefson GD, Garvey MJ: The neuroleptic syndrome and central dopamine metabolites. J Clin Psychopharmacol 4:150–153, 1984

Toru M, Matusda O, Makiguchi K, et al: Neuroleptic malignant syndrome-like state following a withdrawal of antiparkinsonian drugs. J Nerv Ment Dis 169:324–327, 1981

Ungvari GA: Treatment of neuroleptic malignant syndrome with dopamine hydrochloride: a case report. Pharmacopsychiatry 20:120–121, 1987

Warner RRP: Serotonin irritation syndrome (letter to the editor). J Clin Psychiatry 48:217, 1987

Yamawaki S: A consideration on the pathophysiology of "syndrome malin"—three cases of successful treatment with dantrolene. Japanese Journal of Psychiatric Treatment 1:413–422, 1986

Yamawaki S, Lai H, Horita A: Dopaminergic and serotonergic mechanisms of thermoregulation: mediation of thermal effects of apomorphine and dopamine. J Pharmacol Exp Ther 227:383–388, 1983

Yamawaki S, Yanagawa K, Morio M, et al: Possible central effect of dantrolene sodium in neuroleptic malignant syndrome. J Clin Psychopharmacol 6:378–379, 1986

Yamawaki S, Yano E, Kato T, et al: Animal model of neuroleptic malignant syndrome—abnormality of intracellular calcium mobilization in hypothalamus in rats. Platform presentation to the XVI Collegium Internationale Neuro-Psychopharmacologicum Congress, Munich, Germany, Aug 15–19, 1988

Child and Adolescent Medical Psychiatry

Chapter 13

Psychopharmacology in Medically Ill Children and Adolescents

Betty Pfefferbaum, M.D.

While few studies have documented the effectiveness of psychoactive drugs in children with physical illnesses, clinicians frequently use these drugs with success. A wide array of symptoms, including anxiety, depression, sleep disturbance, nausea, pain, and delirium, occur in physically ill children and are responsive to the same psychopharmacological interventions as similar symptoms in adults. Benzodiazepines, tricyclic antidepressants, neuroleptics, and stimulants have been used in children.

Two trends are worth noting: Benzodiazepines, once unpopular with child psychiatrists, are becoming drugs of choice in the treatment of anxiety in physically ill children and are also being used to treat emesis and as adjuvants to analgesics. Stimulants, which have long been used to treat attention deficit disorders, may have an important place in the management of depression in physically ill children who do not tolerate tricyclics or in whom a rapid response is crucial.

Pediatricians and child psychiatrists retain a strong bias toward using psychotherapy and behavioral therapies and demonstrate considerable resistance to psychopharmacologic interventions. The use of psychopharmacologic agents in children is further complicated by a variety of factors, including imprecise diagnostic classification schemes,

455

normal changes in physical characteristics of children as they mature, and heightened concern about the legal and ethical issues related to experimentation and informed consent in minors.

Because there are few systematic studies of the use of psychoactive agents in children with medical illnesses, the clinician working with physically ill children is required to base treatment decisions on knowledge about the use of such agents in physically healthy children and in adults. In this chapter, I present guidelines for the use of psychotropic medications in general and for the use of some specific drug classes in medically ill children. I also review research and clinical experience with the use of benzodiazepines, tricyclic antidepressants, neuroleptics, and stimulants in the treatment of secondary psychiatric problems in physically ill children. This chapter does not cover the use of psychoactive agents to treat primary medical (e.g., ulcers), neurological (e.g., seizures), or psychiatric (e.g., bipolar mood disorders) conditions. However, their use in treating physical symptoms, such as nausea and pain, that have strong psychological components, will be addressed. Case examples are used to illustrate some of the subtleties of prescribing psychotropics for physically ill children.

GENERAL PRINCIPLES FOR PRESCRIBING PSYCHOTROPIC DRUGS

Nonpharmacologic interventions should always be considered as treatment options to use instead of, or in conjunction with, pharmacological treatments. A number of general principles ideally influence decisions regarding the use of psychopharmacologic agents. A careful history, including a history of medication use and sensitivity, and a mental status examination should precede drug administration. The physician is encouraged to use, and become familiar with, one or two drugs in each class. Preferably, these should be well-established agents that have been investigated in children, because newer agents may have unusual, adverse, or toxic effects that are not yet known.

While relatively new agents such as the anxiolytic buspirone or the antidepressants fluoxetine and bupropion apparently have fewer toxic side effects than tricyclic antidepressants, their histories of use have not been long enough to conclusively establish their overall level of safety. The risks of these substances cannot be accurately determined until they have been investigated in large numbers of patients.

Use of them in children before accumulating extensive experience in adults should be discouraged except in research contexts.

Target symptoms should be identified and monitored to determine drug effect. Initial doses should be as low as possible to enable the physician to identify idiosyncratic reactions. Side effects are minimized if doses are increased in small increments, and benefit is maximized if drug administration is titrated against target symptoms and side effects. The maximum dose should be the lowest effective dose. The drug should be discontinued as soon as possible after target symptoms have abated, except when the psychiatric symptoms represent a definite primary psychiatric disorder, such as schizophrenia or a mood disorder. Before discontinuing a drug, it is wise to taper the dosage to avoid precipitating withdrawal or rebound symptoms or the recurrence of original symptoms.

It is imperative that the child psychiatrist work closely with the pediatrician managing the child's physical illness. Furthermore, the beneficial and adverse effects of a particular drug should be considered before treatment with psychoactive medication is initiated. Because there has been little documentation of the use of psychoactive drugs in children, the child psychiatrist or pediatrician should discuss potential problems with a pediatric specialist. For example, a cardiologist should be consulted if the child's primary illness is cardiac or if cardiotoxic drugs have significantly affected cardiovascular status; a neurologist should be consulted before giving antidepressants or antipsychotics, which lower the seizure threshold, to a child with known seizures. Since experience with, and literature on, the use of psychoactive agents in physically ill children is so limited, such consultations are emphasized for both medical and legal reasons.

Measures of system functioning, such as a complete blood count with differential and platelet count; liver function tests such as serum glutamic-oxaloacetic transaminase (SGOT), serum glutamic-pyruvic transaminase (SGPT), alkaline phosphatase, and bilirubin; and urinalysis, blood urea nitrogen (BUN) and creatinine clearance should be obtained before administering any psychoactive drug to a physically ill child or adolescent. An ECG or EEG should be obtained if there is concern about cardiac or neurologic status or if the drugs being used predispose to cardiac or neurologic dysfunction.

It is imperative that the child and the child's family, as well as the consulting pediatrician, understand the goals of the psychopharmacologic intervention, know the target symptoms and side effects that will be monitored, appreciate the risk-benefit profile, and be comfortable with the intervention. It is important not to overwhelm the child and the child's parents with so much information about side effects that they refuse a valuable treatment out of anxiety alone. On the other hand, they need to understand that the administration of drugs is not without risks. In some situations, a trial of psychotherapy or behavioral intervention is a reasonable initial intervention.

Some psychiatric symptoms, such as those associated with delirium, are so disorganizing that psychopharmacologic intervention is essential. When a child's mood or anxiety contribute to noncompliance with medical management, psychopharmacologic intervention is attractive but not urgent, and a concerted effort with nondrug treatment should be tried first. The decision to use psychoactive agents in nonemergency situations should be reached only after all concerned parties understand the goals and plan and support the intervention. In the case of older children or adolescents, the patient should be included in the decision.

LEGAL ISSUES

Legal issues associated with the use of drugs increasingly present concern. Many psychopharmacologic agents that might prove useful in managing psychiatric symptomatology in physically ill children have not been investigated in children and have not been approved by the Food and Drug Administration for use in children. The clinician is encouraged to engage in a careful pretreatment dialogue about the use of a drug with both the child and parents. Nye (1980) identifies three requirements of valid informed consent: the consenter should be told the nature of the condition being treated, treatment alternatives, and the probable success of treatment; the foreseeable risks (including side effects) and benefits of the proposed treatment and alternatives; and the potential risks if no treatment is provided.

In a book dealing with the rights and responsibilities of children, the Group for the Advancement of Psychiatry (1989) provided guidelines regarding ages at which children should be expected to understand informed consent. They suggested that a child with a mental age of 7 or older assent to participate in research; informed consent should be required for children older than age 14. By preschool age, children understand the concept of illness, and they should be included in treatment decisions using age-appropriate language and information modified in content. While a child cannot be expected to understand the intricacies of optimal and adverse effects, it can be beneficial to discuss even with a young child the positive and negative ways in which the medication is expected to act. Such discussions enhance trust and allow the child to feel a sense of autonomy and self-respect.

In addition, the psychiatrist should document the need for the drug, attempts to determine the lowest effective dose, risks and benefits, the discussion of these with the child and parents, and their decision about whether to use the drug (Mills and Daniels 1987). Periodic reassessment to determine whether medication is needed or whether side effects have appeared is essential.

ABSORPTION, DISTRIBUTION, METABOLISM, AND EXCRETION

Maturational changes potentially alter the metabolism and excretion and, less frequently, the absorption and distribution of drugs (Kauffman and Habersang 1978). Pharmacokinetic studies in children have been completed on relatively few drugs. Theoretical conclusions coupled with the data available from the studies that do exist provide information that may be helpful when prescribing drugs for children.

Many factors, including gastric emptying time, acidity of the intestines, the presence of food, and effects of disease, influence gastric absorption. Since these factors stabilize after the neonatal period, gastrointestinal absorption varies little with age after that time. Drug distribution, which does change with age, is based on rates of absorption, membrane penetration, and perfusion, volume and composition of body compartments, and protein and tissue binding. Water-soluble drugs have their greatest volume of distribution during the neonatal period and early infancy. Maturational changes affecting fat-soluble drugs are more variable (World Health Organization 1987).

Most drugs are metabolized in the liver through biotransformation, a process related to hepatic enzyme activity, hepatic blood flow, and protein binding (Rane 1980). Oral drugs that are absorbed by the gastrointestinal tract pass through the liver and are metabolized before entering the general circulation. This process, the "first pass" effect of the liver, explains the relatively low bioavailability of oral forms of some drugs compared to parenteral forms. The rate at which the liver metabolizes a drug may be increased in children, resulting in a shorter half-life for that drug (Blau 1978).

Drug excretion occurs mainly through the kidneys, though some drugs are eliminated through the intestines, lungs, and other body fluids. The various mechanisms of elimination mature at different rates. It is difficult to predict renal excretion by age, but for the most part, renal excretion is lower in neonates than in adults, and doses and dosing intervals should be adjusted accordingly (Braunlich 1977).

Various disease states may influence the biological processes related to drug administration. In addition, medications given to treat a primary illness may interact with medications given for secondary psychiatric symptomatology by altering their rate and degree of absorption, distribution, metabolism, or excretion. Information on potential drug-drug and disease-drug interactions should be reviewed before administering psychoactive drugs to physically ill children.

Gastrointestinal diseases such as cystic fibrosis, which is often accompanied by malabsorption; acute gastroenteritis; celiac disease; and Crohn's disease may impair drug absorption. Doses and intervals should be determined with this in mind. Liver disease frequently affects metabolism. Unfortunately, there are no studies of drug metabolism in children with acute and chronic hepatic disease, and standard liver function tests such as SGOT, SGPT, alkaline phosphatase, and bilirubin do not adequately reflect changes in hepatic drug metabolism and distribution. Therefore, it is essential to carefully monitor clinical response as well as liver function tests when administering drugs to patients with liver disease (Kauffman and Habersang 1978). As the technology for determining blood levels improves for these agents, the use of such techniques may prove helpful.

Renal disease may influence excretion. The rate of renal elimination of drugs is related to the glomerular filtration rate, which can be estimated by measuring creatinine clearance (Kauffman and Habersang 1978). Studies indicate that in adults with uremia, blood levels of benzodiazepines may be decreased but levels of tricyclic antidepressants and probably phenothiazines are similar to those of physically healthy individuals. In most situations, decreased glomerular filtration will not result in toxic levels of psychotropic agents. Nevertheless, it is reasonable to use lower doses and extended dosing intervals, at least initially, and to follow increases in dose or changes in dosing schedule with careful monitoring for clinical effects and side effects (Meyers 1989).

Thyroid disease, fever, dehydration, and malnutrition may also influence the biological processes associated with metabolism and excretion. While few studies have documented the point at which such conditions have significant effect, it is prudent to exercise caution by carefully monitoring clinical effect and using it as a basis for altering the dose or dosing interval. Nowhere is it more important to focus on individual response than in the physically ill child.

BENZODIAZEPINES

While anxiolytics, particularly benzodiazepines, have been used for many years in the treatment of a variety of symptoms in adults, they have been less popular among child psychiatrists. In a study of prescribing practices, child psychiatrists were asked to rank medications they would consider for a variety of childhood disorders. Benzodiazepines were infrequent choices for any disorder (Pfefferbaum and Overall 1984). Pediatricians, anesthesiologists, radiologists, and a host of other clinicians, on the other hand, use these drugs routinely to manage anxiety and other symptoms in physically ill children. The development of new drugs of this class, better understanding of and classification of anxiety disorders, and concerns about potentially serious side effects of other drugs, such as neuroleptics, have led to increased interest in benzodiazepines. A number of recent studies have examined the use of various benzodiazepines in physically healthy and ill children (Jay et al. 1987; Petti et al. 1982; Pfefferbaum et al. 1987b; Van Hoff and Olszewski 1988).

Both antipsychotics and tricyclic antidepressants have been used for the treatment of anxiety in children, but benzodiazepines compare favorably to them on a number of measures: benzodiazepines are more specific for anxiety relief; they have rapid onset of therapeutic action; they have relatively low toxicity; and they are less apt to cause serious adverse effects. Concern about the potential for abuse of benzodiazepines, however, has limited their use.

Benzodiazepines with short half-lives, such as oxazepam and lorazepam, do not have active metabolites and are eliminated more quickly than those with long half-lives. They must be administered more frequently. Long-acting benzodiazepines, such as diazepam, have active metabolites. The withdrawal effects of agents with longer half-lives are milder but continue over a longer period. When the drugs are administered repeatedly for a week or longer, these differences should be considered, but they are of little importance in single-dose applications (Salzman 1989).

Absorption of benzodiazepines following oral administration is variable. Alprazolam, chlordiazepoxide, lorazepam, and oxazepam are absorbed relatively slowly, but diazepam reaches peak concentrations in about 1 hour in adults and as quickly as 15–30 minutes in children (Baldessarini 1985). The drugs are metabolized primarily by hepatic biotransformation, and severe liver disease can increase the half-life of diazepam by two to five times (Baldessarini 1985). The half-life of diazepam is increased in infants, who have lower rates of biotransformation than older children and adults.

However, once liver enzymes reach adult capacity and excretory capacity matures during the first year of life, children appear to metabolize the drug at higher rates than adults (Coffey et al. 1983). More frequent dosing may therefore be appropriate when using these drugs to treat children (Rapoport et al. 1978). The pharmacokinetics of these drugs are similar in adolescents and adults (McDermott et al. 1989).

Medical treatment situations requiring invasive procedures provide an ideal model for the study and use of benzodiazepines for the relief of acute situational and anticipatory anxiety. Diazepam and the newer, popular, shorter-acting benzodiazepines, such as alprazolam, lorazepam, and oxazepam, are commonly used by the oral or intravenous route to calm children and adolescents who must undergo painful and frightening medical procedures. The drugs are favored for their rapid action, calming effects, and amnestic properties. They are given about 1 hour (for oral administration) or immediately (for intravenous use) before the procedure and may also be given the day or night preceding the procedure if anticipatory anxiety is a problem.

Low doses of diazepam were compared with cognitive-behavioral strategies and traditional treatment in a sample of 56 leukemic children between the ages of 3 and 13 who were undergoing invasive procedures. Treatment with diazepam was associated with decreased diastolic blood pressure but not decreased pulse, pain, or behavioral distress. The authors concluded that the antianxiety agent acted to reduce anticipatory anxiety but not behavioral distress (Jay et al. 1987).

Pfefferbaum et al. (1987b) studied the use of alprazolam in childhood cancer patients and reported beneficial results with very low doses (0.003–0.025 mg/kg tid) given for 3 days prior to treatment procedures. Midazolam, another short-acting benzodiazepine, has been investigated in children for use as a preanesthetic induction agent, but the efficacy of the drug is in some dispute (Diament and Stanley 1988; Salonen et al. 1987). Salonen et al. (1987) studied the pharmacokinetics of midazolam in 21 children undergoing elective surgery and found the elimination half-life was shorter than in adult patients.

Benzodiazepines are also excellent agents to treat episodes of severe anxiety during the course of an illness and may also be used to promote sleep in children whose anxiety interferes with rest. The following example illustrates appropriate use of benzodiazepines in a medically ill teenager.

> Cathy, 13 years old, had been tense and difficult to manage since being hospitalized for a hemipelvectomy. About 10 days after surgery, she became extremely upset upon hearing about discharge plans and began screaming, pulling her hair, banging her head, and refusing to cooperate with her care. She responded to a single 2-mg po dose of lorazepam.
>
> A trial of amitriptyline was initiated because she had experienced considerable anxiety since hospitalization, she was sad and withdrawn, and she experienced initial insomnia. Unfortunately, her parents were so concerned about the side effects of the tricyclic that they discontinued it as soon as she was discharged. Cathy continued to have episodes of severe anxiety. Eventually, she was given lorazepam on a schedule of 2 mg po every 6 hours, to which the episodes responded.

Finally, benzodiazepines are being used and investigated in children with cancer in the treatment of nausea and vomiting—symptoms that are thought to be strongly influenced by anxiety and other psychological factors. Van Hoff and Olszewski (1988) compared the use of lorazepam (0.05 mg/kg) to methylprednisolone, phenothiazines, or both in children ages 3–15 and found the drug to be about as beneficial as standard antiemetic treatment for children over age 6. The drug was well tolerated. Side effects included sedation in children of all ages and visual hallucinations in children under age 6.

Benzodiazepines have anxiolytic, sedative-hypnotic, muscle-relaxant and anticonvulsant properties. Their side effects have not generally been considered serious and include sedation, slurred speech, diplopia, ataxia, and tremor. Some individuals report feeling drugged and some become depressed while on these drugs. Dependence on benzodiazepines is a well-known problem, and abrupt withdrawal may lead to symptom recurrence or rebound symptoms. Withdrawal symptoms include anxiety, sleep disturbance, irritability, sweating, decreased concentration, nausea, weight loss, palpitations, muscular pains, tremor, seizures, and psychosis. Serious withdrawal symptoms are uncommon but may occur days after abrupt discontinuation of the drug (Baldessarini 1985).

Although rare, benzodiazepine toxicity presenting as behavioral disinhibition or psychosis has been reported in both adults and children and can be alarming (Einarson and Yoder 1982; Pfefferbaum et al. 1987a;

Van Hoff and Olszewski 1988). Van Hoff and Olszewski (1988) reported that children experienced "nonfrightening" hallucinations after receiving lorazepam prophylactically for nausea; it is difficult to imagine, however, that hallucinations would not cause concern in the patient, family, and staff.

The following case example illustrates several points, including the unsuitability of benzodiazepine hypnotics for some children.

> David, 14 years old, was in treatment for osteogenic sarcoma. He had a history of attention-deficit disorder with hyperactivity, conduct disorder, and learning problems. He also had perceptual problems and subtle paranoia. David had undergone unsuccessful treatment trials with methylphenidate and dextroamphetamine. At the time he was seen for the cancer, he was taking pemoline 37.5 mg po in the morning and 18.75 mg po in the afternoon. He was prescribed 0.25 mg po triazolam for insomnia after low doses of tricyclics were ineffective. David slept about 4 hours after the first dose, but the next night he experienced visual hallucinations and insomnia most likely secondary to triazolam. Finally, he was successfully treated with chlorpromazine 50 mg po at bedtime and 10 mg po in the afternoon. His afternoon dose of pemoline was discontinued because of concern that it may have contributed to insomnia.

A careful history, including information about previous drug reactions and a mental status examination should precede trials of psychoactive drugs. Of particular concern in this case was the choice of benzodiazepine. Triazolam is a relatively new agent that has not been studied or used frequently in children, especially those with physical illness. While this child's reaction could have occurred with any benzodiazepine, an agent that had been used more extensively in children might have been a wiser choice. It is also possible that adverse effects like those experienced by this patient are more likely to occur in individuals who suffer preexisting disorders such as mental retardation, attention-deficit disorder, or brain damage or in those receiving other psychoactive agents.

TRICYCLIC ANTIDEPRESSANTS

Depressive symptomatology frequently accompanies medical conditions and their treatments. Symptoms associated with depression, such as anorexia, fatigue, and sleep disturbance, often mimic symptoms associated with illness or treatment side effects, at times making it difficult to determine whether a depressive illness actually exists.

Further complicating treatment is the commonly held attitude that anxiety and depression are to be expected in the course of physical illness and warrant no intervention. Just because such symptoms are a natural and reasonable consequence does not mean that they should not be treated. While reassurance, support, and insight may be beneficial, the ill child may also require antidepressant medication for relief of serious or long-standing depressive symptoms.

Tricyclic antidepressants are now widely used in the management of children with a variety of psychiatric disorders, despite the fact that only a few studies of small populations have demonstrated their efficacy, and their effectiveness over placebo in healthy children has not been unequivocally established (Ambrosini 1987; Rapoport 1987). Kashani et al. (1984) administered low doses (no greater than 1.5 mg/kg per day) of amitriptyline to physically healthy depressed children in a crossover, placebo-controlled study and found a trend for superior efficacy of the drug.

Petti and Law (1982) also demonstrated superiority of imipramine over placebo in a small sample of children. Preskorn et al. (1982) found tricyclic treatment response in children whose depression was unresponsive to outpatient psychotherapy and brief hospitalization. Puig-Antich et al. (1987) found similar overall response rates with imipramine and placebo in a double-blind study of prepubertal depression, but found that the maintenance plasma level of imipramine plus desipramine positively predicted clinical response. Pfefferbaum-Levine et al. (1983) reported clinical improvement with low doses of tricyclics (less than 2 mg/kg per day) in a small series of child and adolescent cancer patients.

While the most obvious use for tricyclic antidepressants is for depressive symptomatology of some severity and duration, these drugs have also been used in the treatment of chronic anxiety, panic, school refusal, hyperactivity, attention problems, conduct disorders, chronic pain, eating disorders, and substance abuse. Tricyclics are also being used and studied for use in the treatment of ulcers, allergies, and skin disorders. Gastrointestinal diseases, including duodenal ulcer, gastric ulcer, and irritable bowel syndromes, generally respond to lower doses than used for the treatment of depression. Amitriptyline and doxepin are potent antihistamines and are being used for allergic and dermatologic disorders.

It is sometimes difficult to distinguish the specific effect of an intervention, and drug choices may be based on any number of factors. A knowledge of all potential drug effects is beneficial, as illustrated by the following case example.

A pediatric allergist requested consultation from a child psychiatrist in the treatment of a 9-year-old boy with chronic eczema whose body was covered with excoriated skin lesions. He lived with his mother, stepfather, and younger sibling in a household marked by considerable conflict. The child was depressed and withdrawn. The family resisted psychotherapeutic intervention. Because of the combined symptoms of pruritus and depression, the physicians initiated a trial of amitriptyline 10 mg po bid. The child responded, and the dose was increased to 25 mg po bid. The child's response was dramatic. He was discharged from the hospital with plans to be followed up in outpatient psychotherapy. The family failed to attend psychotherapy and eventually discontinued use of amitriptyline. The child was thereafter seen periodically by the allergist for exacerbations of the skin condition.

This case demonstrates several points. Because tricyclic antidepressants are used to treat nonpsychiatric disorders, it is important to understand the full range of properties they exhibit. They may be used for a variety of coexisting symptoms. The delicate interplay between psychological and physiological symptoms may be startling. In this case, both the allergist and the psychiatrist wondered which disease was primary and whether benefit resulted from amitriptyline's antidepressant or antihistaminic effect or both. Finally, successful pharmacological management alone may be insufficient in overall treatment of both psychological and physiological disorders.

Tricyclics have been demonstrated to have analgesic properties that some believe are primary (Fields 1987). They may also decrease the subjective experience of pain by affecting a host of symptoms such as anxiety, depression, or sleep disturbance. Their beneficial use has been demonstrated in the treatment of postherpetic neuralgia, diabetic neuropathy, tension headache, migraine headache, rheumatoid arthritis, chronic low-back pain, and cancer (Fields 1987).

Analgesic response may be rapid and may occur at doses lower than those used to treat depression. One teenager emerged from surgery in excruciating pain and suffering from severe depression, anxiety, and sleep disturbance. Initially, low doses of a short-acting benzodiazepine were used to treat the anxiety. When the anxiety became more pervasive and severe, amitriptyline was initiated. When the dose was titrated to 75 mg po at bedtime, the patient showed remarkable progress with respect to all symptoms. He was even able to acknowledge and discern that anxiety heightened his feelings of pain. While such insight did not alleviate the pain, it did facilitate management.

Tricyclics must be administered with caution and monitored carefully for beneficial and adverse effects. Since most of the drugs in this category are sedating, it is wise to begin with an initial dose at bedtime, starting with the lowest available dose and increasing it as far as it is tolerated until beneficial effects are demonstrated. Untoward side effects may limit any further increase and are an important factor in determining the eventual dose and schedule.

Although doses up to 5 mg/kg per day may be necessary to achieve antidepressant effect in physically healthy children, one small series indicated that some children with cancer responded to doses of less than 2 mg/kg per day (Pfefferbaum-Levine et al. 1983). These results are in keeping with experience in adult oncology patients, who tend to respond faster and to lower doses of tricyclic antidepressants than physically healthy adults (Massie and Holland 1984). Patients with advanced liver and renal disease also require lower doses (Fava and Sonino 1987).

Side Effects

A number of side effects occur with tricyclics. These should be discussed with the child, the parents, and the pediatrician before initiating treatment. Anticholinergic side effects, including dry mouth, blurred vision, urinary retention, and constipation, are bothersome but not usually serious, and they are reversible. Other side effects include tremor, sweating, and appetite and weight changes. Even when they have been alerted to the possibility of these effects, some children and adolescents find them intolerable and refuse to continue taking the drugs. Drying of bronchial secretions may pose problems for patients with pulmonary disorders such as asthma. Agranulocytosis is also a rare adverse effect.

Orthostatic hypotension may present more serious problems in the physically ill, especially patients with reduced blood volume and patients for whom a fall could be particularly serious, such as children with hemophilia. Whether pretreatment orthostatic changes predict orthostatic changes secondary to tricyclic treatment is not definitely established (Jefferson 1989). Nonetheless, it is advisable to alert children and their parents about this side effect and use special caution in patients with cardiovascular problems or decreased blood volume. One teenage cancer patient given tricyclics fell while away from the hospital on a pass. Fearing an extension of his brain tumor, he returned to the hospital to learn that orthostatic hypotension was responsible for the dizziness and fall. Had he been alerted to this potential side effect and given instructions to sit or lie down if he felt dizzy, he could have avoided returning to the hospital. More important, he would have been spared the anxiety associated with what he considered an alarming change in his course.

Tricyclic antidepressants are contraindicated in patients with certain cardiac diseases, though many cardiac conditions do not preclude the use of these drugs (Jefferson 1989). Few studies have documented the cardiovascular effects of tricyclics in children. Consultation with a cardiologist is strongly advised when tricyclics are to be given to children with impaired cardiovascular functioning or to children receiving medical therapies that could also affect their cardiac status. Daily doses above 3.5 mg/kg in physically healthy children warrant monitoring with periodic ECGs (McDermott et al. 1989).

Because children have a smaller lipid compartment than adults and drugs do not bind to albumin to the same degree as in adults, they may be at greater risk than adults of developing cardiovascular toxicity as a result of tricyclics (Schroeder et al. 1989). Schroeder et al. (1989) studied the cardiovascular effects of desipramine in a series of children treated for attention-deficit disorder, affective disturbance, and eating disorders. Serial heart rate, blood pressure, ECG, and 24-hour ambulatory cardiac activity were monitored both before treatment and at 4 and 8 weeks during treatment. The maximum dose of desipramine used was 5 mg/kg per day. Increased heart rate and increased Q-T interval were found at 4 and 8 weeks. No dysrhythmias or clinically significant changes in blood pressure occurred.

An EEG should precede the administration of tricyclics in children with central nervous system disease regardless of whether they have seizures. Stoudemire and Fogel (1987) assert that tricyclics are not contraindicated in patients with seizures if adequate levels of anticonvulsants are maintained, seizures are controlled, and tricyclics are discontinued if they exacerbate seizures. Nonetheless, the use of these drugs in children with seizures should be initiated in collaboration with a neurologic consultant.

Choice of tricyclic should take into consideration the drugs' side effects. Amitriptyline and imipramine produce more tachycardia, postural hypotension, and quinidine-like effects than does nortriptyline. Desipramine may be preferred for patients with seizures as it may not lower the seizure threshold as much as other tricyclics. For disorders in which serotonin is thought to be an important mediator, such as migraine headaches and chronic pain, antidepressants with a relatively high affinity for serotonin, such as amitriptyline, nortriptyline, and doxepin, may be drugs of choice. When allergy is present, amitriptyline, nortriptyline, and doxepin may be chosen. Patients with diarrhea may benefit from amitriptyline, doxepin, and imipramine because of their anticholinergic side effects. Desipramine may be preferred for those who are constipated. Patients with peptic ulcer may benefit from amitriptyline, doxepin, or imipramine (Richardson and Richelson 1984; Richelson 1983).

The half-lives of tricyclics are of intermediate length, ranging from 6 to 28 hours (Richardson and Richelson 1984). Individuals vary widely in their absorption, distribution, and excretion of antidepressants such that individual metabolism varies by 10- to 30-fold and there are marked interindividual variations in plasma level. Therefore, the drug dosage must be individualized. Tricyclics are metabolized primarily by the liver and excreted by the kidneys. The tricyclics are highly lipid soluble and have wide distribution. Hepatic biotransformation is increased in children, making more frequent administration of the drug necessary (Combrinck-Graham et al. 1980).

Geller et al. (1987) in a series of studies tested the hypothesis that the pharmacokinetics of nortriptyline is similar in children and adults. The results indicate that the drug has a significantly shorter half-life and significantly greater apparent oral clearance in children under the age of 12 than in adolescents. It is recommended that the drug be given in divided doses to children and adolescents.

A recent investigation studied the effects of desipramine on liver function tests in children and adolescents with attention-deficit disorder and major depression. SGOT, alkaline phosphatase, and total bilirubin were measured at baseline and monthly thereafter during a 3- to 24-month treatment period. There were no statistically or clinically significant increases, with the exception of single-enzyme values slightly elevated above laboratory standards in some patients. These were not considered to reflect liver dysfunction and did not have associated clinical findings (Hoge and Biederman 1987).

Blood Levels

The clinical importance of blood levels of tricyclics has not been definitely established. For some tricyclics, such as nortriptyline and imipramine, therapeutic blood levels are well defined. Weller et al. (1982) found a sixfold variation in total plasma levels (imipramine plus desipramine) in children treated with imipramine. Puig-Antich et al. (1979) found that blood levels, but not dose, distinguished imipramine responders; patients with levels greater than 146 ng/ml had significantly better results. Preskorn et al. (1982) and Weller et al. (1982) reported that total plasma levels between 125 and 225 ng/ml of imipramine plus desipramine produced maximal improvement.

While the meaning of blood levels of tricyclics in children is not clearly established, it has been recommended that levels be obtained and followed in the following situations: 1) when patients fail to respond to the expected dose and duration of treatment; 2) when using a tricyclic for which a therapeutic window exists; 3) when drug toxicity is suspected or may be confused with an underlying medical disorder; 4) when the patient's clinical condition changes unfavorably; 5) when drug interactions may be present or suspected; 6) when patients are very young; 7) when poor compliance is suspected; 8) when concurrent cardiovascular, hepatic, or renal disorders are present; or 9) when the required dose exceeds the recommended limit (Orsulak 1986).

If tricyclics are used to treat anxiety or pain, they may be discontinued once symptoms abate. If they are used to treat persistent, severe depression, the child should remain on the drug well beyond the disappearance of symptoms. Abrupt withdrawal may result in withdrawal or relapse symptoms that can be avoided by tapering the drug over several weeks. These principles are illustrated by the following case example.

Sally, 15 years old, was in treatment for cancer. Shortly after being diagnosed, she became despondent and withdrawn and refused to interact with anyone except her immediate family members. She had frequent crying spells, anorexia, and nightmares. Sally did not respond to psychotherapy or to attempts by staff to engage her in activities. A trial of imipramine was initiated, and she had an excellent response at a dose of 75 mg po per day (1.5 mg/kg per day). Blood levels were 73 ng/ml of imipramine and 167 ng/ml of desipramine. Sally had been receiving imipramine for about 6 months when the decision was made to discontinue the drug. It was tapered slowly but nonetheless, she became very sad, withdrawn, and anorexic as the drug was withdrawn. She responded well when the previous dose was reinstituted.

NEUROLEPTICS (MAJOR TRANQUILIZERS)

Neuroleptics may be used in the management of a variety of conditions arising in the course of a medical illness: severe anxiety, organic brain syndromes, nausea, and pain. Severe emotional reactions may occur during invasive procedures or with acute change in medical status; sometimes they have no obvious explanation. Concern about potentially serious adverse effects of neuroleptics now makes benzodiazepines the drugs of choice for the treatment of anxiety occurring during the course of a medical illness. However, neuroleptics also have a role in the treatment of anxiety, particularly anxiety that reaches panic proportions, is accompanied by severe agitation, or has psychotic features.

In many situations, a single low dose of an antipsychotic agent is effective. In other situations it is necessary to treat the child with repeated doses. Because of their potentially serious adverse effects, these drugs are not ideal for chronic use, but they should not be denied to those patients in need of treatment who respond to them. When treating episodes of severe anxiety or agitation, low doses are recommended: 5–25 mg of chlorpromazine per dose or 0.5–2 mg of haloperidol per dose are often sufficient depending on the child's response. While these drugs are commonly administered, alone or in combination with other agents, for the prophylactic management of anxiety associated with invasive procedures, some children do not like their effects and do better with benzodiazepines or with no medication at all. The individual child's response and preference are important factors in determining which drug, if any, is used.

Anxiety may accompany other symptoms, such as pain. One 7-year-old amputee suffered severe anxiety, phantom limb pain, sleep disturbance, and nightmares every evening after his discharge from the hospital. Treatment with a low dose of chlorpromazine, 5 mg po in the evening and again at bedtime, diminished his pain and anxiety and allowed him to sleep. Whether the chlorpromazine was effective because of analgesic or antianxiety properties, or both, is unclear. A benzodiazepine might have been equally effective and would now be considered the drug of first choice.

The mechanism by which neuroleptics affect pain has not been definitely established. They may have primary analgesic effects; they may potentiate analgesic effects of other agents; or they may diminish other symptoms associated with pain. The sedating effects of most neuroleptics make them desirable in some situations and undesirable in others. Their antiemetic effects are beneficial in patients given narcotics for pain, although they may aggravate the respiratory depression caused by narcotics. The choice of agent is best based on the drug's profile and the physician's familiarity with the drug. Schechter (1984) recommends using 2 mg/kg per day of chlorpromazine or 0.05–0.075 mg/kg per day of haloperidol for relief of pain. The use of neuroleptics in a medically ill child is illustrated below.

> A 10-year-old child awoke after brain surgery with agitated hyperactive behavior, anxiety, and pressured speech. He complained that the pain was more severe than after his previous brain surgery. Hydromorphone given for pain was discontinued after his parents informed the staff of a previous, similar adverse behavioral reaction to methadone. Subsequently, the child became self-destructive, thrashing about and banging his head, and was given haloperidol 2 mg iv.
>
> On awakening, his hyperactive behavior and pressured speech recurred. He reported sensations of pain at the surgical site. Additional doses of haloperidol, 0.5 mg iv, were administered along with diphenhydramine 25 mg po every 4–6 hours for sedation and as a prophylactic for extrapyramidal side effects. The patient's complaints of pain and fear of pain ceased, and he began to behave normally.

The antiemetic properties of neuroleptics make them useful for the treatment of vomiting accompanying migraine headaches, cancer chemotherapy, postoperative recovery (including vomiting provoked by narcotic analgesics), and other conditions or treatments. They may be given prophylactically to prepare for anticipated nausea. However, one study (Zeltzer et al. 1984) found paradoxical effects when prochlorperazine or chlorpromazine were given prophylactically to control nausea and vomiting related to cancer chemotherapy. Children served as their own controls during trials with and without the drugs. The children as a group actually demonstrated more symptoms and behaviors related to nausea and vomiting during trials in which the phenothiazines were used. Children are known to be highly suggestible regarding emesis and may have thought they should feel more nauseated when the drugs were given. This study should not be construed as unequivocal proof that prophylactic treatment of emesis is ineffective. Rather, the clinician is advised to consider each child and each situation individually to determine whether an antiemetic would be beneficial and, if so, which to use. Droperidol, a butyrophenone, has been used as an adjuvant in anesthesia and as an antiemetic (Marshall and Wollman 1985). Doses of 0.025–0.075 mg/kg have been used successfully in the treatment of postanesthetic vomiting in children undergoing surgery for strabismus (Christensen et al. 1989; Eustis et al. 1987; Nicolson et al. 1988), though the lowest effective dose of droperidol is in question (Abramowitz et al. 1983; Apt 1987). Droperidol is thought to have more rapid onset, shorter duration of action, and lower incidence of extrapyramidal symptoms than haloperidol (Cassem 1984; Liston 1989).

While some clinicians prefer to treat delirium with drugs from other classes, antipsychotics have an important place in the management of delirium, especially when psychotic features predominate. Antipsychotics may be necessary for sedation or to correct disorganized thinking or self-destructive or aggressive behavior. Usually, the doses needed to treat organic mental disorders are considerably lower than those necessary to treat functional psychoses. Many clinicians prefer high-potency agents such as haloperidol, which are less sedating and less apt to lower blood pressure and seizure threshold than low-potency phenothiazines (Baldessarini 1985). Side effects include sedation, hypotension, and extrapyramidal symptoms. In a study of 112 children with cardiovascular and respiratory side effects, the children had a mild drop in blood pressure but no statistically significant changes in pulse or respiratory rate (Butt and Mets 1988). Several cases examples illustrate the use of antipsychotics to treat manifestations of delirium in children.

A 7-year-old boy with medulloblastoma required treatment with dexamethasone, which even in low doses caused visual and tactile hallucinations that alarmed the child and his family. Because dexamethasone was considered essential in the management of his primary illness, chlorpromazine was added with excellent results. Although the hallucinations did not abate entirely, they became less frightening.

Victor, a 13-year-old with aplastic anemia, developed a severe infection of his arm. The arm was covered so he would not see the unsightly lesion. He was anxious and severely agitated and eventually began to hallucinate, describing motorcycles racing toward him and waterfalls rushing in from the walls. After receiving a total of 250 mg po of chlorpromazine without benefit, he was given 25 mg iv, which sedated him and controlled the hallucinations.

Cathy, a 16-year-old undergoing bone marrow transplantation for acute lymphocytic leukemia, developed herpetic infections and was in severe pain. Fearing that death was imminent, she resisted sleep and became severely agitated and hypervigilant and thrashed about on her bed. She was finally sedated with 25 mg iv of chlorpromazine. A dosage of approximately 200 mg/day kept her comfortable during the terminal phase of her illness.

The choice of a neuroleptic depends in large part on the familiarity of the psychiatrist and pediatrician with the various drugs and their knowledge about potential side effects. The most popular neuroleptics in the pediatric setting appear to be chlorpromazine, thioridazine, and haloperidol. The use of chlorpromazine is discouraged by some because of its potential to produce agranulocytosis; however, some pediatricians, familiar with its use as a sedative and an antiemetic are comfortable with it. Haloperidol is favored by many because it is less sedating and acts rapidly; others fear its potential for extrapyramidal side effects. Except when used to treat schizophrenia, the doses of neuroleptics used in physically ill children usually are so low that acute side effects are rarely a major problem.

Side effects may occur, however, and include sedation, allergic reactions, skin rashes, agranulocytosis, jaundice and hepatic damage, retinopathy and photosensitivity, anticholinergic effects, galactorrhea, tachycardia, decreased blood pressure and ECG changes, extrapyramidal symptoms, tardive dyskinesia, neuroleptic-induced catatonia and neuroleptic malignant syndrome, impaired cognition and learning, and even psychosis or depression. They may also lower the seizure threshold. Dystonic reactions may occur with any of these drugs and are not necessarily dose related (World Health Organization 1987). Dystonic reactions may respond to a decrease in dose, but usually require treatment with diphenhydramine or benztropine. Prophylactic use of these antiparkinsonian agents is not recommended because of their usually unwanted anticholinergic effects.

Because of the potential for neuroleptics to produce EEG changes and to lower the seizure threshold, it is wise to obtain neurologic consultation before using these drugs in children with significant central nervous system diseases or previously abnormal EEGs. Unless a child is psychotic, it is usually possible to find therapeutic alternatives to antipsychotics, thereby avoiding these drugs in children with central nervous system pathology. A review by Itil (1980) provides useful information about the epileptogenic nature of these drugs in adults. Neuroleptics with more prominent extrapyramidal side effects tend to be less epileptogenic. Patients with normal EEGs without detectable organic CNS dysfunction and no history of seizures can be considered essentially risk free.

Patients with symptoms or a history of organic brain dysfunction or epilepsy and patients with abnormal EEGs should be carefully evaluated before being given psychotropic drugs. Agents with strong epileptogenic properties, such as chlorpromazine, should be avoided. If an antipsychotic is necessary, the dose should be increased gradually, and very high doses, sudden dose changes, or unnecessarily prolonged treatment should be avoided. These patients should receive EEGs after treatment as a screen for neurotoxicity. Patients without previous organic brain dysfunction who have EEG abnormalities while on neuroleptic drugs should be carefully reevaluated neurologically. EEG abnormalities during the course of neuroleptic drug treatment in the absence of abnormal clinical findings or seizures are of less concern than those associated with definite neurological disorder. EEGs and neurological examinations should be repeated regularly for patients at risk on prolonged treatment; anticonvulsant medication should be considered for overt seizures or epileptiform EEG abnormalities (Itil 1980).

The recognition of tardive dyskinesia as a serious consequence of the use of neuroleptic agents has resulted in increasing concern. Gualtieri et al. (1980) described a number of movement disorders associated with neuroleptics, including extrapyramidal symptoms, tardive dyskinesia, and withdrawal dyskinesias. While the dose of antipsychotics is usually quite low and the duration of treatment is usually brief in physically ill children, dose and length of treatment are not necessarily predictive of the occurrence of these movement disorders. A study of neurologists' experiences with patients who develop movement disorders indicates that neuroleptic-induced movement disorders during and after drug treatment occur with significant frequency in children (Silverstein and Johnston 1987). Therefore, alternatives should be used when possible.

When neuroleptics are to be used, patients and their parents need to be told of the risk of tardive dyskinesia and of the absence of definitive treatments for it. Children on neuroleptics should be examined regularly and systematically for involuntary movements, and the results of the examinations should be documented.

STIMULANTS

Stimulants were introduced many years ago and have enjoyed extraordinary success in the treatment of attention-deficit and hyperactivity disorders in children. Since the introduction of tricyclic antidepressants and monoamine oxidase inhibitors, their use in the treatment of depression has been unpopular. The fact that stimulants (other than pemoline) are designated Schedule II drugs by the Drug Enforcement Administration and concern about their addictive potential have made many physicians hesitant to use them. However, recently there has been a resurgence of interest in these drugs to manage depression in the medically ill and elderly and as adjuvant analgesic agents.

Studies of depressed geriatric and medically ill patients provide information on the indications for and efficacy of stimulant treatment. Reports and studies address the use of only dextroamphetamine and methylphenidate, but there may also be situations in which pemoline is indicated. Stimulants should be considered for short-term use in depressed medically ill patients for whom the anticholinergic and cardiovascular effects of tricyclics are contraindicated, for patients with cardiovascular disorders, and for patients in whom rapid improvement is critical (see also Chapter 2).

Woods et al. (1986) reviewed medical records of 66 medically ill patients who underwent 71 therapeutic trials of stimulants. The average age of patients was 72 years, with a range of 37–87 years, and diagnoses included major depression, adjustment disorder with depressed mood, organic affective syndrome, and dementia. Both dextroamphetamine and methylphenidate were used in trials lasting between 1 and 87 days, with a mean length of trial of 8.9 days. Improvement occurred in 52, or 73%, of the trials; the improvement was marked or moderate in 34, or 48%, of the trials. Improvement occurred rapidly and was evident in a wide range of functional areas, including mood, motivation, concentration, activity level, appetite, and sleep. Relapse occurred in only 5 patients, 4 of whom had diagnoses of major depression. Five patients, or 7%, developed side effects that led to the discontinuation of the medication. Two patients with dementia became more confused; 1 patient developed sinus tachycardia and diaphoresis; 1 patient developed nausea; and 1 developed a rash. None of the side effects were considered severe, and all were reversible.

Fernandez et al. (1987) treated 30 depressed cancer patients, ages 30 years and older, with methylphenidate. Psychiatric diagnoses included major depression, adjustment disorder with depression, dementia with depressed mood, organic affective syndrome, and organic personality disorder. Methylphenidate was given three times daily at 7 A.M., 10 A.M., and 1 P.M. Ten patients showed marked improvement, and 13 showed moderate improvement. One patient with dementia experienced confusion and agitation; another developed tachycardia and chest pain. These problems disappeared when the drug was discontinued and did not return when it was reinstituted at a lower dose. In 11 of the patients, recurrence or rebound symptoms occurred when attempts were made to discontinue the drug. No tolerance or abuse had occurred as long as 1 year after beginning treatment.

Favoring the use of stimulants is their rapid onset of action and their lack of serious adverse side effects. Whether the drugs are clinically effective in a given patient can be decided rapidly. The drugs can be given two or three times a day, but the final dose should be administered by early or mid-afternoon to prevent interference with sleep (Ayd 1985). Side effects and toxic effects of stimulants include irritability, agitation, anxiety, insomnia, confusion, tremor, aggressive behavior, depression, psychosis, appetite and weight changes, abdominal pain, headache, tachycardia and dysrhythmias, and changes in blood pressure. Stimulants do not increase seizure activity (Prugh 1983; Tesar 1982). Side effects generally occur within the first few days of treatment, are reversible, and usually are less bothersome than those associated with tricyclics. While tolerance and abuse may occur, most reports of stimulant use in medically ill adults have not found them to be serious concerns (Satel and Nelson 1989).

Amphetamines and methylphenidate are rapidly absorbed, and peak concentrations are reached 1–3 hours after oral administration. Distribution of amphetamines is extensive, and they undergo considerable biotransformation (Combrinck-Graham et al. 1980). Since their use for treating depression in medically ill children has not been investigated, certain points of caution are advised. Very low doses of 5 mg or less are appropriate initial therapy and should be given early in the day. Response should be evident within a few days. Headache, abdominal pain, and loss of appetite have been observed in children on stimulants but are usually reversible if the dose is decreased. Rebound depression in the late afternoon or evening can also occur and is more problematic; if adjustments in dose and schedule are not effective, the drug may need to be discontinued.

In addition to their use for the treatment of depression in the medically ill, stimulants may be used as adjuvants in the treatment of pain. These agents, however, have little if any analgesic effect when used alone (Tesar 1982). Forrest et al. (1977) compared the analgesic effect of dextroamphetamine and morphine with morphine alone for the treatment of postoperative pain in adults and found the combination was more effective. There is no evidence, however, that this combination is effective for pain relief over an extended period (Fields

1987). Stimulants may also be effective in pediatric populations. Schechter (1984) recommends doses of 2–10 mg/day of dextroamphetamine. As in other situations, the initial dose should be very low but can be increased as tolerated.

Kaufmann and Murray (1982) and Walling and Pfefferbaum (1990) have reported the use of stimulants in individual teenagers with medical illnesses. However, there are no known studies systematically investigating the use of these drugs in medically ill children and teenagers. Their successful use in medically ill and elderly adults, rapid onset of action, relatively benign profile of side effects, and extensive testing in physically healthy children with attention-deficit disorder argue in favor of their use in selected situations.

REFERENCES

Abramowitz MD, Oh TH, Epstein BS, et al: The antiemetic effect of droperidol following outpatient strabismus surgery in children. Anesthesiology 59:579–583, 1983

Ambrosini PJ: Pharmacotherapy in child and adolescent major depressive disorder, in Psychopharmacology: The Third Generation of Progress. Edited by Meltzer HY. New York, Raven, 1987, pp 1247–1254

Apt L: Discussion. J Pediatr Ophthalmol Strabismus 24:168–169, 1987

Ayd FJ: Psychostimulant therapy for depressed medically ill patients. Psychiatric Annals 15:462–465, 1985

Baldessarini RJ: Drugs and the treatment of psychiatric disorders, in The Pharmacological Basis of Therapeutics. Edited by Gilman AG, Goodman LS, Rall TW, et al. New York, Macmillan, 1985, pp 387–445

Blau S: A guide to the use of psychotropic medication in children and adolescents. J Clin Psychiatry 39:766–772, 1978

Braunlich H: Kidney development: drug elimination mechanisms, in Drug Disposition During Development. Edited by Morselli PL. New York, Spectrum, 1977, pp 89–100

Butt AD, Mets B: Cardiovascular and respiratory effects of oral premedication with trimeprazine and droperidol in children. S Afr Med J 73:582–583, 1988

Cassem NH: Critical care psychiatry, in Textbook of Critical Care. Edited by Shoemaker WC, Thompson WL, Holbrook PR. Philadelphia, PA, WB Saunders, 1984, pp 981–989

Christensen S, Farrow-Gillespie A, Lerman J: Incidence of emesis and postanesthetic recovery after strabismus surgery in children: a comparison of droperidol and lidocaine. Anesthesiology 70:251–254, 1989

Coffey B, Shader RI, Greenblatt DJ: Pharmacokinetics of benzodiazepines and psychostimulants in children. J Clin Psychopharmacol 3:217–225, 1983

Combrinck-Graham L, Gursky EJ, Saccar CL: Psychoactive agents, in Pediatric Pharmacology: Therapeutic Principles in Practice. Edited by Yaffe SJ. New York, Grune & Stratton, 1980, pp 455–478

Diament MJ, Stanley P: The use of midazolam for sedation of infants and children. AJR 150:377–378, 1988

Einarson TR, Yoder ES: Triazolam psychosis—a syndrome? Drug Intell Clin Pharm 16:330–331, 1982

Eustis S, Lerman J, Smith DR: Effect of droperidol pretreatment on post-anesthetic vomiting in children undergoing strabismus surgery: the minimum effective dose. J Pediatr Ophthalmol Strabismus 24:165–168, 1987

Fava GA, Sonino N: The use of antidepressant drugs in the medically ill. Psychiatric Annals 17:42–44, 1987

Fernandez F, Adams F, Holmes VF, et al: Methylphenidate for depressive disorders in cancer patients. Psychosomatics 28:455–461, 1987

Fields HL: Pain. New York, McGraw-Hill, 1987

Forrest WH, Brown BW, Brown CR, et al: Dextroamphetamine with morphine for the treatment of postoperative pain. N Engl J Med 296:712–715, 1977

Geller B, Cooper TB, Schluchter MD, et al: Child and adolescent nortriptyline single dose pharmacokinetic parameters: final report. J Clin Psychopharmacol 7:321–323, 1987

Group for the Advancement of Psychiatry: How Old Is Old Enough? The Ages of Rights and Responsibilities. New York, Brunner/Mazel, 1989, pp 53–73

Gualtieri CT, Barnhill J, McGimsey J, et al: Tardive dyskinesia and other movement disorders in children treated with psychotrophic drugs. J Am Acad Child Psychiatry 19:491–510, 1980

Hoge SK, Biederman J: Liver function tests during treatment with desipramine in children and adolescents. J Clin Psychopharmacol 7:87–89, 1987

Itil TM, Soldatos C: Epileptogenic side effects of psychotropic drugs. JAMA 244:1460–1463, 1980

Jay SM, Elliott CH, Katz E, et al: Cognitive-behavioral and pharmacologic interventions for children's distress during painful medical procedures. J Consult Clin Psychol 55:860–865, 1987

Jefferson JW: Cardiovascular effects and toxicity of anxiolytics and antidepressants. J Clin Psychiatry 50:368–378, 1989

Kashani J, Shekim WO, Reid JC: Amitriptyline in children with major depressive disorder: a double-blind crossover pilot study. J Am Acad Child Psychiatry 23:348–351, 1984

Kauffman RE, Habersang R: Modification of dosage regimens in disease states of childhood, in Clinical Pharmacology and Therapeutics: A Pediatric Perspective. Edited by Mirkin BL. Chicago, IL, Year Book Medical, 1978, pp 73–88

Kaufmann MW, Murray GB: The use of d-amphetamine in medically ill depressed patients. J Clin Psychiatry 43:463–464, 1982

Liston EH: Delirium, in Treatments of Psychiatric Disorders: A Task Force Report of the American Psychiatric Association, Vol 1. Washington, DC, American Psychiatric Association, 1989, pp 804–815

Marshall BE, Wollman H: General anesthetics, in The Pharmacological Basis of Therapeutics. Edited by Gilman AG, Goodman LS, Rall TW, et al. New York, Macmillan, 1985, pp 276–301

Massie MJ, Holland JC: Psychiatry and oncology, in Psychiatry Update: The American Psychiatric Association Annual Review, Vol 3. Edited by Grinspoon L. Washington, DC, American Psychiatric Association Press, 1984, pp 239–256

McDermott JF, Werry J, Petti T, et al: Anxiety disorders of childhood or adolescence, in Treatments of Psychiatric Disorders: A Task Force Report of the American Psychiatric Association, Vol 1. Washington, DC, American Psychiatric Association, 1989, pp 401–446

Meyers BS: The patient with renal disease, in Treatments of Psychiatric Disorders: A Task Force Report of the American Psychiatric Association, Vol 1. Washington, DC, American Psychiatric Association, 1989, pp 915–929

Mills MJ, Daniels ML: Medical-legal issues, in Principles of Medical Psychiatry. Edited by Stoudemire A, Fogel BS. Orlando, FL, Grune & Stratton, 1987, pp 463–474

Nicolson SC, Kaya KM, Betts EK: The effect of preoperative oral droperidol on the incidence of postoperative emesis after paediatric strabismus surgery. Can J Anaesth 35:364–367, 1988

Nye SG: Legal issues in the practice of child psychiatry, in Child Psychiatry and the Law. Edited by Schetky DH, Benedek EP. New York, Brunner/Mazel, 1980, pp 266–286

Orsulak PJ: Therapeutic monitoring of antidepressant drugs: current methodology and applications. J Clin Psychiatry 47:39–50, 1986

Petti TA, Law W: Imipramine treatment of depressed children: a double blind-pilot study. J Clin Psychopharmacol 2:107–110, 1982

Petti TA, Fish B, Shapiro T, et al: Effects of chlordiazepoxide in disturbed children: a pilot study. J Clin Psychopharmacol 2:270–273, 1982

Pfefferbaum B, Overall JE: Decisions about drug treatment in children. J Am Acad Child Psychiatry 23:209–214, 1984

Pfefferbaum B, Butler PM, Mullins D, et al: Two cases of benzodiazepine toxicity in children. J Clin Psychiatry 48:450–452, 1987a

Pfefferbaum B, Overall JE, Boren HA, et al: Alprazolam in the treatment of anticipatory and acute situational anxiety in children with cancer. J Am Acad Child Adolesc Psychiatry 26:532–535, 1987b

Pfefferbaum-Levine B, Kumor K, Cangir A, et al: Tricyclic antidepressants for children with cancer. Am J Psychiatry 140:1074–1076, 1983

Preskorn SH, Weller EB, Weller RA: Depression in children: relationship between plasma imipramine levels and response. J Clin Psychiatry 43:450–453, 1982

Prugh DG: The Psychosocial Aspects of Pediatrics. Philadelphia, PA, Lea & Febiger, 1983

Puig-Antich J, Perel JM, Lupatkin W, et al: Plasma levels of imipramine (IMI) and desmethylimipramine (DMI) and clinical response in prepubertal major depressive disorder. J Am Acad Child Psychiatry 18:616–627, 1979

Puig-Antich J, Perel JM, Lupatkin W, et al: Imipramine in prepubertal major depressive disorders. Arch Gen Psychiatry 44:81–89, 1987

Rane A: Basic principles of drug disposition and action in infants and children, in Pediatric Pharmacology: Therapeutic Principles in Practice. Edited by Yaffe SJ. New York, Grune & Stratton, 1980, pp 7–28

Rapoport JL: Pediatric psychopharmacology: the last decade, in Psychopharmacology: The Third Generation of Progress. Edited by Meltzer HY. New York, Raven, 1987, pp 1211–1214

Rapoport JL, Mikkelsen EJ, Werry JS: Antimanic, antianxiety, hallucinogenic, and miscellaneous drugs, in Pediatric Psychopharmacology: The Use of Behavior Modifying Drugs in Children. Edited by Werry JS. New York, Brunner/Mazel, 1978, pp 316–355

Richardson JW, Richelson E: Antidepressants: a clinical update for medical practitioners. Mayo Clin Proc 59:330–337, 1984

Richelson E: Tricyclic antidepressants: therapy for ulcer and other novel uses. Modern Medicine 51(10):74–84, 1983

Roose SP, Glassman AH, Giardina EGV, et al: Tricyclic antidepressants in depressed patients with cardiac conduction disease. Arch Gen Psychiatry 44:273–275, 1987

Salonen M, Kanto J, Iisalo E, et al: Midazolam as an induction agent in children: a pharmacokinetic and clinical study. Anesth Analg 66:625–628, 1987

Salzman C: Treatment with antianxiety agents, in Treatments of Psychiatric Disorders: A Task Force Report of the American Psychiatric Association, Vol 2. Washington, DC, American Psychiatric Association, 1989, pp 2036–2052

Satel SL, Nelson JC: Stimulants in the treatment of depression: a critical overview. J Clin Psychiatry 50:241–249, 1989

Schechter NL: Recurrent pains in children: an overview and an approach. Pediatr Clin North Am 31:949–968, 1984

Schroeder JS, Mullin AV, Elliott GR, et al: Cardiovascular effects of desipramine in children. J Am Acad Child Adolesc Psychiatry 28:376–379, 1989

Silverstein FS, Johnston MV: Risks of neuroleptic drugs in children. J Child Neurol 2:41–43, 1987

Stoudemire A, Fogel BS: Psychopharmacology in the medically ill, in Principles of Medical Psychiatry. Edited by Stoudemire A, Fogel BS. Orlando, FL, Grune & Stratton, 1987, pp 79–112

Tesar GE: The role of stimulants in general medicine. Drug Therapy 12:186–195, 1982

Van Hoff J, Olszewski D: Lorazepam for the control of chemotherapy-related nausea and vomiting in children. J Pediatr 113:146–149, 1988

Walling VR, Pfefferbaum B: The use of methylphenidate in a depressed adolescent with AIDS. J Dev Behav Pediatr 11:195–197, 1990

Weller EB, Weller RA, Preskorn SH, et al: Steady-state plasma imipramine levels in prepubertal depressed children. Am J Psychiatry 139:506–508, 1982

Woods SW, Tesar GE, Murray GB, et al: Psychostimulant treatment of depressive disorders secondary to medical illness. J Clin Psychiatry 47:12–15, 1986

World Health Organization: Drugs for Children. Edited by Rylance G. Denmark, World Health Organization, 1987

Zeltzer L, LeBaron S, Zeltzer PM: Paradoxical effects of prophylactic phenothiazine antiemetics in children receiving chemotherapy. J Clin Oncol 2:930–936, 1984

Chapter 14

Family Therapy in the Context of Childhood Medical Illness

Jane Jacobs, Ed.D.

Rapid advances in technology have resulted in a larger group of children who survive previously life-threatening childhood illnesses; approximately 7.5 million (12%) of all children have some chronic medical condition, and about 10% of these children suffer from severe or disabling chronic disorders (Hobbs et al. 1985). Ironically, the survival of large numbers of seriously ill children has created difficulties for their families, who must shoulder extensive responsibilities of caring for a chronically ill or disabled child.

The psychiatrist is often in a strategic position to provide specialized interventions for families facing difficulties related to caretaking. The psychiatrist may intervene directly or through consultation to the pediatricians, pediatric specialists, and family physicians who provide primary medical care to the ill child.

COMMON PROBLEMS OF FAMILIES WITH ILL CHILDREN

The presence of a chronic medical illness does not automatically result in severe distress for family members. However, it often signif-

Table 14-1.   Common family problems with childhood medical illness

---

I. Intrafamilial problems
  A. Organizational
    1. Inflexibility in problem solving (instrumental rigidity)
    2. Inability to express conflict or grief (affective constraint)
    3. Reorganization of the family around the illness
  B. Developmental
    1. Constraints on the child's development
    2. Delays or disruption of the family's life cycle (e.g., siblings leaving home)

II. Family interface problems
  A. The family and the medical care team
  B. The family and the child's peer group
  C. Financial problems

---

icantly affects critical areas of family adjustment and performance. For example, while divorce is not more common in families with a chronically ill child than in those with a healthy child, parents of children with serious medical problems report higher levels of disagreement and express more marital dissatisfaction (Sabbeth and Leventhal 1984).

Similarly, siblings of chronically ill children do not show pervasive psychiatric symptomatology compared with children with healthy siblings, but they do have greater difficulties in social adjustment, for example, in managing aggression (Breslau et al. 1981), and in overcoming social isolation (Vance et al. 1980).

Chronic medical illness is likely to trigger or exacerbate organizational and developmental problems within the family. When problems arise, the family's response depends in part on the action of others, including the medical care system, the child's school and peer group, and the various sources of financial support for the child's care. Major illness-related problems for caretaking families can therefore be subdivided into "intrafamilial problems" and "family interface problems" (Table 14-1).

Intrafamilial Problems

Organizational issues.   Many observers have noted the power of chronic disorders to disrupt family regulatory processes (Campbell 1986; Gonzalez et al. 1989; Jacobs and Steinglass, in press; Penn 1983; Ramsey 1989; Rolland 1987; Sheinberg 1983; Steinglass and Horan 1988). These disruptions affect both the affective and the instrumental (problem-solving) domains of family life. In the affective domain, a problematic degree of constraint may begin to pervade family interaction. Fearing that conflict or intense affect will exacerbate the child's symptoms, family members impose a new level of emotional constriction on the system. This constraint curtails not only the necessary expression of differences among family members but also the intense feelings of grief family members inevitably experience in the face of a child's chronic illness.

In the instrumental area, the family may develop greater rigidity in its problem-solving strategies. A "walking on eggshells" mentality takes hold in this area of family life as well; members fear that experimenting with new solutions may lead to dangerous mistakes. Family members may form alliances or "coalitions" to oppose any new approaches to treatment, whether they are suggested by a health professional or a dissenting member of the family.

The construct of "family burden" has been used to describe both the objective amount of family time devoted to the illness and the subjective distress experienced in connection with caretaking responsibilities. The family members may allow the illness to become the dominant force in the family as more and more time, energy, and money are devoted to the care of the ill child. There is a risk that in many aspects of family life—the expression of feelings, the negotiation of tasks, and the setting of priorities—the family will reorganize around the illness and give insufficient weight to the needs of other members of the family (Gonzalez et al. 1989).

In the case of divorced and single-parent families, the burden on family resources is considerably more intense. Reduced adult availability and conflicts over parental responsibilities make it even more difficult for families to maintain their equilibrium in the face of the illness's demands.

Developmental issues. Chronic medical illness can engender developmental problems both in the ill child and in the family that is caring for the child (Whitt 1982). Complications relating to the child occur when the illness disrupts a key developmental process or when family members protect the child from pursuing new personal challenges due to concern about the illness. Family developmental deviation occurs when important life cycle processes are delayed or omitted because of concerns about the illness. For example, young adult siblings of the ill child may feel pressure not to leave the home because of caretaking demands or financial constraints brought on by the illness. The illness may lead the parents to decide not to have more children because of the burden of illness or because of concerns about genetic transmission. In the case of a terminal or debilitating illness, the family may have difficulty picturing its own future or planning future events because of its inability to contemplate a time when the child will be institutionalized or will die.

Family Interface Problems

The family and the medical care team. In the course of managing the long-term care of a child with serious medical problems, the immediate family and the medical team form an enduring caregiving system. The intensity of attachments between the family and the medical team and their effect on the child's illness are often underestimated (Reiss and Kaplan-De-Nour 1989). Changes in the illness, within the family, and in the composition or organization of the medical staff cause small perturbations in these relationships.

Two common problems arise within the caregiving system formed by the family and medical team. The first concerns the priorities of the professional caregivers. Medical care providers, who become attached to the ill child, emphasize everything the family can do to promote the recovery of the patient. The family, which becomes dependent on the medical providers, usually strives to comply with their advice. This exclusive focus on the patient fails to take non-illness-related family priorities into account and reinforces the family's tendency to organize itself solely around the illness. The second problem arises from the difficulty experienced by family members and medical caregivers in accepting the child's illness and, by definition, the limits of what they can do. Both groups, faced with the initial diagnosis, with relapses, or with deterioration, must work through a variety of feelings that may include anxiety, anger, guilt, and grief. Family members may avoid dealing with their feelings by not listening to information provided by the medical care team, by maintaining unrealistic expectations of the medical team, or by harboring resentments toward health professionals for perceived mistakes and insensitivities. Either the medical team as a whole may be attacked, or the team may be split in the family's perception into "good" and "bad" caregivers.

Physicians may be narcissistically wounded by their inability to prevent recurrent illness or disability. Consequently, they may unwittingly contribute to the problem by not talking to parents frankly about their child's prognosis in a way that permits everyone to express disappointment.

The family and the child's peer group.   An important challenge for families with a medically ill child is the reintegration of the child into his or her social network. Spending time in the hospital or sick at home often disrupts peer relationships and may leave the child with visible signs of illness. Restrictions on activity may inhibit the child from rejoining friends. The child's fears may not be unfounded; his or her friends may be frightened or repulsed by the physical consequences of the illness.

Depending on the child's age, the parents may have to intercede directly with the child's teachers, classmates, or friends. Problems may arise as parents struggle to allow their children an appropriate degree of autonomy in negotiating their somewhat mercurial social sphere. Hostility in the child's social environment may serve as a stimulus for parents to protect the child excessively from important developmental challenges, including age-appropriate differentiation of the child from the family.

Financial problems.   Financial burden is one of the greatest sources of distress for families with a medically ill child. A financial crisis may arise either from uncovered medical or rehabilitation expenses, from loss of income due to curtailed parental employment, or often both (Hobbs et al. 1985). Public and private reimbursement entities typically pay for hospitalization and emergency services but rarely for maintenance functions such as transportation to specialty care facilities, special equipment needed at home, child care, social services, and respite care. Such reimbursement priorities reinforce the family's tendency to organize around the illness by making heroic caretaking strategies necessary.

The lack of reimbursement for maintenance services leaves the family with difficult financial and moral choices about the proper allocation of family resources. The primary caretaker, often the mother, must decide whether to cut back on paid employment to care for the child herself, or to continue working to pay for private support services. The difficulty of making such morally complex decisions raises the level of distress in the family. Rigidly organized families, for example, those with narrowly defined sex roles, may be unable to approach this dilemma effectively.

FAMILY ASSESSMENT

Assessment of families with a child with a serious medical illness should include evaluation in three major dimensions: illness charac-

Table 14-2. Dimensions of family assessment

I. Illness characteristics
   A. Illness phase
      1. Acute
      2. Chronic
   B. Specific illness features
      1. Unpredictability
      2. Need for intensive monitoring
      3. Uncertain prognosis
      4. Extensive developmental constriction
      5. Disfigurement and stigmatization

II. Child developmental factors
   A. Emotional development
   B. Cognitive development

III. Family response
   A. Fit between family style and demands of the illness
   B. Preservation of preillness activities, pleasures, and traditions
   C. Developmental issues of family members
   D. Family beliefs
   E. "Toxic intergenerational themes"

---

teristics, child developmental factors, and family response (Table 14-2).

Illness Characteristics

The primary focus of this discussion are childhood illnesses that are either chronic or relapsing and remitting, as they make the greatest demands on the family. Relevant illness characteristics include illness phase (acute or chronic, relapse or remission) and specific illness characteristics such as prognosis, predictability, disability, and disfigurement (Gonzalez et al. 1989; Jacobs 1989; Rolland 1987).

Illness phase. The tasks faced by family members dealing with the acute and chronic phases of childhood illnesses are different; behaviors and attitudes that are adaptive in one phase can be ineffective or even counterproductive in another. The *acute phase* of childhood medical illness includes the diagnostic procedures and medical interventions aimed at controlling symptoms, preventing further progression of the disease, and in some illnesses, such as cancer, inducing a remission. The primary tasks for a family dealing with the acute phase of an illness are to incorporate accurate information about the disorder

Table 14-3. Elements of adaptive response to a child's illness

I. Acute phase
  A. Obtaining and integrating information about the child's illness
  B. Explaining the illness to the sick child and to the siblings
  C. Mobilizing extended family and friends for support
  D. Coping with anxiety and depression about the illness
  E. Reallocating family resources

II. Chronic phase
  A. Adhering to regimens of diet, medications, and activity
  B. Carrying out maintenance and prophylactic treatments
  C. Providing support and rehabilitation when needed
  D. Containing and routinizing illness management
  E. Restoring pre-illness family routines, priorities, and traditions

as quickly as possible and to mobilize resources to deal with the ensuing medical crisis.

Family resources of time, money, and effort need to be reallocated to attend to the needs of the ill child even at considerable cost to other family priorities. One or both parents often miss work or neglect major household responsibilities in order to keep medical appointments, make inquiries about the illness, or provide direct care for the child. While this high level of mobilization is not "normal," it is adaptive. A temporary narrowing of the family's focus is a phase-specific necessity for adequately responding to a family crisis.

Assessment of a family's response to an acute episode of serious illness should focus on family members' ability to comprehend the nature of the illness and to appropriately allocate family resources for efficacious management of the medical condition (Table 14-3). Specific elements include 1) the family's ability to obtain and integrate critical information about the disorder; 2) the parents' ability to explain the illness to the sick child and to their other children in an age-appropriate manner; 3) the family's ability to mobilize extended family and friends for emotional and pragmatic support; 4) the family members' ability to deal appropriately with anxiety and depression about the illness; and 5) the family members' ability to reallocate family resources on a temporary basis to attend to the illness.

The *chronic phase* begins after initial treatments have controlled the disease process to the extent possible. For many illnesses, the chronic phase involves minimizing exacerbations through medications, diet, restrictions on patient activity, or treatments (sometimes involving elective hospitalizations). For other illnesses, chronic care involves providing social supports and rehabilitative interventions to mitigate disability from a stable or deteriorating medical condition. The care-taking tasks during the chronic phase may be great or small, but by a certain point the nature of caretaking tasks is known.

It is critical during the chronic phase of childhood illness that family members find ways to routinize and contain illness manage-ment and to prevent the illness and the sick child from completely dominating the family. A family's successful adaptation to the chronic phase involves protecting important family routines, priorities, and traditions that preceded the illness. The elements that comprise this adaptation process are discussed in greater detail later in this section under "Family Response."

Specific illness features. There is a growing literature on the psy-chosocial effects of specific medical disorders on children and families (Brunnquell and Hall 1982; Heisler and Friedman 1981; Hobbs and Perrin 1985; Rolland 1984; Whitt 1984). Rolland (1984) has emphasized the usefulness of classifying illnesses by similarities in onset, course, and prognosis. It is helpful to characterize childhood medical disorders according to the following salient features that pose particular chal-lenges to the family:

1. *Unpredictability.* Although rarely life threatening, acute ep-isodes of pediatric asthma, hemophilia, and sickle cell ane-mia are highly unpredictable. Therefore, family members never know when the child will have to miss school or social events, when they will have to cancel a long-planned activ-ity, or when they will have to pay for an emergency medical treatment.

2. *Need for intensive monitoring.* Children with renal disease and juvenile diabetes require close daily supervision, in-cluding daily injections, frequent blood or urine tests, a strict dietary regimen, and exercise restrictions. With the medical stakes so high, the parents and the ill child often have dif-ficulty deciding how much autonomous responsibility the child should have for self-care. When the patient is an ad-olescent, excessive parental assumption of responsibility poses a threat to the child's successful completion of a teenager's central developmental task.

3. *Uncertain prognosis.* End-stage renal disease, childhood cancer, and congenital heart disease may make the long-term survival of the child uncertain. This ambiguity can lead the family to avoid any discussion of the illness and,

at times, to be unable to conceptualize its future. Alternatively, the family may maintain an inappropriately high level of vigilance after the acute treatment period is over. For example, the family may avoid all situations believed to even minimally increase the risk of infection or injury.

4. *Extensive developmental constriction.* Such conditions as spina bifida, which may include mental retardation, fecal and urinary incontinence, and partial or complete loss of coordination in the lower extremities, inflict a pervasive emotional and financial burden on the family. Virtually all family plans and routines are in some way affected by the constant attention required by the ill child. Siblings may feel guilty about enjoying social activities or demanding parental attention. Young adult siblings may be reluctant to move away from the family, and no longer share the family's burden.

5. *Disfiguring and stigmatizing conditions.* Craniofacial anomalies and other disfiguring conditions may cause special problems for the attachment process between the child and the family and for the child's socialization with his or her peer group. Although some craniofacial anomalies are correctable with multiple surgeries, the parents' ambivalence about the child often is a source of intense guilt and sometimes is a barrier to the provision of adequate care. The social stigma associated with conditions such as acquired immunodeficiency syndrome (AIDS) may reduce the child's social support, discourage siblings from socializing with friends at home, and exacerbate parental isolation.

Child's developmental stage. The psychological impact of illness on a child depends on the child's specific developmental stage (Bibace and Walsh 1981; Brunnquell and Hall 1982; Drotar et al. 1984; Heisler and Friedman 1981; Mattsson 1972; Perrin and Gerrity 1981; Prugh and Eckhardt 1980; Whitt 1984). For example, surgical procedures or loss or disfigurement of body parts have different meanings for children at different ages. For children under the age of 7, such events may trigger fears of punishment by mutilation. For latency-aged children, these losses may interfere with the child's ability to master critical tasks of dealing with the physical environment and with peers. For adolescents, bodily injury is usually experienced as a narcissistic wound.

Loss of mobility is generally difficult for younger children because motoric movement is so important for the discharge of tension; for toddlers, specifically, interference with emerging physical autonomy may cause intense distress. Adolescents most often experience immobility as a disruption in their contacts with their peer network. Repeated hospitalizations or emergency procedures also cause distress for different reasons at different ages. Young children are particularly sensitive to disruptions in their routines, and adolescents are often painfully aware of the financial and emotional cost of their illness to family members.

The psychiatrist may help the family determine how well the child understands the nature of the illness. An appreciation of children's cognitive development aids in this task. Children under age 6 generally cannot understand the relationship between physical symptoms and processes taking place in unseen organs; they respond best to reassurance and to concrete descriptions of actions that may alleviate the symptoms. Children at the stage of concrete operations (ages 7 through 12) can grasp the relationship between sets of intangible events, i.e., the relationship between germs, viruses, and organ dysfunctions. Children at the stage of formal operations (ages 12 and up) are able to understand the more complex unfolding of systemic relationships such as the processes underlying multiple organ deterioration in diabetes or the breaking off of cancer cells and subsequent recurrence of the disease in another site.

Family Response

Family response to chronic pediatric illness is a product of the "fit" between the particular demands of the disorder and the family's characteristic belief systems and behavioral strategies. A family that is invested in the orderliness of its routines, for example, may have a great deal of difficulty adjusting to the unpredictability of episodic asthma attacks. Assessment of family response should consider both the family's behavior and the family's beliefs.

Behavioral assessment of the family should examine the family's ability to balance illness-care responsibilities and nonillness activities. The clinician should ask how well family members are able to preserve pre-illness activities, pleasures, and relationships in the face of the illness's demands. A review of a typical day in the family's life in concrete behavioral terms before and after the appearance of the illness helps clarify the nature of any changes. Two research tools provide particularly helpful adjuncts to a clinical interview. The Impact-on-Family Scale (Stein and Riessman 1980), is a questionnaire designed to measure the impact of childhood medical illness on parents; it addresses the individual parent's subjective sense of burden as well as the financial, intrafamilial, and social effects of the illness. The Psychosocial Adjustment to Illness Scale (Derogatis 1986) is a semistructured interview that assesses emotional, family, and social adjustment in a patient or family member; because of its language it is best used with adolescents and adults.

Family routines and rituals, such as dinnertime, vacations, and holidays, are concrete, accessible markers for assessing the extent to which the family has been able to maintain important family traditions in the face of an illness. The Ritual Interview (Wolin et al. 1988), originally developed to assess the protection of routines and rituals in alcoholic families, can easily be adapted to assess the preservation of family routines in families with a physically ill child.

The adaptability of the family's problem-solving strategies and affective style to the demands of the illness should also be assessed. No known instrument specifically assesses the "fit" between a family's style and the particular demands of an illness. However, instruments can be helpful in describing the family's response patterns; these can then be assessed for their efficacy in dealing with the specific illness phase and characteristics.

Two particularly valuable instruments for this purpose are the Family Assessment Device (Epstein et al. 1983), which elicits behaviorally based information about family affective and instrumental processes, and the Card Sort Procedure (Reiss et al. 1986), a family observational tool that has successfully predicted survival rates in end-stage renal patients. A third instrument, the Coping Health Inventory for Parents (McCubbin et al. 1983), assesses family coping strategies with medically ill children. A summary of standard instruments helpful in the behavioral assessment of family response is presented in Table 14-4.

Developmental issues of family members other than the ill child deserve attention. While older siblings may find it difficult to leave home because of a sense of duty to the family, younger siblings may be pressured into a hyperresponsible position. Parents' adult development may also be impaired; efforts to advance occupationally, form new interests, or develop generativity in nonfamily contexts may be limited by the burden of care for the ill child. Women who had deferred career development while caring for young children may find that their future personal options are greatly restricted by the ill child's ongoing need for maternal attention.

Finally, the cognitive dimensions of the child's development should

Table 14-4.   Questionnaires and interviews used in assessment of families in which a child has a chronic illness

Instrument	Type	Administration time (minutes)	Target area
Impact on Family Scale (Stein and Riessman 1980)	Questionnaire	10	Family burden
Psychosocial Adaptation to Illness Scale (PAIS) (Derogatis 1986)	Semistructured interview	30	Patient/family adjustment
Ritual Interview (Wolin et al. 1988)	Semistructured interview	50	Family-ritual protection
Family Assessment Device (Epstein et al. 1983)	Questionnaire	30	Family problem solving/ communication
Card Sort Procedure (Reiss et al. 1986)	Observation	45	Shared perceptions
Coping Health Inventory for Parents (McCubbin et al. 1983)	Questionnaire	10	Coping strategies

be considered. Every family has a core identity that is composed of a set of beliefs about those core qualities that make the family special (Jacobs 1989; Jacobs and Steinglass, in press). Sometimes the appearance of a chronic illness defies a core element in a family's belief system. For example, a family that has prided itself in overcoming obstacles through its own competence can be devastated by the persistence of an illness that it cannot eradicate. "Toxic intergenerational themes" often interfere with the management of the child's medical illness. For example, a parent who was traumatized by his parent's alcoholic rages may become overcontrolling in managing his child's diabetes. Family belief systems deserve particularly careful evaluation when a family's maladaptive response to a child's illness is refractory to educational and supportive interventions and does not seem to be completely explained by features of the illness or the child's development.

FAMILY INTERVENTIONS

Clinical theory and methods in the treatment of families with a medically ill child have changed substantially in recent years. Earlier theoretical models of families and medical illness emphasized the major role of pathogenic family processes in the development and severity of the medical condition (Coyne and Anderson 1988; Minuchin et al. 1978; Purcell et al. 1969). The best known was that of the "psychosomatic family," adapted from individually based psychosomatic theory (Alexander 1950); this model asserted that particular family processes predispose a target family member to produce a somatic response to stress.

The classic work articulating the psychosomatic family model was by Minuchin and his group, who studied families of children with brittle diabetes, anorexia, and intractable asthma (Minuchin et al. 1978). Minuchin specified four features of the psychosomatic family: 1) enmeshment and overinvolvement among family members; 2) overprotectiveness among family members; 3) rigidity or resistance to change; and 4) lack of conflict resolution.

In an influential series of experiments with families of children with insulin-dependent diabetes mellitus, Minuchin and colleagues (1978) reported a family "crossover" phenomenon that they believed was linked to the disease process in the child. Using free fatty acid (FFA) levels to measure arousal, Minuchin studied arousal levels in diabetic children who entered a room while their parents were having a disagreement. He observed that in certain families, the more-aroused parent would calm down and the child would become more aroused. Because elevated FFA levels are associated with diabetic ketoacidosis, Minuchin concluded that problems in the management of conflict within the family were responsible for the emergence or exacerbation of diabetes in the child. Minuchin and his group (1978) also conducted family therapy trials with families of anorexic children; they reported that the intervention, which helped the family to keep the child out of parental conflicts, alleviated symptoms successfully (1978).

Although Minuchin has never published key methodological details pertaining to the FFA experiments and has not systematically tested the family therapy intervention with other illnesses, the generic concept of the psychosomatic family remains popular among family therapists. Other practitioners working with families with a member with chronic illness have observed family characteristics similar to those described by Minuchin (Gonzalez et al. 1989; Penn 1983; Sheinberg 1983). Minuchin's emphasis on pathogenic processes, however, has left the impression that such gross somatic phenomena as acute asthmatic episodes can be generated by family dysfunction alone.

A more comprehensive biopsychosocial model underlies current treatment approaches for families with a medically ill child. This model conceptualizes medical illness as an external stressor to which the family members respond with varying degrees of competence. The family is not seen as inherently pathogenic; however, preexisting patterns of behavior in the family influence the degree to which the new challenge is mastered. The critical difference is that preexisting biological realities of the illness are accepted as "givens" with which the family must cope.

The biopsychosocial model, exemplified in the successful trials of structured family interventions in the management of schizophrenia (Anderson et al. 1986b; Falloon et al. 1984), focuses on using educational and behavioral interventions to promote successful management of the illness. The illness remains the focus of attention as families learn both to promote recovery and to pursue other family priorities. Family therapists concerned with the treatment of medical disorders increasingly have adopted this approach. Interest has focused around identifying generic issues that arise in families in response to serious illness as well as issues that are specific to particular illnesses.

SUPPORT OR THERAPY?

Families having difficulty coping with a medically ill child may come to the attention of a pediatrician in several ways. The most common include the following:

1. *Problems with medical care.* Persistent problems with adherence to treatment, lack of improvement in the medical condition despite apparent compliance, and frequent, inappropriate, or adversarial contacts with medical staff are all signs of family dysfunction.

2. *Psychiatric symptomatology in the patient.* This may include signs of depression or anxiety, unaccustomed antisocial behavior, decreased school performance, and medically unexplained weight loss or sleep problems.

3. *Symptomatology in the family.* Persistent disagreements or misunderstandings between parents regarding the child's medical care, frequent parental illness, parental sleepless-

ness or weight changes, and problems with siblings are probable signs of family distress.

Depending on the degree of dysfunction, three levels of intervention may be considered for families having difficulty with their medically ill child. They include educational and supportive intervention by members of the pediatric staff, time-limited psychoeducational intervention, and formal family therapy.

Education and Support by the Medical Team

Families commonly experience transient distress around three specific events: initial diagnosis (often the greatest crisis period), relapse, and the time when the child with a chronic condition reaches the "ceiling of recovery." At these times, families with a medically ill child are far more likely to accept psychosocial intervention from members of their child's own medical team than from external specialists. The psychiatrist, functioning as a consultant, can help pediatricians, nurses, and social work staff to provide effective supportive interventions for families experiencing transient distress.

One of the most common transient problems is inadequate understanding of the illness and its implications because of excessive anxiety that has interfered with family members' ability to process medical information. A careful review of the factual information may be sufficient to correct this problem. The consultant, at times, can help by discouraging the medical team from providing excessively detailed information to families too soon after they hear a distressing diagnosis.

Additional supportive functions that usually can be carried out by the medical team with psychiatric backup include helping family members express and accept feelings of grief and anger and helping families reallocate or supplement family resources to accommodate the requirements of the illness. In addition to listening supportively and nonjudgmentally, staff can provide information about financial or nursing assistance, or suggestions about the reallocation of duties among parents and older children. In most cases, 1 or 2 hours with a pediatrician, nurse, or social worker is adequate to address these issues.

Time-Limited Psychoeducation

At an intermediate level, families can be offered a brief educational intervention aimed at management of a specific illness or at mastery

Table 14-5.   Interventions for families with a seriously ill child

Reference	Illness	Intervention	Study type
Golden et al. 1985	Diabetes	Individualized education, insulin adjustment	Randomized control ($n = 44$)
Brownell et al. 1983	Obesity	Family/individual education and support	Randomized control ($n = 42$)
Clark et al. 1981	Asthma	Self-management education	Randomized control ($n = 300$)
Gonzalez et al. 1989	Generic	Multiple-family group psychoeducation	Randomized control ($n = 31$)
Lask and Matthew 1979	Asthma	Family therapy	Randomized control ($n = 33$)
Minuchin et al. 1975	Diabetes, asthma	Family therapy	No control ($n = 48$)

of generic illness-related issues. Interventions of this type have been shown to be effective in randomized controlled trials (Table 14-5). An example is an eight-session, multiple-family discussion group that focuses on generic issues facing families with a medically ill member (Gonzalez et al. 1989). Through a highly structured format, two discussion leaders guide a group of four to five families through a series of discussions that highlight the typical challenges facing families with a chronically ill member. The leaders provide the families with useful principles and metaphors with which to articulate their experience, and the families are encouraged to call on their own experiences to help other families with illness-related problems.

The theoretical framework for the multiple-family discussion group is the notion of the family's reorganization around the illness. For example, group leaders describe the illness as an "unwanted intruder" on family life, a "2-year-old terrorist" who shows up uninvited to a family meal and interrupts conversations and knocks over glasses. The family with such a "terrorist" in its midst must become more conscious of its valued traditions and plans and strive to maintain them despite the disruption of the illness. Successful adaptation to chronic illness involves a twofold process: accepting the reality of the illness (making a place for the illness) and protecting family traditions in the face of the illness (putting the illness in its place).

The discussion group consists of three structured components that systematically provide families with an opportunity to explore how these principles apply to them, as well as to help other families to address these questions. Group leaders follow a detailed treatment manual that gives instructions for conducting each session (Gonzalez et al. 1986). Each component employs an innovative "group-within-a-group" format. In the first stage, called the "educational component," the "patient" family members (including children) are asked to sit in a circle and, with the guidance of a group leader, to talk with each other about living with a chronic illness in a family. The "nonpatient" family members are asked to listen quietly and later to respond to what they have heard.

In the second session, the process is reversed, as "patient" members listen to a conversation among "nonpatient" members from every family. The purpose of this exercise is to help family members think systemically about the impact of the illness, i.e., to think about the characteristic roles played by patients and family members in the face of serious medical illness. The third session consists of a didactic meeting in which the leaders describe the concept of family reorganization around an illness and the principle of maintaining important family traditions and priorities; family members are urged to think of examples of how the illness has intruded on its priorities.

In the "family issues" component, families take turns describing in detail an important family issue that has emerged in relation to the illness. In this component the individual family is the "group within a group"; the purpose of the exercise is to help each family articulate how the illness has disrupted an important aspect of family life. Group members then add additional observations to the formulation and offer suggestions for addressing each family's dilemma. An underlying principle of these discussions is to identify valued features of family life that have been disrupted because of the illness; group members help other families to recapture these core elements while adapting to the reality of the illness.

An example of this process is the case of a 12-year-old boy with diabetes whose family had excelled in sports for many generations. Ultimately, the boy was required to use an insulin pump and to limit physical activity. Depression settled over the family as they curtailed their sports activities and avoided expressing their disappointment in the "heir apparent." In the family issues component the leader asked the family members to name personal attributes they associated with athletic competition; these included toughness, discipline, and skill. The other families began to point out the ways in which the diabetic boy exhibited all these traits superbly in his management of his illness: he had an optimistic attitude about his own future, he was in good control of his diabetes, and he had explained his illness so skillfully to his school friends that they accepted his limitations with tremendous support and even occasional humor. Gradually the family realized that the boy was fulfilling the values of athletic competition in a different way. They then began to develop a broader definition of their identity that very definitely included the boy.

In the "affective component," families explore the ways in which the illness has disrupted the affective rules by which the family operates. In this case, the leaders select the most psychologically minded family member for the group-within-a-group to discuss this somewhat sophisticated concept. Commonly, it emerges that the family member who has usually expressed important feelings for the family has become a caretaker for the patient and fears that emotional upheavals may trigger a relapse. Critical expressions of conflict go underground as the family tries not to rock the boat. Once this pattern is revealed, the remaining family members, now quite outspoken, advise each other on ways to protect the free expression of feeling.

Formal Family Therapy

There have been relatively few controlled trials of family therapy with medically ill children (see Table 14-5). Studies of the use of structural family therapy in cases of brittle diabetes, intractable asthma, and anorexia nervosa have reported impressive results (Minuchin et al. 1975), but most had no control group and lacked critical methodological details. In one of the few randomized trials of family therapy with a somatic illness (Lask and Matthew 1979), children with moderate to severe asthma whose families developed coping strategies for wheezing behavior had less daily wheezing and lower residual gas volume than a group of families who received no psychosocial intervention. The existing literature suggests that highly specific behavioral interventions targeted toward management of illness behavior were the most effective family interventions for reducing illness symptoms (Anderson et al. 1986a; Brownell et al. 1983; Clark et al. 1981; Lask and Matthew 1979). Interventions that protected nonillness family priorities (Gonzalez et al. 1989) were most effective in alleviating family distress.

The absence of rigorous empirical evidence of the efficacy of more open-ended, process-oriented family therapy with this population should not be considered a definitive statement of the superiority of focused behavioral interventions, but rather a reflection of the fact that the former type of intervention has not been adequately tested.

Family therapy is best used in cases in which a time-limited psychoeducational intervention has revealed issues needing further work, and in cases in which the family itself sees the importance of pursuing particular issues in greater depth. These usually are cases in which the illness has become embedded in a persistent dysfunctional pattern of family communication or behavior that is impervious to education and support alone. Based on what has been learned from empirical studies of behaviorally focused models, family therapy interventions should include an illness-related definition of the problem, treatment objectives grounded in successful management of the illness, and progressive treatment interventions.

Illness-related definition of the problem.   Although the presenting problem is typically reframed as a broader systemic issue in traditional family therapy, families facing chronic illness often experience this conceptual leap as blaming and irrelevant. The therapist is advised to use the assessment framework described earlier in the chapter to assess problematic behavioral sequences around the illness, the impact of the illness on core family beliefs and traditions, and the relationship between the family and the medical care team. These systematic inquiries should lead to a formulation that directly links the problem to the presence of the illness in the family.

Treatment objectives grounded in successful management of the illness.   Even if illness management problems are reflections of more general family problems, the illness is usually the major family preoccupation at the time of referral; an initial successful experience in managing the illness will provide family members with confidence in the therapy process as well as a greater capacity to grapple with more complex emotional issues. The overall objective can be conceptualized as a successful balance between attending to requirements of the illness and maintaining non-illness-related family priorities. To address these issues meaningfully, however, the family must engage in difficult judgments about "how much is enough" to give to the illness. The contextual approach of Boszormenyi-Nagy and Spark (1973), which deals with issues of fairness and indebtedness, offers useful concepts and terminology for therapists addressing these judgments.

Progressive treatment interventions.   The focus of the interventions should progress from specific problems to more general issues, beginning with reallocation of caretaking responsibilities. Particularly for families who are not psychologically minded, an initial focused intervention that alleviates family burden is usually most effective. Common interventions in this category include involving the more peripheral parent in the care of the child, delegating limited and age-appropriate responsibilities to siblings, and giving increased responsibility to the child for her or his own care. In families experiencing an excessive degree of burden, the assignment of caretaking responsibilities is often tied to a dysfunctional family pattern. Frequently, the primary caretaker has taken on full responsibility for the child's recovery process, while the child and the other parent have abrogated responsibility for maximizing the child's self-care. The therapist must help the family reallocate care responsibility to the child to an age-appropriate degree, while explaining the benefits of doing so to all family members and holding each family member responsible for his or her role in the reallocation.

Once caretaking responsibilities have been reallocated, the therapy addresses the larger implications of the illness for the family, in particular the family's recapturing of its own priorities and its balancing of illness- and non-illness-related activities over the long term. Based on a careful assessment of illness phase and characteristics, the developmental stage of the child, and the family response, the therapist helps the family see the illness in the context of the family's current and future needs and plans. When families are unable to take this step after an initial educational intervention, it is usually because the management of the illness in embedded in a "toxic" family issue.

For example, a mother may feel blamed for her child's illness because of a genetic vulnerability on her side of the family; this blaming process reawakens an old family issue in which her husband's family disapproved of the marriage. The mother and father both covertly believe that the mother "owes" it to the child and the family to be the child's major caretaker. The therapist must help family members to work through these systemic issues in order to disconnect, or "disembed," the illness management process.

Creating a powerful family ritual can be an effective way of disengaging the family from excessive involvement with illness management. An example is the case of a family whose 12-year-old daughter had been successfully treated for Hodgkin's disease. The family was now struggling with the transition from the acute treatment phase to an open-ended posttreatment stage. In this case the family needed to acknowledge the end of the acute phase and to take the risk of imagining the future with their daughter present (despite their fears of relapse and loss). In one such case the therapist helped the family create a ritual in which the daughter assembled her cancer paraphernalia (e.g., the cap used for radiation, medication containers) and, with her family's help, decided what to do with each article. Some were given to friends she had made on the cancer unit, some were thrown away, and some were kept as reminders of a momentous event in her life. The therapist then encouraged the family to plan an important family event (in this case a family trip to Europe for the following year) that made it necessary for the family to give the illness a new and more minor position in family life.

SUMMARY

In this chapter, I have reviewed the major problems facing families with a medically ill child, provided a model for family assessment, and described three levels of family intervention for this population. A growing literature of controlled trials of family interventions suggest that this area deserves increased attention by psychiatrists in the medical setting.

REFERENCES

Alexander F: Psychosomatic Medicine: Its Principles and Applications. New York, WW Norton, 1950

Anderson C, Reiss DJ, Hogarty GE: Schizophrenia and the Family: A Practitioner's Guide to Psychoeducation and Management. New York, Guilford, 1986a

Anderson CM, Griffin S, Rossi A, et al: A comparative study of the impact of education vs. process groups for families of patients with affective disorders. Fam Process 25:185–205, 1986b

Bibace R, Walsh M (eds): Children's conceptions of health, illness, and bodily functions. New Dir Child Dev 14, 1981

Boszormenyi-Nagy I, Spark G: Invisible Loyalties: Reciprocity in Intergenerational Family Therapy. New York, Harper & Row, 1973

Breslau N, Weitzman M, Messenger K: Psychologic functioning of siblings of disabled children. Pediatrics 67:344–353, 1981

Brownell KD, Kelman JH, Stunkard AJ: Treatment of obese children with and without their mothers: changes in weight and blood pressure. Pediatrics 71:515–523, 1983

Brunnquell D, Hall MD: Issues in the psychological care of pediatric oncology patients. Am J Orthopsychiatry 52:32–44, 1982

Campbell TL: Family's impact on health: a critical review. Family Systems Medicine 4:135–200, 1986

Clark NM, Feldman CH, Evans D, et al: The effectiveness of education for family management of asthma in children: a preliminary report. Health Educ Q 8:166–174, 1981

Coyne J, Anderson B: The "psychosomatic family" reconsidered: diabetes in context. Journal of Marital and Family Therapy 14:113–123, 1988

Derogatis LR: Psychosocial Adaptation to Illness Scale (PAIS). Psychosomatics 30:77–91, 1986

Drotar D, Crawford P, Bush M: The family context of childhood chronic illness: implications for psychosocial intervention, in Chronic Illness and Disability Through the Life Span: Effects on Self and Family. Edited by Eisenberg M, Sutkin L, Jansen M. New York, Springer, 1984

Epstein N, Baldwin L, Bishop S: The McMaster Family Assessment Device. Journal of Marital and Family Therapy 9:171–180, 1983

Falloon I, Boyd J, McGill C: Family Care of Schizophrenia. New York, Guilford, 1984

Golden MP, Herrold AJ, Orr DP: An approach to prevention of recurrent diabetic ketoacidosis in the pediatric population. J Pediatr 107(2):195–200, 1985

Gonzalez S, Steinglass P, Reiss D: Family-Centered Interventions for the Chronically Disabled: The 8-Session Multiple Family Discussion Group Program (treatment manual). Washington, DC, George Washington University Rehabilitation Research and Training Center, 1986

Gonzalez S, Steinglass P, Reiss D: Putting the illness in its place. Fam Process 28:69–87, 1989

Heisler AB, Friedman SB: Social and psychological considerations in chronic disease: with particular reference to the management of seizure disorders. J Pediatr Psychol 6:239–250, 1981

Hobbs N, Perrin J (eds): Issues in the Care of Children With Chronic Illness: A Sourcebook on Problems, Services, and Policies. San Francisco, CA, Jossey-Bass, 1985

Hobbs N, Perrin J, Ireys H: Chronically Ill Children and Their Families: Problems, Prospects, and Proposals from the Vanderbilt Study. New York, Jossey-Bass, 1985

Jacobs J: Family resilience in the context of chronic medical illness. Presented at the American Family Therapy Association annual conference, Colorado Springs, CO, June 1989

Jacobs J, Steinglass P: Risk and resilience in family response to alcohol use, in Developmental Issues in Alcohol Use. Edited by Brooks P, Gaines L. (in press)

Lask B, Matthew D: Childhood asthma: a controlled trial of family psychotherapy. Arch Dis Child 54:116–119, 1979

Mattsson A: Long-term physical illness in children: a challenge to psychosocial adaptation. Pediatrics 50:801–811, 1972

McCubbin H, McCubbin J, Cauble A, et al: Coping health inventory for parents. Journal of Marriage and the Family 45:359–370, 1983

Minuchin S, Baker L, Rosman BL, et al: A conceptual model of psychosomatic illness in children: family organization and family therapy. Arch Gen Psychiatry 32:1031–1038, 1975

Minuchin S, Rosman BL, Baker L: Psychosomatic Families. Cambridge, Harvard University Press, 1978

Penn P: Coalitions and binding interactions in families with chronic illness. Family Systems Medicine 1:16–25, 1983

Perrin EC, Gerrity PS: There's a demon in your belly: children's understanding of illness. Pediatrics 67:841–849, 1981

Prugh DG, Eckhardt LO: Stages and phases in the response of children and adolescents to illness or injury, in Advances in Behavioral Pediatrics, Vol 1. Edited by Camp BW. Greenwich, CT, JAI Press, 1980, pp 181–194

Purcell K, Brady K, Chai H, et al: The effects of asthma in children of experimental separation from the family. Psychosom Med 31:144–163, 1969

Ramsey CN (ed): Family Systems in Medicine. New York, Guilford, 1989

Reiss D, Kaplan-De-Nour A: The family and medical team in chronic illness: a transactional and developmental perspective, in Family Systems in Medicine. Edited by Ramsey CN. New York, Guilford, 1989, pp 435–444

Reiss D, Gonzalez S, Kramer N: Family process, chronic illness, and death: on the weakness of strong bonds. Arch Gen Psychiatry 43:795–804, 1986

Rolland J: Toward a psychosocial typology of chronic illness. Family Systems Medicine 2:245–262, 1984

Rolland J: Chronic illness and the life cycle: a conceptual framework. Fam Process 26:203–221, 1987

Sabbeth B, Leventhal J: Marital adjustment to chronic medical illness: a critique of the literature. Pediatrics 73:763–768, 1984

Sheinberg M: The family and chronic illness: a treatment diary. Family Systems Medicine 1:26–36, 1983

Stein R, Riessman C: The development of an impact on family scale: preliminary findings. Med Care 18:465–472, 1980

Steinglass P, Horan E: Families and chronic medical illness, in Chronic Disorders and the Family. Edited by Walsh F, Anderson C. New York, Haworth, 1988, pp 127–142

Vance JC, Fazan, Satterwhite, et al: Effects of nephrotic syndrome on the family: a controlled study. Pediatrics 65:948–955, 1980

Whitt JK: Children's understanding of illness: Developmental considerations and pediatric intervention, in Advances in Behavioral Pediatrics, Vol 3.

Edited by Wolraich M, Routh DK. Greenwich, CT, JAI Press, 1982, pp 163–201

Whitt JK: Children's adaptation to chronic illness and handicapping conditions, in Chronic Illness and Disability Through the Life Span. Edited by Eisenberg M, Sutkin L, Jansen M. New York, Springer, 1984, pp 69–129

Wolin S, Bennett L, Jacobs J: Assessing family rituals, in Rituals in Families and Family Therapy. Edited by Imber-Black E, Roberts J, Whiting R. New York, WW Norton, 1988, pp 230–256

Chapter 15

Pharmacotherapy of Severe Psychiatric Disorders in Mentally Retarded Individuals

Carl Feinstein, M.D.
David Levoy, M.D.

In this chapter, we review the diagnosis and pharmacotherapy of the major psychiatric disorders in mentally retarded individuals. First, however, it is necessary to review certain basic facts and issues concerning psychiatric care of the mentally retarded, particularly as they relate to the challenge of formulating accurate psychiatric diagnoses. In this population, as in others, the foundation of scientific clinical practice depends on accurate initial diagnosis and reliable and valid criteria for measuring improvement in psychiatric status.

OVERVIEW

Mental retardation is a chronic mental disability characterized by a significant and generalized deficit in intellectual functioning. DSM-III-R (American Psychiatric Association 1987) criteria for diagnosis include an IQ below 70 on a standardized test and significant impairments in adaptive behavior.

Slightly more than 1% of the total population suffers from some degree of this disability. Within this group, 85% are mildly retarded (IQ between 50–55 and 70), 10% are moderately retarded (IQ between 35–40 and 50–55), 3–4% are severely retarded (IQ between 20–25 and 35–40), and 1–2% are profoundly retarded (IQ below 20–25). (Szymanski and Crocker 1985).

Mentally retarded people form a heterogeneous group. The retardation itself derives from many different organic and hereditary etiologies and is influenced by a wide range of sociocultural factors. Specific neurological diagnoses are made more often in patients with moderate and more severe retardation. The range of temperaments and personalities among retarded individuals is equivalent to that among cognitively normal people. In the past two decades, public attitudes toward mentally retarded people have undergone major changes. Segregation and isolation of retarded adults in custodial institutions have been supplanted by significant efforts aimed at returning these individuals to community-based living, educational, and vocational settings. Federal laws, such as PL-94-142 and PL-99-457, guarantee the right of retarded and other disabled children to an appropriate education in the least restrictive environment.

The prevalence of behavior problems and psychiatric disorders among mentally retarded individuals is far higher than that for the general population. Indeed, most epidemiologic studies have found that psychiatric disorders occur four to six times more frequently in mentally retarded individuals than in the general population, or at a rate of about 30–60% (Corbett 1979; Jacobson 1982; Matson and Barrett 1982; Russell 1985; Szymanski and Crocker 1989). Up to 32,000 mentally retarded patients are admitted to ambulatory mental health services each year, and a high percentage of institutionalized retarded individuals suffer from serious psychiatric disturbance (Manderscheid et al. 1988; Szymanski and Crocker 1985).

Despite the immense mental health needs of the retarded population, there is a shortage of psychiatrists available to provide these services. In addition, the long-standing pattern of mental health service delivery to this population has fostered an overly constricted role for the psychiatrist on the multidisciplinary team. During the past 50 years, highly skilled nonmedical professionals specializing in direct assessment, education, and behavioral management of retarded persons assumed primary diagnostic and therapeutic responsibility. In most cases, the psychiatrist functioned as a part-time consultant whose responsibility was largely confined to the prescription of psychotropic medications, often based on little or no direct observation of the patient.

This pattern of practice, along with similar roles for nonpsychiatric physicians, contributed to what is now generally acknowledged as widespread overuse of psychotropic drugs in this population. It also increased the isolation of psychiatric efforts with retarded individuals from the mainstream of psychiatric practice, interfered with the development of subspecialty expertise, and impeded the development of a scientifically sophisticated clinical research base.

DIAGNOSIS

The diagnosis of psychiatric disorders in the mentally retarded requires a biopsychosocial approach and is a complex and challenging task for several reasons. First, there is a tendency for clinicians less experienced with this population to dismiss abnormal behavioral patterns as due to the cognitive deficiency, ignoring the possibility of a concurrent psychiatric disorder. This phenomenon has been aptly called "diagnostic overshadowing" (Reiss et al. 1982). Second, difficulties in language, self-evaluation, and concept development in retarded individuals make it more difficult for the psychiatrist to obtain an accurate history to identify precipitating or stressful events and to evaluate thought disorder. The mentally retarded patient is also generally less facile in reporting subjective distress, poor self-esteem, and subjective mood disturbances, such as anxiety, dysphoria, and euphoria (Feinstein et al. 1988; Gualtieri et al. 1989).

Third, it appears that some of the neurobehavioral syndromes and aberrant behaviors seen in retarded individuals do not fit neatly into current classifications of psychiatric disorders. This issue presents especially perplexing diagnostic problems. A growing body of literature documents that most well-validated psychiatric disorders that occur in the general population also occur in retarded individuals (Matson and Barrett 1982; Menolascino 1988; Myers 1987b; Reid 1982; Szymanski and Crocker 1985). However, the presentation of these disorders may, in some cases, also include behavioral features that are very rarely seen in nonretarded individuals. Stereotypic behaviors, self-injurious behaviors, and aggressive tantrums are widely variable but extremely common symptom clusters in retarded individuals that are often manifestations of better validated syndromes. However, they may also be free-standing, concurrent conditions.

These behaviors may, in turn, derive from cognitive and communicative insufficiency, severe environmental deprivation, or psychosocial developmental delay (Donnelan et al. 1984; Feinstein et al. 1988; Szymanski and Doherty 1989a, 1989b). Alternatively, they may represent neuropathic features related to the brain pathology that resulted in retardation (Gualtieri et al. 1989). It appears that unique neurobiologic mechanisms or deficits in social cognition, levels of disinhibition, and self-awareness of a degree not often seen in nonretarded individuals result in aberrant behaviors that lie beyond the range of psychopathology seen in cognitively normal individuals. Nevertheless, the psychiatrist is well advised to seek underlying causes and to carefully rule out major well-validated diagnostic categories before targeting isolated behaviors for pharmacotherapeutic interventions.

Last but not least, it is difficult to fully appreciate the chronic stress with which retarded individuals must cope. Sources of stress include social isolation, stigmatization, and diminution of opportunities for social, sexual, recreational, and work fulfillment far beyond those that confront most nonretarded individuals. When the retarded person's physical appearance, social habitus, or language identifies him or her as mentally deficient, even routine social interactions with nonretarded individuals are continuously distorted by the subjective discomfort and unfavorable responses of others.

Elements of the Psychiatric Evaluation

The evaluation of psychopathology in the mentally retarded individual involves the same basic psychiatric techniques used in the nonretarded population, although greater reliance on gathering clinical history from family and caretakers may be necessary. However, interviewing and observing the patient remains critically important. Ancillary evaluation data, such as behavior rating scales, can be helpful but are no substitute for first-hand evaluation of the patient. Rating instruments that may be helpful for general evaluation of adaptive functioning are the Vineland Scales of Social Maturity (Sparrow et al. 1984) and the Adaptive Behavior Scale (Fogelman 1975; Nihira et al. 1975). The Aberrant Behavior Checklist collects information about a wide range of symptoms (Aman and Singh 1985). The Emotional Disorder Rating Scale (EDRS) is a useful rating scale for affective symptoms (Feinstein et al. 1988). The Psychopathology Instrument for Mentally

Retarded Adults (PIMRA) (Kazdin et al. 1983) is a well-validated structured psychiatric interview.

The history from family, caregivers, and others who know the patient well is also of vital importance. As with any psychiatric evaluation, there should be careful scrutiny paid to context, including exploration of recent losses, stressors, frustrations in communication or social relationships, and shortcomings in the individual's support system or caretaking environment.

The psychiatrist should review the patient's past psychiatric history, including previous treatments, as well as family psychiatric history, medical history, and developmental history. The basis for the diagnosis of mental retardation should always be reviewed. The psychiatrist should attempt to determine how and when the diagnosis was made, attempt to identify underlying neurologic, genetic, and metabolic disorders, and characterize the patient's past and present cognitive, physical, adaptive, and social functioning. Adaptive and cognitive deficits that seem pronounced during the school years may become less significant in adolescence and adulthood.

Medical workup. The medical workup, particularly the initial workup, of retarded patients with psychiatric disorder is critical. It should always include a careful medical history and physical examination, and particular attention should be paid to neurological findings such as stigmata of neurocutaneous syndromes, evidence of movement disorders, and evidence of lateralizing motor signs or cerebral palsy. Chromosomal studies, including testing for fragile X chromosome, should be done, unless such testing was done within the past few years. Older studies no longer reflect the state of the art in this area.

Other necessary tests include thyroid function, electrolytes, blood urea nitrogen, creatinine, liver function, metabolic screening, amino acid studies (unless previously performed), lead level, free erythrocyte protoporphyrin (especially for children susceptible to lead toxicity), complete blood count, and urinalysis. An EEG and brain imaging studies may be helpful in some cases, especially where there is a deteriorating course. These can also serve as a baseline for future studies should later evaluation be necessary. The dexamethasone suppression test (DST) may be considered whenever affective disorder is suspected, but the clinical presentation is atypical, or when there is a pattern of self-injurious or aggressive outbursts associated with affective symptoms. When treating patients with Down's syndrome, a condition associated with numerous medical problems, the psychiatrist should be particularly aware of cardiac anomalies (a particularly careful cardiac

workup is necessary before starting tricyclic antidepressants) and at-
lantoaxial instability (should the patient require physical restraints).

The patient's course may deteriorate if the condition is degenerative or for iatrogenic reasons, for example, as a result of excessive or
inappropriate neuroleptic treatment, side effects of anticonvulsants, or
adverse drug interactions (Rivinus et al. 1989).

Individual interview.   The individual diagnostic interview is often the most difficult obstacle for the psychiatrist who is not used to
the evaluation of mentally retarded individuals. This difficulty is frequently due to anxiety over preconceived differences in this population
and may be confounded by untested assumptions that the retarded
person cannot provide useful or valid information about his or her
problem.

Of vital importance in the individual assessment is the establishment of rapport with the patient. Rapport will be influenced by the
level of cognition and the level of social development. Mildly and
moderately mentally retarded individuals generally are capable of relating fairly well at a verbal level, if language is kept simple and complicated phrasing is avoided. Infantile autism and other pervasive
developmental disorders often involve mental retardation. These developmental disorders are underdiagnosed in adult retarded populations. Social development is uniquely impaired in these individuals.

Mental age alone is not an adequate guide for gauging the developmental level at which to aim in the interview (Szymanski and Crocker
1985). Mildly retarded adult individuals with the mental age of a child
should not be interviewed as one would interview a child. While reduction in complexity of language is appropriate, the tone of voice and
both nonverbal behavior and social behavior of the interviewer should
be tied more closely to the patient's chronological age. There is substantial evidence that most mildly or moderately retarded individuals
can provide useful information about their problems and symptoms,
if they are appropriately interviewed (Kazdin et al. 1983). For the patient
who is nonverbal or has difficulty with the verbal interview, nonverbal
interactions should be used to assess capacity for social interaction.
The patient's use of alternative communication systems, such as ges-
turing, sign language, and symbol boards, should be ascertained.

Assessment of Specific Disorders

Mood disorders.   All forms of mood disorder occur in the mentally
retarded population. Though hard data are lacking because of meth-

odological problems in research assessment, depression and other affective disorders are relatively common in the mentally retarded (Matson and Barrett 1982; Sovner and Hurley 1983). Mentally retarded individuals are less likely to seek or to be referred for help for subjective dysphoria. Depression and social withdrawal in the absence of problematic behavior is often ignored by caretakers. When affectively disordered retarded individuals have disruptive symptoms, there is a tendency to focus on the problem behaviors without paying sufficient attention to the underlying affective disturbance. The core symptoms of depression among retarded individuals are, however, the same as those for the nonretarded population, and DSM-III-R remains a helpful diagnostic guideline.

Somatic complaints and the full range of cognitive symptoms of depression, including guilt, derogatory self-statements, self-doubt and increased dependence on others, thoughts of death and morbid ruminations, and hopelessness, may occur. Psychotic depressive features, including mood-congruent or incongruent delusions and hallucinations, also occur and have been well described in the literature. Suicidal ideation and behavior may be a serious concern (Kaminer et al. 1987). In the less verbal patient, fearfulness, a sad facial expression, a sad tone of voice, decreased interest in previously preferred activities (which can include a change in response to behavioral "rewards"), and social withdrawal may be observed. Psychomotor slowing or agitation and difficulty with concentration may be seen even in the most severely retarded, who may become unable to perform their usual activities of daily living or "prevocational" tasks such as simple sorting of objects. Vegetative symptoms, such as significant weight gain or loss, appetite changes, and sleep disturbances, frequently can be found. Deterioration in self-care and regression in function may be prominent. Depression may be connected to more florid behavioral symptoms directly (e.g., increased noncompliance), or indirectly (e.g., failure of behavioral programming due to decreased interest in reinforcers).

Self-injurious behavior, which may range from mild to severely mutilative and life threatening, is a very common and serious problem in mentally retarded individuals (Hill et al. 1985; Singh and Millichamp 1985). Many different etiologic factors, ranging from organic (severity of retardation, specific neurobehavioral syndromes, serotonin levels, endogenous opiate mechanisms, and seizure disorders) to socioemotional (communicative frustrations, deprivation anxiety, learned behavior) have been implicated and may apply to subsets of afflicted patients (Schroeder 1989). However, self-injurious behavior is fairly frequent in depressed retarded patients and, along with aggressive outbursts, has been specifically seen in depressed mentally retarded patients with positive DSTs (Beckwith et al. 1985; Pirodsky et al. 1985; Ruedrich et al. 1987). Increased preoccupation with self-stimulatory behavior, such as repetitive stereotypies involving tactile or visual stimulation, may also indicate underlying depression.

Bipolar disorder has been well described in retarded individuals (Gualtieri 1989a; Kaminer et al. 1986; Myers 1987b; Naylor et al. 1974; Reid 1972; Reid and Naglov 1976; Sovner and Hurley 1983). Unlike depressive withdrawal, manic episodes tend to produce more disruption in caretaking, school, or workplace environments. Verbal patients may present with pressured speech, flight of ideas, or grandiose ideas and statements, and psychomotor agitation, aggressiveness or self-injurious behavior, and insomnia may be apparent in all patients. A significant increase in risk-taking behavior may occur. Florid psychotic features may be present.

In diagnosing both depression and mania, it is crucial to determine that the patient's mood has changed markedly from baseline. Occasionally, the pattern of such changes will reveal a cyclical mood disorder such as menstrually related mood disorder (Kaminer et al. 1988), seasonal affective disorder, or a rapid-cycling bipolar disorder. Family history is also an important component in the diagnosis of affective disorders in the mentally retarded (Gualtieri 1989a).

Ancillary tools for the evaluation of affective disorder include the DST and several rating scales and there is some evidence for the usefulness of DST in supporting the diagnosis of major depression in mentally retarded individuals (Beckwith et al. 1985; Ruedrich et al. 1987). Rating scales that may be useful include the Beck Depression Inventory and the Depression Self-Rating Scale (Beck et al. 1987), the Self-report Depression Questionnaire (Reynolds and Baker 1988), the PIMRA (Kazdin et al. 1983; Senatore et al. 1985), and the Emotional Disorders Rating Scale (Feinstein et al. 1988).

The Aberrant Behavior Checklist (Aman et al. 1985) is a rating scale of general symptoms, including affective symptoms, and is particularly useful when other behavioral problems occur together with affective disorder. All but the Beck scales have been developed specifically for retarded populations. The Beck scales have not been specifically validated for retarded persons but probably are valid in mildly retarded individuals.

Psychotic disorders.   Psychosis in mentally retarded individuals may be symptomatic of a mood disorder or of any of the psychotic disorders described in DSM-III-R. Care must be taken to distinguish between mentally retarded patients with psychosis and those with pervasive developmental disorders. This requires taking a systematic developmental history and defining the social deficit. Patients with pervasive developmental disorder have a disproportionate impairment in social functioning relative to cognitive level. For individuals with low IQ this is a difficult distinction to make. Furthermore, a small percentage of children with pervasive developmental disorder do develop clinical conditions indistinguishable from schizophrenia as adults. As a rule, a functional psychosis is not diagnosed unless new psychotic psychopathology, clearly distinct from the patient's baseline adaptive deficit, can be demonstrated.

The full range of schizophrenic symptoms has been described in mentally retarded persons (Menolascino 1988; Menolascino et al. 1985a). These include hallucinations, paranoia, bizarre rituals and behavior, delusions, withdrawal, and blunting of affect. A history of deterioration from a higher level of functioning, even if the original level was impaired, is an important indicator. For the most severely retarded, the evaluation of paranoid disorder is difficult, making symptoms associated with paranoid disorder, such as ideas of reference and persecutory delusions, less diagnostically useful (Reid 1982). Brief reactive psychosis and schizoaffective disorder may be properly diagnosed based on the temporal cause and pattern of mood disturbance.

In the assessment, care must be taken not to misidentify misperceptions or misunderstandings of a situation that derive from cognitive limitations as delusions or hallucinations. Conversely, the pitfall of "diagnostic overshadowing," in which psychotic ideation or behavior is ascribed to the mental retardation itself, should also be avoided. Schizophrenia in the retarded frequently is accompanied by a variety of highly problematic behaviors, including stereotypies, self-injurious behavior, and destructiveness and aggression. These symptoms should not detract from a thorough assessment of underlying psychosis.

Anxiety disorders.   Anxiety is common in retarded individuals (Levine 1985; Ollendick and Ollendick 1982). In one study, 4% percent of acute inpatient admissions of mentally retarded patients were noted to have a DSM-III (American Psychiatric Association 1980) anxiety disorder (Menolascino 1988). However, a much higher percentage of retarded individuals experience anxiety and engage in avoidant or compulsive behavior that may mimic psychosis. Many retarded individuals have difficulty verbalizing feelings of anxiety. However, physiological symptoms such as hyperventilation, cardiovascular changes, and diaphoresis are important indicators (Feinstein et al. 1988). Often, anxiety must be inferred from the history and from observation of behavior.

Panic reactions, phobias, and performance anxiety all may lead quickly to discharge in the form of self-injurious or aggressive outbursts or stereotypic motor behaviors. In some instances, the outward cause or precipitant of the distress may be a particular situation or a demand to perform a disliked activity. However, it is commonly the case that by the time psychiatric consultation is sought, the discharge behavior has been reinforced by the removal of the provoking agent, and the avoidant behavior has generalized to a wider arena. This may result in a pattern of phobic avoidance similar to that of normal-IQ patients with recurrent panic attacks. At times, repeatedly reinforced anxiety discharge behaviors may result in a pattern of severe behavioral outbursts resembling a psychotic disorder. Thus, anxiety disorders in the retarded may lead to behavior disturbances equivalent in severity and generalization to affective disorders or schizophrenia.

Role of Organic Factors in Evaluation

Organic factors play a major role in the diagnosis of psychiatric disorders in the mentally retarded population. Numerous congenital syndromes are associated with mental retardation and may also increase vulnerability to psychiatric disorders (Szymanski and Crocker 1985). In Menolascino's study (1988) of 543 mentally retarded individuals, more than 34% were found to have significant medical difficulties, including epilepsy, cerebral palsy, diabetes, and hypothyroidism. Seizure disorders were the most common, affecting over 21% of the patients.

Seizure disorders are quite common in mentally retarded individuals. Approximately 11% living outside institutions and 33% of those institutionalized receive anticonvulsant drugs (Gadow and Kalachnik 1981). The coexistence of mental retardation and seizures is often due to a shared etiology involving brain injury or maldevelopment. Seizures may lead directly to disturbed behavior in the form of organic mental disorder such as an episodic dyscontrol syndrome. They may also lead indirectly to psychiatric disorders by acutely and recurrently disrupting cognition or by leading to chronic cognitive deterioration. Anticonvulsant therapy adequate to control generalized convulsions may still allow for partial seizures that can disrupt cognitive and emotional function. Investigation of the adequacy of seizure control can be aided by EEG; however, it must be remembered that nonspecific EEG abnormalities are common in mental retardation, even among individuals who do not have a seizure disorder.

Another route by which seizure disorders affect the psychiatric status of mentally retarded individuals is through the adverse effects of seizure medications. The most common problem is anticonvulsant toxicity. In one study, 16% of mentally retarded patients receiving carbamazepine and 28% of those receiving phenytoin were noted to have toxic levels (Aman et al. 1986). Even at therapeutic levels, anticonvulsants may contribute to behavioral symptoms, including attention deficit, hyperactivity, and psychosis (Rivinus et al. 1989). Phenobarbital and similar antiseizure medications with sedative-hypnotic properties can be particularly problematic because they produce affective symptoms such as irritability and tearfulness and may cause sleep difficulties (Aman and Singh 1988). Chronic therapy with phenytoin and phenobarbital may be associated with cognitive deterioration (Corbett et al. 1985). Treatment of the epileptic mentally retarded individual with a disturbance of mood or behavior must include attempts to assure maximum possible seizure control and evaluation and avoidance of anticonvulsant toxicity. Use of barbiturates should be minimized because of their adverse effects on learning (Corbett et al. 1985).

Unfortunately, it is well documented that overprescription, overdosage, and polypharmacy with a wide range of psychotropic medications in the retarded population are major contributors to organically based psychiatric symptoms (Aman and Singh 1988; Bates et al. 1986; Keppel and Gualtieri 1989). The rate of psychotropic drug use is 30–50% among the institutionally retarded, and for adult outpatients the range is probably 26–36% (Aman and Singh 1988).

Unplanned polypharmacy is common and often leads to confusing symptom pictures that include primary symptoms, side effects of more than one drug, and difficulty assessing drug interactions (Sovner and Hurley 1982). Excessive neuroleptics can aggravate psychopathology and complicate accurate diagnosis by disrupting already impaired cognitive functioning, by causing psychomotor retardation, by mimicking depression through parkinsonian effects such as masked facies, and by creating restlessness or agitation related to akathisia. The combination of neuroleptics and lithium may produce confusion, even at usual therapeutic doses. Anticholinergic toxicity from antidepressants can also depress cognitive function. The antianxiety and sedative-hypnotic agents can produce a "paradoxical" reaction involving disinhibition with agitation (Fahs 1989). Both long- and short-acting benzodiazepines can produce this reaction.

PSYCHOTROPIC DRUG TREATMENT

Neuroleptics

Neuroleptics have been widely used for several decades in the treatment of psychiatric disorders in mentally retarded individuals. During this time, an extensive literature has documented treatment responses and side effects (Aman and Singh 1988). Despite clear indications for the use of at least some of these agents, there is great danger that short-term treatment will turn into inadequately monitored long-term use, especially given the risk of long-term tardive dyskinesia and other adverse outcomes (Aman 1989a). The choice of neuroleptic is complicated by a lack of controlled studies that targeted clinically well-defined populations and documented clinical response. Nevertheless, a number of recent studies have examined the relative effectiveness of different drugs using more reliable indicators of clinical response (Aman 1989a; Campbell 1985; Gualtieri and Keppel 1985; Menolascino et al. 1986).

It is also important to note that many treatment effects reported may be due to nonspecific suppression of aggressive or autoaggressive behavior or to a specific reduction of stereotyped motor behaviors rather than to any overall improvement in mental status (Heistad and Zimmermann 1979; Singh and Aman 1981).

In this review, we specifically discuss chlorpromazine, haloperidol, thioridazine, and thiothixene because they have the most representation in the treatment literature. Many other neuroleptics are used with the dually diagnosed mentally retarded population. There is no strong reason to maintain on theoretical grounds that other neuroleptics with similar properties and mechanisms of action should be less effective. However, in view of the disturbing trends of inadequately controlled drug use previously discussed for this population, it seems wisest to proceed along the best documented path, until controlled studies indicate special advantages of other drugs. Drugs with less empirical support for efficacy in retarded patients should be considered when response to established agents has been poor and the severity of the disorder dictates further therapeutic efforts. For those seeking further information, Schroeder (1988) has recently reviewed the literature concerning the full range of neuroleptics.

Chlorpromazine.   The neuroleptic with the longest history of use in mentally retarded patients is chlorpromazine. Numerous anecdotal and uncontrolled studies have reported effectiveness in treating aggression, self-injurious behavior, stereotyped movements, and hyperactivity (Aman 1989a; Freeman 1970; Sprague and Werry 1971). However, better controlled studies tend to report efficacy only in reducing stereotyped movements (Aman et al. 1984). Chlorpromazine, however, has been shown to depress cognitive functioning to a greater degree than certain other neuroleptics. Therefore, pending reports of more specific indications for its use, it should not be considered a first-line drug for retarded patients (Aman 1989a; Campbell 1985).

Haloperidol. This neuroleptic is increasingly used with dual-diagnosis retarded patients (Aman 1989a; Grabowski 1973). Its desirable features are its high potency and relatively low sedative effect. At least one well-controlled study using low doses of haloperidol with autistic children has shown significant improvement in social withdrawal, stereotypies, hyperactivity, negativism, and labile affect without reduction in cognitive performance (Campbell 1985). Another study, unfortunately uncontrolled, reported low doses (0.5–6 mg per day) of haloperidol to be effective in reducing self-injurious behavior in severely retarded patients without any evidence of sedation (Mikkelsen 1986). More recently, however, Aman (1989a) could not demonstrate efficacy in a well-controlled study employing low or moderate doses of haloperidol in an institutionalized population that had been chronically treated with neuroleptics.

In summary, haloperidol has shown some promise as a neuroleptic for use in the mentally retarded population, specifically in treating stereotyped behavior and aggression. Specific antipsychotic effects, however, have not been well documented. It may have a particular advantage because of relative lack of sedation at low doses.

Thioridazine. Another neuroleptic that has been widely used and studied in the treatment of retarded patients is thioridazine. Several studies, some well controlled, have reported it to be effective for stereotyped and self-stimulatory behaviors, self-injury, bizarre behaviors, social withdrawal, overactivity, aggression, and emotional lability (Aman 1989a; Menolascino et al. 1985a, 1985b; Singh and Aman 1981). However, these reports have also documented sedation and depressed cognition. Nonetheless, thioridazine has more scientific support than any other neuroleptic agent for use in the mentally retarded and should be considered a first-line drug.

Thiothixene. An increasingly used antipsychotic in mentally retarded patients is thiothixene. Menolascino et al. (1985a, 1985b) reported it to be as effective as thioridazine, but with a shorter onset of action and less sedation. These authors also reported that optimum doses for both drugs were lower for mentally retarded schizophrenic patients than for schizophrenic patients of normal intelligence. The mean daily effective dose was 225 mg for thioridazine and 30 mg for thiothixene.

In summary, thiothixene, a drug midway on the continuum of potency versus sedation, shows promise as a first-line drug for treating schizophrenic and other psychotic disorders in mentally retarded patients, although further studies are needed.

Adverse effects.   The adverse effects of neuroleptics among retarded individuals are the same as those found in the nonretarded population, with the added complication that subjective reports of side effects may be more difficult to elicit from retarded patients. Adverse effects include oversedation, cognitive dysfunction, parkinsonism, dyskinesias, akathisia, neuroleptic malignant syndrome, and tardive dyskinesia (Physicians' Desk Reference 1990).

The assessment of dyskinetic movements, including tardive dyskinesia, in developmentally disabled individuals can be complex. Since tic disorders and stereotypic behaviors occur frequently in the mentally retarded population and may be temporarily suppressed by neuroleptic treatment, there is potential for much confusion between movement disorders associated with mental retardation and tardive dyskinesia (Golden 1988).

Assessment of involuntary movements can be aided by using structured examinations and rating scales, such as the Abnormal Involuntary Movement Scale (Guy 1976). The DISCUS, along with its predecessor, the DIS-CO, is the only dyskinesia scale that has been systematically studied in the developmentally disabled population (Kalachnik et al. 1983; Sprague et al. 1989). The DISCUS includes 15 separate ratings from 0 to 4 for dyskinetic movements in seven body regions.

In cases of preexisting movement disorder, videotaping the patient performing usual activities or during a rating evaluation, before medication treatment, and at intervals after initiation of treatment can aid in evaluating drug effects. The videotapes also provide a permanent record that may be helpful if legal issues ever arise.

Combined use of neuroleptics and phenytoin is common, and phenytoin-induced movement disorders may resemble tardive dyskinesia. Current estimates of the rate of tardive dyskinesia in mentally retarded patients receiving neuroleptics chronically range from 20.4 to 36% (Gualtieri et al. 1986; Richardson et al. 1986).

Parkinsonism and akathisia in the mentally retarded generally are treated in a similar manner as in the nonretarded population. Amantadine may be preferable to anticholinergic antiparkinsonian drugs because of its milder cognitive side effects. Identification of these side effects may be more difficult, as retarded patients may have more difficulty describing the subjective symptoms involved. The physician needs to ask about these symptoms in a simple, clear manner, while paying special attention to motoric signs of these disorders. When treating side effects, it is always preferable to reduce the neuroleptic dosage than to add a new drug to mitigate side effects.

Neuroleptics must be used cautiously and with good indications in the mentally retarded due to the risks involved. In a recent study, 13 of 38 mentally retarded patients were found to have tardive dyskinesia, but in only 3 were the symptoms of the tardive dyskinesia apparent during the neuroleptic treatment. The other cases were revealed during systematic efforts to withdraw the patients from neuroleptics (Gualtieri et al. 1986). These same authors also observed symptoms of nausea, vomiting, anorexia, weight loss, and diaphoresis in response to neuroleptic withdrawal. Acute behavioral deteriorations during the acute phase of withdrawal were also reported.

Optimum doses of neuroleptics are frequently lower for mentally retarded schizophrenic patients than for nonretarded schizophrenic patients. Use of less anticholinergic and less sedating agents is also preferable in this already cognitively impaired population. This preference creates a paradox with respect to thioridazine—while the drug has been extensively tested in mentally retarded persons, it is a low-potency, sedating, and highly anticholinergic agent. Our practice is to use thioridazine mainly in situations where a low dose is likely to be effective and where sedation would be acceptable. For long-term outpatient treatment of schizophrenia, a higher-potency agent is preferable.

When treating retarded individuals, the psychiatrist who is attuned to the relative risks and benefits of neuroleptic medication is likely to discontinue neuroleptic regimens more often than initiate them. The physician should review the history correctly, including the indications that led to neuroleptic treatment and benefits and problems associated with treatment. A careful examination for side effects, including dyskinesia, parkinsonism, akathisia, and oversedation, should be conducted.

If the relative problems associated with neuroleptic treatment outweigh the benefits or if no clear indication for neuroleptic treatment can be established, the neuroleptic should be discontinued. This should be done by tapering the dose by 10% every 2–4 weeks, so as to avoid insomnia, agitation, cholinergic rebound, and other withdrawal effects. In cases of polypharmacy, medications should be discontinued gradually, one at a time.

Withdrawal of possibly unnecessary neuroleptics. Not infrequently, psychiatrists encounter mentally retarded patients who have been on neuroleptics for several years without a well-established indication. The initial approach in such cases is to gather additional history from the family or other caretaker and to examine available medical records. If these do not help establish an indication, gradual withdrawal of the neuroleptic is advisable. The rate of withdrawal is crucial, because excessively rapid withdrawal of long-term neuroleptic therapy may itself produce physical and mental symptoms, even when there was no good indication for the drug in the first place.

A conservative approach is to begin withdrawal at the rate of 10–15% of the total dose per month. If definite psychotic symptoms emerge, the neuroleptic should be raised to the lowest dose necessary to suppress them.

Antidepressants

The tricyclic antidepressants have not been extensively used for the treatment of depressive disorders in mentally retarded patients. A single uncontrolled study (Pilkington 1962) reported improvement in some depressed retarded children in response to imipramine. However, Aman and associates (1986) conducted a double-blind, placebo-controlled crossover trial of imipramine in 10 profoundly retarded patients with depressive or assaultive or self-injurious behavior and reported that the patients became clinically worse. There have been a few reports of positive response to amitriptyline, but, in these cases, depression was not specifically targeted for treatment. Anecdotal reports of favorable response to the most recent generation of novel antidepressants circulate from time to time, specifically with regard to bupropion. However, there are no published studies as yet on the use of these agents.

Desipramine has been reported to be effective in noncognitively impaired children with attention-deficit disorder (Biederman et al. 1986), and imipramine has been reported to be useful in the treatment of adults with panic disorder (Liebowitz 1985). Since these are common problems among retarded individuals, further studies of the use of these tricyclic antidepressants in this population seem warranted.

One reason for the lack of published studies is that the existence of depression in retarded individuals and a methodology for assessing it have been well described only in the last decade. Further, there is continuing uncertainty about the precise relationship between self-injurious and aggressive behavior on the one hand, and depression and panic disorder on the other. Further studies are needed of the effectiveness of tricyclic antidepressants in depressed retarded patients, and in those suffering from attention-deficit disorder or panic disorder.

Until further data are available, we have found that it is best to proceed clinically with antidepressant treatment in much the same manner as one would in the nonretarded population. Specific risks to be considered in retarded patients are seizures and mental status changes due to anticholinergic effects. Also, patients with Down's syndrome may be at particular risk for cardiac conduction problems due to cardiac anomalies associated with Down's syndrome.

Lithium

Numerous clinical case reports and recent controlled studies have documented the effectiveness of lithium for the treatment of a wide variety of disorders in mentally retarded patients, including mania and depression, aggressiveness, and self-injurious behavior (Dostal and Zvotsky 1970; Gualtieri 1989b; Hasan and Mooney 1979; Kaminer et al. 1986; Kelly et al. 1976; Naylor et al. 1974; Reid and Leonard 1977; Rivinus and Harmatz 1979; Sovner and Hurley 1988b). As reviewed previously, this clustering of affective symptoms with aggressive and autoaggressive behaviors and the finding of dexamethasone non-suppression in aggressive and autoaggressive patients are topics of considerable importance.

While greater elucidation of the mechanisms of treatment response to these different symptoms is critical, lithium is a first-line medication in the treatment of both mood disorder and behavioral outbursts. An evaluation of family history for the presence of bipolar disorder in patients with aggressive or self-injurious outbursts should be routine. For those patients with phasic or cyclical outbursts, especially those with a family history of bipolar disorder, a trial of lithium may be worthwhile. Despite reports that lithium produces EEG changes, a history of seizures or abnormal EEGs does not contraindicate lithium use, or necessarily imply that an anticonvulsant will work better for behavioral control (see Chapters 2 and 5).

Anticonvulsants

Anticonvulsants are widely prescribed for the treatment of seizure disorders in mentally retarded patients. It is well established that mentally retarded individuals with seizure disorders have a higher rate of behavioral disturbance than those without seizure disorders (Eyman et al. 1970; Martin and Agran 1985). In addition, the efficacy of carbamazepine in the treatment of major mood disorders is now well documented (Post 1988). This confluence of different indications for the use of anticonvulsants in mentally retarded patients has recently resulted in considerable progress in establishing their efficacy for this population.

Carbamazepine has been reported to be effective for a variety of psychiatric disturbances in retarded patients, including self-injurious behavior, motor tics, hyperactivity, affective disorder, and stereotyped acts (Rivinus et al. 1989). Reid et al. (1981), in a well-controlled study, found that carbamazepine treatment resulted in significant improvement in a group of overactive retarded patients, especially if the overactivity was accompanied by elevated mood. Work by Sovner and Hurley (1988a) suggests that carbamazepine has a specific antidepressant effect in some mentally retarded patients. The same authors have also reported preliminary observations that valproic acid may be useful for the same indications (see also McElroy et al. 1987; Sovner 1989).

The findings for carbamazepine and valproic acid require replication before they can be considered first-choice medications for the treatment of psychiatric disorders in mentally retarded individuals without seizure disorders. However, therapeutic trials are warranted in treatment-resistant patients or when chronic neuroleptic therapy is the only other alternative. Whenever possible, these anticonvulsants should replace neuroleptics or other drugs. The practical approach to substitution would depend on whether the drugs already in place show partial benefit. If they do, anticonvulsants should be added and the other agents subsequently withdrawn if the anticonvulsants helped. If they show no benefit, the ineffective agent or agents would be tapered and discontinued before starting a trial of anticonvulsants.

Antianxiety and Sedative-Hypnotic Agents

Antianxiety and sedative-hypnotic drugs have historically been used frequently in mentally retarded patients, but there is little empirical support for their efficacy (Fahs 1989). Among this class of drugs, the benzodiazepines have been most commonly prescribed, although meprobamate, diphenhydramine, and hydroxyzine are also commonly used (Hill et al. 1985; Intagliata and Rinck 1985) despite the absence of clinical studies documenting their effectiveness. Buspirone has received considerable anecdotal mention as a treatment for anxiety and agitation in the mentally retarded population, but it is not yet commonly used, and there have been no published controlled studies of its efficacy.

The benzodiazepines are used primarily for the control of hyperactive, aggressive, or agitated behavior, either intermittently explosive or chronic. Although clinicians report occasional positive responses (Freinhar 1985), there are no controlled studies confirming their effectiveness in long-term use. They play a role when short-term sedation or short-term treatment of insomnia is required. However, paradoxical responses, characterized by disinhibition, increased motor activity, restlessness, and agitation, are fairly common (Fahs 1989). Retarded individuals who may be at particular risk for paradoxical reactions include those with lower mental age and histories of perinatal trauma, self-injurious behavior, and aggressive behavior. The incidence may approach 70% for those with both self-injurious and stereotypic behaviors (Barron and Sandman 1985). Caution must be exercised in the use of these drugs, because they create physiologic dependence, and withdrawal may result in exacerbations of behavior problems as serious as those initially targeted for treatment. Triazolam in particular has been associated with anterograde amnesia and dissociated reactions.

Beta-Adrenergic Blockers

There is accumulating evidence that beta-blocking drugs such as propranolol and nadolol are effective in treating panic attacks and chronic anxiety in mentally retarded patients. Doses in one study of severely and profoundly mentally retarded individuals ranged from 40 to 240 mg per day of propranolol, in divided doses, and the longer-acting nadolol, given once a day. Therapeutic dosages of more than 520 mg have been reported in other populations (Ratey et al. 1986). Treatment should, however, be started at smaller doses, such as 20 mg per day.

In most younger patients, asthma and related disorders are the main contraindication to treatment with beta-blockers. In older patients or younger patients with congenital heart disease, the drugs' negative inotropic effect on the heart must be considered. Open clinical trials with beta-blockers have yielded encouraging patterns of clinical improvement in patients with violent, aggressive, or self-injurious outbursts, which have been postulated to be manifestations of panic or high anxiety levels (Jenkins and Maruta 1987; Ratey et al. 1986, 1987). The mechanism of action of beta-blockers is unclear, but one popular hypothesis is that rather than acting centrally, they reduce peripheral autonomic manifestations of anxiety (Noyes 1985; Ratey et al., in press). Other than their effect in lowering blood pressure and pulse rate, which usually is tolerated well in younger, healthy subjects, they are relatively safe. Reports of depressive responses to beta-blockers in cognitively normal patients have not yet been replicated for retarded patients; however, monitoring of depressed mood should be considered.

Clonidine

There appears to be a significant subgroup of mentally retarded individuals for whom Tourette's disorder (multiple motor or vocal tics or both) leads to behavior problems and emotional outbursts. Clonidine, although somewhat less effective than haloperidol or pimozide in the treatment of tics, plays a useful role in the treatment of these patients (Leckman et al. 1988). It has the advantage of not carrying a risk of tardive dyskinesia. Clonidine also has been found in a controlled study to be effective in the treatment of at least a subset of children with attention-deficit hyperactivity disorder (Hunt et al. 1985) and may have a beneficial effect on obsessive-compulsive behavior. Because clonidine may cause hypotension and sedation, it must be given in divided doses and should be initiated at low dosages.

Psychostimulants

Psychostimulants such as methylphenidate and dextroamphetamine are commonly used in the treatment of hyperactivity in mentally retarded children who live at home (Gadow and Kalachnik 1981). However, for unclear reasons, they are rarely tried in institutionalized adults (Aman and Singh 1988). The psychostimulants are relatively safe drugs, and their treatment and side effects have been well studied (Donnelly 1989). There have been a large number of well-designed studies of the effects of psychostimulants on mentally retarded individuals (Aman 1982, 1989b; Gualtieri and Hicks 1990). In general, these studies indicate that psychostimulants are more likely to be effective in treating attention-deficit disorder in patients with milder cognitive deficits and are much less likely to be effective and may even have negative effects in severely or profoundly retarded patients. Patients with moderate retardation occasionally benefit, but do less well in general than those with mild retardation.

Opiate Antagonists

The opiate antagonists naloxone and naltrexone have been the subjects of numerous recent clinical trials in the treatment of severe self-injurious behavior in retarded and autistic retarded patients (Rivinus et al. 1989). The rationale for the use of opiate antagonists is based on hypothesized elevations in endogenous brain opiates in these patients (Barrett et al. 1989; Sandman et al. 1983). According to these authors, elevated brain opiate supports self-injurious behavior either by producing insensitivity to pain or by creating a euphoric effect in response to self-inflicted pain.

Naloxone, a short-acting opiate antagonist requiring intravenous administration, has not been consistently effective in open clinical trials. However, several well-designed single case studies, and a few recent open but methodologically sound group studies, have shown naltrexone, a long-acting, orally administered opiate antagonist, to be effective in reducing self-injurious behavior (Barrett et al. 1989; Bernstein et al. 1987; Campbell et al. 1988; Herman et al. 1987; Walters et al. 1989). Still, at least one study (Szymanski et al. 1987) reported a negative result. Group, double-blind, crossover drug placebo studies are urgently needed to assess the value of this promising new treatment approach.

Dosing of naltrexone is similar to that used for opiate dependence, i.e., 50 mg per day. Its most medically relevant, though rare, side effect is hepatotoxicity.

Elevations of transaminases were seen in 5 of 26 patients treated with 300 mg of naltrexone per day (Physicians' Desk Reference 1990). While the incidence of liver abnormalities is thought to be much lower at 50 mg per day, patients with preexisting liver disease may be at risk even at this dosage of naltrexone. In view of the relative lack of experience with naltrexone in the mentally retarded population, we recommend that liver function tests be monitored monthly for the first 3 months of naltrexone therapy and the drug discontinued if significant abnormalities develop.

Preexisting liver disease is a relative contraindication to the drug, as is upcoming surgery (because pharmacologic pain control would become problematic). Optic atrophy and seizures associated with naltrexone in a brain-damaged, profoundly retarded child have been reported (Barrett et al. 1989). This patient had previously received chlorpromazine. Evidence of optic atrophy from ophthalmologic or brain imaging studies is also, therefore, a relative contraindication. A second case of partial loss of vision occurring during combined naltrexone-chlorpromazine therapy was recently communicated to us. Until further clarification of this possible drug interaction is available, it is not advisable to combine naltrexone with current or recently discontinued phenothiazines.

Newer Medications

More recent additions to the general psychiatry pharmacologic armamentarium such as buspirone, clozapine, fluoxetine, and bupropion theoretically may be of use and can be cautiously considered in certain cases of mental retardation. Anecdotal reports suggest that buspirone may help with anxiety, clozapine with psychosis, fluoxetine with depression and obsessive-compulsive disorder, and bupropion with depression. As there are no controlled studies that clearly demonstrate the efficacy of these newer medications in the mentally retarded population, they should usually be considered after more established treatments have failed.

INFORMED CONSENT IN MENTALLY RETARDED PATIENTS

To successfully provide informed consent, the patient must understand the purpose of the treatment, the description of the treatment process, the risks of treatment, and alternatives to the proposed treatment, including no treatment (Popper 1987).

Many mildly and even moderately mentally retarded adults may be able to participate fully in the process of informed consent. However, if there is a doubt as to the patient's ability to make a decision concerning medication, legal measures such as a formal determination of competence to make the decision and some form of substituted judgment process should be considered. The patient's family should be involved if at all possible.

Because of the high risk of tardive dyskinesia posed by neuroleptics, and their widespread overprescription to retarded patients, special care must be taken to obtain informed consent when neuroleptics are prescribed, including a bias toward using formal substitute judgment if the patient is incompetent.

The issues to consider in the use of psychopharmacology in children and adolescents, discussed in Chapter 13, are relevant to many retarded adults, whose cognitive development may be at an adolescent level.

SUMMARY

The scientific practice of pharmacotherapy in mentally retarded patients depends on a sound foundation of knowledge concerning the biological, cognitive, sociodevelopmental, and sociological aspects of mental retardation itself. Accurate and complete diagnostic evaluations, including the direct assessment of the mentally retarded patient, are essential to the formulation of a safe and effective pharmacotherapeutic treatment plan. Accurate diagnosis is a complex undertaking, due to the complicated interaction between syndromes of severe psychiatric disorder, the particular neurobehavioral features of mental retardation, and the uniquely stressful and stigmatized status of the retarded individual in our society.

Pharmacotherapy should be but one element in a multidimensional treatment plan that includes appropriate interpersonal, behavioral, and educational interventions. When medication is used, it should be continually monitored according to a structured plan to minimize unnecessary chronic use of drugs, especially neuroleptics. Careful attention should be paid to the potential for development of tardive dyskinesia. Clinical research in the pharmacotherapy of retarded individuals still lags behind that of noncognitively impaired individuals. Nevertheless, considerable progress in establishing a scientific clinical basis for effective and specific pharmacotherapy for this underserved population has been made.

REFERENCES

Aman MG: Stimulant drug effects in developmental disorders and hyperactivity: toward a resolution of disparate findings. J Autism Dev Disord 12:385–398, 1982

Aman MG: Neuroleptics, in Treatments of Psychiatric Disorders, Vol 1. Edited by the American Psychiatric Association Task Force on Treatments of Psychiatric Disorders. Washington, DC, American Psychiatric Association, 1989a, pp 71–77

Aman MG: Psychostimulant drugs, in Treatments of Psychiatric Disorders, Vol 1. Edited by the American Psychiatric Association Task Force on Treatments of Psychiatric Disorders. Washington, DC, American Psychiatric Association, 1989b, pp 91–93

Aman MG, Singh NN: Aberrant Behavior Checklist. Canterbury, New Zealand, University of Canterbury, 1985

Aman MG, Singh NN: Patterns of drug use, methodologic considerations, measurement techniques, and future trends, in Psychopharmacology of the Developmental Disabilities. Edited by Aman MG, Singh NN. New York, Springer Verlag, 1988

Aman MG, White AJ, Field CJ: Chlorpromazine effects on stereotypic and conditioned behaviour of severely retarded patients—a pilot study. J Ment Defic Res 28:253–260, 1984

Aman MG, Singh NN, Steward AW, et al: The Aberrant Behavior Checklist: a behavior rating scale for the assessment of treatment effects. Am J Ment Defic 89:485–491, 1985

Aman MG, Paxton JW, Field CJ, et al: Prevalence of toxic anticonvulsant drug concentrations in mentally retarded individuals with epilepsy. Am J Ment Defic 90:643–650, 1986

American Psychiatric Association: Diagnostic and Statistical Manual of Mental Disorders, 3rd Edition. Washington, DC, American Psychiatric Association, 1980

American Psychiatric Association: Diagnostic and Statistical Manual of Mental Disorders, 3rd Edition, Revised. Washington, DC, American Psychiatric Association, 1987

Barrett RP, Feinstein C, Hole W: Effects of naloxone and naltrexone on self-injury: a double-blind, placebo-controlled analysis. American Journal of Mental Retardation 93:644–656, 1989

Barron J, Sandman CA: Paradoxical excitement to sedative/hypnotics in mentally retarded clients. Am J Ment Defic 90:124–129, 1985

Bates WJ, Smeltzer DJ, Arnoczky SM: Appropriate and inappropriate use of psychotherapeutic medications for institutionalized mentally retarded persons. Am J Ment Defic 90:363–370, 1986

Beck DC, Carlson GA, Russell AT, et al: Use of depression rating instruments in developmentally and educationally delayed adolescents. J Am Acad Child Adolesc Psychiatry 26:97–100, 1987

Beckwith BE, Parker L, Pawlarczyk D, et al: The dexamethasone suppression test in depressed retarded adults: preliminary findings. Biol Psychiatry 20:825–831, 1985

Bernstein GA, Hughes JR, Mitchell JE, et al: Effects of narcotic antagonists on self-injurious behavior: a single-case study. J Am Acad Child Adolesc Psychiatry 26:886–889, 1987

Biederman J, Gastfriend D, Jellinek MS: Desipramine in the treatment of children with attention deficit disorder. J Clin Psychopharmacol 6:359–363, 1986

Campbell M: Schizophrenic disorders and pervasive developmental disorders/infantile autism, in Diagnosis and Psychopharmacology of Childhood and Adolescent Disorders. Edited by Weiner JM. New York, John Wiley, 1985

Campbell M, Adams P, Small AM, et al: Naltrexone in infantile autism. Psychopharmacol Bull 24:135–139, 1988

Corbett JA: Psychiatry morbidity and mental retardation, in Psychiatric Illness and Mental Handicap. Edited by James FE, Smith RP. London, Gaskell, 1979

Corbett JA, Trimble MR, Nichol TC: Behavioral and cognitive impairments in children with epilepsy: the long-term effects of anticonvulsant therapy. J Am Acad Child Psychiatry 24:17–23, 1985

Donnellan AM, Anderson JL, Mesaros RA: An observational study of stereotypic behavior and proximity related to the occurrence of autistic child-family member interactions. J Autism Dev Disord 14:205–210, 1984

Donnelly M: Attention-deficit hyperactivity disorder and conduct disorder, in Treatments of Psychiatric Disorders, Vol 1. Edited by the American Psychiatric Association Task Force on Treatments of Psychiatric Disorders. Washington, DC, American Psychiatric Association, 1989, pp 365–398

Dostal T, Zvotsky P: Antiaggressive effect of lithium salts in severely mentally retarded adolescents. International Psychopsychiatry 5:302–307, 1970

Eyman RK, Moore BC, Capes L, et al: Maladaptive behavior of institutional retardates with seizures. Am J Ment Defic 74:651–659, 1970

Fahs JJ: Antianxiety and sedative-hypnotic agents, in Treatments of Psychiatric Disorders, Vol 1. Edited by the American Psychiatric Association Task Force on Treatments of Psychiatric Disorders. Washington, DC, American Psychiatric Association, 1989, pp 85–91

Feinstein C, Kaminer Y, Barrett R, et al: The assessment of mood and affect in developmentally disabled children and adolescents: the Emotional Disorders Rating Scale. Res Dev Disabil 9:109–121, 1988

Fogelman CJ (ed): AAMD Adaptive Behavior Scale Manual, 1975 Revision. Washington, DC, American Association on Mental Deficiency, 1975

Freeman RD: Psychopharmacology and the retarded child, in Psychiatric Approaches to Mental Retardation. Edited by Menolascino FJ. New York, Basic Books, 1970

Freinhar JP: Clonazepam treatment of a mentally retarded woman. Am J Psychiatry 142:1513–1516, 1985

Gadow KD, Kalachnik J: Prevalence and pattern of drug treatment for behavior and seizure disorders of TMR students. Am J Ment Defic 85:588–595, 1981

Golden GS: Tardive dyskinesia and developmental disabilities, in Psychopharmacology of the Developmental Disabilities. Edited by Aman MG, Singh NN. New York, Springer Verlag, 1988

Grabowski SW: Haloperidol for control of severe emotional reaction in mentally retarded patients. Diseases of the Nervous System 34:315–317, 1973

Gualtieri CT: Affective disorders, in Treatments of Psychiatric Disorders, Vol 1. Edited by the American Psychiatric Association Task Force on Treatments of Psychiatric Disorders. Washington, DC, American Psychiatric Association, 1989a, pp 10–14

Gualtieri CT: Antidepressant drugs and lithium, in Treatments of Psychiatric Disorders, Vol 1. Edited by the American Psychiatric Association Task Force on Treatments of Psychiatric Disorders. Washington, DC, American Psychiatric Association, 1989b, pp 77–85

Gualtieri CT, Hicks RE: The neuropsychology of stimulant effects in attention deficit disorder, in Attention Deficit Disorder, Vol 3. Edited by Bloomingdale L. New York, Spectrum, 1990

Gualtieri CT, Keppel JM: Psychopharmacology in the mentally retarded and a few related issues. Psychopharmacol Bull 21:304–309, 1985

Gualtieri CT, Schroeder SR, Hicks RE, et al: Tardive dyskinesia in young mentally retarded individuals. Arch Gen Psychiatry 43:335–340, 1986

Gualtieri CT, Matson JL, Keppel JM: Psychopathology in the mentally retarded, in Treatments of Psychiatric Disorders, Vol 1. Edited by the American Psychiatric Association Task Force on Treatments of Psychiatric Disorders. Washington, DC, American Psychiatric Association, 1989, pp 4–8

Guy W: ECDEU assessment for psychopharmacology, revised (DHHS Publ No ADM-76-338). Rockville, MD, National Institute of Mental Health, Psychopharmacology Research Branch, 1976

Hasan MK, Mooney RP: Three cases of manic-depressive illness in mentally retarded adults. Am J Psychiatry 136:1069–1071, 1979

Heistad GT, Zimmermann RL: Double-blind assessment of Mellaril in a mentally retarded population using detailed evaluations. Psychopharmacol Bull 15:86–88, 1979

Herman BH, Hammock MK, Arthur-Smith A, et al: Naltrexone decreases self-injurious behavior. Ann Neurol 22:550–552, 1987

Hill BK, Balow EA, Bruininks RH: A national study of prescribed drugs in institutions and community residential facilities for mentally retarded people. Psychopharmacol Bull 21:179–284, 1985

Hunt RD, Mindera RB, Cohen DJ: Clonidine benefits children with attention deficit disorder and hyperactivity: report of a double-blind placebo-controlled crossover therapeutic trial. J Am Acad Child Psychiatry 24:617–629, 1985

Intagliata J, Rinck C: Psychoactive drug use in public and community residential facilities for mentally retarded persons. Psychopharmacol Bull 21:268–278, 1985

Jacobson JW: Problem behavior and psychiatric impairment within a developmentally disabled population, I: behavior frequency. Applied Research in Mental Retardation 3:121–139, 1982

Jenkins SC, Maruta T: Therapeutic use of propranolol for intermittent explosive disorder. Mayo Clin Proc 62:204–214, 1987

Kalachnik JE, Miller RF, Jamison AG, et al: Results of a system to monitor effects of psychotropic medication in an applied setting. Psychopharmacol Bull 19:12–15, 1983

Kaminer Y, Feinstein C, Barrett R: A relationship between pervasive developmental disorders and affective disorders. J Am Acad Child Psychiatry 25:434–435, 1986

Kaminer Y, Feinstein C, Barrett R: Suicidal behavior in mentally retarded adolescents: an overlooked problem. Child Psychiatry Hum Dev 18:90–94, 1987

Kaminer Y, Feinstein C, Barrett RP, et al: Menstrually related mood disorders in developmentally disabled adolescents: review and current state. Child Psychiatry Hum Dev 18:239–249, 1988

Kazdin AE, Matson JL, Senatore V: Assessment of depression in the mentally retarded. Am J Psychiatry 140:1040–1043, 1983

Kelly JT, Koch M, Buegel D: Lithium carbonate in juvenile manic-depressive illness. Diseases of the Nervous System 37:90–92, 1976

Keppel JM, Gualtieri CT: Monitoring psychopharmacology in programs for the retarded, in Treatments of Psychiatric Disorders, Vol 1. Edited by the American Psychiatric Association Task Force on Treatments of Psychiatric Disorders. Washington, DC, American Psychiatric Association, 1989, pp 68–71

Leckman JF, Walkup JT, Cohen DJ: Clonidine treatment of Tourette's disorder, in Tourette's Syndrome and Tic Disorders: Clinical Understanding and Treatment. Edited by Cohen DJ, Bruun RD, Leckman JF. New York, John Wiley, 1988

Levine HG: Situational anxiety and everyday life experience of mildly mentally retarded adults. Am J Ment Defic 90:27–33, 1985

Liebowitz MR: Imipramine in the treatment of panic disorder and its complications. Psychiatr Clin North Am 8:37–47, 1985

Manderscheid RW, Wurster CR, Rosenstein MJ, et al: Data collection at the National Institute of Mental Health, in Mental Retardation and Mental

Health: Classification, Diagnosis, Treatment, Services. Edited by Stark JA, Menolascino FJ, Albarelli MH, et al. New York, Springer Verlag, 1988

Martin JE, Agran M: Psychotropic and anticonvulsant drug use by mentally retarded adults across community residential and vocational placements. Applied Research in Mental Retardation 6:33–49, 1985

Matson JL, Barrett RP: Psychopathology in the Mentally Retarded. Edited by Matson JL, Barrett RP. New York, Grune & Stratton, 1982

McElroy SL, Keck PE, Pope HG: Sodium valproate: its use in primary psychiatry disorders. J Clin Psychopharmacol 7:16–24, 1987

Menolascino FJ: Mental illness in the mentally retarded: diagnostic and treatment issues, in Mental Retardation and Mental Health: Classification, Diagnosis, Treatment, Services. Edited by Stark JA, Menolascino FJ, Albarelli MH, et al. New York, Springer Verlag, 1988

Menolascino FJ, Ruedrich S, Golden C, et al: Diagnosis and pharmacotherapy of schizophrenia in the retarded. Psychopharmacol Bull 21:316–322, 1985a

Menolascino FJ, Ruedrich S, Golden C, et al: Schizophrenia in the mentally retarded. Psychiatic Hospital 12:21–25, 1985b

Menolascino FJ, Wilson J, Golden CJ, et al: Medications and treatment of schizophrenia in persons with mental retardation. Ment Retard 24:277–283, 1986

Mikkelsen EJ: Low dose haloperidol for stereotypic self-injurious behavior in the mentally retarded. N Engl J Med 315:398–399, 1986

Myers BA: Conduct disorders of adolescents with developmental disabilities. Ment Retard 25:335–340, 1987a

Myers BA: Psychiatric problems in adolescents with developmental disabilities. J Am Acad Child Adolesc Psychiatry 26:74–79, 1987b

Naylor GJ, Donald JM, LePoidevin D, et al: A double blind trial of long-term lithium therapy in mental defectives. Br J Psychiatry 124:52–57, 1974

Nihira J, Foster R, Shehaus M, et al: American Association on Mental Deficiency Adaptive Behavior Scales, Revised. Washington, DC, American Association on Mental Deficiency, 1975

Noyes R: Beta-adrenergic blocking drugs in anxiety and stress. Psychiatr Clin North Am 8:119–132, 1985

Ollendick TH, Ollendick DG: Anxiety disorders, in Psychopathology in the Mentally Retarded. Edited by Matson JL, Barrett RP. New York, Grune & Stratton, 1982

Physicians' Desk Reference, 44th Edition. Oradell, NJ, Medical Economics, 1990

Pilkington TL: A report on Tofranil in mental deficiency. Am J Ment Defic 66:729–732, 1962

Pirodsky DM, Gibbs JW, Hesse RA, et al: Use of the dexamethasone suppression test to detect depressive disorders of mentally retarded individuals. Am J Ment Defic 90:245–252, 1985

Popper C: Medical unknowns and ethical consent: prescribing psychotropic medications for children in the face of uncertainty, in Psychiatric Pharmacosciences of Children and Adolescents. Edited by Popper C. Washington, DC, American Psychiatric Press, 1987

Post RM: Time course of clinical effects of carbamazepine: implications for mechanisms of action. J Clin Psychiatry 49:35–48, 1988

Ratey JJ, Mikkelsen EJ, Smith GB, et al: Beta-blockers in the severely and profoundly retarded. J Clin Psychopharmacol 6:103–107, 1986

Ratey JJ, Mikkelsen EJ, Smith GB, et al: Open trial effects of beta-blockers on speech and social behaviors in eight autistic adults. J Autism Dev Disord 17:439–446, 1987

Ratey JJ, Bemporad J, Sorgi P, et al: The effects of beta-blockers on speech and social behaviors: results of an open trial in eight autistic adults. J Autism Dev Disord (in press)

Reid AH: Psychoses in adult mental defectives, manic depressive psychosis. Br J Psychiatry 120:205–212, 1972

Reid AH: The Psychiatry of Mental Handicap. Oxford, Blackwell Scientific, 1982

Reid AH, Leonard A: Lithium treatment of cyclical vomiting in a mentally defective patient. Br J Psychiatry 130:316–318, 1977

Reid AH, Naglov GJ: Short-cycle manic depressive psychoses in mental defectives: a clinical and physiologic study. J Ment Defic Res 20:67–76, 1976

Reid AH, Naylor GS, Kay DSG: A double-blind placebo controlled crossover trial of carbamazepine in overactive severely mentally handicapped patients. Psychol Med 11:109–113, 1981

Reiss S, Levitan GW, Szyszko J: Emotional disturbance and mental retardation: diagnostic overshadowing. Am J Ment Defic 86:567–574, 1982

Reynolds WM, Baker JA: Assessment of depression in persons with mental retardation. American Journal of Mental Retardation 93:1:93–103, 1988

Richardson MA, Haugland G, Pass R, et al: The prevalence of tardive dyskinesia in a mentally retarded population. Psychopharmacol Bull 22:243–249, 1986

Rivinus TM, Harmatz JS: Diagnosis and lithium treatment of affective disorder in the retarded: five cases. Am J Psychiatry 136:551–554, 1979

Rivinus TM, Grofer LM, Feinstein C, et al: Psychopharmacology in the mentally retarded individual: new approaches, new directions. Journal of the Multihandicapped Person 2:1–23, 1989

Ruedrich SL, Wadle CV, Hahn RK, et al: Neuroendocrine investigation of depression in mentally retarded patients. J Nerv Ment Dis 173:85–89,1987

Russell AT: The mentally retarded emotionally disturbed child and adolescent, in Children With Emotional Disorders and Developmental Disabilities. Edited by Sigman M. New York, Grune & Stratton, 1985

Sandman CA, Datta PC, Barron J, et al: Naloxone attenuates self-abuse behavior in developmentally disabled clients. Applied Research in Mental Retardation 4:5–11, 1983

Schroeder SR: Neuroleptic medications for persons with developmental disabilities, in Psychopharmacology of the Developmental Disabilities. Edited by Aman MG, Singh NN. New York, Springer Verlag, 1988

Schroeder SR: Abnormal stereotyped behaviors, in Treatments of Psychiatric Disorders, Vol 1. Edited by the American Psychiatric Association Task Force on Treatments of Psychiatric Disorders. Washington, DC, American Psychiatric Association, 1989, pp 44–49

Senatore V, Matson J, Kazdin A: An inventory to assess psychopathology of mentally retarded adults. Am J Ment Defic 89:459–466, 1985

Singh NN, Aman MG: Effects of thioridazine dosage on the behavior of severely mentally retarded persons. Am J Ment Defic 85:580–587, 1981

Singh NN, Millichamp CJ: Pharmacological treatment of self-injurious behavior in mentally retarded persons. J Autism Dev Disord 15:257–267, 1985

Sovner R: The use of valproate in the treatment of mentally retarded persons with typical and atypical bipolar disorders. J Clin Psychiatry 50:40–43, 1989

Sovner R, Hurley A: Psychotropic drug interaction with anticonvulsants. Psychiatric Aspects of Mental Retardation 1:17–22, 1982

Sovner R, Hurley A: Do the mentally retarded suffer from affective illness? Arch Gen Psychiatry 40:61–67, 1983

Sovner R, Hurley A: Drug profiles, IV: carbamazepine and valproate. Psychiatric Aspects of Mental Retardation 7: 1988a

Sovner R, Hurley A: The management of chronic behavior disorders in mentally retarded adults with lithium carbonate. J Nerv Ment Dis 169:191–195, 1988b

Sparrow SS, Balla DA, Cicchetti DUR: Vineland Adaptive Behavior Scales. Circle Pines, MN, American Guidance Service, 1984

Sprague RL, Werry JS: Methodology of psychopharmacological studies with the retarded, in International Review of Research in Mental Retardation, Vol 5. Edited by Ellis NR. New York, Academic, 1971

Sprague RL, Kalachnik JE, Shaw KM: Psychometric properties of the Dyskinesia Identification System: Condenser User Scale (DISCUS). Ment Retard 27:141–148, 1989

Szymanski LS, Crocker AC: Mental retardation, in Comprehensive Textbook of Psychiatry, 4th Edition. Edited by Kaplan and Sadock. Baltimore, MD, Williams & Wilkins, 1985, pp 1635–1671

Szymanski LS, Doherty M: Behavioral and psychiatric disorders, mildly and moderately retarded persons, in Developmental Disabilities. Edited by Rubin IL, Crocker AC. Philadelphia, PA, Lea & Febiger, 1989a

Szymanski LS, Doherty M: Developmental Disabilities: Delivery of Medical

Care for Children and Adults. Edited by Rubin IL, Crocker AC. Philadelphia, PA, Lea & Febiger, 1989b

Szymanski LS, Kedesky J, Sulkes S, et al: Naltrexone in treatment of self-injurious behavior: a clinical study. Res Dev Disabil 8:179–190, 1987

Walters AS, Barrett RP, Feinstein C, et al: A case report of naltrexone treatment of self-injury and social withdrawal in autism. J Autism Dev Disord 20(2):169–176, 1990

Section V

Special Topics

Chapter 16

Pharmacological and Behavioral Treatment of Nicotine Dependence: Nicotine as a Drug of Abuse

Michael G. Goldstein, M.D.
Raymond Niaura, Ph.D.
David B. Abrams, Ph.D.

In 1980, with the publication of the diagnostic criteria for tobacco dependence in DSM-III (American Psychiatric Association 1980), cigarette smoking and other forms of tobacco use were officially identified as psychiatric problems. Psychiatrists, however, remained rather uninterested in the problems associated with cigarette smoking and other forms of tobacco use until quite recently, when several new developments stimulated them and other physicians to become more involved in research on and treatment of tobacco use disorders.

The authors would like to express their appreciation to John R. Hughes, M.D., for his helpful feedback and suggestions on an early version of the manuscript and to Lori Kravetz for her secretarial assistance.

This chapter was supported in part by the National Institute on Drug Abuse, Grant No. DA05623 to M.G.G.; the National Cancer Institute, Grant No. CA38309 to D.B.A.; the National Cancer Institute Cancer Prevention Research Consortium, Grant No. PO1 CA50087 to James O. Prochaska, D.B.A., Wayne Velicer, and M.G.G.; and the National Heart Lung and Blood Institute, Grant No. HL32318 to D.B.A.

These new developments include the identification of nicotine as a powerful psychoactive drug with high addictive potential (U.S. Department of Health and Human Services [U.S. DHHS] 1988), inclusion of nicotine dependence among other psychoactive substance abuse disorders in DSM-III-R (American Psychiatric Association 1987), the development of several promising pharmacologic agents to treat nicotine dependence (Jarvik and Henningfield 1988), the association of nicotine dependence with other psychiatric disorders (Davis 1984; Hughes et al. 1986a), and the growing awareness of the health hazards of smoking as well as of passive smoke exposure.

The overall goal of this chapter is to increase the reader's knowledge and skill in the diagnosis and treatment of nicotine dependence. The chapter begins with an overview of the scope of the nicotine dependence problem and its relationship to other psychiatric disorders, including other substance use disorders. A discussion follows of the characteristics of nicotine that have led to its identification as a psychoactive drug, the metabolic consequences of cigarette smoking, the criteria for diagnosing and assessing nicotine dependence, and principles and strategies for effectively treating nicotine dependence. Both pharmacologic and nonpharmacologic treatment strategies will be described.

SCOPE OF THE PROBLEM

Despite a steady decline in the prevalence of cigarette smoking since the late 1960s, cigarette smoking remains the most important contributor to premature death in the United States. Currently, about 50 million adults, or about 28% of the U.S. population, smoke cigarettes, down from 38% in 1976 (U.S. DHHS 1988). The total number of adults who have quit smoking has increased from approximately 30 million in 1976 to 40 million in 1988 (U.S. DHHS 1988). However, the proportion of "ever smokers" who are now former smokers is increasing at a yearly rate of less than 1%, suggesting that smoking prevalence will remain high well beyond the year 2000 (Pierce et al. 1989).

Several factors contribute to the relatively slow decline in smoking prevalence. Though more than 90% of smokers surveyed say that they want to quit smoking (Gallup Opinion Index 1974), only a fraction (15%) are actively attempting to quit, either on their own or with the help of some form of aid or program (Prochaska and DiClemente 1983). High relapse rates also contribute to the slow overall rate of change of smoking prevalence. Almost 80% of smokers who quit will relapse within a year (Hunt and Bespalec 1974; Schwartz 1987). Moreover, relapse appears to be very common in the earliest stages of attempted abstinence. As many as 30% of smokers who quit without assistance relapse within 72 hours (Garvey 1988). Formal treatment for nicotine dependence produces slightly higher 1-year abstinence rates of about 20–30% (Schwartz 1987). Thus, the 1-year outcome of formal treatment leaves considerable room for improvement.

As the prevalence of smoking in the general population declines, the percentage of "hard-core" smokers increases, a phenomenon that may slow the rate of decline of smoking (DiFranza and Guerrera 1989; Pierce et al. 1989). A growing body of evidence, reviewed below, suggests that development of physical dependence on nicotine in chronic smokers serves to maintain smoking and promote smoking relapse. Thus, nicotine dependence may be a central characteristic of a growing group of smokers, one that erodes the motivation to quit smoking and promotes relapse when abstinence is attempted. Recognition of the importance of nicotine dependence in the maintenance of smoking has led to increased efforts to identify effective, dependence-based treatments for smoking cessation. These will be described in the sections on treatment below.

CIGARETTE SMOKING AND PSYCHIATRIC DISORDERS

A number of studies have established that psychiatric patients, especially those with psychoses or with other psychoactive substance use disorders, are much more likely to smoke than the general population or even than nonpsychiatric patients. Table 16-1 summarizes some of this literature.

More recently, concern has been focused more specifically on the association of smoking with depression and with other substance abuse, both in general and in psychiatric populations, and on the implications of these associations for treatment. Some studies have demonstrated significant relationships between self-reported depression and the frequency of smoking. For example, Leon et al. (1979) found that in a nonpsychiatric sample, scores on the depression subscale of the Minnesota Multiphasic Personality Inventory (MMPI) indicated that smokers were more depressed than nonsmokers.

In a community study, Waal-Manning and de Hamel (1978) reported that self-reported depression was significantly related to smok-

Table 16-1. Smoking prevalence in psychiatric patients and general U.S. population

Population	Rate (%)	References
Psychiatric inpatients		
VA inpatients	83	O'Farrell et al. 1983
Alcoholics	>80	Maletzky and Klotter 1974; Walton 1972; Battjes 1988
Drug abusers	>85	Rounsaville et al. 1985; Burling and Ziff 1988
Psychiatric outpatients		
Schizophrenia	88	Hughes et al. 1986b; U.S. DHHS 1988
Mania	70	
Other	45–49	
General U.S. population	28	

ing behavior in both males and females even after controlling for age and obesity. Frederick et al. (1988) recently reported that the prevalence of depression in a community sample (measured with the Center for Epidemiologic Studies Depression Symptom Scale) was almost two times higher in female smokers than in female nonsmokers. Glassman et al. (1990) recently reported similar results from the Epidemiologic Catchment Area Survey which measured the prevalence and incidence of psychiatric disorders in a community-based sample, using a structured clinical interview. In a 9-year longitudinal study of adolescents, self-reported depression in adolescence predicted subsequent frequency and duration of smoking during young adulthood (Kandel and Davies 1986). Though smoking and depression are correlated, other studies controlling for the possibly confounding effects of age, income, sex, and employment have failed to find a relationship between self-reported depression and smoking (Frerichs et al. 1981; Haines et al. 1980). So, the precise nature and causal significance of the relationship between depression and smoking remain to be defined.

Whether or not depression causes smoking in some individuals, mood disorder may play a role in precipitating a relapse of smoking after attempted abstinence. Epidemiological data from the Epidemiologic Catchment Area study also suggest that a lifetime diagnosis of depression predicts an inability to stop smoking (Glassman et al. 1990). Glassman et al. (1988) found that a history of depression significantly predicted poorer smoking abstinence rates after treatment (33%) compared with abstinence rates for patients without a history of depression (57%), independent of the effects of treatment or sex. Moreover, none of the patients was depressed on entering the study. Glassman and colleagues (1989a) have also reported that smokers with a history of depression commonly develop depressive symptoms when they attempt abstinence. Finally, another study has found that self-reported depression predicted smoking relapse during the second and third weeks of attempted abstinence (West et al., in press). These studies suggest that a past history of depression or current depressive symptoms increase susceptibility to smoking relapse. There is also preliminary evidence that pretreatment with antidepressants may prevent the development of abstinence-related depressive symptoms in smokers with a past history of a depressive disorder (Glassman et al. 1989b).

Alcohol use and abuse and quite possibly abuse of other drugs are also associated with difficulty in giving up smoking. Drinking alcohol is reported to be a significant precipitant of smoking relapse in the general population (Shiffman 1986). Moreover, alcoholics are considerably less likely to be successful than nonalcoholics in their attempts to quit smoking (DiFranza and Guerrera, in press). However, at least half of alcoholics express a strong desire to attend a smoking treatment program (Kozlowski et al. 1989), and many have made multiple attempts at quitting (Bobo et al. 1987).

The increased prevalence of smoking among patients with psychiatric disorders has important implications for treatment of both the psychiatric disorder and nicotine dependence. A careful assessment of patients who seek help with stopping smoking is warranted to uncover possible psychiatric comorbidity, since prolonged abstinence may not be possible until the psychiatric disorder is treated.

NICOTINE AS A PSYCHOTROPIC DRUG

Pharmacokinetics and Pharmacodynamics of Nicotine

Nicotine is readily absorbed from tobacco smoke in the lungs and from smokeless tobacco in the mouth and nose (U.S. DHHS 1988) (see Figure 16-1). Nicotine rapidly accumulates in the brain after cigarette smoking. Within 1 minute, maximum brain concentrations are reached (U.S. DHHS 1988). The rapid accumulation of nicotine in the brain combined with nicotine's effects on brain activity and function provide optimal reinforcement for the development of drug dependence (U.S. DHHS 1988). With regular use, levels of nicotine accumulate in the

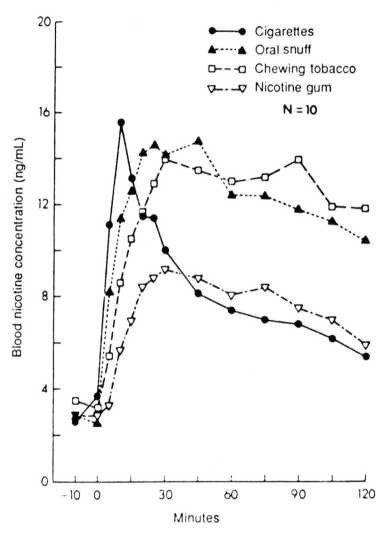

Figure 16-1. Blood nicotine concentrations during and after smoking cigarettes, using oral snuff, chewing tobacco, and chewing nicotine gum.
Source. Reprinted with permission from U.S. Department of Health and Human Services: The Health Consequences of Smoking: Nicotine Addiction: A Report to the Surgeon General (DHHS Publ No CDC-88-8406). Rockville, MD, Office on Smoking and Health, Public Health Service, U.S. Department of Health and Human Services, 1988.

body during the day and persist overnight. Thus, daily tobacco users are exposed to the effects of nicotine 24 hours a day, which increases the likelihood that pharmacologic tolerance will develop (U.S. DHHS 1988).

Acute and chronic tolerance develop to many effects of nicotine (U.S. DHHS 1988). The development of chronic tolerance contributes to an increase in cigarette consumption, as individuals smoke more to obtain desired effects of nicotine (Henningfield et al. 1985; U.S. DHHS 1988).

Nicotine is a powerful pharmacologic agent with a wide variety of stimulant and depressant effects involving the central and peripheral nervous, cardiovascular, endocrine, and other systems (U.S. DHHS 1988). These effects contribute to nicotine self-administration.

Peripheral nervous system effects include skeletal muscle relaxation (U.S. DHHS 1988). Central nervous system effects include electrocortical activation and increases in brain serotonin, endogenous opioid peptides, pituitary hormones, catecholamines, and vasopressin (Pomerleau and Pomerleau 1984; U.S. DHHS 1988). The rewarding properties of nicotine may be related to nicotine's stimulatory effects on dopaminergic pathways in the mesolimbic system (Clarke 1989; Fuxe et al. 1987; Pert and Clarke 1987; U.S. DHHS 1988).

Effects on attention, memory, and learning. Nicotine has been shown to increase attention, memory, and learning in smokers, especially when the environment exerts a relatively low demand (e.g., while performing clerical work or long-distance driving) and stimulation is most desirable (U.S. DHHS 1988). Nicotine appears to improve general attentional processing capacity, producing improved selective and sustained attention and improved ability to disregard irrelevant stimuli (U.S. DHHS 1988). The mechanism for these effects appears to be nicotine's effect on cholinergic pathways controlling electrocortical activation and arousal (Wesnes 1987).

The effects of nicotine on memory, learning, and performance are less clear because studies have not always controlled for the effects of deprivation, and some studies have found that nicotine may actually impair immediate memory (U.S. DHHS 1988). However, many smokers report that smoking helps them to think and perform; these effects promote continued smoking as well as relapse after quitting (U.S. DHHS 1988).

Effects on mood regulation, affect, and stress. Nicotine also has anxiolytic and antinociceptive effects (U.S. DHHS 1988). Evidence from surveys and experimental studies suggests that smokers smoke more during stressful situations or in situations involving negative mood and also that nicotine consumption is associated with decreases in negative affect (U.S. DHHS 1988). Nicotine may be most effective in reducing negative affect in situations involving anticipatory anxiety or ambiguous stressors (U.S. DHHS 1988). However, because the great majority of studies did not control for the effects of nicotine deprivation, which itself may produce negative affects, these results must be interpreted with caution (U.S. DHHS 1988). When delivered by intravenous or inhaled route to experimental subjects with a history of using a variety of dependence drugs, nicotine produces an increase in euphoria, and the effect is dose related (Henningfield et al. 1985) (see Figure 16-2). High doses of nicotine can produce cocainelike stimulant effects (Henningfield et al. 1985).

Nicotine's mood-regulating effects may be mediated by several mechanisms (U.S. DHHS 1988), including alleviation of withdrawal symptoms, increases in neuromodulators (Pomerleau and Pomerleau 1984), biphasic effects on the sympathetic nervous system (initial stimulation followed by decreased activity), antinociceptive actions (Fertig et al. 1986), increased activation of the left cerebral hemisphere (Gilbert 1985), reduction of hypothalamic consummatory drive (Grunberg and Baum 1985; Jarvik 1987), indirect effects secondary to nicotine-induced body sensations (Rose 1988), and effects on cognitive functioning (Wesnes 1987). Nicotine effects vary greatly between individuals and within the same individual over time (U.S. DHHS 1988). Differences depend on the setting in which the smoking occurs, the current state of the individual (e.g., whether he or she is smoking, nicotine-deprived, tolerant, stressed, nonstressed) and individual differences in dependence, genetics, and learning history (Pomerleau and Pomerleau 1987; U.S. DHHS 1988). The implications of these differences for treatment are described below.

Addictive properties.   The characteristics and patterns of chronic nicotine use have much in common with the use of other psychotropic drugs (Henningfield 1984; Jarvik and Henningfield 1988; U.S. DHHS 1988). As with other psychotropic drugs that produce addiction, humans will self-administer nicotine in the laboratory to reproduce desired effects and will respond to nicotine as a positive reinforcer (Henningfield 1984; Jarvik and Henningfield 1988; U.S. DHHS 1988). Patterns of relapse of smoking after smoking cessation are quite similar to the relapse patterns noted after treatment for other forms of drug abuse and dependence (Henningfield 1984; Hunt et al. 1971; U.S. DHHS

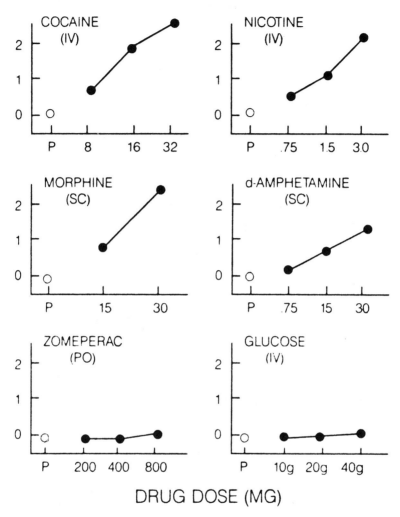

Figure 16-2. Euphoria scores of nicotine and other psychoactive drugs (higher score = higher level of euphoria). *Source.* Reprinted with permission from U.S. Department of Health and Human Services: The Health Consequences of Smoking: Nicotine Addiction: A Report to the Surgeon General (DHHS Publ No CDC-88-8406). Rockville, MD, Office on Smoking and Health, Public Health Service, U.S. Department of Health and Human Services, 1988.

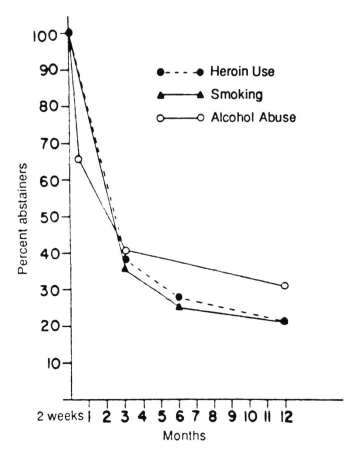

Figure 16-3.   Patterns of relapse after smoking cessation compared with relapse rates for other psychoactive substance use disorders. *Source.* Reprinted with permission from U.S. Department of Health and Human Services: The Health Consequences of Smoking: Nicotine Addiction: A Report to the Surgeon General (DHHS Publ No CDC-88-8406). Rockville, MD, Office on Smoking and Health, Public Health Service, U.S. Department of Health and Human Services, 1988.

1988) (Figure 16-3). Nicotine also can produce the physiological changes associated with physical dependence, including tolerance and withdrawal states (Henningfield 1986; U.S. DHHS 1988). (See "Nicotine Dependence" section below for more details.)

Nicotine meets the criteria for classification as an addicting drug, which are 1) the presence of highly controlled and compulsive patterns of drug taking; 2) the presence of psychoactive effects that contribute to use; and 3) the drug's capability of functioning as a reinforcer that can strengthen behavior, leading to further drug ingestion (Henningfield 1984, 1986; U.S. DHHS 1988). Moreover, nicotine use has additional properties that are associated with drug addiction: stereotypic patterns of use, use despite harmful effects, relapse following abstinence, recurrent drug cravings, development of tolerance and physical dependence, and pleasant or euphoric effects (Henningfield 1984, 1986; U.S. DHHS 1988).

METABOLIC CONSEQUENCES OF CIGARETTE SMOKING

Smoking and Body Weight

Recently, attention has focused on the relationships among smoking, nicotine, and body weight as potential mediators of smoking initiation, maintenance, and relapse. There is substantial evidence of an inverse relationship between cigarette smoking and body weight (U.S. DHHS 1988) and evidence to suggest that some people, especially women, smoke to prevent weight gain (Klesges and Klesges 1988; Russell and Epstein 1988; U.S. DHHS 1988). Moreover, weight gain accompanying smoking cessation may trigger a relapse of smoking (Klesges and Klesges 1988; U.S. DHHS 1988), although some studies have found positive correlations between weight gain during abstinence and 1-year abstinence rates (Hall et al. 1986; Hughes et al., in press).

The mechanisms that may underlie the relationship between smoking and body weight include a nicotine-induced increase in energy use (Benowitz 1988; U.S. DHHS 1988) and nicotine-induced suppression of food intake, especially carbohydrates (Benowitz 1988; Grunberg 1985; Jarvik 1987; U.S. DHHS 1988). The latter mechanism may be especially important in women, as both animal and human studies have found that female smokers who quit smoking increase their dietary intake significantly more than male smokers (U.S. DHHS 1988).

Table 16-2. Drugs whose metabolism is accelerated by cigarette smoking

Antipyrine	Lidocaine
Caffeine	Oxazepam
Clomipramine	Pentazocine
Clorazepate	Phenacetin
Desmethyldiazepam	Propranolol
Imipramine	Theophylline

Effects on Drug Metabolism and Pharmacodynamics

Smoking is known to accelerate the metabolism of many drugs (Benowitz 1988, 1989). Table 16-2 lists those drugs whose metabolism is significantly accelerated by smoking. It should be noted that the list includes several psychoactive drugs (i.e., imipramine, clomipramine, clorazepate, oxazepam, desmethyldiazepam, and pentazocine). The metabolic effects of smoking are likely due to nicotine as well to as other constituents of cigarettes, including polyaromatic hydrocarbons (Benowitz 1988).

Because cigarette smoking's effects on metabolism are complex, it is difficult to generalize about the effects of cigarette smoking or nicotine use on entire classes of drugs (Benowitz 1988, 1989). For example, though cigarette smoking increases the metabolism of imipramine, it has minimal or no effect on the metabolism of nortriptyline (Benowitz 1988, 1989). Moreover, although smoking accelerates the metabolism of such benzodiazepines as clorazepate, oxazepam, and desmethyldiazepam, it does not significantly alter the metabolism of chlordiazepoxide, diazepam, and lorazepam (Benowitz 1988, 1989). Smoking may also increase the metabolism of some neuroleptics, though this has not been carefully studied (Benowitz 1989). Phenytoin levels are not significantly altered by smoking, but the effects of smoking on the metabolism of other anticonvulsants has also not been well studied (Benowitz 1988, 1989). The relationships between smoking or nicotine use and the metabolism of other psychoactive drugs are likely to be clarified, as this important issue increasingly is being addressed in pharmacologic studies.

In addition to its metabolic effects, nicotine use also results in pharmacodynamic interactions that may potentiate or interfere with the effects of other drugs. For example, nicotine's stimulatory effects may counteract the sedative effects of phenothiazines and benzodiazepines (Benowitz 1988, 1989). The clinical implications of the effects of smoking and nicotine on drug metabolism and pharmacodynamics are important but often overlooked.

Because smoking may increase metabolism and decrease the effectiveness of several psychoactive drugs, higher dosages of these drugs may be needed in patients who smoke. A recent study of schizophrenic patients found that smokers received significantly more neuroleptics than nonsmokers, even after statistically controlling for severity of illness, age, weight, sex, and alcohol and caffeine intake (Bansil et al. 1989). Moreover, when smokers taking psychotropic drugs quit smoking or significantly reduce their smoking rate, drug toxicity may occur. As psychiatric inpatient units move toward becoming smoke-free environments, psychiatric patients may be forced to stop smoking. In this setting, the interactions between smoking and psychotropic drug levels and effects become even more salient.

Another implication of these pharmacologic effects is that the increased smoking rates among psychiatric patients may result from patients' attempts to overcome some of the undesirable properties of psychoactive drugs. Because of the complex metabolic and pharmacodynamic effects of smoking, we recommend obtaining drug levels of psychotropics in patients who also smoke when there is evidence for drug toxicity, or if the patient fails to respond to psychoactive drug treatment.

NICOTINE DEPENDENCE

As noted in the preceding section, evidence has converged from several sources to suggest that nicotine is an addicting or dependence-producing drug. It was recently included in the most recent edition of the Diagnostic and Statistical Manual of Mental Disorders (DSM-III-R) among the drugs that may produce psychoactive substance dependence. The diagnostic criteria for psychoactive substance dependence are reproduced in Table 16-3. The diagnosis of nicotine dependence by these criteria requires persistence of the problem for at least 1 month and evidence of any three of the nine criteria.

The criteria that apply most directly to nicotine use include 1) having a persistent desire or making unsuccessful attempts to quit or reduce use, 2) spending a great deal of time in activities necessary to get the substance or taking the substance (e.g., chain smoking), 3) continuing to use the substance despite having a physical problem that is caused or exacerbated by the use of the substance, 4) developing withdrawal

Table 16-3.   DSM-III-R diagnostic criteria for psychoactive substance
dependence

Psychoactive substance dependence

A. At least three of the following:

1. Substance often taken in larger amounts or over a longer period than the
person intended
2. Persistent desire or one or more unsuccessful efforts to cut down or control
substance use
3. A great deal of time spent in activities necessary to get the substance (e.g.,
theft), taking the substance (e.g., chain smoking), or recovering from its effects
4. Frequent intoxication or withdrawal symptoms when expected to fulfill major
role obligations at work, school, or home (e.g., does not go to work because
hung over, goes to school or work "high," intoxicated while taking care of his
or her children), or when substance use is physically hazardous (e.g., drives
when intoxicated)
5. Important social, occupational, or recreational activities given up or reduced
because of substance use
6. Continued substance use despite knowledge of having a persistent or recurrent
social, psychological, or physical problem that is caused or exacerbated by the
use of the substance (e.g., keeps using heroin despite family arguments about
it, cocaine-induced depression, or having an ulcer made worse by drinking)
7. Marked tolerance: need for markedly increased amounts of the substance (i.e.,
at least a 50% increase) in order to achieve intoxication or desired effect, or
markedly diminished effect with continued use of the same amount

Note: The following items may not apply to cannabis, hallucinogens, or
phencyclidine (PCP):

8. Characteristic withdrawal symptoms (see specific withdrawal syndromes under
psychoactive substance-induced organic mental disorders)
9. Substance often taken to relieve or avoid withdrawal symptoms

B. Some symptoms of the disturbance have persisted for at least 1 month or have
occurred repeatedly over a longer period of time.

Source.   Reprinted with permission from the *Diagnostic and Statistical Manual of Mental Disorders,*
3rd Edition, Revised. Copyright 1987 American Psychiatric Association.

symptoms while attempting to quit, and 5) taking the substance often
to relieve or avoid withdrawal symptoms.

The nicotine withdrawal syndrome is now fairly well characterized
(Hughes and Hatsukami 1986). The DSM-III-R criteria for nicotine
withdrawal are listed in Table 16-4. The syndrome includes craving or
urges to use nicotine; irritability, frustration or anger; anxiety; difficulty concentrating; restlessness; decreased heart rate; and increased
appetite or weight gain. DSM-III-R requires that at least four of these
signs be present for a diagnosis of nicotine withdrawal. When these

Table 16-4. DSM-III-R diagnostic criteria for nicotine withdrawal

A. Daily use of nicotine for at least several weeks.

B. Abrupt cessation of nicotine use, or reduction in the amount of nicotine used, followed within 24 hours by at least four of the following signs:
1. Craving for nicotine
2. Irritability, frustration, or anger
3. Anxiety
4. Difficulty concentrating
5. Restlessness
6. Decreased heart rate
7. Increased appetite or weight gain

Source. Reprinted with permission from the *Diagnostic and Statistical Manual of Mental Disorders, 3rd Edition, Revised.* Copyright 1987 American Psychiatric Association.

criteria are revised in DSM-IV, it is likely that disrupted sleep, impatience, and depression or dysphoric mood will be added (J. Hughes, March 1989, personal communication).

The signs and symptoms of the nicotine withdrawal syndrome can appear within 2 hours after the last use of tobacco, usually peak between 24 and 48 hours after cessation, and last from a few days to a few weeks (Hughes et al. 1990; Hughes et al., in press). Recently, Hughes et al. (in press) found that most withdrawal symptoms resolve by 1 month, although craving, hunger, and increased weight continue for 6 months in many former smokers. However, there is a great deal of individual variation in both the symptomatic pattern and time course of withdrawal symptoms. While a history of previous withdrawal symptoms is important to the diagnosis of nicotine dependence, the patient's future experiences during attempted abstinence cannot always be predicted.

In addition to experiencing the characteristics described in the DSM-III-R diagnostic criteria, many patients also describe patterns of compulsive use or tobacco seeking. For example, some smokers will often go out of their way to ensure that they have a steady supply of cigarettes. In extreme cases, they will smoke butts found in ashtrays if they have run out of cigarettes.

Another aspect of nicotine dependence relates to the notion of nicotine regulation. Some evidence suggests that smokers will consciously or unconsciously compensate and adjust their smoking patterns to maintain their usual plasma levels of nicotine (Moss and Prue 1982; Russell 1987; U.S. DHHS 1988). For example, individuals who switch to cigarettes with lower nicotine than their usual brand will often smoke more cigarettes or smoke them more effectively to extract a greater amount of nicotine.

Tolerance is also listed among the criteria for psychoactive substance dependence. Though there is considerable evidence for the development of tolerance among chronic cigarette smokers, clinical assessment of tolerance is difficult because self-reports may be unreliable, and laboratory evaluation of tolerance is still in the developmental stage.

General Considerations for Treatment

Stages of Change

Before attempting to intervene with smokers to provide treatment for nicotine dependence, it is essential to determine whether they are seriously considering quitting smoking. As noted in the introductory section of this chapter, only a fraction of smokers are ready to take action either on their own or with the help of some form of aid or program (Prochaska and DiClemente, 1983).

Prochaska and DiClemente (1986) have found that smokers move through several stages of change during the process of quitting smoking: 1) precontemplation, a stage of unawareness or denial of smoking as a problem; 2) contemplation, a stage of ambivalence, when pros and cons for quitting are weighed without definite commitment to taking action; 3) action, characterized by serious attempts to quit smoking; and 4) maintenance, characterized by successful change but also activity to monitor behavior to prevent relapse (see Figure 16-4). Individuals are likely to benefit from different interventions matched to their stage of change (Prochaska and DiClemente 1986). For example, consciousness raising is most useful for individuals in the contemplation stage, while pharmacologic agents are most likely to benefit individuals in the action stage.

The Role of the Psychiatrist

Because smoking is highly prevalent among patients with psychiatric disorders, general psychiatrists are likely to encounter many nicotine-dependent patients. Many of these patients are likely to be in the precontemplation or contemplation stage of change and will be resistant to being treated for nicotine dependence. In contrast, psychiatrists who develop expertise in the treatment of nicotine depen-

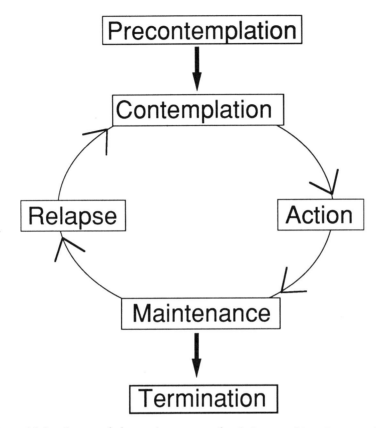

Figure 16-4. Stages of change in process of quitting smoking. Reprinted with permission from Prochaska JO, DiClemente CC: Towards a comprehensive model of change, in Treating Addictive Disorders: Processes of Change. Edited by Miller WR, Heather N. New York, Plenum, 1986.

dence tend to see self-referred patients and those referred by primary-care physicians specifically for treatment of this disorder.

The discussion of nicotine-dependence treatment strategies that follows focuses primarily on the treatment of smokers who are actively trying to quit smoking and who, therefore, are in the action stage of change. Self-help strategies (Schwartz 1987), brief or minimal physician-delivered interventions (Goldstein et al. 1990; Kottke et al. 1988; Ockene 1987; Orleans 1985; Stokes and Rigotti 1988) and work site and community interventions (Schwartz 1987; U.S. DHHS 1985) will not be discussed in detail in this chapter. Many of these strategies are designed to move patients from early stages of change to the action stage (Goldstein et al. 1990; Prochaska and DiClemente 1986).

The general psychiatrist who becomes skilled in the treatment of nicotine dependence may also wish to provide consultation to primary-care physicians about how they might increase their effectiveness. Research has shown that physician intervention in the primary-care setting is effective (Goldstein et al. 1990; Kottke et al. 1988; Ockene 1987; Orleans 1985; Stokes and Rigotti 1988). A recent meta-analysis of 39 controlled trials of smoking-cessation interventions in medical practice found that patients who received smoking-cessation interventions had 5.8% higher 1-year abstinence rates than controls (Kottke et al. 1988). Strategies that increase the likelihood of success include face-to-face interventions, the combination of physician and nonphysician counselors, multiple sessions, and multiple intervention modalities (Kottke et al. 1988; Ockene 1987).

Cohen and colleagues (1987) recently found that physicians who were reminded to ask patients about smoking by stickers attached to patients charts were more likely to inquire about smoking, to give advice to patients to stop smoking, and to spend more time counseling patients about stopping smoking than physicians who did not receive this intervention. The results of these studies suggest that psychiatrists can help primary-care physicians to be more effective in several ways: by increasing their awareness of the data demonstrating the effectiveness of physician interventions; by encouraging them to provide repeated, multiple interventions; by involving office staff in the effort; and by encouraging them to utilize reminder systems and other organizational aids to increase their consistency in delivering antismoking interventions.

Psychiatrists can also help train physicians in brief counseling skills and inform them about the use of pharmacological adjuncts to treatment. Primary-care physicians should also be referred to the excellent resources that have recently been developed to help them provide effective antismoking interventions. (See the discussion of resources in the section "Step-by-Step Approach to Treatment," below.) Kristeller and Ockene (1987) have recently described a strategy for assessment and treatment of smoking on a general hospital psychiatry consultation service.

Though previous sections of this chapter have emphasized the biological aspects of nicotine dependence, psychological and behavioral factors also play a crucial role in the dependence process (Abrams and Wilson 1986; Lichtenstein 1982; Schacter 1979). As a result, a combined biobehavioral approach to treatment of nicotine dependence is generally more effective than either behavioral or pharmacological treatment alone, especially for the heavily addicted smoker or the smoker who has failed to remain abstinent after multiple attempts to quit (Abrams and Wilson 1986; Goldstein et al. 1989; U.S. DHHS 1988). The high frequency of psychiatric comorbidity also increases the need for an integrated approach to treatment.

The strategies described below require a skilled treatment provider. Though many of these interventions are usually provided in the context of a formal nicotine-dependence treatment program, they can also be utilized in an individual practitioner's office.

Evaluation

This section describes a detailed evaluation process to guide the choice of a treatment program that is best matched to the needs of the patient. The two principal goals of this evaluation process are to characterize the severity of nicotine dependence and to identify psychiatric comorbidity that is likely to complicate treatment. Identification of specific behavioral and psychological factors that contribute to maintenance of smoking (reasons for smoking) will also be discussed. A list of assessment strategies is included in Table 16-5.

Assessing the Level of Nicotine Dependence

A reasonable first step in evaluating the diagnosis of nicotine dependence is to interview the patient and to obtain a detailed smoking history. Because most smokers will have already made one or more unsuccessful efforts to cut down or quit smoking, it is useful to inquire about previous attempts to quit to document signs and symptoms during abstinence, the duration of withdrawal symptoms, and reasons for resuming smoking. If smoking again relieved any or all of their symptoms, the likelihood is greater that they had experienced nicotine withdrawal.

Symptoms may also have been apparent when the patient switched to a low-tar, low-nicotine cigarette or after the patient stopped using smokeless tobacco products or nicotine gum. It may also be useful to assess the intensity of withdrawal symptoms during a prescribed period of abstinence of 1–3 days.

Nicotine withdrawal symptoms can be monitored using one of many available scales (Hughes and Hatsukami 1986; Shiffman et al. 1979). Simultaneous monitoring of depressive symptoms may also be

Table 16-5.   Evaluation of patients with nicotine dependence

---

- **Assessing the level of nicotine dependence**

    Smoking history
    Nicotine intake
       Smoking rate
       Nicotine content of brand
    Self-reported smoking pattern
       Self-reported severity and pattern of withdrawal
       Time to first cigarette in the morning
       Evidence for nicotine regulation

    Measures of nicotine intake
    Nicotine or cotinine assays
    Alveolar carbon monoxide level

    Fagerstrom Tolerance Questionnaire

    Prescribed abstinence period

- **Assessing reasons for smoking**

    Smoking typology scales

    Self-monitoring of smoking
    Cues or triggers associated with smoking

- **Assessment of comorbidity**

    Current or past psychiatric disorder
    Other psychoactive substance use disorder
    Schizophrenia
    Mood disorder
    Anxiety disorder

    Psychoactive drug use

    Obesity or history of weight gain with cessation of smoking

---

useful, particularly in patients with histories of depression. Measures of nicotine intake may provide some index of the degree of nicotine dependence. These include self-reported smoking rate and nicotine content of cigarettes, biochemical assays of nicotine and its metabolites, and alveolar carbon monoxide levels (an indirect measure). Cotinine, a metabolite of nicotine, has a half-life of roughly 20 hours (Benowitz 1988) and can be measured in any body fluid. Higher levels of cotinine in body fluids reflect greater nicotine intake. Cotinine determination may provide a more accurate reflection of nicotine intake than self-reported smoking rate, because of problems with recall and because actual levels of nicotine exposure will vary due to various other factors (e.g., nicotine content of cigarette, effective extraction of nicotine from cigarettes). Higher cotinine levels are related to nicotine tolerance and to withdrawal symptoms during periods of tobacco abstinence (Pomerleau et al. 1983) and were predictive in one study of relapse of smoking (Hall et al. 1984b).

Cotinine assays can be most conveniently obtained on saliva samples, though blood and urine also may be used. To obtain a saliva sample for cotinine assay, the patient must first rinse his or her mouth and then expectorate approximately 2 ml of saliva into a standard polystyrene tube. Samples should be frozen at approximately 0°F and shipped frozen for analysis. The price per assay may range between $10 and $60, depending on the laboratory and the type of assay conducted. Because of the relatively high cost of analysis and a turnaround time of 1 to several weeks, cotinine analysis may not be a feasible method for determining nicotine intake for most clinicians. Efforts are currently under way to produce inexpensive and easy to use cotinine screening kits to classify individuals into gross categories of intake (i.e., low, moderate, or high). Such kits are likely to become available over the next few years, but their usefulness in a clinical context will have to be demonstrated.

A less expensive alternative to using cotinine assays to assess nicotine exposure is analysis of expired alveolar carbon monoxide. Devices to measure concentrations of carbon monoxide (parts per million) in breath samples are readily available and relatively inexpensive. Two devices, the EC50 (Vitalograph, Inc., Lenexa, Kansas) and the Ecolyzer 2000 (National Draeger, Pittsburgh, Pennsylvania), show good correlations ($r \geq .95$) with carboxyhemoglobin concentrations in venous blood (Jarvis et al. 1986). The EC50 is somewhat less expensive, more portable, and easier to use than the Ecolyzer 2000, making it a good choice for clinicians. The patient need only breathe into the machine, and the entire assessment can be completed in less than 1 minute. Studies have pointed to the value of carbon monoxide measurement as a predictor of the severity of nicotine withdrawal symptoms (West and Russell 1985a). More studies are needed, though, to determine the relationship between the carbon monoxide level and the level of nicotine intake.

Perhaps the most common measure of nicotine dependence in current use is the Fagerstrom Tolerance Questionnaire (FTQ) (Fagerstrom 1978; Table 16-6). The FTQ is a seven-item self-administered form that identifies behaviors thought to reflect nicotine dependence (e.g., high smoking rate, and nicotine level of cigarette brand, and smoking when ill or soon after awakening). Evidence suggests that scores on the FTQ

Table 16-6. Fagerstrom Tolerance Questionnaire

For questions 1–6, please write the number of your answer on the blank line to the right.

1. Do you find it difficult to refrain from smoking in places where it
   is forbidden; e.g., in church, at the library, in cinemas, etc.?   _____
           0. NO   1. YES

2. Do you smoke more during the first 2 hours of your day than
   during the rest of the day?   _____
           0. NO   1. YES

3. Do you smoke if you are so ill that you are in bed most of the day?_____
           0. NO   1. YES

4. When you are smoking, do you inhale: _____
           0. Never
           1. Sometimes
           2. Always

5. How many minutes after you wake do you smoke your first
   cigarette?   _____

6. How many cigarettes a day do you smoke?   _____

For questions 7 and 8, please write your answer on the blank line below each question.

7. Which cigarette of the day would you hate most to give up?
   (Please be specific) _____

8. a. What is your usual brand of cigarettes?
      Brand: _____

   b. Check off all the following that apply to your brand:

___regular	___menthol	___hard pack	___nonfiltered
___lights	___nonmenthol	___soft pack	___filtered
___ultralights	___kings	___100's	___120's

Source. Reprinted with permission from Fagerstrom K-O: Measuring degree of physical dependence to tobacco smoking with reference to individualization of treatment. Addict Behav 3:235–241, 1978.

are related to withdrawal symptoms (Fagerstrom 1980; Fagerstrom and Schneider 1989; Killen et al. 1988) and success in smoking cessation (Fagerstrom 1982; Fagerstrom and Schneider 1989; Hughes 1984; Pinto et al. 1987).

The FTQ also appears to predict differential responsiveness to nicotine gum treatments for smoking cessation (Fagerstrom 1988). The scale can be administered within several minutes and is easily scored. Time to first cigarette in the morning, a specific question on the FTQ, is an indirect measure of withdrawal following overnight abstinence and appears to be a better predictor of outcome after attempted smoking cessation than the total FTQ score (Lichtenstein and Mermelstein 1986). Another measure of nicotine dependence, the Horn-Russell Nicotine Dependence Scale, was useful in predicting differential response to nicotine gum in a recently reported trial in Denmark (Tonnesen et al. 1988a).

Assessment of nicotine regulation provides additional evidence about nicotine dependence. Thus, an individual may tell you that he smoked more cigarettes after switching to a cigarette with a lower nicotine yield. Assessment of tolerance to nicotine is difficult to accomplish via self-report (Porchet et al. 1988; Russell 1988). Most smokers report at least some subjective and physiological effects after smoking the first cigarette of the day.

In summary, assessment of the level of nicotine dependence can be accomplished using a variety of methods with varying levels of invasiveness and cost. Though much valuable information can be obtained from a carefully obtained smoking history, use of self-monitoring strategies, questionnaires, and biochemical measures can provide additional information to help guide treatment decisions.

Assessing Reasons for Smoking

Smoking typology scales, which classify individuals' reasons for smoking (e.g., for management of affect, to satisfy craving, out of habit, for stimulation, or automatically) (Frith 1971; Ikard et al. 1969; Mausner and Platt 1971; McKennel 1970), can be used to assess aspects of nicotine dependence as well as psychological and behavioral factors that may contribute to smoking behavior. Studies have noted positive relationships between scores on some of these subscales and withdrawal distress (Niaura et al. 1989; West and Russell 1985), and some of the scales have been related to successful smoking cessation (Pomerleau et al. 1978). We recommend, in addition to using smoking typology scales, detailed functional analysis of each patient's reasons for smoking. The patient is instructed to monitor his or her level of smoking over a few days, recording in a diary the perceived reasons for smoking each cigarette. Other useful information can be monitored simultaneously, including the time of day and the situation in which smoking took place. The clinician and patient review the self-monitoring record to make note of frequent or powerful cues or "triggers" for smoking.

Assessing Comorbidity

In addition to assessing the patient's level of nicotine dependence, it is extremely important to determine whether there is evidence of psychiatric comorbidity. As described earlier, there is an association between smoking and other psychiatric disorders (Battjes 1988; Davis 1984; Hughes et al. 1986a; O'Farrell et al. 1983; Rounsaville et al. 1985). The presence or past history of major psychiatric disorder is likely to make smoking cessation more difficult (DiFranza and Guerrera, in press; Glassman et al. 1988). Moreover, smoking cessation may precipitate a relapse of an underlying psychiatric disorder, especially depression (Glassman et al. 1989b). Identification of psychiatric comorbidity facilitates monitoring and early treatment of exacerbations or relapses of psychiatric disorders.

Also, as noted in the section on the pharmacodynamics of nicotine, nicotine interacts with many psychoactive drugs and may affect their metabolism (Benowitz 1988, 1989). Adjustment of these medications may be needed during smoking cessation.

Finally, though not usually considered as psychiatric comorbidity, the presence of obesity, excessive weight gain during previous smoking-cessation attempts, or excessive concern about weight gain after cessation is likely to negatively influence the outcome of any smoking-cessation treatment program. Attention to these problems during smoking-cessation treatment is likely to improve long-term smoking-cessation outcome. Though there is little research-based data on the treatment of nicotine dependence in individuals with psychiatric comorbidity, identification, monitoring, and treatment of comorbidity are essential components of the management of such patients.

Pharmacologic Treatment

Pharmacologic treatments for nicotine dependence can be characterized using the same typology that has been developed for treating other forms of drug dependence (Jarvik and Henningfield 1988; U.S. DHHS 1988). The four categories of pharmacologic treatment, based on the pharmacologic strategy employed, are listed in Table 16-7. Each of these strategies will be described in some detail, using specific pharmacologic agents as examples.

Table 16-7. Pharmacologic treatments for nicotine dependence

- **Nicotine replacement or substitution**

  Nicotine resin complex
  Nicotine patch
  Nasal nicotine solution
  Nicotine aerosol rods
  Lobeline
  Stimulants

- **Nonspecific pharmacotherapy**

  Clonidine
  Antidepressants
    Doxepin
    Fluoxetine
  Buspirone
  Treatment of weight gain

- **Blockade therapy**

  Mecamylamine

- **Deterrent therapy**

  Silver acetate

Nicotine Replacement or Substitution Therapy

The principle of replacement therapy is to provide the patient with a more manageable and safer form of the drug to ameliorate withdrawal symptoms and allow the patient to gradually discontinue use of the drug (Jarvik and Henningfield 1988; U.S. DHHS 1988). Replacement therapy also provides an opportunity to develop strategies to deal with behavioral or learned components of the drug dependence while controlling the physiologic "need" for the drug. Moreover, if the method of administration of the replacement drug is sufficiently different than the method associated with the development of drug dependence, the learned associations between cues associated with drug administration and the drug's physiologic effects can be broken.

For example, the use of nicotine resin complex over a prolonged period may decrease the craving that previously occurred when a patient talked on the telephone and handled a cigarette. Because tolerance to nicotine is maintained during replacement therapy, the reinforcing effects of the replacement form of the drug are minimized. Several nicotine replacement strategies will be discussed below. The only nicotine replacement agent presently available in the United States is nicotine resin complex.

Nicotine resin complex. Also known as nicotine polacrilex (Nicorette) or nicotine gum, nicotine resin complex is the only form of nicotine replacement that has been approved for use by the Food and Drug Administration. Nicotine resin complex is effective in attenuating nicotine withdrawal symptoms (Fagerstrom 1988; Lam et al. 1987; U.S. DHHS 1988). Several controlled trials have found that when combined with a formal treatment program, nicotine resin complex is more effective than placebo in promoting abstinence from smoking (Fagerstrom 1988; Grabowski and Hall 1985; Lam et al. 1987; Lichtenstein 1986; Schwartz 1987; U.S. DHHS 1988).

However, nicotine resin complex appears to have limited effectiveness in producing long-term abstinence when provided with little or no counseling, especially in physicians' offices (Fagerstrom 1988; Hughes et al. 1989b; Schwartz 1987; U.S. DHHS 1988). That may be due to several factors, including improper and ineffective use, decreased compliance, and increased reliance on the drug at the expense of developing behavioral strategies for dealing with urges to smoke. Thus, formal relapse prevention training may be crucial when nicotine resin complex is used. This statement is supported by research associating nicotine resin complex use with significantly increased rates of short-term, but not long-term, abstinence (Hall et al. 1985; Harackiewicz et al. 1988; Hughes et al. 1989; U.S. DHHS 1988) and a study that demonstrated improved outcome when relapse prevention skills training was added to a treatment program that included nicotine resin complex (Goldstein et al. 1989). Evidence also suggests that nicotine resin complex is most effective for smokers who are more heavily dependent on nicotine (Fagerstrom and Melin 1985; Jarvik and Schneider 1984; Tonnesen et al. 1988a, 1988b; U.S. DHHS 1988).

Several issues related to the use of nicotine resin complex remain unresolved. The 4-mg dose may be more effective for the heavily dependent smoker (Kornitzer et al. 1987; Tonnesen et al. 1988a, 1988b), but this possibility has not been adequately tested. Theoretically, a fixed schedule of nicotine gum administration might be more likely to be effective in reducing withdrawal symptoms and aiding abstinence in the highly dependent smoker. However, there is presently only suggestive evidence to support this hypothesis (Fortmann et al. 1988; Goldstein et al. 1989).

The properties of nicotine resin complex require that patients be provided with very specific instructions about proper use. These in-

Table 16-8. Instructions for patients using nicotine resin complex (seven S's)

- Stop smoking cigarettes—do not smoke and chew.
- Substitute gum for cigarettes—at each urge to smoke.
- Slowly chew—only a few chews, then "park" the gum.
- Several pieces per day—about one piece for every two cigarettes.
- Stay on the gum for 2–3 months.
- Staged reduction—decrease use over several weeks.
- Stop using the gum.

Source. Adapted from the treatment protocol developed for the Warterloo Smoking Project, J.A. Best and D. Wilson, principal investigators, Waterloo University and McMaster University, National Cancer Institute, Smoking, Tobacco and Cancer Program, 1988.

structions are outlined in Table 16-8. Side effects of nicotine resin complex are common but are usually well tolerated, especially when patients receive instructions regarding proper use. Hiccups, nausea, anorexia, oral soreness, jaw soreness, and gastrointestinal distress are the most frequent side effects (Fortmann et al. 1988). Individuals who utilize nicotine resin complex to stop smoking may become physically dependent on the gum and experience withdrawal when they abstain from chewing it (Hughes et al. 1986a; West and Russell 1985b). However, only 6–9% of subjects who receive nicotine resin complex in specialty clinics continue to use the gum 1 year after treatment (West and Russell 1986). Among those who successfully abstain from cigarettes, 34–54% use the gum for more than 6 months (Hughes et al. 1986b), and about 25% continue to use the gum after 1 year (Hajek 1988). These individuals may require slow tapering of the gum use over a longer period of time or the use of other pharmacologic treatments to treat withdrawal.

Nicotine patch, nasal nicotine solution, and nicotine aerosol rods. Several systems for delivering nicotine are currently being developed or tested. The most promising new nicotine delivery system is the nicotine transdermal patch, which delivers nicotine through the skin. Early studies demonstrated that craving was reduced when a nicotine patch was used (Rose et al. 1985). A recent report suggests that the patch reduced cigarette smoking in psychiatric patients (Hartman et al. 1989). A controlled trial, in Europe, of a nicotine patch that provides a 24-hour infusion of nicotine found that the patch produced significant improvement in 1-, 2-, and 3-month abstinence rates (Abelin et al. 1989). No significant behavioral or psychological treatment was provided, and longer-term abstinence rates were not reported. Buchkremer et al. (1989), in another European sample, found that nicotine patches produced significantly higher abstinence rates than placebo during treatment but not at the end of treatment. In that study, all subjects attended weekly behavioral group sessions. Patches were discontinued 2 weeks before the end of treatment.

Nicotine patches are presently undergoing further clinical trials in the United States and Europe and will not be available for general use for some time.

Nicotine nasal solution has been tested in England by Russell and colleagues (1983). Though it showed promise in reducing withdrawal and aiding abstinence, nasal irritation and embarrassment regarding its use has limited further development (U.S. DHHS 1988). However, a nasally inhaled aerosol preparation developed by Perkins and co-workers (1986) is better tolerated and can provide excellent control over dose delivery. In a pilot clinical trial, nasal nicotine solution, applied as a droplet in the nose, was well tolerated and showed promise as an aid to smoking cessation (Jarvis et al. 1989).

Aerosolized rods, developed by the tobacco industry as smokeless cigarettes, can also deliver nicotine in significant doses, but only when puffed intensively (Russell et al. 1987; U.S. DHHS 1988). Sublingual nicotine tablets have also been used as a research tool (Jarvik and Henningfield 1988). Overall, nicotine aerosols, rods, and sublingual tablets have not yet been shown to be effective aids to smoking cessation.

Other nicotine replacement strategies.   Lobeline, a weak nicotine receptor agonist found in many over-the-counter aids for quitting smoking, is of unproven efficacy for the treatment of tobacco dependence (Jarvik and Henningfield 1988; Schwartz 1987). Stimulants have also been tried as a substitute for nicotine, but there is no evidence of significant efficacy and, in one study, administration of *d*-amphetamine resulted in increased pleasure from smoking and higher smoking rates (Jarvik and Henningfield 1988).

Other Pharmacotherapy

In addition to nicotine replacement therapy, several other pharmacologic strategies have been developed to treat manifestations of the nicotine withdrawal syndrome. (See "Nicotine Dependence," above, for a description of the withdrawal syndrome.) Medications intended to symptomatically reduce withdrawal discomfort (e.g., sedatives, anticholinergics, and sympathomimetics) have generally been found to be ineffective compared with placebos (Jarvik and Henningfield 1988;

U.S. DHHS 1988). In some cases, provision of sedatives or stimulants has actually led to increases in smoking (Jarvik and Henningfield 1988). Moreover, there is a risk in prescribing potentially addictive drugs to treat nicotine dependence (Jarvik and Henningfield 1988).

More recently, efforts to manage withdrawal have focused on preventing or attenuating the entire withdrawal syndrome, rather than simply treating the symptoms. These strategies will be described below. The role of these newer pharmacotherapies, including clonidine and antidepressants, in the treatment of nicotine dependence is likely to expand in the near future as they are studied further. Use of other pharmacologic agents to specifically treat associated or coexisting psychiatric disorders will also help to increase the successfulness of nicotine dependence treatment.

Clonidine. Clonidine is a centrally acting antihypertensive agent that has been shown to be effective in preventing symptoms associated with opiate withdrawal (Gold et al. 1980; Washton and Resnick 1981) and alcohol withdrawal (Baumgartner and Rowen 1987; Manhem et al. 1985; Wilkins et al. 1983). Recently, clonidine has also been shown to attenuate the nicotine withdrawal syndrome (Glassman et al. 1984, 1986; Ornish et al. 1988). Clonidine is thought to reduce withdrawal symptoms by inhibiting activity of the locus coeruleus, which regulates noradrenergic activity (Aghajanian 1978; Foote et al. 1983; Glassman et al. 1986; Issac 1980). Noradrenergic overactivity is a characteristic of withdrawal states from various drugs (Ashton 1984; Brown 1982; U.S. DHHS 1988), and noradrenergic overactivity is also believed to be responsible for some of the symptoms of nicotine withdrawal, especially anxiety and craving (Glassman et al. 1986).

Clonidine has also shown promise as an adjunct to smoking-cessation treatment (Glassman et al. 1988; Wei and Young 1988). Glassman and colleagues (1988) demonstrated in a randomized, double-blind, placebo-controlled trial that treatment with oral clonidine significantly improved 6-month smoking-cessation treatment outcomes compared with placebo (27% and 5% smoking abstinence rates, respectively). Clonidine's effect on 4-week outcomes in this study was significant for women, but not for men. Wei and Young (1988) reported that clonidine was significantly more effective after 4.5 months of treatment (57% abstinence rate) than either diazepam (37%) or placebo (37%) in a double-blind trial conducted in China.

Because all patients in both Glassman et al.'s and Wei and Young's studies also received behavioral treatment for smoking cessation, one cannot conclude from these results that clonidine used alone is effective as a treatment for smoking cessation. Indeed, when clonidine was dispensed without behavioral treatment in another study, a significant benefit over placebo was found at 1 week, but not at 4, 8, or 12 weeks, after the initiation of treatment (Davison et al. 1988). Because of its effects on nicotine withdrawal, clonidine is most likely to be effective in heavy, dependent smokers who are more likely to exhibit severe withdrawal upon smoking cessation (Glassman et al. 1986; Pomerleau et al. 1986). As is the case for nicotine resin complex (Goldstein et al. 1989), clonidine's effect on long-term smoking-cessation outcome is likely to be greatest when the drug is combined with behavioral skills training. The use of a transdermal preparation of clonidine may further increase its efficacy, as this delivery system provides therapeutic levels at a steady state for several days with fewer side effects than the oral preparation (Ornish et al. 1988; Weber and Drayer 1984). Though transdermal clonidine effectively attenuates nicotine withdrawal symptoms (Ornish et al. 1988), its efficacy as a smoking-cessation treatment has not yet been tested.

Antidepressants. The theoretical basis for considering antidepressants as a treatment for nicotine dependence comes from several sources. First, as noted previously, a history of depression is associated with increased difficulty with smoking cessation (Glassman et al. 1988, 1989a). Second, depressive symptoms commonly occur during nicotine withdrawal (Hughes et al. 1990) (Table 16-4), especially when there is a past history of depression (Glassman et al. 1989a). Third, nicotine appears to be a powerful regulator of affect (U.S. DHHS 1988). Finally, antidepressants have been quite useful in ameliorating the withdrawal state associated with cocaine, a psychoactive drug that shares stimulant properties with nicotine (Gawin and Kleber 1987).

At present, doxepin hydrochloride is the only antidepressant that has been shown to be effective in attenuating withdrawal symptoms after smoking cessation (Edwards et al. 1988). Pilot data suggest that doxepin also has some benefit as an adjunct to smoking cessation (Edwards et al. 1989a, 1989b). Fluoxetine, an antidepressant with serotonergic effects, is currently being evaluated as an adjunct to behavioral treatment for smoking cessation in a multicenter controlled trial (D. Wheadon, July 1989, personal communication).

We currently recommend that antidepressants be considered as an adjunct to smoking-cessation treatment when 1) there is a past history of a major depressive episode or dysthymia; 2) previous smoking-cessation attempts were associated with prominent depressive symptoms, especially if they persisted beyond the first 2 weeks of abstinence; and

3) multiple attempts at cessation using intensive behavioral interventions and other pharmacologic agents have failed.

Buspirone and other anxiolytics. Buspirone, a novel anxiolytic with presynaptic dopaminergic activity, reduced craving for cigarettes, minimized withdrawal anxiety and fatigue, and led to reduced smoking in an open, uncontrolled pilot study (Gawin et al. 1989). Buspirone might prove to be especially useful as an adjunct to treatment in patients who have a coexisting anxiety disorder, especially generalized anxiety disorder, or in patients who develop pronounced or persistent anxiety symptoms after smoking cessation. Patients with coexisting panic disorder or obsessive-compulsive disorder may also benefit from adjunctive treatment with an antidepressant with proven efficacy for these disorders (e.g., imipramine and fluoxetine, respectively). The use of benzodiazepines for a patient with a coexisting anxiety disorder is not recommended (unless all else has failed) because they have no proven efficacy (Schwartz 1987; Wei and Young 1988).

Treatment of weight gain. As noted previously, there is substantial evidence that some people, especially women, smoke to prevent weight gain (Klesges and Klesges 1988; Russell and Epstein 1988; U.S. DHHS 1988). Moreover, the weight gain that frequently accompanies smoking cessation may trigger smoking relapse (Klesges and Klesges 1988; U.S. DHHS 1988). When the evaluation identifies weight gain as an issue, behavioral treatment interventions that focus on weight management are likely to increase the effectiveness of treatment. A description of behavioral treatment interventions for weight management is beyond the scope of this chapter but may be found in reviews by Abrams (1984) and Brownell (1986). Pharmacologic agents that have the potential to limit weight gain may also be considered as adjuncts to treatment. There is some evidence that the use of nicotine gum during smoking cessation limits postcessation weight gain (Klesges et al. 1989), and it is also conceivable that stimulants or stimulating antidepressants, such as fluoxetine and bupropion, may prove to be useful adjuncts to treatment for these patients. Fenfluramine, which is FDA-approved as an anorectic agent for short-term use, might also be considered. However, none of these agents has been formally studied in the context of smoking cessation.

Blockade therapy. The goal of blockade therapy is to reduce or eliminate any rewarding pharmacologic effects that would occur if an individual resumed use of the drug after becoming abstinent (Jarvik and Henningfield 1988; U.S. DHHS 1988). The prototypical blockade therapy is the use of naltrexone for opiate dependence. Mecamylamine, a nicotine antagonist that acts both peripherally and centrally, has been shown to block the nicotine-mediated reinforcing consequences of cigarette smoking (Stolerman 1986; U.S. DHHS 1988). However, it has not been tested in a clinical trial as an aid to maintain abstinence. Its use in this regard is limited by its ganglionic blocking activity, which produces several unwanted side effects (U.S. DHHS 1988).

Deterrent therapy. Deterrent therapy is based on the idea that pretreatment with an agent that transforms nicotine use from a rewarding to an adverse experience would decrease relapse (Jarvik and Henningfield 1988; U.S. DHHS 1988). Disulfiram treatment of alcoholism is the pharmacologic analogy for this form of treatment. Presently, silver acetate preparations are available as deterrent treatments for smoking. Sulfide salts, which are very distasteful, are produced whenever sulfides, present in tobacco smoke, come in contact with silver acetate residue in the mouth (Jarvik and Henningfield 1988; U.S. DHHS 1988).

Silver acetate gum, a currently available preparation, has to be chewed upon awakening and then several times throughout the day. Its efficacy was recently tested in a double-blind, placebo-controlled trial (Malcolm et al. 1986). At the end of 3 weeks of treatment, active silver acetate was significantly more effective in achieving abstinence than placebo (11% versus 4%). However, at 4-month follow-up, differences between active silver acetate and placebo gum were no longer significant (Malcolm et al. 1986).

Behavioral and Other Nonpharmacologic Treatments

Behavioral treatment strategies are essential to the long-term success of the treatment of nicotine dependence (Abrams and Wilson 1986; U.S. DHHS 1988). Several recent reviews comprehensively describe behavioral and other nonpharmacological interventions for treating smokers (Abrams and Wilson 1986; Fielding 1985; Goldstein et al. 1990; Health and Public Policy Committee, American College of Physicians 1986; Lichtenstein 1986; Ockene 1987; Schwartz 1987; Stokes and Rigotti 1988; U.S. DHHS 1988).

In the following sections, we provide an overview of several be-

Table 16-9. Behavioral treatments for nicotine dependence

- **Nicotine fading**

- **Aversive techniques**

  Rapid smoking
  Smoke holding
  Mild electric shock
  Covert sensitization

- **Cognitive-behavioral strategies**

  Self-monitoring of smoking behavior
  Goal setting and self-reinforcement
  Stimulus control
  Coping skills training
    Cognitive restructuring and other cognitive techniques
    Assertiveness training
    Problem solving
    Time management
    Relaxation training
    Relapse-prevention training

- **Social support**

- **Hypnosis**

- **Acupuncture**

- **Multicomponent programs and groups**

havioral interventions, which are listed in Table 16-9. As noted previously, we have elected not to focus on self-help, brief, or minimal interventions in this review. Most of the behavioral interventions described below can be combined to meet the needs of the patient.

Nicotine Fading

Nicotine fading is a substitute for pharmacologic treatment to manage nicotine withdrawal symptoms. It involves switching to a brand of cigarettes with lower nicotine content and then reducing the number of cigarettes smoked per day on a systematic basis over a period of 3–5 weeks (Foxx and Brown 1979). Subjects using this strategy are usually asked to monitor and plot their nicotine intake as they "fade." They discontinue smoking when they have reached a level of nicotine intake that is 10–25% of their initial level.

Aversive Techniques

Aversive strategies have generally been among the most effective of all behavioral strategies used for smoking-cessation treatment (Abrams and Wilson 1986; Schwartz 1987; U.S. DHHS 1988). *Rapid smoking* involves having smokers inhale every 6 seconds until they begin to feel ill (Hall et al. 1984a). This strategy, repeated several times over several sessions, has been found to be effective and safe, even in patients with medical disorders, when medical supervision is provided (Hall et al. 1984a). *Smoke holding* (holding smoke in the mouth while continuing to breathe) is safer and also effective (Schwartz 1987). The use of *mild electric shock* as a punishing stimulus and *covert sensitization* (imagined noxious scenes and thoughts paired with imagined smoking) have been found to be somewhat less effective than aversive techniques that use smoke (Schwartz 1987).

Cognitive-Behavioral Strategies

Cognitive-behavioral strategies are based on learning theory and actively involve the patient in the assessment and treatment plan (Abrams and Wilson 1986; U.S. DHHS 1988). Often several specific behavior change components are combined.

Self-monitoring of smoking behavior is a basic component of most behavior modification treatment programs. During evaluation, self-monitoring helps the therapist, as well as the patient, to identify environmental, cognitive, and affective cues for smoking (Schwartz 1987; Shiffman 1985). These cues, or triggers, can then be addressed directly using other components of the treatment process. Even without the addition of other treatment components, self-monitoring often leads to decreased smoking rates.

Goal setting and self-reinforcement, also known as contingency contracting, involves rewarding patients for not smoking or punishing them for smoking or both. Generally, reward works best, especially when the patient participates in setting up the reward paradigm.

Stimulus control strategies involve either removing or altering cues for smoking (e.g., removing ashtrays, sitting in a different seat at the dinner table), avoiding trigger situations (e.g., avoiding alcohol intake) or setting up barriers to smoking (sitting in a no-smoking area).

Coping skills training is a an important component of most behavior modification treatment plans for nicotine dependence. Its inclusion in treatment is based on the assumption that smokers will need to develop new skills or hone old ones to help them to maintain effective functioning in the absence of nicotine (Shiffman 1985; U.S. DHHS 1988). Coping responses may be directed at either the urge to smoke or a precipitating stressor. Several coping strategies may be taught to the patient, who is then encouraged to practice the skills and use them in imagined and real trigger situations. A list of coping skills that can be taught or reinforced as a component of treatment are listed in Table 16-9.

Cognitive skills provide the patient with a strategy for identifying maladaptive cognitions that may accompany smoking (e.g., "I need this cigarette") or that serve as triggers to smoking (e.g., "I'm a failure"). Thought-stopping techniques and cognitive restructuring techniques can then be applied to alter maladaptive thought patterns (Abrams and Wilson 1986; Beck 1976). Development of problem-solving skills provides the patient with an increased capacity to cope with unanticipated or new triggers after the treatment program ends.

When used as a relapse prevention strategy, patients are encouraged to anticipate "high-risk" relapse situations and prepare coping strategies to manage the triggers associated with relapse (Marlatt and Gordon 1985). For example, a smoker who has identified anxiety at work as a high-risk relapse situation might practice a relaxation technique as a coping strategy and plan to use it when anxiety increases in the work environment. Alternatively, the patient might be taught specific time management techniques to help cope with everyday work-related time pressures. Relapse-prevention training also includes helping the individual to avoid or manage negative emotional states associated with "slips" (Marlatt and Gordon 1985). In this way, slips are less likely to become full-blown relapses.

Social Support

Although evidence suggests that social support influences outcome after smoking-cessation attempts (Schwartz 1987; U.S. DHHS 1988), interventions to increase patients' social support during treatment for nicotine dependence have met with mixed results (Lichtenstein et al. 1986; U.S. DHHS 1988). Nevertheless, inclusion of spouses in treatment and teaching them how to be supportive of patients' attempts to quit have shown promise (McIntyre-Kingsolver et al. 1986).

Hypnosis

Hypnosis, when applied to smoking cessation, produces only modest results when used alone (Schwartz 1987). It appears to be most effective when hypnosis is provided by a skilled hypnotherapist, the patient is highly susceptible to hypnotic induction, there are several hours of treatment over several sessions, the relationship with the therapist is intense, hypnotic suggestions are personalized, and there is either adjunctive counseling or follow-up (Holroyd 1980; Schwartz 1987). Brown and Fromm (1987) have provided a comprehensive description of the use of hypnosis as an adjunct to other behavioral interventions for the treatment of nicotine dependence.

Acupuncture

Acupuncture is an ancient Chinese science that utilizes needles or staples to treat various conditions, including smoking. The needles or staples are placed in specific locations, or "points," that are thought to provide connections with the body's regulatory systems (Schwartz 1987). The ear is a common site for needle or staple insertion because it is believed to connect to the "neurovegetative system," which controls appetitive behavior (Schwartz 1987). Schwartz (1987), in a recent review, found no convincing evidence that acupuncture either relieves withdrawal symptoms after smoking cessation or significantly improves smoking-cessation outcome when used alone. However, it may have a positive placebo effect and deserves consideration as an adjunct in highly dependent smokers who cannot or will not try pharmacologic interventions (Schwartz 1987). See Choy and colleagues (1978) for a description of the technique of auricular acupuncture.

Multicomponent Programs and Groups

Programs that include multiple components have success rates that are generally greater than programs utilizing only one or two strategies (Abrams and Wilson 1986; Lichtenstein 1986; Schwartz 1987; U.S. DHHS 1988). However, the relative strengths and weaknesses of various combinations of behavioral and other nonpharmacological interventions remain unresolved. In general, it appears that programs that combine strategies to help the patient quit (e.g., nicotine fading and aversive strategies) with strategies to help the patient maintain abstinence (e.g., relapse-prevention training and social support) have the best outcomes (Schwartz 1987; Tiffany et al. 1986; U.S. DHHS 1988). However, including more strategies in a given program may overwhelm subjects and reduce adherence to treatment (U.S. DHHS 1988). As noted previously, the combination of behavioral and pharmacologic interventions also appears to have greater efficacy than either treatment alone, especially for patients with high levels of nicotine dependence (Goldstein et al. 1989; U.S. DHHS 1988).

Group treatment settings have frequently been used to deliver multicomponent treatment. This approach takes advantage of the social support component of group treatment, is less costly than individual treatment, and facilitates the involvement of multiple therapists who may have overlapping but distinct therapeutic skills (e.g., a psychiatrist skilled in pharmacologic interventions and a psychologist skilled in behavioral interventions). However, we are not aware of any studies that have compared the effectiveness of group versus individual nicotine-dependence treatment that controlled for program content and therapist contact time. A description of group treatment technique is beyond the scope of this chapter. A manual for group treatment combining coping skills training with use of nicotine resin complex (Goldstein et al. 1989) is available from the authors; contact Michael G. Goldstein, M.D., The Miriam Hospital, 164 Summit Avenue, Providence, RI 02906.

Table 16-10 provides a summary of follow-up abstinence rates according to different intervention methods for studies published during the years 1959–1985. The table provides only a general guide to the efficacy of various treatment modalities. The variability in results reflects methodological differences among the trials as well as varying definitions of abstinence. Moreover, many of these studies used self-reported abstinence rather than relying on biochemical measures. Therefore, the table should be interpreted with caution. Investigators interested in the effectiveness of a particular treatment should review the individual studies and evaluate results based on the quality and rigor of the experimental design and methods employed. The table also does not provide information concerning the efficacy of treatments tested after 1985. However, recent studies concerning the effects of nicotine gum, other medications, and physician interventions are reviewed elsewhere in this chapter.

STEP-BY-STEP APPROACH TO TREATMENT

This section describes a step-by-step approach to treatment of nicotine dependence for the general psychiatrist in an outpatient clinic

Table 16-10.   Summary of 6-month follow-up abstinence rates of smoking cessation trials by method (1959–1985)

Intervention method	Number of trials	Abstinence rate (%)	
		Range	Median
Self-help	11	0–33	17
Educational	7	13–50	36
Group	15	0–54	24
Medication*	7	0–47	18
Nicotine resin complex	3	17–33	23
Nicotine resin complex and behavioral treatment	3	23–50	35
Hypnosis			
Individual	11	0–60	25
Group	10	8–68	34
Acupuncture	7	5–61	18
Physician advice/counseling	3	5–12	5
Physician intervention more than counseling	3	23–40	29
Physician intervention			
Pulmonary patients	10	10–51	24
Cardiac patients	5	21–69	44
Rapid smoking	12	7–62	25.5
Rapid smoking plus other procedures	21	8–67	38
Satiation smoking	11	14–76	38
Regular-paced aversive smoking	13	0–56	29
Nicotine fading	7	26–46	27
Contingency contracting	9	25–76	46
Multiple component programs	13	18–52	32

*Medications included lobeline hydrochloride, meprobamate, amphetamine, silver acetate, methylphenidate, diazepam, and hydroxyzine.
Source. Adapted from Schwartz 1987.

or office setting. Though we have oversimplified the approach to increase clarity, we believe this strategy is clinically useful. It is anticipated that this treatment would be provided in 6–10 weekly individual sessions, each lasting 30–50 minutes. After an initial assessment, individual treatment sessions would include behavioral interventions, as well as psychotherapy aimed at associated psychiatric disorders, if present. If successful smoking cessation is achieved, monthly 15-minute follow-up sessions are suggested for the next 6–12 months.

Step 1: Assessment

The first step in the treatment process is a careful assessment of the severity of nicotine dependence, psychiatric comorbidity, and other psychological and behavioral factors contributing to nicotine use (e.g., reasons for smoking). Evaluation of nicotine dependence is described in considerable detail above. After assessment, patients can be characterized as having high or low nicotine dependence, with or without associated psychiatric comorbidity, yielding four groups (Figure 16-5).

Step 2: Initial Treatment

Initial treatment involves choosing a treatment plan that is matched to the specific needs of the patient. All patients should be offered some form of behavioral treatment since studies have demonstrated that pharmacologic treatments have very limited efficacy when used alone (Hughes et al. 1989; Schwartz 1987; U.S. DHHS 1988). If the evaluation identifies high levels of nicotine dependence, we recommend adding a pharmacologic intervention to help the patient manage withdrawal symptoms and craving. Response to pharmacologic agents during previous attempts to quit helps to guide the choice of a specific pharmacologic agent. Nicotine resin complex is usually our first choice if the patient has not previously tried nicotine resin complex or used it incorrectly, if there are no contraindications to its use (i.e., a recent myocardial infarction, pregnancy, or significant dental or gum disease), and if there is no associated psychiatric comorbidity.

If a highly dependent patient has failed to quit smoking while correctly using nicotine resin complex, we advise utilizing clonidine hydrochloride in oral or patch form (if there are no contraindications to its use). If the patient has been unsuccessful despite well-supervised treatment with nicotine resin complex and clonidine, one of the newer pharmacologic therapies, such as antidepressants or buspirone, can be tried.

If psychiatric comorbidity is uncovered by the assessment, we recommend choosing a behavioral treatment plus a pharmacologic agent that specifically addresses the associated psychiatric disorder. When a patient is currently being treated with a psychoactive agent for an associated psychiatric disorder, it may be necessary to adjust the dose of the agent in anticipation of an exacerbation or recurrence of the underlying disorder. In addition, a change in metabolism or pharmacodynamics may result from smoking cessation. If the patient is not currently on a psychoactive agent to treat an associated psychiatric disorder, adding such an agent should be considered, especially if psychiatric symptoms have developed during previous attempts to quit smoking.

Step 1. Assessment

| Nicotine Dependence = Low, Psychiatric co-morbidity | Nicotine Dependence = High, Psychiatric co-morbidity | Nicotine Dependence = High, No psychiatric co-morbidity | Nicotine Dependence = Low, No psychiatric co-morbidity |

Step 2. Initial Treatment

| Behavioral treatment + Specific Agent for Associated Co-Morbidity | Behavioral treatment + Nicotine resin complex / Clonidine hydrochloride / Other agent + Specific Agent for Associated Co-Morbidity | Behavioral treatment + Nicotine resin complex / Clonidine hydrochloride / Other agent | Behavioral treatment |

Nicotine resin complex:
- If no previous use or
- If previously used successfully or
- If previously used unsuccessfully but incorrectly
- If not contraindicated

or

Clonidine hydrochloride

or

Other agent (see text)

Specific Agent for Associated Co-Morbidity

Step 3. Reassessment

| Quit Successfully No Relapse | Quit Successfully Late Relapse | Quit Successfully Early Relapse | Unable to Quit or Severe Withdrawal |

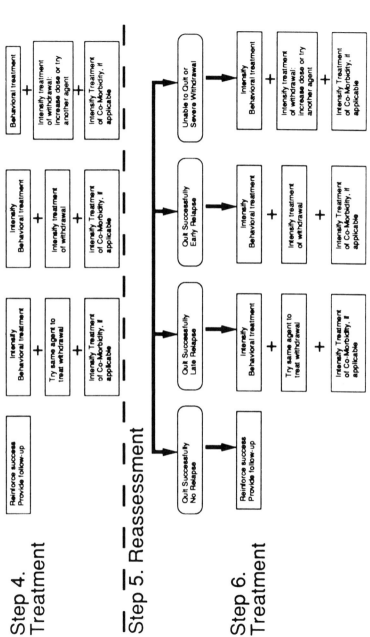

Figure 16-5. Step-by-step approach to treatment of nicotine dependence.

If both high nicotine dependence and psychiatric comorbidity are present, the patient may require separate agents to treat withdrawal and comorbidity. However, as discussed in the section on pharmacologic treatment above, several agents used to treat anxiety and depression have also shown some promise as treatments of nicotine withdrawal. If studies demonstrate the effectiveness of these agents as treatments of withdrawal, it may be possible to use these agents (e.g., doxepin, buspirone) as the sole pharmacologic treatment for patients with both high dependence and associated psychiatric comorbidity. Patients with neither high levels of nicotine dependence nor psychiatric morbidity should initially be treated with behavioral treatments alone.

Step 3: Reassessment

The third step is a reassessment based on the results of initial treatment. Subjects can be characterized along a continuum that reflects the difficulty they have had with quitting smoking and remaining abstinent.

Step 4: Treatment

The fourth step involves adjusting treatment to match the problems that emerge from the initial treatment attempt. Subjects who have been unable to remain abstinent during the first 48 hours after attempting to quit smoking may be suffering from severe withdrawal or experiencing an acute exacerbation of their underlying psychiatric disorder. For these patients, pharmacologic treatment of withdrawal should be initiated, or if already in place, intensified either by using higher doses of the initial agent or by using another drug. More intensive treatment of the associated psychiatric disorder may also be needed.

Patients who have quit successfully but relapse within the first 2 weeks after quitting have different needs. This group of patients may have experienced prolonged withdrawal symptoms, subacute exacerbation of an associated psychiatric condition, or trouble coping with cues for smoking or the consequences of not smoking. They are likely to require adjustment of the pharmacologic intervention used to treat withdrawal symptoms as well as intensification of the behavioral interventions to address the triggers of relapse. Again, more intensive treatment of comorbidity may be required.

Those patients who relapse to smoking after more than 2 weeks of abstinence probably do not require more intensive pharmacologic treatment of withdrawal but will require more help to deal with the behavioral and psychological aspects of smoking. They also may require more intensive treatment of associated psychiatric disorders, if they were exacerbated during abstinence from smoking. Weight gain is a common reason for late relapse and may need to be specifically addressed.

Finally, those patients who both quit successfully and remain abstinent throughout treatment will benefit from follow-up visits to allow the practitioner to reinforce the patients' success and monitor mental state for several months after smoking cessation. Medication, if used, will require monitoring and tapering as well. Nicotine gum should be tapered over several weeks and discontinued after about 3 months. It is unclear how long clonidine and other agents should be prescribed, but we prefer to limit their use to 4 weeks if the patient is successful in quitting. Treatment of associated or emergent psychiatric disorders may require longer treatment and follow-up. Relapse-prevention strategies should be reviewed during these visits to increase the patient's self-efficacy and confidence.

Step 5: Further Reassessment

The fifth step is another reassessment based on the results of subsequent treatment. Subjects can again be characterized along a continuum that reflects the difficulty they have had with quitting smoking and remaining abstinent.

Step 6: Treatment Adjustments

The sixth step involves adjusting treatment to match the problems that emerge from the subsequent treatment attempt. The only difference between the fourth and sixth steps is that we recommend intensifying behavioral treatment for all subjects who have not been able to remain abstinent. The fifth and sixth steps are repeated until the patient successfully remains abstinent.

REFERRAL TO A SPECIALIZED
TREATMENT PROGRAM

Patients who are not able to remain abstinent after repeated trials of office-based treatment using the step-by-step model described above are certainly candidates for referral to a specialized, formal nicotine-dependence treatment program. Those patients assessed to have low levels of nicotine dependence and no psychiatric comorbidity are most likely to benefit from standard behavioral treatment programs offered in the community. Patients with high levels of nicotine dependence who remain refractory to office-based treatment including pharmacological agents may require referral to a specialized program that can provide both pharmacological and intensive behavioral treatment modalities.

There are only a small number of interdisciplinary nicotine-dependence treatment programs that offer both pharmacologic and behavioral treatment. However, the behavioral medicine and substance-abuse treatment communities are presently developing such programs throughout the country.

The Miriam Hospital Behavioral Medicine Clinic in Providence, RI, is an example of an interdisciplinary program providing integrated and comprehensive care to patients with nicotine dependence. In this model, psychiatrists, psychologists, and social workers perform initial evaluations. New cases are presented and staffed during a team meeting. A psychiatrist evaluates every patient who has high levels of nicotine dependence or psychiatric comorbidity. Usually, a psychologist or social worker provides behavioral and psychological treatment, while medications, if indicated, are managed by a psychiatrist. Behavioral treatment is provided individually or in groups. The choice of group versus individual treatment is primarily based on the patient's preferences. Group treatment is less costly, but also less flexible and less intensive. Groups are particularly useful for those patients who lack a social network that is supportive of not smoking.

Psychiatrists in general practice may wish to develop a relationship with a local behavioral medicine program where patients can be sent for more intensive behavioral treatment while the psychiatrist continues to prescribe adjunctive pharmacologic agents. Recently, an inpatient program to treat nicotine dependence, developed in conjunction with a substance-abuse treatment program, was developed at the Mayo Clinic (R. Hurt, September 1989, personal communication). More are sure to follow, especially if treatment for nicotine dependence becomes reimbursable by third-party insurers.

RESOURCES

Resources have been developed to assist physicians in providing interventions to their patients who smoke, including 1) educational materials for patients, in the form of pamphlets, self-help manuals, audiotapes, and videotapes; 2) materials to facilitate the identification and tracking of smokers; and 3) manuals and kits designed to assist physicians in their office practice to develop an integrated approach to smoking-cessation interventions. Excellent manuals or kits are available from the National Cancer Institute (NCI), the American Academy of Family Physicians, and Marion/Merrell Dow, which markets nicotine resin complex in the United States.

The NCI manual is particularly helpful for primary-care physicians in office practice. It provides specific guidelines for developing an office-based smoking-cessation program consisting of five steps: 1) select an office smoking-cessation coordinator; 2) create a nonsmoking office environment; 3) identify all smoking patients in the practice; 4) develop smoking-cessation plans for patients; and 5) provide follow-up support to maximize patients' success. Step 4 contains a simple smoking-cessation counseling strategy that physicians can use with every patient. Though this manual is designed for primary-care physicians, it is also likely to be very useful for psychiatrists wishing to provide only minimal behavioral interventions to their patients who smoke. Moreover, psychiatrists providing consultation to primary-care physicians can utilize the NCI manual as a teaching tool to help primary-care physicians provide clear and effective smoking-cessation interventions.

Among the other specific resources that are available, the self-help manuals developed by the American Lung Association (ALA) (Davis et al. 1984) are particularly useful as adjuncts to treatment. The ALA also has developed videotapes for patients. The American Cancer Society, the American Heart Association, and NCI also have developed educational materials for patients. For those seeking formal training in smoking-cessation counseling, the American Society of Addiction Medicine holds a 3-day workshop on treating nicotine dependence each fall. Books written to help the physician to learn behavioral counseling strategies are also available (Russell 1986).

Information on how to order physician resources/manuals from the National Cancer Institute, the American Academy of Family Physicians, the American Lung Association, the American Cancer Society, and the American Heart Association can be found in the reference section of this chapter.

REFERENCES

Abelin T, Muller P, Buehler A, et al: Controlled trial of transdermal nicotine patch in tobacco withdrawal. Lancet 1:7–10, 1989

Abrams DB: Current status and clinical developments in the behavioral treatment of obesity, in New Directions in Behavior Therapy. Edited by Franks CM. New York, Haworth Press, 1984, pp 21–55

Abrams DB, Wilson GT: Clinical advances in treatment of smoking and alcohol addiction, in Psychiatry Update: The American Psychiatric Association Annual Review, Vol 5. Edited by Frances AJ, Hales RE. Washington, DC, American Psychiatric Press, 1986

Aghajanian GK: Tolerance of locus coeruleus neurons to morphine and suppression of withdrawal response by clonidine. Nature 276:186–188, 1978

American Academy of Family Physicians: AAFP Stop Smoking Kit. Kansas City, MO, American Academy of Family Physicians, 1987 (1-800-274-2237)

American Cancer Society: Smart Move. Atlanta, GA, American Cancer Society, 1988 (404-320-3333)

American Heart Association: Calling It Quits. Dallas, TX, American Heart Association, 1984 (214-822-9380)

American Lung Association: Freedom From Smoking for You and Your Family. New York, American Lung Association, 1987 (212-315-8700)

American Psychiatric Association: Diagnostic and Statistical Manual of Mental Disorders, 3rd Edition. Washington, DC, American Psychiatric Association, 1980

American Psychiatric Association: Diagnostic and Statistical Manual of Mental Disorders, 3rd Edition, Revised. Washington, DC, American Psychiatric Association, 1987

Ashton H: Benzodiazepine withdrawal: an unfinished story. Br Med J 288:1135–1140, 1984

Bansil RK, Hymowitz N, Keller S, et al: Cigarette smoking and neuroleptics. Paper presented at the annual meeting of the American Psychiatric Association, San Francisco, CA, May 1989

Battjes RJ: Smoking as an issue in alcohol and drug abuse treatment. Addict Behav 13:225–230, 1988

Baumgartner GR, Rowen RC: Clonidine vs chlordiazepoxide in the management of acute alcohol withdrawal syndrome. Arch Intern Med 147:1223–1226, 1987

Beck AT: Cognitive Therapy and the Emotional Disorders. New York, International Universities Press, 1976

Benowitz NL: Pharmacologic aspects of cigarette smoking and nicotine addiction. N Engl J Med 319:1318–1330, 1988

Benowitz NL: Nicotine interactions with psychiatric medications. Paper presented at the annual meeting of the American Psychiatric Association, San Francisco, CA, May 1989

Bobo JK, Gilchrist LD, Schilling RF II, et al: Cigarette smoking cessation attempts by recovering alcoholics. Addict Behav 12:209–215, 1987

Brown CG: The alcohol withdrawal syndrome. Ann Emerg Med 11:276–280, 1982

Brown D, Fromm E: Hypnosis and Behavioral Medicine. Hillsdale, New Jersey, Lawrence Erlbaum, 1987

Brownell KD: Public health approaches to obesity and its management. Ann Rev Public Health 7:521–533, 1986

Buchkremer G, Bents H, Horstmann M, et al: Combination of behavioral smoking cessation with transdermal nicotine substitution. Addict Behav 14:229–238, 1989

Burling TA, Ziff DC: Tobacco smoking: a comparison between alcohol and drug abuse inpatients. Addict Behav 13:185–190, 1988

Choy DSJ, Purnell F, Jaffe R: Auricular acupuncture for cessation of smoking, in Progress in Smoking Cessation: Proceedings of the International Conference on Smoking Cessation. Edited by Schwartz JL. New York, American Cancer Society, 1978, pp 329–334

Clarke PBS: Nicotinic receptors and mechanisms in the brain. Paper presented at the annual meeting of the American Psychiatric Association, San Francisco, CA, May 1989

Cohen SJ, Christen AG, Katz BP, et al: Counseling medical and dental patients about cigarette smoking: the impact of nicotine gum and chart reminders. Am J Public Health 77:313–316, 1987

Davis AL, Faust R, Ordentlich M: Self-help smoking cessation and maintenance programs: a comparative study with 12 month follow-up by the American Lung Association. Am J Public Health 74:1212–1217, 1984

Davis DI: Differences in the use of substances of abuse by psychiatric patients compared with medical and surgical patients. J Nerv Ment Dis 172:654–657, 1984

Davison R, Kaplan K, Fintel D, et al: The effect of clonidine on the cessation of cigarette smoking. Clin Pharmacol Ther 44:265–267, 1988

DiFranza JR, Guerrera MP: Hard core smokers (letter). JAMA 261:2634, 1989

DiFranza JR, Guerrera MP: Alcoholism and smoking. J Stud Alcohol (in press)

Edwards NB, Murphy JK, Downs AD, et al: Antidepressants and nicotine withdrawal symptoms. Paper presented at the annual meeting of the American Psychiatric Association, Montreal, Canada, May 1988

Edwards NB, Downs AD, Murphy JK, et al: Brief doxepin therapy for smoking cessation. Paper presented at the annual meeting of the American Psychiatric Association, San Francisco, CA, May 1989a

Edwards NB, Murphy JK, Downs AD, et al: Doxepin as an adjunct to smoking cessation: a double-blind pilot study. Am J Psychiatry 146:373–376, 1989b

Fagerstrom K-O: Measuring degree of physical dependence to tobacco smoking with reference to individualization of treatment. Addict Behav 3:235–241, 1978

Fagerstrom K-O: Physical dependence on nicotine as a determinant of success in smoking cessation. World Smoking and Health 5:22–23, 1980

Fagerstrom K-O: A comparison of psychological and pharmacological treatment in smoking cessation. J Behav Med 5:343–351, 1982

Fagerstrom K-O: Efficacy of nicotine chewing gum: a review, in Nicotine Replacement: A Critical Evaluation. Edited by Pomerleau O, Pomerleau CS. New York, Alan R Liss, 1988, pp 109–128

Fagerstrom K-O, Melin B: Nicotine chewing gum in smoking cessation: efficiency, nicotine dependence, therapy duration, and clinical recommendations, in Pharmacologic Adjuncts to Smoking Cessation (DHHS Publ No ADM-85-1333). Edited by Grabowski J, Hall SM. Washington, DC, U.S. Government Printing Office, 1985, pp 102–109

Fagerstrom K-O, Schneider NG: Measuring nicotine dependence: a review of the Fagerstrom Tolerance Questionnaire. J Behav Med 12:159–182, 1989

Fertig JB, Pomerleau OF, Sanders B: Nicotine-produced antinociception in minimally deprived smokers and ex-smokers. Addict Behav 11:239–248, 1986

Fielding JE: Smoking: health effects and control. N Engl J Med 313:491–498, 555–561, 1985

Foote SL, Bloom FE, Aston-Jones G: Nucleus locus ceruleus: new evidence of anatomical and physiological specificity. Physiol Rev 63:844–914, 1983

Fortmann SP, Killen JD, Telch MJ, et al: Minimal contact treatment for smoking cessation: a placebo controlled trial of nicotine polacrilex and self-directed relapse prevention: initial results of the Stanford Stop Smoking Project. JAMA 260:1575–1580, 1988

Foxx RM, Brown RA: Nicotine fading and self-monitoring for cigarette abstinence or controlled smoking. J Appl Behav Anal 12:111–125, 1979

Frederick T, Frerichs RR, Clark VA: Personal health habits and symptoms of depression at the community level. Prev Med 17:173–182, 1988

Frerichs RR, Aneshensel CS, Clark VA, et al: Smoking and depression: a community survey. Am J Public Health 71:637–640, 1981

Frith CD: Smoking behavior and its relation to the smoker's immediate experience. Br J Soc Clin Psychol 10:73–78, 1971

Fuxe K, Anderson K, Eneroth P, et al: Effects of nicotine and exposure to cigarette smoke on discrete dopamine and noradrenaline nerve terminal systems of the telencephalon and diencephalon of the rat: relationship to reward mechanisms and distribution of nicotine binding sites in brain, in Tobacco Smoking and Nicotine: A Neurobiological Approach. Edited by Martin WR, Van Loon GR, Iwamoto ET, et al. New York, Plenum, 1987, pp 225–262

Gallup Opinion Index, #108. June 1974, pp 20–21

Garvey AJ: Factors related to relapse after smoking cessation. Paper presented at the annual meeting of the Society of Behavioral Medicine, Boston, MA, April 1988

Gawin FH, Kleber H: Issues in cocaine abuse treatment research, in Cocaine: Clinical and Biobehavioral Aspects. Edited by Fisher S, Raskin A, Uhlenhuth EH. New York, Oxford University Press, 1987, pp 174–192

Gawin FH, Compton M, Byck R: Buspirone reduces smoking. Arch Gen Psychiatry 46:288–289, 1989

Gilbert DG: Nicotine's effects on lateralized EEG and emotion. Paper presented at the annual meeting of the Society of Behavioral Medicine, Boston, MA, April 1988

Glassman AH, Jackson WK, Walsh BT, et al: Cigarette craving, smoking withdrawal, and clonidine. Science 226:864–866, 1984

Glassman AH, Stetner F, Raizman P: Clonidine and cigarette smoking withdrawal, in The Pharmacologic Treatment of Tobacco Dependence: Proceedings of the World Congress, November 4–5, 1985. Edited by Ockene JK. Cambridge, MA, Institute for the Study of Smoking Behavior and Policy, 1986, pp 174–180

Glassman AH, Stetner F, Walsh BT, et al: Heavy smokers, smoking cessation, and clonidine. JAMA 259:2863–2866, 1988

Glassman AH, Covey LS, Stetner F: Smoking cessation, depression, and antidepressants. Paper presented at the annual meeting of the American Psychiatric Association, San Francisco, CA, May 1989a

Glassman AH, Covey LS, Stetner F: Smoking, smoking cessation, and depression. Paper presented at the annual meeting of the American Psychiatric Association, San Francisco, CA, May 1989b

Glassman AH, Helzer JE, Covey LS, et al: Smoking, smoking cessation and depression. JAMA 264:1546–1549, 1990

Gold MS, Pottash AC, Sweeney DR: Opiate withdrawal using clonidine. JAMA 243:343–346, 1980

Goldstein MG, Niaura R, Abrams DB, et al: Effects of behavioral skills training and schedule of nicotine gum administration on smoking cessation. Am J Psychiatry 146:56–60, 1989

Goldstein MG, Guise BJ, Ruggiero L, et al: Behavioral medicine strategies for medical patients, in Clinical Psychiatry for Medical Students. Edited by Stoudemire A. Philadelphia, PA, JB Lippincott, 1990, pp 609–629

Grabowski J, Hall SM: Tobacco use, treatment strategies, and pharmacological adjuncts: an overview, in Pharmacologic Adjuncts in Smoking Cessation (NIDA Research Monograph 53; DHHS Publ No ADM-85-1333). Edited by Grabowski J, Hall SM. Rockville, MD, Alcohol, Drug Abuse, and Mental Health Administration, 1985, pp 102–109

Grunberg NE: Nicotine, cigarette smoking, and body weight. Br J Addict 80:369–377, 1985

Grunberg NE, Baum A: Biological commonalities of stress and substance abuse, in Coping and Substance Abuse. Edited by Shiffman S, Wills TA. Orlando, FL, Academic, 1985, pp 25–62

Haines AP, Imeson JD, Meade TW: Psychoneurotic profiles of smokers and non-smokers. Br Med J 280:1422, 1980

Hall RG, Sachs DPL, Hall SM, et al: Two-year efficacy and safety of rapid smoking therapy in patients with cardiac and pulmonary disease. J Consult Clin Psychol 52:574–581, 1984a

Hall SM, Herning R, Jones RT, et al: Blood cotinine levels as indicators of smoking treatment outcome. Clin Pharmacol Ther 35:810–814, 1984b

Hall SM, Tunstall C, Rugg D, et al: Nicotine gum and behavioral treatment in smoking cessation. J Consult Clin Psychol 53:256–258, 1985

Hall SM, Ginsberg D, Jones RT: Smoking cessation and weight gain. J Consult Clin Psychol 54:342–346, 1986

Harackiewicz JM, Blair LW, Sansone C, et al: Nicotine gum and self-help manuals in smoking cessation: an evaluation in a medical context. Addict Behav 13:319–390, 1988

Hartman N, Jarvik ME, Wilkins JN: Reduction of cigarette smoking by use of a nicotine patch. Arch Gen Psychiatry 46:289, 1989

Health and Public Policy Committee, American College of Physicians: Methods for stopping cigarette smoking. Ann Intern Med 105:281–291, 1986

Henningfield JE: Pharmacologic basis and treatment of cigarette smoking. J Clin Psychiatry 45:24–34, 1984

Henningfield JE: How tobacco produces drug dependence, in The Pharmacologic Treatment of Tobacco Dependence: Proceedings of the World Congress, November 4–5, 1985. Edited by Ockene JK. Cambridge, MA, Institute for the Study of Smoking Behavior and Policy, 1986, pp 19–31

Henningfield JE, Miyasato K, Jasinske DR: Abuse liability and pharmacodynamic characteristics of intravenous and inhaled nicotine. J Pharmacol Exp Ther 234:1–12, 1985

Holroyd J: Hypnosis treatment for smoking: an evaluative review. Int J Clin Exp Hypn 28:341–367, 1980

Hughes JR: Identification of the dependent smoker: validity and clinical utility. Behavioral Medicine Abstracts 5:202–204, 1984

Hughes JR, Hatsukami D: Signs and symptoms of tobacco withdrawal. Arch Gen Psychiatry 43:289–294, 1986

Hughes JR, Hatsukami DK, Mitchell JE, et al: Prevalence of smoking among psychiatric outpatients. Am J Psychiatry 143:993–997, 1986a

Hughes JR, Hatsukami DK, Skoog KP: Physical dependence on nicotine in gum: a placebo substitution trial. JAMA 255:3277–3279, 1986b

Hughes JR, Gust SW, Keenan RM, et al: Nicotine vs placebo gum in general medical practice. JAMA 261:1300–1305, 1989

Hughes JR, Higgins ST, Hatsukami DK: Effects of abstinence from tobacco, in Recent Advances in Alcohol and Drug Problems. Edited by Kozlowski LT, Annis H, Cappell HD, et al. New York, Plenum, 1990, pp 317–398

Hughes JR, Gust SW, Skoog K, et al: Symptoms of tobacco withdrawal: a replication and extension. Arch Gen Psychiatry (in press)

Hunt WA, Bespalec DA: An evaluation of current methods of modifying smoking behavior. J Clin Psychol 30:431–438, 1974

Hunt WA, Barnett LW, Branch LG: Relapse rates in addiction programs. J Clin Psychol 27:455–456, 1971

Ikard FF, Green D, Horn D: A scale to differentiate between types of smoking as related to the management of affect. Int J Addict 4:649–659, 1969

Issac L: Clonidine in the central nervous system: site and mechanism of hypotensive action. J Cardiovasc Pharmacol 2 (suppl):S5–S19, 1980

Jarvik ME: Does smoking decrease eating and eating increase smoking? in Tobacco, Smoking and Nicotine: A Neurobiological Approach. Edited by Martin WR, Van Loon GR, Iwamoto ET, et al. New York, Plenum, 1987, pp 389–400

Jarvik ME, Henningfield JE: Pharmacologic treatment of tobacco dependence. Pharmacol Biochem Behav 30:279–294, 1988

Jarvik ME, Schneider NG: Degree of addiction and the effectiveness of nicotine gum therapy for smoking. Am J Psychiatry 141:790–791, 1984

Jarvis MJ, Belcher M, Vesey C, et al: Low cost carbon monoxide monitors in smoking assessment. Thorax 41:867–886, 1986

Jarvis MJ, Hajek P, Russell MAH, et al: Br J Addict 82:983–988, 1989

Kandel DB, Davies M: Adult sequelae of adolescent depressive symptoms. Arch Gen Psychiatry 43:255–262, 1986

Killen J, Fortmann S, Telch M, et al: Are heavy smokers different from light smokers? A comparison after 48 hours without cigarettes. JAMA 260:1581–1585, 1988

Klesges RC, Klesges LM: Cigarette smoking as a dietary strategy in a university population. International Journal of Eating Disorders 7:413–419, 1988

Klesges RC, Meyers AW, Klesges LM, et al: Smoking, body weight, and their effects on smoking behavior: a comprehensive review of the literature. Psychol Bull 106:204–230, 1989

Kornitzer M, Kittel F, Dramaix M, et al: A double-blind study of 2 mg vs 4 mg nicotine chewing gum in an industrial setting. J Psychosom Res 31:171–176, 1987

Kottke TE, Battista RN, DeFriesse GH, et al: Attributes of successful smoking cessation interventions in medical practice. JAMA 259:2882–2889, 1988

Kozlowski LT, Wilkinson A, Skinner W, et al: Comparing tobacco cigarette dependence with other drug dependencies: greater or equal "difficulty quitting" and "urges to use," but less "pleasure" from cigarettes. JAMA 261:898–901, 1989

Kristeller JL, Ockene JK: Assessment and treatment of smoking on a consultation service, in Psychiatry. Edited by Michels R, Cavenar JO Jr. Philadelphia, PA, JB Lippincott, 1987, pp 1–13

Lam W, Sacks HS, Sze PC, et al: Meta-analysis of randomised controlled trials of nicotine chewing-gum. Lancet 2:27–30, 1987

Leon GR, Kolotkin R, Korgeski G: MacAndrew addiction scale and other MMPI characteristics associated with obesity, anorexia and smoking behavior. Addict Behav 4:401–407, 1979

Lichtenstein E: The smoking problem: a behavioral perspective. J Consult Clin Psychol 50:804–819, 1982

Lichtenstein E: Clinic-based cessation strategies, in The Pharmacologic Treatment of Tobacco Dependence: Proceedings of the World Congress, November 4–5, 1985. Edited by Ockene JK. Cambridge, MA, Institute for the Study of Smoking Behavior and Policy, 1986, pp 205–217

Lichtenstein E, Mermelstein RJ: Some methodological caution in the use of the tolerance questionnaire. Addict Behav 11:439–442, 1986

Lichtenstein E, Glasgow RE, Abrams DB: Social support in smoking cessation: in search of effective interventions. Behavior Therapy 17:607–619, 1986

Malcolm R, Currey HS, Mitchell MA, et al: Silver acetate as a deterrent to smoking. Chest 90:107–111, 1986

Maletzky BM, Klotter J: Smoking and alcoholism. Am J Psychiatry 131:445–447, 1974

Manhem P, Nilsson LH, Moberg AL, et al: Alcohol withdrawal: effects of clonidine treatment on sympathetic activity, the renin-aldosterone system, and clinical symptoms. Alcoholism 9:238–243, 1985

Marlatt GA, Gordon J: Relapse Prevention. New York, Guilford, 1985

Mausner B, Platt ES: Smoking: A Behavioral Analysis. New York, Pergamon, 1971

McIntyre-Kingsolver K, Lichtenstein E, Mermelstein RJ: Spouse training in a multicomponent smoking-cessation program. Behavior Therapy 17:67–74, 1986

McKennel AC: Smoking motivation factors. Br J Soc Clin Psychol 9:8–22, 1970

Moss RA, Prue DM: Research on nicotine regulation. Behavior Therapy 13:31–46, 1982

National Cancer Institute: Clearing the Air: How to Quit Smoking and Stay Quit for Keeps. Bethesda, MD, National Cancer Institute, Office of Cancer Communications, 1988 (1-800-4CANCER)

National Cancer Institute: How to help your patients stop smoking: a National Cancer Institute manual for physicians (NIH Publ No 90-3064). Washington, DC, U.S. Government Printing Office (or National Cancer Institute, Office of Cancer Communications, 1-800-4CANCER)

Niaura R, Goldstein MG, Ward KD, et al: Reasons for smoking and residual withdrawal symptoms when using nicotine chewing gum. Br J Addict 84:681–687, 1989

O'Farrell TJ, Connors GJ, Upper D: Addictive behaviors among hospitalized psychiatric patients. Addict Behav 18:329–333, 1983

Ockene JK: Physician-delivered interventions for smoking cessation: strategies for increasing effectiveness. Prev Med 16:723–737, 1987

Orleans CT: Understanding and promoting smoking cessation: overview and guidelines for physician intervention. Annu Rev Med 36:51–61, 1985

Ornish SA, Zisook S, McAdams LA: Effects of transdermal clonidine treatment on withdrawal symptoms associated with cigarette smoking: a randomized controlled trial. Arch Intern Med 148:2027–2031, 1988

Perkins KA, Epstein LH, Stiller R, et al: An aerosol spray alternative to cigarette smoking in the study of the behavioral and physiological effects of nicotine. Behavior Research Methods, Instruments, and Computers 18:420–426, 1986

Pert A, Clarke PBS: Nicotinic modulation of dopaminergic transmission: functional implications, in Tobacco, Smoking, and Nicotine: A Neurobiological Approach. Edited by Martin WR, Van Loon GR, Iwamoto ET, et al. New York, Plenum, 1987, pp 169–189

Pierce JP, Fiore MC, Novotny TE, et al: Trends in smoking in the United States: projections to the year 2000. JAMA 261:61–65, 1989

Pinto RP, Abrams DB, Monti PM, et al: Nicotine dependence and likelihood of quitting smoking. Addict Behav 12:371–374, 1987

Pomerleau OF, Pomerleau CS: Neuroregulators and the reinforcement of smoking: towards a biobehavioral explanation. Neurosci Biobehav Rev 8:503–513, 1984

Pomerleau OF, Pomerleau CS: A biobehavioral view of substance abuse and addiction. Journal of Drug Issues 17:111–131, 1987

Pomerleau O, Adkins D, Pertschuck M: Predictors of outcome and recidivism in smoking cessation treatment. Addict Behav 3:65–70, 1978

Pomerleau OF, Fertig JB, Shanahan SO: Nicotine dependence in cigarette smoking: an empirically-based, multivariate model. Pharmacol Biochem Behav 19:291–299, 1983

Pomerleau OF, Bell CS, Benowitz NL, et al: Task force 4: nicotine and smoking relapse. Health Psychol 5 (suppl):41–51, 1986

Porchet HC, Benowitz NL, Sheiner LB: Pharmacodynamic model of tolerance: application to nicotine. J Pharmacol Exp Ther 244:231–236, 1988

Prochaska JO, DiClemente CC: Stages and processes of self-change of smoking: toward an integrative model of change. J Consult Clin Psychol 51:390–395, 1983

Prochaska JO, DiClemente CC: Towards a comprehensive model of change, in Treating Addictive Disorders: Processes of Change. Edited by Miller WR, Heather N. New York, Plenum, 1986, pp 3–27

Rose JE: The role of upper airway stimulation in smoking, in Nicotine Replacement: A Critical Evaluation. Edited by Pomerleau OF, Pomerleau CS. New York, Alan R Liss, 1988, pp 95–106

Rose JE, Herskovic JE, Trilling Y, et al: Transdermal nicotine reduces cigarette craving and nicotine preference. Clin Pharmacol Ther 38:450–456, 1985

Rounsaville BJ, Kosten TR, Weissman MM, et al: Evaluating and treating depressive disorders in opiate addicts (DHHS Publ No ADM-85-1406). Washington, DC, U.S. Government Printing Office, 1985

Russell MAH: Nicotine intake and its regulation by smokers, in Tobacco, Smoking and Nicotine: A Neurobiological Approach. Edited by Martin WR, Van Loon GR, Iwamoto ET, et al. New York, Plenum, 1987, pp 25–50

Russell MAH: Nicotine replacement: the role of blood nicotine levels, their rate of change, and nicotine tolerance, in Nicotine Replacement: A Critical Evaluation. Edited by Pomerleau O, Pomerleau CS. New York, Alan R Liss, 1988, pp 63–94

Russell MAH, Jarvis MJ, Feyerabend C, et al: Nasal nicotine solution: a potential aid to giving up smoking? Br Med J 286:683–684, 1983

Russell MAH, Jarvis MJ, Sutherland G, et al: Nicotine replacement in smoking cessation: absorption of nicotine vapor from smoke-free cigarettes. JAMA 257:3262–3265, 1987

Russell ML: Behavioral Counseling in Medicine: Strategies for Modifying At-Risk Behaviour. New York, Oxford University Press, 1986

Russell PO, Epstein LH: Smoking, in Handbook of Behavioral Medicine for Women. Edited by Blechman EA, Brownell KD. New York, Pergamon, 1988, pp 369–383

Schacter S: Pharmacological and psychological determinants of smoking. Ann Intern Med 88:104–114, 1979

Schwartz JL: Review and Evaluation of Smoking Cessation Methods: The United States and Canada, 1978–1985. Bethesda, MD, National Institutes of Health, 1987

Shiffman S: Coping with temptations to smoke, in Coping and Substance Use. Edited by Wills TA, Shiffman S. Orlando, FL, Academic, 1985, pp 223–242

Shiffman S: A cluster-analytic typology of smoking relapse episodes. Addict Behav 11:295–307, 1986

Shiffman SM: The tobacco withdrawal syndrome, in Cigarette Smoking as a Dependence Process (DHHS Publ No ADM-79-800). Edited by Krasnegor KA. Washington, DC, U.S. Government Printing Office, 1979, pp 158–185

Stokes J, Rigotti NA: The health consequences of cigarette smoking and the internist's role in smoking cessation. Adv Intern Med 33:431–460, 1988

Stolerman IP: Could nicotine antagonists be used in smoking cessation? Br J Addict 81:47–53, 1986

Tiffany ST, Martin EM, Baker TB: Treatments for cigarette smoking: an evaluation of the contributions of aversion and counseling procedures. Behav Res Ther 24:437–452, 1986

Tonnesen P, Fryd V, Hansen M, et al: Effect of nicotine chewing gum in combination with group counseling on the cessation of smoking. N Engl J Med 318:15–18, 1988a

Tonnesen P, Fryd V, Hansen M, et al: Two and four mg nicotine chewing gum in combination with group counseling in smoking cessation: an open, randomized, controlled trial with a 22 month follow-up. Addict Behav 13:17–27, 1988b

U.S. Department of Health and Human Services: The Health Consequence of Smoking: Nicotine Addiction: A Report of the Surgeon General (DHHS Publ No CDC-88-8406). Rockville, MD, Office on Smoking and Health, Public Health Service, U.S. Department of Health and Human Services, 1988

Waal-Manning HJ, de Hamel FA: Smoking habit and psychometric scores: a community study. N Z Med J 88:188–191, 1978

Walton RG: Smoking and alcoholism: a brief report. Am J Psychiatry 128:1455–1456, 1972

Washton AM, Resnick RB: Clonidine in opiate withdrawal: review and appraisal of clinical findings. Pharmacotherapy 1:140–146, 1981

Weber MA, Drayer JIM: Clinical experience with rate-controlled delivery of antihypertensive therapy by a transdermal system. Am Heart J 108:231–236, 1984

Wei H, Young D: Effect of clonidine on cigarette cessation and in the alleviation of withdrawal symptoms. Br J Addict 83:1221–1226, 1988

Wesnes K: Nicotine increases mental efficiency: but how? in Tobacco, Smoking, and Nicotine: A Neurobiological Approach. Edited by Martin WR, Van Loon GR, Iwamoto ET, et al. New York, Plenum, 1987, pp 63–80

West RJ, Russell MAH: Pre-abstinence smoke intake and smoking motivation as predictors of severity of cigarette withdrawal symptoms. Psychopharmacology 87:334–336, 1985a

West RJ, Russell MAH: Effects of withdrawal from long-term nicotine gum use. Psychol Med 15:891–893, 1985b

West RJ, Russell MAH: Dependence on nicotine chewing gum. JAMA 256:3214–3215, 1986

West RJ, Hajek P, Belcher M: Severity of withdrawal symptoms as a predictor of outcome of an attempt to quit smoking. Psychol Med (in press)

Wilkins AJ, Jenkins WJ, Steiner JA: Efficacy of clonidine in treatment of alcohol withdrawal state. Psychopharmacology 81:78–80, 1983

Chapter 17

Psychiatric Aspects of Medical Disability

Arthur T. Meyerson, M.D.
Beryl Lawn, M.D.

In this chapter, we address three areas of interest in regard to psychiatric components of disabling physical illness. First, we describe a typology of biological, psychological, and social factors relevant to an individual's psychiatric status as it bears on and complicates the disabling effects of a medical illness. Second, we attempt to provide guidelines for physicians for evaluating the disability of patients who are applying for benefits under the Supplemental Security Income and Social Security Disability Insurance systems, the Veterans Administration Disability Benefits Program, and worker's compensation programs. Finally, we address the difficult clinical issue of malingering, which occurs with some frequency in entitlement programs covering the physically and mentally disabled.

A TYPOLOGY OF DISABILITY

Each human being responds to life events, stressors, physical illnesses, and injuries with a characteristic, complex set of responses. The following set of clinical vignettes illustrates the range of phenomena that may occur when individuals respond to potentially disabling physical illness.

Patient 1. A 44-year-old white, Protestant, married physician, the father of three teenage children, suffered an occlusion of the anterior descending coronary artery. After 3 weeks in the hospital, he returned home on a regimen of aspirin, a low-cholesterol diet, and a systematic exercise program. When his cardiologist saw him for a 2-month follow-up visit, the patient had returned to his practice and had lost 7 pounds. He described the resumption of his sexual life, usual parenting activities, and leisure-time pursuits. Although he was still somewhat anxious about his prognosis, he required no psychotropic medication or formal treatment other than medical follow-up.

Patient 2. Another 44-year-old white, Protestant, married physician, father of three, suffered an occlusion of the anterior descending coronary artery. After 3 weeks in the hospital, he also returned home on a regimen of aspirin, a low-cholesterol diet, and a systematic exercise program. However, at the 2-month follow-up visit to the cardiologist, the patient and his wife reported that he constantly feels tired, stays in bed, avoids exercise and sexual activity, and had made only sporadic visits to his office but had not seen patients. On interview, the patient reported being terrified of a fatal recurrence of the myocardial infarction (MI). In addition, he is having difficulty sleeping, eats irregularly and not in accord with his diet, cannot enjoy formerly pleasurable activities, and feels his active life is over and that he is "no longer a man." On inquiry he revealed that he has a family history of mood disorder and a personal history of severe depression in adolescence following the loss of a girl-friend.

The examining physician finds no difference in the cardiac status of patients 1 and 2, yet four months later, patient 2 is still unable to return to work or to resume his functions as an effective father and husband.

Patient 1 appears to have had an adaptive response to his MI. He is fearful but requires only minimal counseling and support from his cardiologist. Patient 2, who possibly suffers from a major depressive episode, warrants formal psychiatric treatment.

Patient 3. A 37-year-old, white, Protestant, Appalachian man, who is married with three children, has worked as an ore-crusher operator for 16 years. He visited his local physician to complain of low-back pain that occurred whenever he shifted the crusher's levers or lifted anything at work. The symptoms began 2 months before, after he lifted a heavy piece of equipment. On examination, the physician found no objective evidence of spinal disease or other disabling pathology. However, the patient's wife presented the physician with a set of forms to apply for worker's compensation, carefully completed by her and signed by her husband. Although the physician recommended physical therapy and further tests, the patient's family appeared to resent this as an interference with the patient's "rights" to disability payments and status.

The physician was aware that the patient's father, father-in-law, and several neighbors were all on some form of disability payment. The patient, his family, and neighbors appeared to feel that he was entitled to benefits even though objective findings were absent. No psychiatric symptoms were present. The disability payments were viewed as at least as dignified and meritorious a source of income as his original salary. Neither the patient nor his family appeared depressed by his loss of vocational function. Indeed, "the entire community supports the view that such a man is neither expected nor required to work—he has been 'honorably discharged' from the labor force" (Horton 1984, quoted in Brodsky 1987b).

Patient 4. Another 37-year-old, ore-crusher operator, from West Virginia, lost his left (nondominant) little finger in an accident with the crusher 2 weeks before first seeing his physician. The wound was healing well, but the patient complained of generalized anxiety, recurrent flashbacks, sleeplessness, and lack of energy. Some 6 months earlier, the patient had seen a friend killed while operating a similar machine. He reported nightmares, flashbacks, and impaired attention and concentration after his friend's death, which worsened after his finger injury. Despite his doctor's prescription of a benzodiazepine, the symptoms persisted 4 months later. The patient felt unable to return to work, lost 15 pounds, and applied for psychiatric disability.

While Patient 3 can be said to be demonstrating a subculturally reinforced and supported set of disability behaviors, Patient 4 appears to be suffering from a posttraumatic stress disorder. Patient 3 might be malingering but, as we will discuss later, he may be acting in unconscious response to sociocultural influences rather than consciously feigning illness. Not only is Patient 4 not malingering, he has a specific psychiatric disorder that was initiated by his friend's accidental death and exacerbated by his own injury.

Patient 5. A 48-year-old physics professor with two grown children by a loveless first marriage was remarried for 2 years to a 30-year-old woman who idolized him as his mother adored his scientist father. The patient and his beautiful young wife had a 1-year-old son. While walking along a street at noontime, the patient was struck by a car that jumped the curb; both of his legs required amputation just below the knees. Following emergency surgery and healing of his stumps, physical therapy and prostheses were recommended to permit independent ambulation, but the patient refused to comply with these recommendations. Instead, he learned to use a wheelchair quite effectively.

Within 6 weeks of his accident, this extraordinary man had resumed his full professional life of teaching, research, and administration. He and his wife installed ramps to make their house fully accessible to him, and his fellow church members built him a wheelchair-accessible bathroom. He was learning to drive a modified car. However, although vocationally he was now fully functional, he could not resume a full sexual life with his wife. At first he blamed this on the physical limitations imposed by his stumps, but at a psychiatric interview 4 months after the accident, it became apparent that he was impotent in all positions. He had also discontinued active involvement with his infant son. He was irritable, and his wife described feeling "as if he wants me and our son to disappear one minute, but then he becomes clinging and demanding the next."

Thus, despite his remarkable recovery of occupational function, Patient 5 was maritally and sexually disabled. He also had flashbacks, nightmares, and affective lability characteristic of a posttraumatic stress disorder. His symptoms proved amenable to a psychodynamic approach. He was an only child who had been intensely jealous of his father's dominance of the family and his mother's singular devotion to his father. He dealt with his childhood rage with defensive idealization of his father. His first marriage to a cold, remote woman whose behavior toward him was so unlike his mother's behavior toward his father (and more like the mother's behavior toward the patient) appeared to represent an expression of his guilt over Oedipal desires. When he met and married his second wife, he felt "loved by a woman for the first time . . . like my father was loved." The accident appeared to have been experienced as a punishment for the Oedipal triumph represented by the beautiful loving wife and new baby. Thus, he developed a highly specific, interpersonal disability while his work remained remarkably unimpaired.

Patient 5 did not have risk factors for developing a major depression as did Patient 2. He also did not have a pattern of signs and symptoms fully explicable by a posttraumatic stress disorder, as did Patient 4. His disability was not subculturally reinforced as was the case for patient 3. Patient 5 apparently suffered from the coincidence that the onset of his happiness in marriage and fatherhood, which stimulated a sense of Oedipal triumph, was followed closely by a tragic accident. His particular psychological vulnerability was matched by the particular accident, which he perceived as a castration-like punishment. The accident revived his guilt, leading to his dysfunction as a father and a sexual partner.

The case examples above demonstrate the significance of a thorough psychiatric evaluation for those persons who appear to have psychiatric factors relevant to potential or real physical disability. The evaluation requires particular focus on a number of issues, including

1. A personal and family history of psychiatric illness with special attention to mood disorders
2. The development or reactivation of a posttraumatic stress disorder
3. Sociocultural factors in the history or current environment that foster a sense of entitlement and encourage disability status
4. Potential for the physical illness or injury to represent unique psychodynamic stressors given a patient's particular developmental history, personality, and coping style.

Motivation

A number of authors have made significant contributions to our understanding of what determines a given individual's motivation to overcome a potentially disabling injury or illness. Although the patient's diagnosis is important in assessing the severity and prognosis of any injury, motivation may be a key factor in determining outcome. Brodsky (1987b) has studied motivational issues in individuals who have sustained job-related injury. He lists four major groups of factors that are important in determining prognosis: cultural factors, personal factors, work-related factors, and factors inherent in the disability system.

Perhaps the most important cultural factor according to Brodsky is a belief (or lack of belief) in the work ethic, a value system that he believes maintains that "1) A person's duty is to work and to work hard; 2) success in work is evidence of personal worth; 3) the measure of success is money, property, and possessions; and 4) the way to success is industry and thrift" (Brodsky 1987b, p. 50). Socialization for work immediately follows from a belief in the work ethic, according to Brodsky. Not only are children provided with appropriate parental and occupational role models, but they also learn to organize time, follow through on tasks, and delay gratification when necessary. Furthermore, degree of education is often a function of belief in the work ethic. With increased educational accomplishment comes a greater belief in the intrinsic rewards of work, a greater likelihood of enhancing extrinsic rewards of work, and a more intellectually rewarding content of work.

Brodsky also believes that many workers who go on to become disabled perceive themselves as disabled or inadequate (physically, intellectually, or emotionally) before their definitive injury or illness. Disability then becomes their "honorable discharge from the work force" (Horton 1984). Specific personal factors he lists that play into this scenario include job-related "culture shock," job-personality fit, incompetence, personality predisposition, age, and family relationships.

Job-related culture shock encompasses difficulty with the basic "rules of work"—coming in on time, adhering to the task at hand, and accepting criticism constructively. Incompetence may extend to victims of the "Peter Principle"—individuals who have been promoted beyond their level of competence. One of Brodsky's examples of predisposing personality factors is that of the parentified child who goes on to become an apparently self-sufficient adult, but who has ambivalence about dependency and strong unmet dependency needs. Physical disability can both legitimize and gratify these needs. Family relationships can also alter attitudes toward work. Marital conflict or problems with children may lead to a desire to spend more time at home and to a resentment of work. On occasion, a dysfunctional family may actually function better after disabling injury or illness to one member.

Age is relevant in that older employees are less likely to return to work after an injury, especially if they have done unskilled or semiskilled labor.

In addition to the personal factors already discussed, we would add one more: cognitive factors that alter perception of illness. As mentioned by Gallagher and Stewart (1987), these factors might include perception of the illness as a threat, as a challenge to heroic effort, as a release, or as a punishment. In the case of punishment, if it is seen as undeserved, the illness might induce rage; if it is seen as deserved, it might result in relief or in depression. Either of these affective responses could contribute to disability at work or in other roles.

The third major category of factors viewed by Brodsky (1987b) as important in outcome of work-related injury comprises job-related factors. Specifically, low pay; boring, repetitive work; heavy physical work; dangerous work; and an unhealthy work environment were all correlated with poor outcome, as were an authoritarian supervisory style, poor communication, lack of autonomy, favoritism, and sexual or other forms of discrimination.

Last, Brodsky (1987b) mentions characteristics of the disability system itself as relevant to injury outcome. Specifically discussed are the amount of disability payment, litigation, an adversarial employee-employer relationship, and functioning of the "disability subculture." An increase in disability benefits is said to provide an economic incentive to become and remain disabled. Litigation "fixes" the symptoms of a disability pending resolution of the associated lawsuit. An adversarial employee-employer relationship, even in the absence of legal action, can perpetuate a disability: patients become determined to "legitimize" their claims and assert their rights in the face of what they perceive to be an unfeeling or hostile bureaucracy. Finally, the disability subculture of similarly affected individuals often gives the patient a sense of identity, closeness, and support missing elsewhere in his or her life. If these factors are conscious, the patient may be malingering. However, they are often not at all conscious.

Psychological Adjustment to Injury

Before elaborating further on personal factors determining outcome after a disabling injury occurring in a non-work-related setting, some general comments will be made about frequently encountered patterns of psychological response to an acute disabling illness or injury. Gallagher and Stewart (1987) found no characteristic pattern of response based on type of disability. However, increasing severity of disability resulted in increased anger, depression, and anxiety. Younger age at the time of illness or injury was correlated with increased depression.

Krueger (1984) listed several stages of psychological adjustment, not unlike Kubler-Ross's (1969) stages of mourning: shock, denial, depressive reaction, reaction against independence, and adaptation. As with Kubler-Ross's stages, they may not be experienced sequentially; patients may get "stuck" in one stage for prolonged periods, and, not uncommonly, the whole process is repeated several times. Krueger emphasizes that depression is a normal and expected response to loss of a body part or to loss of function, much as it is in bereavement. According to Krueger (1984, p. 9), "If it does not occur, even transiently, an alarm should sound because its absence indicates the reality of the loss has not been emotionally recognized."

Krueger's stages of adjustment are initiated not only by the obvious physical injury (e.g., loss of a limb) but also by the less visible alterations in function (e.g., loss of normal sexual function in a man with a spinal cord injury) or alteration in body image. Many men with spinal cord injury, for example, say they would gladly give up hope of ambulation if only they could be assured of normal sexual function. It is also quite common for acutely disabled patients of either sex to feel like "a neuter," which they often express as "I no longer feel like a man [woman]." As Krueger pointed out, the more the patient's impairment interferes with his or her vocation, recreation, self-esteem, and normal coping mechanisms, the more devastating it will be (Krueger 1981–82).

Table 17-1 lists commonly used coping strategies that Krueger adopted from Weisman (1974). These coping strategies are said to be fairly consistent over time, but increased stress favors the use of the most familiar strategy.

Krueger (1984) observes that

> normal personality traits will be exaggerated at a time of stress, especially in the event of such a massive insult to the individual's bodily and emotional integrity. Any stress causes a heightened use of defense mechanisms. The dependent patient will be more dependent; the conscientious, responsible patient will intensify these defenses in an effort to compensate for the disability. Some traits, for example, the willingness to be dependent and to be taken care of within limits and without marked protest, are more adaptive for the patient role. Other traits work better for rehabilitation efforts; an example is the tendency to

be overly conscientious and to strive for independence. Some traits work for neither, as shown by the borderline patient who has no consistent internal sense of self or goals. (p. 10)

Krueger (1984) goes on to say, "The particular ways in which grief is displayed vary in accordance with the patient's personality as well" (p. 10).

Factors that predict depressive illness in patients after an injury or illness include a past history of depression, a family history of depression, and a predisposition to depression based on history of early parental loss or childhood trauma (Krueger 1981–82).

Castelnuovo-Tedesco (1981) lists several other factors important in determining the psychological consequences of a physical defect, including time of acquisition (congenital, acquired in childhood, or acquired as an adult), size and location of the defect, and course of the illness, i.e., whether it results in the deterioration of the person's health or is progressive in nature. Whether the defect is temporary or permanent or whether it results in the loss of a body part is also important. According to Castelnuovo-Tedesco (1981), the most favorable time for acquiring a disability is after stable adult integration has occurred, and patients with onset of disability in childhood or adolescence are more psychologically vulnerable. However, many children do appear psy-

Table 17-1. Commonly used strategies for coping with disability

- **Affective strategies**

  Passivity, isolation of affect, and not worrying
  Denial and reversal of affect (e.g., laughing it off)
  Sharing feelings and reactions with others

- **Behavioral strategies**

  Displacement and distraction with activities
  Confrontation with one's self and taking concerted actions
  Acting out
  Repetition using the activities that worked for previous stresses
  Avoidance and physical withdrawal from people and stressful situations

- **Cognitive strategies**

  Intellectual: seeking information and intellectual control
  Rationalization by redefinition: accepting and making a virtue out of necessity
  Fatalist: stoic acceptance and preparation for the worst
  Projection and externalization, including blaming others
  Strict compliance with authority: doing what one is told
  Masochistic surrender: seeking blame, atonement, and self-sacrifice

chologically resilient in the face of serious physical illness, as shown, for example, by the work of Fritz and Williams (1988) with childhood cancer patients.

In terms of location of the defect, Castelnuovo-Tedesco (1981) feels the face, hands, and the genitalia are the most significant locations: "Face and genitalia play a specific role in the definition of identity and personal attractiveness; the integrity of the hands, by contrast, influences the perception of one's effectiveness and self-sufficiency" (p. 147). Defects are felt to be most psychologically devastating if they are associated with progressive physical illness. Castelnuovo-Tedesco (1981) notes the importance of parental attitudes to disability (if acquired in childhood); the parents' response is a mirror to the child, so that the child sees himself or herself as the parents do. In our experience, this response often occurs with adults and their significant others, such as spouses (Lawn 1989). The patient's symbolic interpretation of the disability, a factor discussed briefly earlier, is also of major importance. "Disproportionate psychopathology may, in fact, be proportionate to the far-reaching view of the defect that the patient has in fantasy" (Castelnuovo-Tedesco 1981, p. 149).

Finally, returning to the issue of motivation, Tucker (1984) makes the interesting and important point that motivation is an interpersonal phenomenon. Tucker writes

> If a patient is consistently devalued, is not given support for progress, and receives a hopeless prognosis, he or she will give up and appear unmotivated. Once such a derogatory label is applied, it is a signal that rehabilitation efforts will fail. But if the person is given positive feedback, the individual's motivation to strive will be enhanced. Potentially, a beneficial cycle or "recipe for motivation" can emerge. A person who is encouraged and respected feels more self-esteem, which facilitates motivation and actual physical progress in rehabilitation. Staff members thereby feel gratified and increase their time and involvement with the patient, all of which brings further rehabilitation participation and ultimately a favorable outcome.
>
> Hope is at the core of motivation. Since the patient is undeniably devastated and overwhelmed, he or she may need to survive initially on borrowed hope from others. Consequently, motivation is redefined as an inter-personal and not purely an internal characteristic. It can significantly be influenced by the rehabilitation staff, the family, and community systems. More-

over, as newcomers to the rehabilitation process, patients are likely to sink or aspire to the level of motivation expected by the veteran professional." (pp. 259–260)

The Role of Psychological Tests

Millon, who has written extensively on the role of psychological testing in evaluating personality traits of disabled adults, considers psychological testing to be useful in two broad categories: "The first centers on identifying personality and psychosocial factors that relate to either the development or exacerbation of various types of physical illness," according to Millon and colleagues (1979). "The second focuses on maximizing treatment efficacy by reference to the patient's preexisting personality or psychological state" (p. 530).

There are few psychodiagnostic instruments specifically applicable to assessing the emotional stability, cognitive outlook, and coping style of the patient seen in rehabilitation settings (Millon et al. 1982). Many of the commonly used instruments, such as the Minnesota Multiphasic Personality Inventory (MMPI; Hathaway and McKinley 1989), the Sixteen Personality Factor Questionnaire (16 PF; Karson and O'Dell 1976), and the Cornell Medical Index (Brodman et al. 1949), designed for use in psychiatric populations are "only tangentially relevant" in the physically disabled population (Millon 1982). The Millon Behavioral Health Inventory (MBHI; Millon et al. 1981, 1982) was created to alleviate this problem. The MBHI is a 150-item, true-false, self-report inventory that addresses major coping styles, sources of psychogenic stressors (e.g., social alienation), psychosomatic vulnerabilities (e.g., gastrointestinal susceptibility and cardiovascular tendency), and prognostic indices.

Several research publications (Millon et al. 1982) document the utility of data derived from the MBHI in predicting speed and level of recovery from major procedures or predicting self-sufficiency following spinal cord injury or amputation. Others feel that our ability to accurately predict disease outcome based on quantifiable personality characteristics is still an imprecise area that needs far more work (L. Derogatis, October 1989, personal communication). A psychological consultation represents a "point-in-time" evaluation; its ability to identify the stressors, psychic strengths, and coping styles necessary to tailor a rehabilitation approach to a particular patient may exceed its predictive validity. "The substantial variations in functioning and well being [of patients with] chronic condition(s) . . . remain to be explained" (Stewart et al. 1989, p. 907).

However, particular psychological instruments such as the Hamilton Rating Scale for Depression (Hamilton 1967), the Symptom Checklist–90—Revised (Derogatis 1983), intelligence scales, and projective tests may help identify the scope and intensity of particular psychological variables such as depression, anxiety, retardation, and psychosis. The literature provides little support for their utility in predicting the degree of disability consequent to a physical illness or injury. As in any approach to complex diagnosis, however, these instruments may be helpful in identifying treatable psychiatric conditions that may complicate any medical illness.

Neuropsychological testing, which is frequently performed in patients with brain injury or neurotoxic exposure, is of limited value in predicting real-life disability or work capacity, except in extreme cases. Results of neuropsychological testing in patients with possible disability should be interpreted only in conjunction with independent evidence that a patient's functional capacities and other medical and psychosocial issues influence the patient's abilities (Faust and Ziskin, in press). Motivational state as well as depression and other psychopathology can influence test performance (Lezak 1983). Furthermore, malingerers can successfully fake abnormal neuropsychological test performance (Faust et al. 1988a, 1988b; Heaton et al. 1978). Despite these limitations, the detailed knowledge of a disabled patient's cognitive strengths and weaknesses may be of great value in planning rehabilitation.

DOCUMENTING PSYCHIATRIC DISABILITY

In addition to appreciating the range of factors that contribute to disability, the practicing clinician must evaluate each patient in accord with the requirements of the specific entitlement or insurance program for which the patient has applied. The requirements for completing an appropriate psychiatric report for a patient applying for Social Security Disability Insurance (SSDI), worker's compensation insurance, or veterans' benefits, respectively, have been reviewed by Krajeski and Lipsett (1987), Brodsky (1987a), and Lipkin (1987).

Establishing the presence of an impairment requires a thorough description of the onset, chief complaint, and course of the present illness, as well as the details of inpatient and outpatient treatment, relevant laboratory findings, including (when appropriate) psychological testing, and a description of any comorbidities. The way in which the present illness impairs functioning should then be addressed, focusing particularly on 1) activities of daily living; 2) appropriate social functioning; 3) deficiencies of concentration, persistence or pace; and 4) deterioration in work or worklike settings (Krajeski and Lipsett 1987). Specific examples of deficiencies in one or more of these areas are far more helpful than nonspecific generalizations, such as "the patient has difficultly relating to others."

The mental status examination should then be performed by the examining psychiatrist; again, Krajeski and Lipsett (1987) stress the importance of citing specific findings rather than general conclusions, such as "there is evidence of mild organicity on cognitive testing." The psychiatrist should then present diagnostic impressions, in DSM-III-R (American Psychiatric Association 1987) terminology, and follow up with a prognostic assessment and recommendations for treatment. Krajeski and Lipsett also recommend detailing any factors that may limit the accuracy of the report, such as poor patient concentration, a language barrier, or apparent malingering. The Supplemental Security Income (SSI) and SSDI regulations allow the applicant to summarize how the effects of the patient's physical and mental disorders justify eligibility for benefits in cases in which neither the physical nor the mental disorder does so on its own.

For worker's compensation evaluation, Brodsky (1987a) lists the following issues as particularly relevant: the presence of a mental disorder, its duration and course, its relation to the patient's employment, the need for psychiatric treatment, the patient's ability to return to work and when, the usefulness of rehabilitation, and the prognosis of the patient's mental disorder. Brodsky suggests reviewing any relevant records before examining the patient to provide clues for the interviewer and to uncover issues that need to be pursued further. He also recommends making clear to the patient at the outset that the examiner is a psychiatrist and that the interview will not be confidential.

The most useful components of the psychiatric examination are 1) a statement by the patient about the nature of the occupation; 2) comments about the present job or last job held; 3) a description of the injury, its treatment and course, and present physical and mental symptoms; 4) a list of the symptoms that in the patient's view are job related; 5) descriptions of attempts to return to work; 6) future work plans; 7) current daily activities; 8) past or present legal problems; and 9) previous work history, with particular emphasis on prior work-related claims (Brodsky 1987a). A formal mental status examination, including evaluation of cognitive impairment, should then be conducted. Diagnostic impressions should be made in DSM-III-R terminology and should include a narrative description of how the diagnosis may affect the patient's work and nonwork life. Possible psychiatric diagnoses that may have existed before the index injury should also be documented.

Finally, the report should address, as thoroughly as possible, all questions asked by the referring agency (Brodsky 1987a). An essential difference between SSI-SSDI and both worker's compensation and veterans' benefits is that the latter two require a direct linkage between the work place or military status and the disability producing physical or mental impairment.

Much of the same information that is relevant for determination of SSDI or worker's compensation eligibility is also important in applications for veterans' benefits. It includes a longitudinal history of the psychiatric illness; a list of current signs and symptoms of illness and effects on all areas of functioning; and reports of the physical examination, laboratory studies, and psychological testing (where applicable). Reports of previous examinations and treatment should be reviewed, as should military records indicating the nature of the stress the patient has undergone (Lipkin 1987).

To be eligible for veterans' benefits, the patient must have developed an illness within 12 months of discharge from the military (Lipkin 1987). Exceptions are made for prisoners of war and for cases of posttraumatic stress disorder, delayed type (Lipkin 1987). A personality disorder is never classified as service related, nor is alcoholism; however, alcohol-related sequelae (such as organic mental disorders) may be considered service related (Lipkin 1987).

Whether a personality disorder is "counted" in assessment of aggregate disability depends on the entitlement program. As just mentioned, it is not considered relevant in a patient applying for veterans' benefits; the same is true for worker's compensation insurance. In SSDI, however, a personality disorder may be included as a legitimate comorbidity.

When a clinician is treating a patient who has a chronic psychiatric illness that amplifies a physical disability, the patient may be tempted to terminate psychiatric treatment on attaining disability status. This is particularly so if improvement of the psychiatric condition might lead to the loss of a financial entitlement. The psychiatrist can include a recommendation for continued treatment and periodic reexamination in reports to entitlement programs. The psychiatrist should fully discuss with the patient whether these issues are potentially interfering with the patient's desire for improvement in psychiatric status.

In treatment planning, the presence of a personality disorder that appears to be contributing to the disabling effects of a physical illness must be unquestionably addressed, since improvement of maladaptive personality traits and behavior may lead to a decrease in the overall disability.

MALINGERING

Clinicians must be prepared to evaluate the likelihood of malingering among patients who apply for benefits under an entitlement or insurance program. Malingering may be difficult to differentiate from somatization disorder, conversion disorder, factitious disorder, and genuine physical illness (Ford and Smith 1987), especially if the malingerer is knowledgeable and a talented actor. The two major points of differentiation are

1. The malingerer feigns an illness to achieve clearly recognizable gains that are not limited to the need to seek medical attention and intervention.
2. The malingerer's physical and psychological symptoms and signs are under conscious control. The malingerer is seeking a realistic gain, such as remuneration, avoidance of legal or other societal obligations, or a prescription for a controlled drug for resale or nonmedical use.

The differential diagnosis begins by ruling out the presence of real medical or major mental illness. Once this is done, malingering must be distinguished from other psychiatric conditions that involve repeated exaggeration or fabrication of illness or injury. Table 17-2 lists features that support a diagnosis of malingering.

Of particular difficulty and concern are patients with genuine physical or mental illness who consciously or unconsciously exaggerate signs and symptoms to reach a level of impairment and disability that would guarantee benefits. The presence of a dependent or antisocial personality disorder or of social factors addressed earlier in this chapter may provide clues as to the possibility of malingering. Symptoms or signs exceeding objective findings (e.g., diagnostic images, psychological testing) are suggestive of either somatization or malingering, but such discrepancies often are encountered in specific medical illnesses, such as systemic lupus erythematosus or multiple sclerosis, and in certain injuries, such as whiplash.

Table 17-2.   Features supporting a diagnosis of malingering

- Vague, ill-defined, and overdramatized symptoms that do not conform to known clinical conditions
- A patient who seeks addicting drugs, financial gain, or the avoidance of onerous conditions (e.g., imprisonment)
- History, examination, and evaluative data that do not support a medical explanation for the patient's complaints
- An uncooperative patient who refuses to accept a clean bill of health or an encouraging prognosis
- Findings that appear compatible with self-inflicted injuries
- A history or records that reveal multiple past episodes of poorly explained injury or undiagnosed illness
- Records or test data that appear to have been tampered with (e.g., presence of erasures or foreign substances in urine)

Hypnosis and Amytal interviews have not proved reliable in differentiating malingering from physical illness or conversion disorder, although they may support the diagnosis of a conversion disorder over physical illness in a patient not suspected of malingering. The problem is that whereas conversion symptoms may be alleviated by a trance, malingerers may feign a trance as well as they do their original symptoms (Meyerson 1989). Also, patients with severe personality disorders may not be easily hypnotized (Spiegel and Spiegel 1978).

Psychiatric intervention for malingering is ineffective; it is also of little help for patients with antisocial personality disorders who amplify symptoms. Patients with factitious and somatization disorders also are rarely responsive to psychiatric intervention. With these important exceptions, most other psychiatric conditions that contribute to disability are treatable. Major depression, posttraumatic stress disorder, and panic disorder are common, readily treatable mental disorders that produce physical symptoms and may aggravate physical disability. Their treatment can return disabled patients to work.

REFERENCES

American Psychiatric Association: Diagnostic and Statistical Manual of Mental Disorders, Third Edition, Revised. Washington, DC, American Psychiatric Association, 1987

Brodman K, Erdmann AJ, Lorge I, et al: The Cornell Medical Index. JAMA 140:530, 1949

Brodsky CM: The psychiatric evaluation in workers' compensation, in Psychiatric Disability: Clinical, Legal, and Administrative Dimensions. Edited by Meyerson AT, Fine T. Washington, DC, American Psychiatric Press, 1987a, pp 313–332

Brodsky CM: Factors influencing work-related disability, in Psychiatric Disability: Clinical, Legal, and Administrative Dimensions. Edited by Meyerson AT, Fine T. Washington, DC, American Psychiatric Press, 1987b, pp 49–65

Castelnuovo-Tedesco P: The psychological consequences of physical trauma and defects. International Review of Psychoanalysis 8:145–154, 1981

Derogatis L: SCL-90-R Manual—II. Towson, MD, Clinical Psychometric Research, 1983

Faust D, Ziskin J: Forensic Neuropsychology: Challenging the Assessment of Brain Damage. Marina Del Rey, CA, Law & Psychology Press (in press)

Faust D, Hart K, Guilmette TJ, et al: Neuropsychologists' capacity to detect adolescent malingerers. Professional Psychology: Research & Practice 19:508–515, 1988a

Faust D, Hart K, Guilmette TJ: Pediatric malingering: the capacity of children to fake believable deficits on neuropsychological testing. J Consult Clin Psychol 56:578–582, 1988b

Ford CV, Smith GR: Somatoform disorders, factitious disorders, and disability syndromes, in Principles of Medical Psychiatry. Edited by Stoudemire A, Fogel BS. Orlando, FL, Grune & Stratton, 1987, pp 205–217

Fritz GK, Williams JR: Issues of adolescent development for survivors of childhood cancer. J Am Acad Child Adolesc Psychiatry 27:712–715, 1988

Gallagher RM, Stewart F: Psychiatric rehabilitation and chronic physical illness, in Psychiatric Disability: Clinical, Legal, and Administrative Dimensions. Edited by Meyerson AT, Fine T. Washington, DC, American Psychiatric Press, 1987, pp 143–182

Hamilton M: Development of a rating scale for primary depressive illness. Br J Soc Clin Psychol 6:278–296, 1967

Hathaway SR, McKinley JC: Minnesota Multiphasic Personality Inventory—2. Minneapolis, MN, University of Minnesota, 1989

Heaton RK, Smith HH, Lehman RA, et al: Prospects for faking believable deficits on neuropsychological testing. J Consult Clin Psychol 46:892–900, 1978

Horton CF: Women have headaches, men have backaches: patterns of illness in an Appalachian community. Soc Sci Med 19:647–654, 1984

Karson S, O'Dell JW: A Guide to the Clinical Use of the 16 PF. Champaign, IL, Institute for Personality & Ability Testing, 1976

Krajeski J, Lipsett M: The psychiatric consultation for Social Security Disability Insurance, in Psychiatric Disability: Clinical, Legal, and Administrative Dimensions. Edited by Meyerson AT, Fine T. Washington, DC, American Psychiatric Press, 1987, pp 287–311

Krueger DW: Emotional rehabilitation of the physical rehabilitation patient. Int J Psychiatry Med 11:183–191, 1981–82

Krueger DW: Psychological rehabilitation of physical trauma and disability, in Rehabilitation Psychology. Edited by Krueger DW. Rockville, MD, Aspen, 1984, pp 3–13

Kubler-Ross E: On Death and Dying. New York, Macmillan, 1969

Lawn B: Experiences of a paraplegic psychiatric resident in an inpatient psychiatric unit. Am J Psychiatry 146:771–774, 1989

Lezak MD: Neuropsychological Assessment, 2nd Edition. New York, Oxford University Press, 1983

Lipkin JO: Psychiatric disability: the Veteran's Administration, in Psychiatric Disability: Clinical, Legal, and Administrative Dimensions. Edited by Meyerson AT, Fine T. Washington, DC, American Psychiatric Press, 1987, pp 333–342

Meyerson AT: Malingering, in Comprehensive Textbook of Psychiatry, 5th Edition. Edited by Kaplan H, Sadock B. Baltimore, MD, Williams & Wilkins, 1989, pp 1396–1399

Millon T, Green CJ, Meagher RB: The MBHI: a new inventory for the psychodiagnostician in medical settings. Professional Psychology, Aug 1979, p 530

Millon T, Green CJ, Meagher RB: Millon Behavior Health Inventory Manual. Minneapolis, National Computer Systems, 1981

Millon T, Green CJ, Meagher RB: A new psychodiagnostic tool for clients in rehabilitation settings: the MBHI. Rehab Psychol 27:23–35, 1982

Spiegel H, Spiegel D: Trance and Treatment. New York, Basic Books, 1978

Stewart AL, Greenfield S, Hays R, et al: Functional status and well-being of patients with chronic conditions. JAMA 262:907, 1989

Tucker JS: Patient staff interaction with the spinal cord patient, in Rehabilitation Psychology. Edited by Krueger DW. Rockville, MD, Aspen, 1984, pp 257–266

Weisman A: The Realization of Death. New York, Jason Aronson, 1974

Chapter 18

Psychotropic Drug Use in Pregnancy: An Update

Lee S. Cohen, M.D.
Vicki L. Heller, M.D.
Jerrold F. Rosenbaum, M.D.

The pregnant psychiatric patient who takes or requires psycho-tropic medication presents a clinical dilemma that places the physician between a teratological rock and a clinical hard place. While reviews describe the known effects of psychotropic drug exposure during pregnancy (Beeley 1986; Calabrese and Gulledge 1985; Hill and Kleinberg 1984a, 1984b; Robinson et al. 1986), only a few authors (Nurnberg and Prudic 1984) have outlined specific treatment guidelines for evaluating and managing the pregnant patient with onset of psychiatric illness during pregnancy, the psychiatric patient maintained on psychotropics who wishes to conceive, or the patient taking psychotropic medication who conceives inadvertently.

Accumulated case reports and reviews over the last decade fail to substantiate putative teratogenic effects of antipsychotic or antide-pressant agents (Edlund and Craig 1984; Idanpaan-Heikkila and Saxen 1973; Kuenssberg and Knox 1972; Milkovich and Van den Berg 1976; Rumeau-Rouguette et al. 1977; Slone et al. 1977). While there has been

Portions of this text were previously published (Cohen LS, Heller VL, Rosenbaum JF: Treatment guidelines for psychotropic drug use in pregnancy. Psychosomatics 30:25–33 1989) and are used with permission.

some linkage of benzodiazepine exposure to an increased risk of oral cleft abnormalities (Aarskog 1975; Laegreid et al. 1987; Saxen 1975; Saxen and Saxen 1975), the evidence linking these agents with gross organ malformation is still weak (Czeizel and Lendvay 1987; Rosenberg et al. 1983; Shiono and Mills 1984). The absence of clear risk, however, does not imply safety. No psychotropic agent, for example, has gained Food and Drug Administration (FDA) approval for use during pregnancy. Further, by clinical consensus, psychotropic agents are avoided in the first trimester of pregnancy, when a developing fetus is most vulnerable to the toxic effects of most exogenous agents (Langman 1975).

An estimated 80% of women take prescribed drugs during pregnancy, and as many as 35% are administered psychoactive agents (Doering and Stewart 1978). The prevalence of drug use during pregnancy underscores the need for thoughtful guidelines to assess the risks and benefits of treating individual patients requiring psychotropics for psychotic illness, unipolar and bipolar depression, and anxiety disorders.

COURSE OF PSYCHIATRIC ILLNESS IN PREGNANCY

Pregnancy has frequently been described as a time of relative psychiatric "well-being" and as playing a "protective role" against the emergence of psychiatric symptoms, but this claim is based on inadequate data (Rosenberg and Silver 1965; Sim 1963; Zajicek 1981) or poor methodology. In a recent prospective study of 99 pregnant women, O'Hara et al. (1986) reported that 10% met criteria for major or minor depression during pregnancy. These researchers also suggested that women with a history of major depression or with first-degree relatives with affective illness may be at particular risk for developing postpartum depression.

The impact of pregnancy on bipolar illness and schizophrenia is uncertain, but bipolar patients may be at particular risk for postpartum depressive episodes (Akiskal et al. 1983; Targum and Gershon 1981), and schizophrenic patients have an estimated 13–20% risk of decompensation postpartum (Protheroe 1961). With regard to the course of anxiety disorders in pregnancy, several authors have described a decrease in frequency of panic attacks in pregnant women (George et al. 1987; Klein 1964), whereas others (Cohen and White 1951; Cohen et al. 1989a, 1989b) have noted persistence, worsening, or emergence of panic symptoms in gravid women and in postpartum patients.

WEIGHING RISKS AND BENEFITS OF PSYCHOTROPIC DRUG USE IN PREGNANCY

Psychotropic drug use in pregnancy should, of course, be limited to those cases in which the risk to the mother and the fetus from the disorder outweigh the risk of drug treatment. The physician, therefore, must be able to quantify the relative risks. Risks associated with pharmacotherapy are of five types: 1) teratogenic potential or the risk of gross organ malformation, 2) behavioral teratogenesis or the potential for enduring impact on neurobehavioral development from in utero drug exposure, 3) direct toxic effects on the fetus, 4) drug effects on labor and delivery, and 5) effects on breast-feeding infants. Such risks need to be weighed against the morbidity (and potential mortality) of psychiatric illness.

Impaired self-care, including the inability to follow appropriate prenatal care, as well as suicidal, impulsive, or potentially dangerous manic behavior are examples of clinical risks that may argue for pharmacotherapy in pregnant patients. Of uncertain clinical effect are the neuroendocrine changes associated with major psychiatric disorders (Carr et al. 1986; Charney and Heninger 1986; Siever and Uhde 1984) or the physiologic consequences (Crandon 1979; Lederman et al. 1985), for example, of untreated panic symptoms on the fetoplacental unit (Cohen et al. 1989a; Omer and Everly 1988). The relevance of untreated psychosis, anxiety, or depression for the maternal attachment process and subsequent psychological development of the child is controversial and, at this time, is a matter of speculation but also of concern (Avant 1981; Brazelton 1975; Cogill et al. 1986; Zahn-Waxler et al. 1984).

While several studies record the incidence of malformations reported in offspring exposed to psychotropics in utero (Kopelman et al. 1975; McBride 1972), we lack precise data from large samples of patients of their teratogenic potential or of the ability of these agents to cause more subtle neurobehavioral sequelae (Asioki and Siekevitz 1988; Shader and Greenblatt 1989; Sivertz et al. 1989). In this state of uncertainty, the physician considering the use of psychotropics in pregnancy must design a treatment plan tailored to the individual patient's overall clinical situation.

GUIDELINES AND CONSIDERATIONS

The following general guidelines have been helpful in our large ambulatory psychopharmacology unit for evaluating psychiatrically ill pregnant patients for whom continuation or institution of pharmacotherapy is being considered.

Planned Pregnancy

For patients with well-diagnosed psychiatric illness who are currently managed on psychotropics, planned pregnancy is extremely important. This must be emphasized to the patient early in treatment (Coverdale and Ruffo 1989). Contraceptive history should be included in evaluations of all women receiving psychotropics. For the psychiatrically ill woman maintained on psychotropics, planned pregnancy provides adequate time for consultation between psychiatrist, obstetrician, patient, and husband or partner, at which time risks and benefits of treatment as well as the potential impact on a couple of pursuing or deferring childbearing can be thoughtfully addressed. Planned pregnancy also allows for gradual nonemergent trials of tapering medication with monitoring of reemergent symptoms and consideration of alternative, potentially less toxic agents.

Unplanned pregnancy often results in an urgent and rapid (though possibly not warranted) discontinuation of medication, which risks the development of rebound or withdrawal symptoms and often leaves the patient more symptomatic or at greater risk for relapse. The impact of rapid withdrawal of medication in a patient with panic disorder, for example, may result in rapid return of severe panic attacks that may threaten the fetoplacental unit. In a case we observed, a woman at term had a panic attack associated with a transient rise in blood pressure and abruptio placentae. An emergency cesarean section was performed following documentation of fetal distress by noninvasive fetal monitoring (Cohen et al. 1989a).

Symptom Control

While maximum control of psychiatric symptoms is the usual goal of treatment, the target of drug therapy in managing the pregnant patient is to control the most threatening symptoms while minimizing pharmacotherapeutic intervention.

Hospitalization

Hospitalization should be reserved as an option at any point during pregnancy if it serves to substitute for pharmacotherapy or higher doses of psychotropic agents. This option should be discussed with the patient and the patient's family as early as possible in the treatment planning process.

Documentation

The decision to use psychotropics in pregnancy requires a systematic process of discussion and planning with patient, partner, psychiatrist, and obstetrician. Thorough documentation of this process before and throughout pregnancy is essential, as is an indication of the patient's competence to understand the issues in question.

PSYCHOSIS IN THE PREGNANT PATIENT

The patient who first becomes psychotic during pregnancy requires a thorough evaluation to rule out organic causes for the change in mental status (Groves and Manschrek 1987). Metabolic derangement, infection, intracranial masses, the presence of toxic substances, and other causes must be eliminated as possible etiologies of an evolving thought disorder. It is a potential clinical error to assume that changes in mental functioning in a pregnant woman are merely "reactive," and a vigorous diagnostic workup should be pursued.

For the chronically psychotic patient already maintained on low doses of antipsychotics, sudden medication discontinuation risks acute decompensation, emergence of impulsivity and other behavioral disruptions, and consequently, the likelihood that the patient will need high doses of neuroleptics to effect recompensation. While available data fail to indict antipsychotics as teratogens (Milkovich and Van den Berg 1976; Rumeau-Rouguette et al. 1977; Slone et al. 1977) or to reveal behavioral sequelae in children of mothers exposed to antipsychotics in pregnancy (Kris 1965; Slone et al. 1977), antipsychotics are best avoided in the first trimester. This recommendation, however, must be weighed against the risk and nature of a relapse of psychosis, particularly in the chronically ill patient who has demonstrated repeated decompensation when not taking these agents. For these severely ill patients, maintenance antipsychotic therapy is a reasonable clinical option.

When the decision has been made to institute or to continue antipsychotic therapy during pregnancy, additional concerns require consideration. Extrapyramidal symptoms lasting up to 6 months in the infant (Hill et al. 1966; Levy and Wisniewski 1974; Tamer et al. 1969) and neonatal jaundice (Scokel and Jones 1962) may follow in utero exposure to antipsychotics. Tapering and discontinuation of antipsychotic medication 10 days to 2 weeks before the estimated date of confinement has been suggested (Calabrese and Gulledge 1985) to minimize these risks, if the clinical situation permits. The more potent piperazine phenothiazines such as trifluoperazine or perphenazine may offer less teratogenic exposure, compared with aliphatic phenothiazines such as chlorpromazine (Rumeau-Rouguette et al. 1977).

BIPOLAR ILLNESS AND PREGNANCY

Patients with bipolar disorder may be more vulnerable to postpartum episodes of depression (Akiskal et al. 1983; Targum and Gershon 1981) than unipolar patients. Little is known, however, about the usual course of bipolar disorder in pregnancy. More clearly established is the teratogenicity of lithium based on the International Register of Lithium Babies begun in 1968. Accumulated reports indicate that offspring of women exposed to lithium at least during the first trimester of pregnancy have increased rates of cardiac anomalies; the greatest number of deformities were of the great heart vessels, most notably Ebstein's anomaly (Weinstein and Goldfield 1975). In one series of 37 patients with this anomaly, approximately half presented with cyanosis and congestive heart failure in the first week of life. Though about half of these neonates died, those who survived the neonatal period tended to do well after corrective surgery (Kirklin and Barratt-Boyes 1986). It has been recently estimated based on unpublished data from the Lithium Register that the risk of Ebstein's anomaly after first-trimester exposure to lithium is 0.1%, or 1 in 1,000 cases of exposure; this may be an overestimate, however, given the bias toward reporting adverse outcome (Elia et al. 1987).

All female patients with bipolar disorder should be informed when begun on lithium about the need for family planning. Discussions with the patient and the obstetrician before attempting to conceive allow for thoughtful selection from the array of treatment options. Patients who plan to discontinue lithium maintenance treatment in order to conceive can discontinue the agent during the menstrual period before the cycle in which they wish to conceive (Gelenberg 1986).

The risk of subsequent relapse is correlated with the number of prior manic episodes. Thus, patients on lithium with a history of one circumscribed episode of mania or rare recurrent episodes may do well with lithium discontinuation and close follow-up. However, a prearranged treatment plan should always be prepared between physician and patient in the event of decompensation.

For the more brittle bipolar patient with a clear need for prophylaxis against recurrent manic episodes, lithium discontinuation places the patient at greater risk for decompensation. Some researchers have suggested that carbamazepine has low teratogenic potential (Nakne et al. 1980; Nidely et al. 1979; Paulson and Paulson 1981; Sullivan and McElhatton 1977) and that its putative antimanic effects make it a possible alternative or adjunctive treatment for severely ill bipolar patients who do not respond to lithium alone (Post et al. 1983). Recent data (Jones et al. 1989) suggest, however, that in utero exposure to carbamazepine appears to be associated with craniofacial anomalies, postnatal growth deficiency, and developmental delay. While there is increasing evidence that valproic acid, too, may be a possible alternative treatment for manic patients who do not respond or who cannot tolerate lithium therapy (McElroy et al. 1988), reports suggest increased rates of spina bifida in offspring exposed to this agent in utero (Lindhout and Schmidt 1986).

Bipolar patients with particular need for prophylaxis may benefit from discontinuation of lithium carbonate only after pregnancy is documented. The rationale for this approach is twofold. First, as it may take months to conceive, continuation of lithium treatment minimizes the time that the patient does not receive appropriate antimanic therapy, thereby decreasing risk of relapse. Second, teratogenic risk associated with drug exposure prior to the first missed menses (corresponding to the first 14 days of development) is small, as toxic insults during this time usually either are completely repaired or result in a nonviable, blighted ovum (Cohen 1988; Dicke 1989).

When a woman with severe bipolar disorder conceives and lithium is discontinued, treatment options during the first trimester vary again with the history of the patient. These include close observation of the patient for symptoms of decompensation or, in more severely ill patients for whom the likelihood and risk of relapse is greater, institution of prophylactic treatment with low doses of antipsychotic (Van Gent and Nabarro 1987). During the second and third trimesters, lithium treatment can be resumed and the antipsychotic slowly tapered depending on the status of the patient at that time.

Despite the clear advantages of planned pregnancy and prearranged emergency programs, unplanned pregnancy is common. The appropriate clinical response varies to some extent with the trimester of pregnancy. Though patients with lithium exposure before week 12 should be advised of the increased risk of cardiac malformation, they can also be reassured about the absence of developmental difficulties noted in follow-up reports of children exposed to lithium in utero (Schou 1976). Fetal cardiac ultrasound at weeks 18–20 is advised for women who have taken lithium in the first trimester to rule out anomalies of the great vessels, particularly Ebstein's anomaly, which is associated with significant morbidity.

A pregnant bipolar patient suffering acute decompensation represents a psychiatric emergency. The risks of mania are well described (Boyd and Weissman 1982), and the added risk to the fetus with an acutely psychotic mother is obvious. First onset of hypomania or mania during pregnancy calls for an evaluation to rule out organic causes (Krauthammer and Klerman 1978). Providing a safe environment for the manic pregnant patient is essential, and hospitalization and pharmacotherapeutic intervention should be considered. Acute treatment options include neuroleptic agents and electroconvulsive therapy (ECT).

Though not widely used currently for manic states, ECT has proven efficacy in the acute treatment of mania (Crowe 1984; Thorpe 1947) and has been used in several cases of psychotic depression in pregnant women without evidence of insult to either mother or fetoplacental unit (Remick and Maurice 1978; Repke and Berger 1984; Wise et al. 1984). Although the number and dose of psychotropic agents should be kept to a minimum, clonazepam, a high-potency benzodiazepine with anticonvulsant (Dreifuss and Susumu 1982), antipanic (Pollack et al. 1986; Spier et al. 1986), and antimanic activity (Chouinard 1985), may be a helpful adjunct to antipsychotic medication, given growing evidence for the utility of adjuvant benzodiazepines in reducing the total dose of antipsychotic medication required (Cohen and Lipinski 1986; Salzman et al. 1986).

Patients who remain on lithium require careful monitoring of plasma levels in light of the changes in renal function noted with pregnancy (Boobis and Lewis 1983; Jeffries and Bochner 1988; Redmond 1985). The drug should be administered in smaller, divided doses. In the third trimester, lithium should be tapered and discontinued, if possible several weeks prior to the estimated date of confinement (Calabrese and Gulledge 1985). Otherwise, at that point the dose of lithium should be reduced by 50%, given that dehydration often associated with labor and the massive shifts in fluid which can accompany delivery result in elevations of lithium levels and possible lithium toxicity. Even lithium levels of 1.0 meq/ml have been associated with neonatal toxicity, including cyanotic states, bradycardia, impaired respiratory function, T wave abnormalities, "floppy babies," and nephrogenic diabetes insipidus (Ananth 1976). Lithium discontinuation or dose reduction can be followed by reinstitution after delivery in light of the vulnerability of the bipolar population to postpartum affective episodes (Reich and Winokur 1970; Targum et al. 1983).

UNIPOLAR DEPRESSION IN PREGNANCY

Reviews of tricyclic antidepressant use in pregnancy fail to show definitive evidence for the teratogenicity of these agents (Idanpaan-Heikkila and Saxen 1973; Kuenssberg and Knox 1972). Fewer data are available about the monoamine oxidase inhibitors (Poulson and Robson 1964) or newer antidepressants such as trazodone, maprotiline, or fluoxetine (Cooper 1989). Studies of neurobehavioral sequelae of antidepressant administration in pregnancy have been limited primarily to animals; these studies reveal decreased exploratory responses, delayed reflex development, and decreased hypothalamic dopamine levels and cortical beta-adrenergic receptors in rats exposed prenatally to imipramine (Coyle 1975a, 1975b; File and Tucker 1984). In one study of 23 children followed up until 2 years of age, in utero exposure to tricyclic antidepressants was not associated with adverse neurobehavioral sequelae (Sivertz et al. 1989).

Data indicating a rate of major or minor depression of 10% in women during pregnancy (O'Hara 1986; O'Hara et al. 1990) do not imply that all depressed pregnant women should be treated with antidepressant agents. While depression may not be uncommon in pregnancy, pharmacotherapeutic interventions should be reserved for the most severe cases of neurovegetative dysfunction, in which decreased appetite, sleep disturbance, psychomotor retardation, and suicidal ideation begin to compromise the well-being of the prospective mother and, by extension, the fetus. Symptom eradication need not be the goal of therapeutic interventions, but attempts should be made to ameliorate the most threatening symptoms. Adjunctive psychotherapy or casework should be pursued to minimize external provocations and to address intrapsychic factors that may be contributing to the patient's distress.

The preferred antidepressants for the pregnant patient requiring pharmacotherapy are secondary amines such as nortriptyline or desipramine (Idanpaan-Heikkila and Saxen 1973), because treatment with these agents also allows for more precise monitoring of relatively well-established therapeutic serum levels. Limited data are available regarding the potential teratogenicity of fluoxetine (Cooper 1989). Regardless, because of the extended half-life of norfluoxetine, the active metabolite of fluoxetine, women who conceive while taking this drug continue to incur in utero exposure to the agent for a minimum of 5 weeks, even if the drug is promptly discontinued.

By contrast, secondary amines are metabolized and cleared quickly. They have relatively few anticholinergic effects and thus minimize the potential for neonates to experience anticholinergic-associated problems, such as transient urinary retention, gastric ileus, and fetal tachycardia (Falterman and Richardson 1980; Prentice and Brown 1989; Shearer et al. 1972). While adequacy of dosing is an important factor in determining treatment response in depressed patients (Quitkin 1985), in the pregnant patient a more suitable interim goal is to find the lowest effective dose and to defer more vigorous treatment until after delivery.

For depressed patients with psychotic symptoms, hospitalization and ECT should be considered. The psychotically depressed patient who is progressively unable to care for herself and who suffers from decreased food intake, guilty ruminations, and self-deprecatory or infanticidal command hallucinations requires aggressive management, including ECT; the risks of withholding treatment in this situation are unacceptable.

ANXIETY DISORDERS IN PREGNANCY

Pregnancy is a time of anxiety for most women. Normative anxiety, however, must be distinguished from symptoms of an anxiety disorder. Anxiety disorders occur in women three times as commonly as men and aggregate in woman of childbearing age (Weissman and Merikangas 1986). Although earlier reports suggested that panic attacks may decrease in pregnancy (George et al. 1987; Klein 1964) recent data (Cohen et al. 1989b) suggest that women with pregravid histories of anxiety disorders may not be "protected" from these symptoms during pregnancy or the postpartum period and that untreated panic symptoms, for example, may pose a risk to the fetoplacental unit (Cohen et al. 1989a). Thus, a carefully tailored treatment plan must be derived both for women treated for anxiety disorders who wish to conceive and for those who develop symptoms during pregnancy.

Patients with anxiety disorders require careful reevaluation of their pharmacotherapeutic regimen before they attempt to conceive. Benzodiazepines and tricyclic antidepressants remain the most frequently used agents for the treatment of anxiety disorders (Klein 1981; Rosenbaum 1982). Given the low teratogenic potential of tricyclic antidepressants, they should constitute the treatment of choice for patients with panic disorder or other anxiety disorders that require pharmacotherapy. Though not contraindicated in pregnancy, the risk of benzodiazepine use in gravid women remains controversial. There have been reports of increased rates of oral clefts after in utero exposure to diazepam (Aarskog 1975; Saxen 1975; Saxen and Saxen 1975) and of a syndrome resembling fetal alcohol syndrome in offspring exposed in utero to benzodiazepines (Laegreid et al. 1987). These reports have been countered by prospective studies that fail to demonstrate increased risk of congenital malformations in benzodiazepine-exposed children (Czeizel and Lendvay 1987; Shiono and Mills 1984).

While alprazolam is frequently used for treatment of panic disorder, there are as yet no systematic reports of the rate of malformations in offspring exposed to alprazolam during pregnancy. Information regarding the teratogenicity of this drug is limited to the manufacturer's case register of voluntary clinician reports of offspring exposed to alprazolam in utero. To date, over 400 cases of alprazolam exposure during pregnancy have been compiled (Barry and St. Clair 1987), and while there have been individual cases of reported malformations, incidence data are not available since the total population exposed is unknown.

Patients with panic disorder maintained on alprazolam who wish to conceive should be tapered on a schedule adjusted to their ability to tolerate decreases in dose. Close attention should be paid to breakthrough symptoms of panic or withdrawal. For patients who are unable to tolerate discontinuation of alprazolam without emergence of severe recurrent symptoms of panic or withdrawal, the addition of a tricyclic may be helpful to treat emergent panic attacks. Similarly, a switch to clonazepam, with its longer duration of action (Herman et al. 1987), may allow the alprazolam-dependent patient who wishes to conceive to wean from benzodiazepine treatment. Last, adjunctive behavioral therapy may be of particular benefit for some patients experiencing difficulty discontinuing antipanic medication (Sanchez-Craig et al. 1987).

The switch to clonazepam in this setting has a twofold rationale.

First, the longer half-life of the drug compared with that of alprazolam affords a more gentle tapering with less "rebound" anxiety. Second, the teratogenic potential of clonazepam appears to be particularly low (Sullivan and McElhatton 1977) in contrast to the relative lack of data regarding teratogenicity for the newer agent, alprazolam, making clonazepam a better choice for the patient who cannot discontinue benzodiazepine therapy without reemergence of panic disorder.

A variety of effects have been reported during the perinatal period in children who have been exposed in utero to benzodiazepines. Transient agitation, hypotonia, decreased respirations and Apgar scores, and difficulty with feeding and temperature regulation have all been described (Calabrese and Gulledge 1985). Neonatal abstinence syndrome has also been reported in newborns of mothers maintained on alprazolam (Barry and St. Clair 1987).

Again, planned pregnancy affords time for thoughtful pharmacotherapeutic strategies in patients maintained on anxiolytic medications; for patients who inadvertently conceive while on these medications, the choices regarding treatment course are difficult. As an example, in a woman chronically maintained on alprazolam, the risks of exposing the fetoplacental unit to a second agent such as a tricyclic antidepressant or another benzodiazepine such as clonazepam may in fact be greater than the risk of low-dose alprazolam.

Behavior therapy may help with phobic avoidance and anticipatory anxiety, allowing use of less medication. It should be emphasized that the goal of managing this population during pregnancy is not necessarily to achieve a comparable level of symptom control as for the nonpregnant patient, but to minimize the risk to the fetus. Moderate phobic avoidance with less pharmacotherapeutic intervention may be acceptable.

The human teratogenic potential of the nonbenzodiazepine anxiolytic buspirone is unknown. Thus, pending further study, clonazepam or a tricyclic would be preferable if drug treatment for anxiety was deemed necessary.

BREAST-FEEDING DURING PSYCHOTROPIC DRUG USE

All psychotropics, including antipsychotics, antidepressants, lithium, and benzodiazepines, are secreted into breast milk by lactating females (Calabrese and Gulledge 1985). Concentrations of drugs in breast milk may vary greatly and depend on the specific characteristics of the drug in question as well as on maternal metabolism (Rivera-Calimlin 1987). The effect of these agents on the neonate is also variable and depends, in part, on the specific drug, its bioavailability, and the maturity of the infant's metabolism and central nervous system.

These variables probably account for the range of reported consequences of individual drugs, from nondetectable effects to symptoms of severe neonatal distress (Anderson and McGuire 1989; Gelenberg 1987). While it is unlikely that clinically appreciable concentrations of drug appear in breast milk of most lactating mothers who take psychotropics, the clinician cannot predict this accurately. Given this uncertainty, unless breast milk can be reliably assayed for the presence of these agents, or the absence of drug can be documented in the baby's serum, then the most thoughtful course for lactating women who require these agents during the postpartum period may be to defer breast-feeding.

The effects of drug in breast milk on the developing brain of the infant are unknown. Although the significance of this issue has been differentially regarded (Committee on Drugs 1989), given the presumed plasticity of the developing brain (Asioki and Siekevitz 1988), the clinician who treats the postpartum patient must weigh again the relative risks of drug exposure against the benefit obtained from breast-feeding. During the postpartum period the treatment of the mother does not imply a need to include the infant in treatment. Thus, patients who require psychotropics should be cautious about breast-feeding until the potential risks to infants are better understood.

CONCLUSIONS

In several reviews over the last decade, antipsychotics, antidepressants, and benzodiazepines have been demonstrated to have low teratogenic potential; yet one cannot assert their safety in pregnancy. Given the rate of psychotropic use in pregnancy and data suggesting the persistence of psychiatric symptoms through pregnancy for some women, the clinician requires guidelines for managing psychiatric disorders in pregnancy. A summary of proposed guidelines for treating psychiatrically ill pregnant patients is outlined in Table 18-1.

For the patients who require psychotropic medication in pregnancy, it is critical to have a prepared clinical approach to drug administration. Clearly, psychotropics can be used in pregnancy without discernible

Table 18-1. Psychotropic drug use in pregnancy

Psychosis

1. Maintenance low-dose antipsychotic therapy for chronically psychotic patients may offset risk of relapse and need for higher doses
2. Medical differential diagnosis and workup for new-onset psychotic states
3. High-potency neuroleptics safer?
4. Medication present in breast milk

Manic-depressive illness

1. Medical differential diagnosis and workup for new-onset manic symptoms
2. Careful contraceptive history
3. Evaluate need for prophylaxis
4. First trimester
   Avoid lithium exposure before week 12; consider fetal cardiac ultrasound at week 20
   Clear need for antimanic prophylaxis: discontinue lithium at documentation of pregnancy
   Consider prophylactic antipsychotics in brittle bipolar women
5. Second and third trimester
   After week 12 and with need for treatment, consider lithium reintroduction
   Discontinue lithium before estimated date of confinement or decrease dose by 50% prior to delivery
   Give lithium in small divided doses
6. Mania during pregnancy
   Hospitalization
   Neuroleptics, adjunctive clonazepam(?), electroconvulsive therapy (ECT)
7. Lithium in breast milk

Unipolar depression

1. Medical differential diagnosis
2. Withhold medication in first trimester if possible
3. Inability to care for self or to provide prenatal care indicates need for somatic therapy
4. Secondary over tertiary amine tricyclics or newer antidepressants
5. ECT for delusional depression
6. Antidepressants in breast milk

Anxiety disorders

1. Medical differential diagnosis
2. Tricyclics are treatment of choice
3. Adjunctive cognitive-behavioral and supportive psychotherapy
4. Withhold medication in first trimester if possible
5. Taper benzodiazepine therapy prior to conception: slow taper vs. change to tricyclic antidepressant
6. If unable to taper short-acting benzodiazepine, consider changing to clonazepam
7. If patient is on an anxiolytic when pregnancy confirmed, attempt to taper
8. Avoid additional drug introduction, particularly in first trimester
9. Benzodiazepines in breast milk

Source. Adapted with permission from Cohen LS, Heller VL, Rosenbaum JF: Treatment guidelines for psychotropic drug use in pregnancy. Psychosomatics 30:25–33, 1989.

adverse consequences. Pending good controlled prospective data on the impact of drugs on fetal and later development, the clinician must continue to act in a state of relative uncertainty as he or she weighs partially calculated risks to manage individual clinical dilemmas.

REFERENCES

Aarskog D: Association between maternal intake of diazepam and oral clefts. Lancet 2:498, 1975

Akiskal HS, Walker P, Puzantian VR, et al: Bipolar outcome in the course of depressive illness: phenomenologic, familiar, and pharmacologic predictors. J Affective Disord 5:115–128, 1983

Ananth J: Side effects of fetus and infant of psychotropic drug use during pregnancy. Pharmacopsychiatry 11:246–260, 1976

Anderson PO, McGuire GG: Neonatal alprazolam withdrawal: possible effects of breast feeding. Drug Intell Clin Pharm 23:614, 1989

Asioki C, Siekevitz AC: Plasticity in brain development. Sci Am 88:56–64, 1988

Avant K: Anxiety as a potential factor affecting maternal attachment. J Obstet Gynecol Neonatal Nurs 10:416–419, 1981

Barry WS, St. Clair SM: Exposure to benzodiazepines in utero (letter). Lancet 1:1436–1437, 1987

Beeley L: Adverse effects of drugs in the first trimester of pregnancy. Clin Obstet Gynecol 13:177–195, 1986

Boobis AR, Lewis PJ: Pharmacokinetics in pregnancy in obstetrics, in Clinical Pharmacology. Edited by Lewis P. Boston, MA, PSG, 1983

Boyd JH, Weissman MM: Epidemiology, in Handbook of Affective Disorders. Edited by Paykel ES. New York, Guilford, 1982

Brazelton TB: Mother-infant reciprocity, in Maternal Attachment and Mothering Disorders: A Roundtable. Edited by Klaus MH, Leger T, Trause MA. North Brunswick, NJ, Johnson & Johnson, 1975

Calabrese JR, Gulledge AD: Psychotropics during pregnancy and lactation: a review. Psychosomatics 26:413–426, 1985

Carr DB, Sheehan DV, Surman OS, et al: Neuroendocrine correlates of lactate-induced anxiety and their response to chronic alprazolam therapy. Am J Psychiatry 143:483–494, 1986

Charney D, Heninger G: Abnormal regulation of noradrenergic function in panic disorder. Arch Gen Psychiatry 43:1042–1054, 1986

Chouinard G: Antimanic effects of clonazepam. Psychosomatics 26 (suppl):7–11, 1985

Cogill SR, Caplan HL, Alexandra H, et al: Impact of maternal depression on cognitive development of young children. Br Med J 292:1165–1167, 1986

Cohen BM, Lipinski JF Jr: Treatment of acute psychosis with non-neuroleptic agents. Psychosomatics 27 (suppl 1):7–16, 1986

Cohen LS: Pregnancy in the bipolar patient. Biological Therapies in Psychiatry 11:42–44, 1988

Cohen LS, Rosenbaum JF, Heller V: Panic attack associated placental abruption: a case report. J Clin Psychiatry 50:7, 1989a

Cohen LS, Rosenbaum JF, Heller VL, et al: Course of panic disorder in 24 pregnant women. Paper presented at the annual meeting of the American Psychiatric Association, San Francisco, CA, May 1989b

Cohen ME, White PD: Life situations, emotions, and neurocirculatory asthenia. Psychosom Med 13(6):335–357, 1951

Committee on Drugs, American Academy of Pediatrics: Transfer of drugs and other chemicals into human milk. Pediatrics 84:924–936, 1989

Cooper GL: The safety of fluoxetine—an update. Br J Psychiatry 153 (suppl 3):77–86, 1989

Coverdale JH, Ruffo JA: Family planning needs of female chronic psychiatric outpatients. Am J Psychiatry 146:1489–1491, 1989

Coyle LR: Changes in developing behavior following prenatal administration of imipramine. Pharmacol Biochem Behav 3:799–807, 1975a

Coyle LR: The interactive effects of prenatal imipramine exposure and postnatal rearing conditions on behavior and histology. Psychopharmacologia 44:253–256, 1975b

Crandon AJ: Maternal anxiety and neonatal wellbeing. J Psychosom Res 23:113–115, 1979

Crowe RR: Electroconvulsive therapy. N Engl J Med 311:163–167, 1984

Czeizel A, Lendvay A: In-utero exposure to benzodiazepines (letter). Lancet 1:628, 1987

Dicke JM: Teratology: principles and practice. Med Clin North Am 73:567–581, 1989

Doering JC, Stewart RB: The extent and character of drug consumption during pregnancy. JAMA 239:843–846, 1978

Dreifuss FE, Susumu S: Clonazepam, in Antiepileptic Drugs, 2nd Edition. Edited by Woodbury DM, Penry JK, Pippenger CE. New York, Raven, 1982

Edlund MJ, Craig TJ: Antipsychotic drug use and birth defects: an epidemiologic reassessment. Compr Psychiatry 25:32–37, 1984

Elia J, Katz IR, Simpson GM: Teratogenicity of psychotherapeutic medications. Psychopharmacol Bull 23:533–537, 1987

Falterman LG, Richardson DJ: Small left colon syndrome associated with maternal ingestion of psychotropics. J Pediatr 97:300–310, 1980

File SE, Tucker JC: Prenatal treatment with clomipramine: effects on the behavior of male and female adolescent rats. Psychopharmacology 82:221–224, 1984

Gelenberg AJ: Pregnancy, psychotropic drugs, and psychiatric disorders. Psychosomatics 27:216–217, 1986

Gelenberg AJ: Antidepressants in milk. Biological Therapies in Psychiatry 10:1, 1987

George DT, Ladenheim JA, Nutt DJ: Effect of pregnancy on panic attacks. Am J Psychiatry 144:1078–1079, 1987

Groves JE, Manschrek TC: Psychotic patients, in Massachusetts General Hospital Handbook of General Hospital Psychiatry. Edited by Hackett TP, Cassem NH. Littleton, MA, PSG, 1987

Herman JB, Rosenbaum JF, Brotman AW: The alprazolam to clonazepam switch for the treatment of panic disorder. J Clin Psychopharmacol 7:175–178, 1987

Hill LM, Kleinberg F: Effects of drugs and chemicals on the fetus and newborn (first of two parts). Mayo Clin Proc 59:707–716, 1984a

Hill LM, Kleinberg F: Effects of drugs and chemicals on the fetus and newborn (second of two parts). Mayo Clin Proc 59:755–765, 1984b

Hill RM, Desmond MM, Kay JL: Extrapyramidal dysfunction in an infant of a schizophrenic mother. J Pediatr 69:589–595, 1966

Idanpaan-Heikkila J, Saxen L: Possible teratogenicity of imipramine-chloropyramine. Lancet 2:282–284, 1973

Jeffries WS, Bochner F: The effect of pregnancy on drug pharmacokinetics. Med J Aust 149:675–677, 1988

Jones KL, Lacro RV, Johnson KA, et al: Pattern of malformations in the children of women treated with carbamazepine during pregnancy. N Engl J Med 320:1661–1666, 1989

Kirklin JW, Barratt-Boyes BG: Ebstein's malformation, in Cardiac Surgery. Edited by Kirklin JW, Barratt-Boyes BG. New York, John Wiley, 1986

Klein D: Delineation of two drug responsive anxiety syndromes. Psychopharmacology 5:397–408, 1964

Klein DF: Anxiety reconceptualized, in Anxiety: New Research and Changing Concepts. Edited by Klein DF, Raskin J. New York, Raven, 1981

Kopelman AE, McCullar FW, Heggeness L: Limb malformations following maternal use of haloperidol. JAMA 231:62–64, 1975

Krauthammer CD, Klerman GL: Secondary mania: manic syndromes associated with antecedent physical illness or drugs. Arch Gen Psychiatry 35:1333–1339, 1978

Kris EB: Children of mothers maintained on pharmacotherapy during pregnancy and postpartum. Current Therapeutic Research 7:785–789, 1965

Kuenssberg EV, Knox JD: Imipramine in pregnancy. Br Med J 2:292, 1972

Laegreid L, Olegard R, Wahlstrom J, et al: Abnormalities in children exposed to benzodiazepines in utero (letter). Lancet 1:108–109, 1987

Langman J: Medical Embryology, 2nd Edition. Baltimore, MD, Williams & Wilkins, 1975

Lederman RP, Lederman E, Work B, et al: Anxiety and epinephrine in multiparous women in labor: relationship to duration of labor and fetal heart rate pattern. Am J Obstet Gynecol 153:870–877, 1985

Levy W, Wisniewski K: Chlorpromazine causing extrapyramidal dysfunction in newborn infants of psychotic mothers. NY State J Med 74:684–685, 1974

Lindhout D, Schmidt D: In utero exposure to valproate and neural defects. Lancet 1:329–393, 1986

McBride WG: Limb deformities associated with ininodibenzyl hydrochloride (letter). Med J Aust 1:492, 1972

McElroy SL, Keck PE, Pope HG, et al: Valproate in the treatment of rapid cycling mood disorder. J Clin Psychopharmacol 8:275–279, 1988

Milkovich L, Van den Berg BJ: An evaluation of the teratogenicity of certain antinauseant drugs. Am J Obstet Gynecol 125:244–248, 1976

Nakne Y, Okuma T, Takahashi R, et al: Multi-institutional study on the teratogenicity and fetal toxicity of antiepileptic drugs: a report of a collaborative study group in Japan. Epilepsia 21:663–680, 1980

Nidely JR, Blake DA, Freeman JM, et al: Carbamazepine levels in pregnancy and lactation. Obstet Gynecol 53:139–140, 1979

Nurnberg HG, Prudic J: Guidelines for treatment of psychosis during pregnancy. Hosp Community Psychiatry 35:67–71, 1984

O'Hara MW: Social support, life events, and depression during pregnancy and the puerperium. Arch Gen Psychiatry 43:569–573, 1986

O'Hara MW, Zekoski EM, Phillips LH, et al: A controlled prospective study of postpartum mood disorders: comparison of childbearing and nonchildbearing women. J Abnorm Psychol 99:3–15, 1990

Omer H, Everly GS: Psychological factors in preterm labor: critical review and theoretical synthesis. Am J Psychiatry 145:1507–1513, 1988

Paulson GW, Paulson RB: Teratogenic effects of anticonvulsants. Arch Neurol 38:140–143, 1981

Pollack MH, Tesar GE, Rosenbaum JF, et al: Clonazepam in the treatment of panic disorder and agoraphobia: a one year follow-up. J Clin Psychopharmacol 6:302–304, 1986

Post RM, Uhde TW, Ballenger JC, et al: Prophylactic efficacy of carbamazepine in manic-depressive illness. Am J Psychiatry 140:1602–1604, 1983

Poulson E, Robson JM: Effect of phenelzine and some related compounds in pregnancy. J Endocrinol 30:205–215, 1964

Prentice A, Brown R: Fetal tachyarrhythmia and maternal antidepressant treatment (letter). Br Med J 298:190, 1989

Protheroe C: Puerperal psychoses: a long-term study, 1927–1961. Br J Psychiatry 115:9–30, 1961

Quitkin FM: The importance of dosage in prescribing antidepressants. Br J Psychiatry 147:593–597, 1985

Redmond GP: Physiological changes during pregnancy and their implications for pharmacological treatment. Clin Invest Med 8:317–322, 1985

Reich T, Winokur G: Postpartum psychosis in patients with manic depressive disease. J Nerv Ment Dis 151:60–68, 1970

Remick RA, Maurice WL: ECT in pregnancy (letter). Am J Psychiatry 135:761–762, 1978

Repke JT, Berger NG: Electroconvulsive therapy in pregnancy. Obstet Gynecol 63 (suppl)39S–40S, 1984

Rivera-Calimlim L: The significance of drugs in breast milk: pharmacokinetic considerations. Clinics in Perinatology 14:51–70, 1987

Robinson GE, Stewart DE, Flak E: The rational use of psychotropic drugs in pregnancy and postpartum. Can J Psychiatry 31:183–190, 1986

Rosenbaum JF: The drug treatment of anxiety. N Engl J Med 306:401–404, 1982

Rosenberg AJ, Silver E: Suicide, psychiatrists, and therapeutic abortion. California Medicine 102:407–411, 1965

Rosenberg L, Mitchell AA, Parsells JL, et al: Lack of relation of oral clefts to diazepam use during pregnancy. N Engl J Med 309:1282–1285, 1983

Rumeau-Rouguette C, Goujard J, Huel G: Possible teratogenic effect of phenothiazines in human beings. Teratology 15:57–64, 1977

Salzman C, Green AI, Rodriguez-Villa F, et al: Benzodiazepines combined with neuroleptics for management of severe disruptive behavior. Psychosomatics 27:17–21, 1986

Sanchez-Craig M, Capell H, Busto U, et al: Cognitive behavioral treatment for benzodiazepine dependence: a comparison of gradual versus abrupt cessation of drug intake. Br J Addict 82:1317–1327, 1987

Saxen I: Association between oral clefts and drugs taken during pregnancy. Int J Epidemiol 4:37–44, 1975

Saxen I, Saxen L: Association between maternal intake of diazepam and oral clefts. Lancet 2:498, 1975

Schou M: What happened later to the lithium babies: a follow-up study of children born without malformations. Acta Psychiatr Scand 54:193–197, 1976

Scokel PW, Jones WD: Infant jaundice after phenothiazine drugs for labour: an enigma. Obstet Gynecol 20:124–127, 1962

Shader RI, Greenblatt DJ: Benzodiazepines and pregnancy: more to say and more to learn. J Clin Psychopharmacol 9:237, 1989

Shearer WT, Schreiner RL, Marshall RE: Urinary retention in a neonate secondary to maternal ingestion of nortriptyline. J Pediatr 81:570–572, 1972

Shiono PH, Mills JL: Oral clefts and diazepam use during pregnancy (letter). N Engl J Med 311:919–920, 1984

Siever L, Uhde T: New studies and perspectives on the noradrenergic receptor system in depression: effects of the alpha-2 adrenergic agonist clonidine. Biol Psychiatry 19:131–156, 1984

Sim M: Abortion and the psychiatrist. Br Med J 5350:145–148, 1963

Sivertz KS, Misri S, Brown M: Tricyclic babies. Paper presented at the annual meeting of the American Psychiatric Association, San Francisco, CA, May 1989

Slone D, Siskind V, Heinonen OP, et al: Antenatal exposure to the phenothiazines in relation to congenital malformations, perinatal mortality rate, birth weight, and intelligence quotient score. Am J Obstet Gynecol 128:486–488, 1977

Spier SA, Tesar GE, Rosenbaum JF, et al: Clonazepam in the treatment of panic disorder and agoraphobia. J Clin Psychiatry 47:238–242, 1986

Sullivan FM, McElhatton PR: A comparison of the teratogenic activity of the antiepileptic drugs carbamazepine, clonazepam, ethosuximide, phenobarbital, phenytoin, and pyrimidone in mice. Toxicol Appl Pharmacol 40:365–378, 1977

Tamer A, McKey R, Arias D, et al: Phenothiazine-induced extrapyramidal dysfunction in the neonate. J Pediatr 7:479–480, 1969

Targum SD, Gershon ES: Pregnancy, genetic counselling and the major psychiatric disorders in genetic diseases, in Genetic Diseases in Pregnancy: Maternal Effects and Fetal Outcome. Edited by Schulman J, Simpson J. New York, Academic, 1981

Targum SD, Davenport YB, Webster MJ: Postpartum mania in bipolar manic depressive patients withdrawn from lithium carbonate. J Nerv Ment Dis 167:572–574, 1983

Thorpe FT: Intensive electrical convulsive therapy in acute mania. Journal of Mental Science 93:89–92, 1947

Van Gent EM, Nabarro G: Haloperidol as an alternative to lithium in pregnant women (letter). Am J Psychiatry 144:1241, 1987

Weinstein MR, Goldfield MD: Administration of lithium during pregnancy, in Lithium Research and Therapy. Edited by Johnson FN. New York, Academic, 1975

Weissman MM, Merikangas KR: The epidemiology of anxiety and panic disorders: an update. J Clin Psychiatry 47 (suppl):11–17, 1986

Wise MG, Ward SC, Townsend-Parchman W, et al: Case report of ECT during high-risk pregnancy. Am J Psychiatry 141:99–101, 1984

Zahn-Waxler C, Cummings EM, Ianoff RJ, et al: Young offspring of depressed patients: a population at risk for affective problems and childhood depression, in Childhood Depression. Edited by Cichetti D, Schneider-Rosen K. San Francisco, CA, Jossey-Bass, 1984, pp 81–105

Zajicek E: Psychiatric problems during pregnancy, in Pregnancy: A Psychological and Social Study. Edited by Wolkind S, Zajicek E. London, Academic, 1981

Index